MW00845602

Efficient Tumor Immunohistochemistry

A Differential Diagnosis-Driven Approach

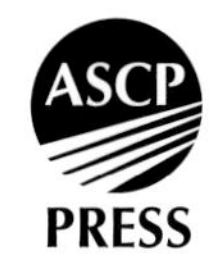

Publishing Team
Erik Tanck (production manager/designer)
Joshua Weikersheimer (publisher)

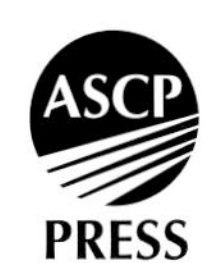

Copyright © 2006 by the American Society for Clinical Pathology. All rights reserved. No part of this publication may be reproduced, stored in a retrieval system, or transmitted in any form or by any means, electronic, mechanical, photocopying, recording, or otherwise, without the prior written permission of the publisher.

printed in Singapore

10 09 08 07 06

ISBN 0-89189-560-4

Efficient Tumor Immunohistochemistry

A Differential Diagnosis-Driven Approach

M. Nadji, MD, M. Nassiri, MD, and A.R. Morales, MD

Department of Pathology
University of Miami Jackson Memorial Hospital
and Sylvester Comprehensive Cancer Center

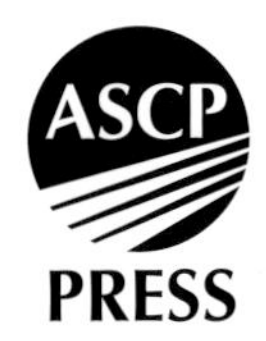

TABLE OF CONTENTS

Preface

Close to a quarter of a century ago, we wrote a monograph titled *Immunoperoxidase Techniques: A Practical Approach to Tumor Diagnosis,* and stated at that time that the practice of pathology has been changed by immunohistochemistry. The writing of that monograph was prompted by the assertion that the lack of a practical manual on the subject prevented pathologists from gaining full benefits of the technique in the daily assessment of surgical tissue samples. Today, immunohistochemistry is an integral part of the daily practice of pathology and there is hardly a day that goes by without the discovery of a new tumor marker. Nor is there a single issue of pathology or other specialty journals that fails to carry an article or a direct reference to immunohistochemistry. In fact, during the last 25 years, more than 165,000 articles and many textbooks have been published on that subject. Consequently, pathologists are challenged to convert the benefits from the florid array of new developments and informations in the field into the daily practice of surgical pathology. As was the case with the original monograph, our intent is to facilitate that task. Therefore, this can be considered as an update on the observations that we have made in the course of the past 25 years by adhering to practicality as the single most important criterion in the resolution of daily diagnostic problems encountered by surgical pathologists. Whenever appropriate, this approach can be complemented by referring to more exhaustive treatises such as Taylor, Clive R and Cote, Richard J, *Immunomicroscopy—A Diagnostic Tool for the Surgical Pathologist*; and Dabbs, David J, *Diagnostic Immunohistochemistry*. Updates on tumor markers may be obtained by visiting the ImmunoQuery Web site, Frisman, Dennis M., www.ipox.com.

Acknowledgments

This manual reflects the application of immunohistochemistry in the resolution of differential diagnostic problems encountered daily in the practice of surgical pathology at the University of Miami Jackson Memorial Hospital and Sylvester Comprehensive Cancer Center. Our practice encompasses cases originated from these institutions as well as those that are referred from colleagues in the United States, primarily from Florida, and also from outside the United States. We therefore acknowledge the benefits derived from more than two decades of interaction with the faculty in our department and our peers in Florida and elsewhere.

We have been most fortunate in maintaining a dedicated, responsible and most competent technical staff in our immunohistochemistry laboratory. Silvia Losa, Blanca Cuenca, Weiyu Wu, and Fay Mucha have provided their skills and commitment to the well being of our patients and to the success of our research endeavors throughout these years. We would like to extend a very special note of gratitude to Alicia Cabrera who confronted the demands of writing and many times revising the manuscript with forbearance, professionalism, and gracious attitude.

The extended efforts of Drs. Parvin Ganjei, Betina Werner and Rima Kanhoush in the preparation of this manual were essential for bringing it about. To Joshua Weikersheimer of the ASCP Press, we owe special thanks for his advice and continuous support. We also like to thank Doug Sweet, Vice President, Celerus Diagnostics, who was instrumental in encouraging us to undertake this project.

Introduction

Immunohistochemistry is now an integral part of every diagnostic pathology laboratory. Its major application is to complement histomorphology in classification of human neoplasms. With the refinement of methodologies, the availability of good quality reagents, and enhancement of the reproducibility of results by introduction of automatic stainers, problems associated with the technical aspects of immunohistochemistry are relatively uncommon. Current limitations of efficient application of immunohistochemistry in diagnostic pathology are mostly analytical, usually related to selection of appropriate markers for a diagnostic problem, as well as the correct interpretation of staining result and its incorporation in the final diagnostic decision. Factors that influence the analytical outcome include scarcity of cell lineage-specific markers, subjectivity of panel selection, lack of practical guidelines, and the experience of the observer.

It is not surprising, therefore, to witness the drastic increase in the number of antibodies used in immunohistochemical panels. However, the indiscriminate use of multiple antibodies without consideration of histomorphology and clinical history—the "shotgun" approach—is neither diagnostically efficient, nor cost-effective. Often, it entangles the pathologists in a confusing web of "positive" and "negative" staining results, leading to indeterminate or incorrect diagnostic conclusions. In practice, however, based on histologic appearance of the tumors, most differential diagnoses in tissue biopsies can be narrowed down to two or three possibilities. Consequently, the choice of antibodies in these situations can also be restricted to two or three.

In this practical handbook we recommend simple guidelines for the resolution of most common—and some uncommon—diagnostic problems by utilization of a limited number of antibodies. This is not an algorithm; it is a "tailor-made" approach that requires the pathologist's input and necessitates his/her active participation by formulating a working differential diagnosis on the basis of clinical information and histomorphology.

Before using the book:

1. The suggested markers are those that we have found most useful. The experienced immunohistochemist may like to use the same set of markers or modify the selection according to his/her preference. The user will find that some of the most commonly utilized immunohistochemical markers are conspicuously absent. We have omitted those we have found to be of limited or no value in a given differential diagnosis, even when they are used in a panel.

2. Not all possible differential diagnostic problems are discussed. This is primarily due to the lack of reliable markers for some common differential diagnoses. For example, there are at least a dozen publications on immunohistochemical separation of renal oncocytomas from chromophobe renal cell carcinomas. None of the several different purported markers in these papers, however, has proved to be useful, at least in our experience.

3. The illustrated images are from cases seen in our own institution or referrals from colleagues in Florida and elsewhere. We have made no attempt to present the most typical examples of each diagnostic entity or the best possible histologic preparations. On the contrary, the majority of illustrations are from cases that may show crushing artifacts, knife nicks, thermal damage, or other changes that most pathologists are familiar with in their daily practice.

4. Some images exhibit positive staining as dark brown, or black, on a green background. This is notable for nuclear antigens because we intensify the color of DAB with a dip in copper sulphate and use fast green as a cytoplasmic counterstain.

5. Finally, we have only discussed and illustrated the immunohistochemistry of human solid tumors. The IHC of hematolymphoid neoplasms is not addressed except when they come into the differential diagnosis of a non-lymphoid neoplasm. The IHC of hematolymphoid neoplasms is a rather vast area and is beyond the scope of this publication..

How to use this book

By evaluating the histomorphology of a tumor, the observer formulates a differential diagnosis. The tumor under study either is completely undifferentiated, or it shows morphologic features that could be shared by one or more neoplasms. Based on the primary observation, the user then consults the book for the recommended "Choice of Markers and the Expected Results." The reaction results in the tables are depicted by symbols in the following manner.

+ **Positive in the majority of cases**
– **Negative in the majority of cases**
S **Sometimes positive**

The tables are followed by "Helpful Hints" where we briefly discuss important points about the technical or analytical aspects of the utilized markers. The user may find this section particularly helpful when dealing with unexpected or discordant results. When needed, one or more key "References"—usually review articles pertaining to the disease or marker/antigen—are included in each section.

We then illustrate each section by one or two "Case Examples" with positive or negative IHC results. In these examples we have included an H&E photograph followed by one to three immunohistochemical stains; usually from the same microscopic fields. Based on the H&E and immunohistochemical reactions a final "Diagnosis" is rendered.

Punch biopsy of a skin lesion

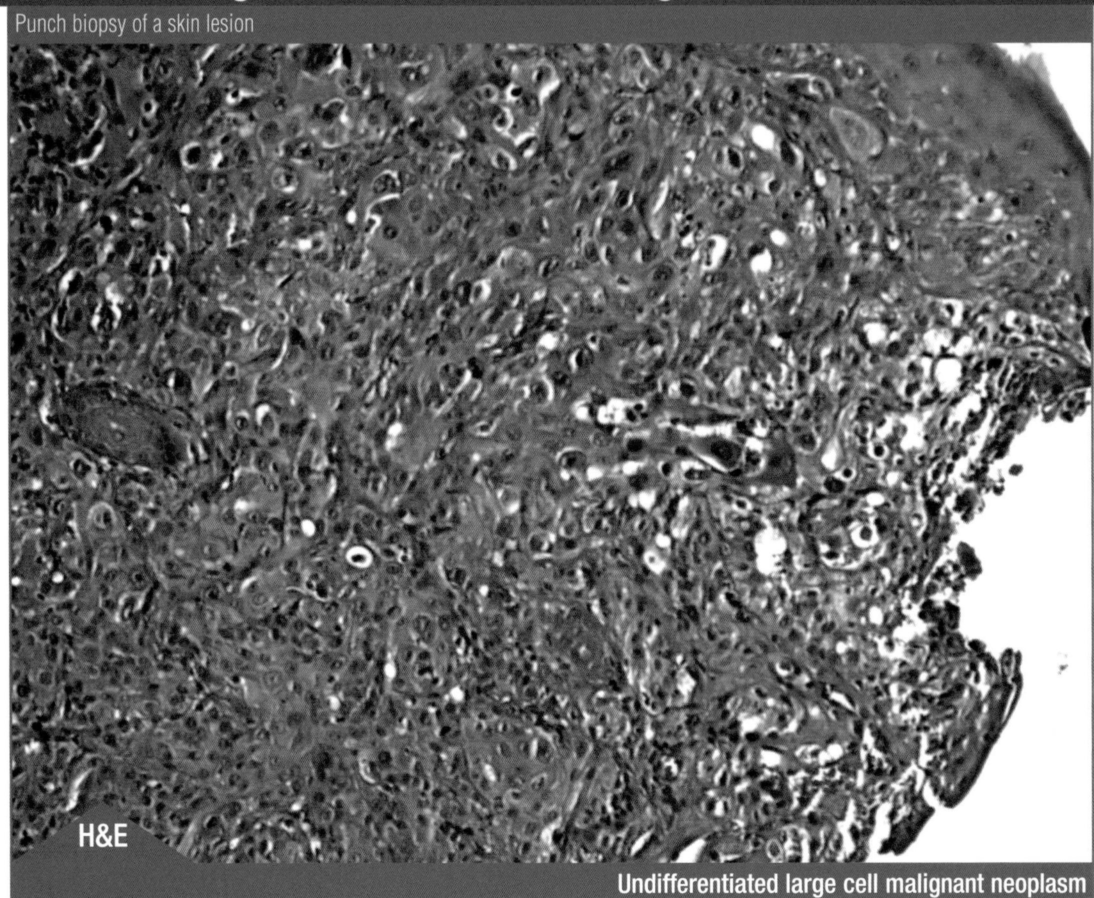

Undifferentiated large cell malignant neoplasm

Large Cell Carcinoma vs Malignant Melanoma			
	Cytokeratin (CK)	S100	HMB-45
Carcinoma	+	S	–
Melanoma	–	+	S

Helpful Hints

Cytokeratin: The cytokeratin antibody for the above differential diagnosis should be broad-spectrum (cytokeratin cocktail). There are twenty different cytokeratin proteins and no single reagent reacts against all of them. In fact, a number of commercially available "broad-spectrum" cytokeratin antibodies have only reactivity against 2-5 cytokeratin types.

S100 protein: Although S100 protein is the most sensitive marker for malignant melanoma; it is by no means the most specific one. A number of non-melanocytic neoplasms could show a positive reaction for S100 protein. Positive staining of occasional carcinomas is usually focal, as opposed to malignant melanomas where the reaction is usually diffuse throughout the tumor. A true positive reaction for S100 protein is both cytoplasmic and nuclear. In the absence of nuclear staining, one should question the validity of results.

HMB-45: Please see next case (p 4).

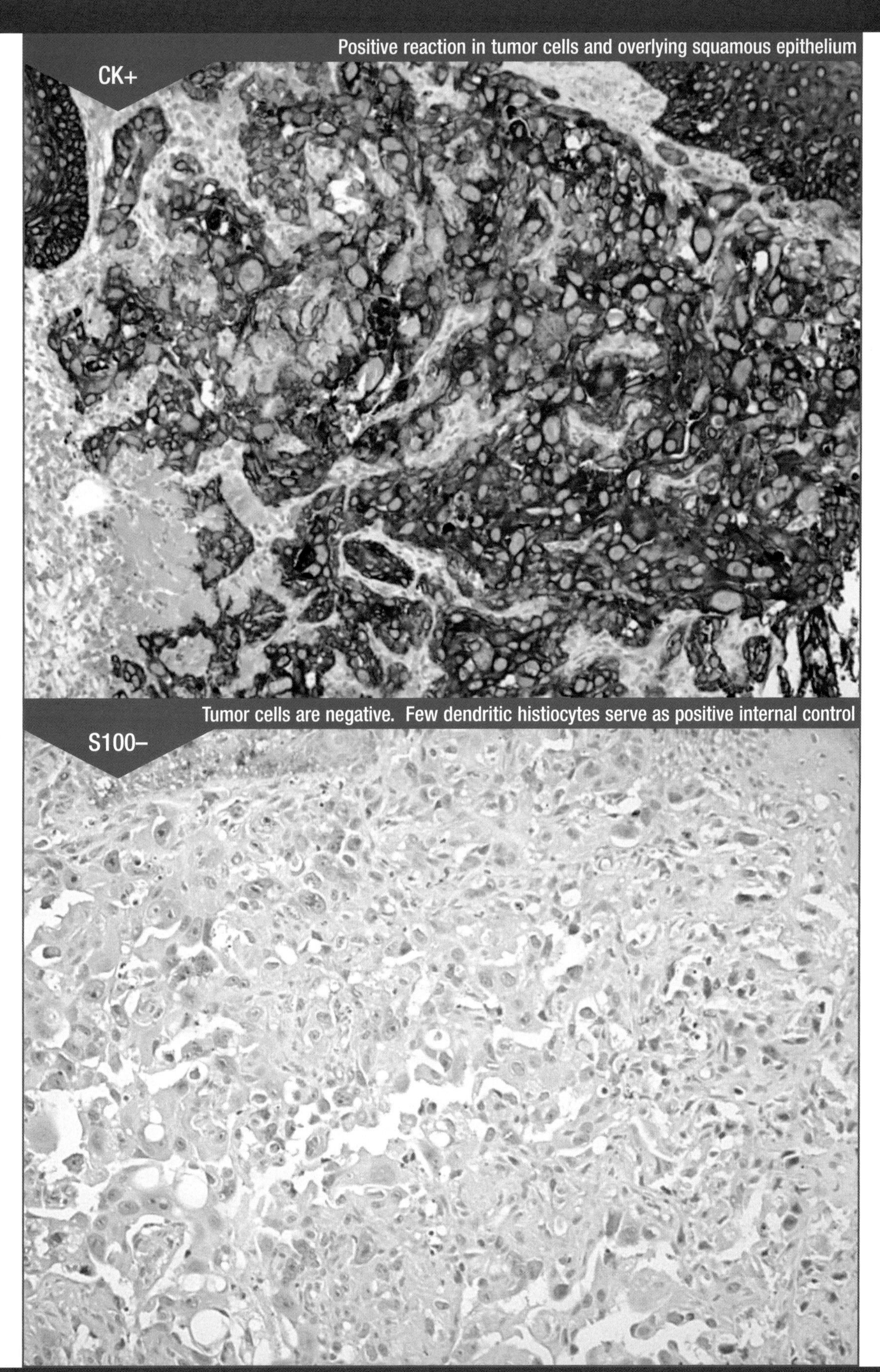

Diagnosis: Poorly Differentiated Carcinoma

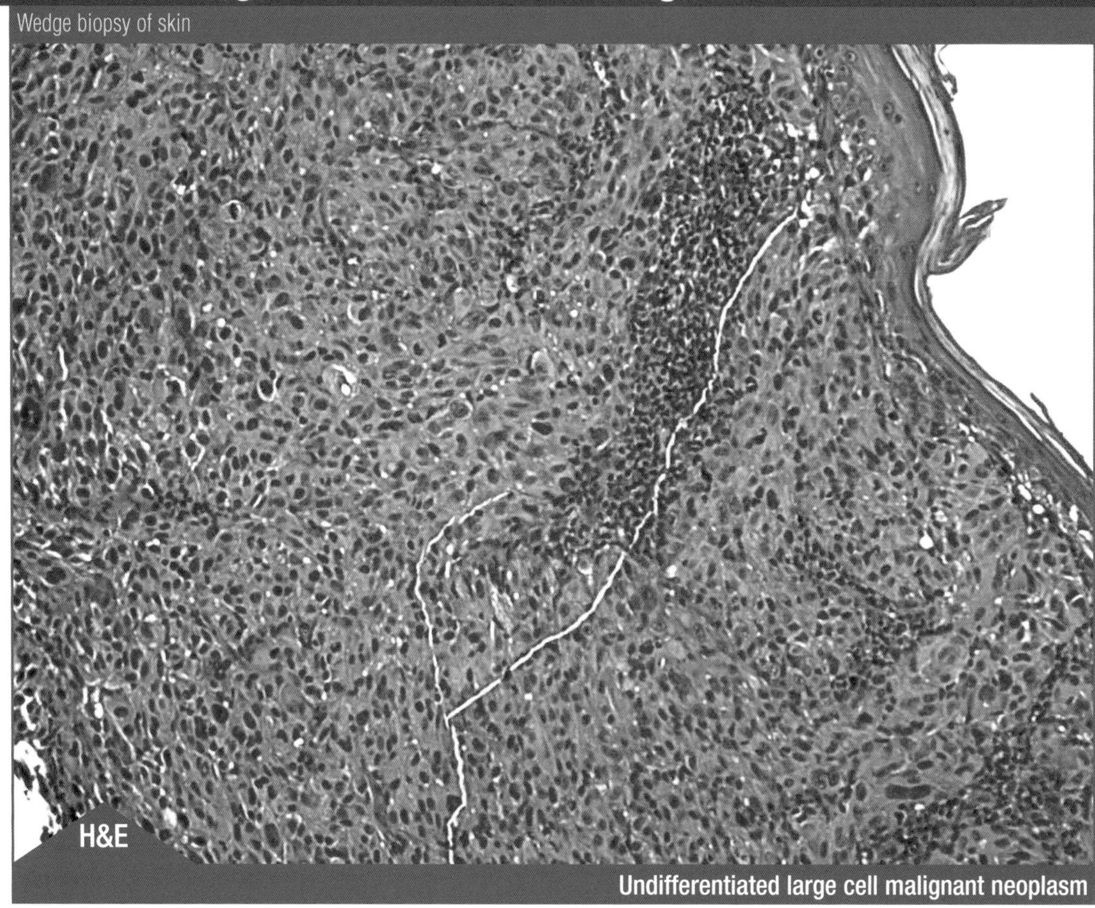

Wedge biopsy of skin

Undifferentiated large cell malignant neoplasm

Large Cell Carcinoma vs Malignant Melanoma			
	Cytokeratin (CK)	S100	HMB-45
Carcinoma	+	S	–
Melanoma	–	+	S

Helpful Hints

Cytokeratin: The cytokeratin antibody for the above differential diagnosis should be broad-spectrum (cytokeratin cocktail).

S100 protein: Although S100 protein is the most sensitive marker for malignant melanoma; it is by no means the most specific one. A number of non-melanocytic neoplasms could show a positive reaction for S100 protein. Positive staining of occasional carcinomas is usually focal, as opposed to malignant melanomas where the reaction is usually diffuse throughout the tumor. A true positive reaction for S100 protein is both cytoplasmic and nuclear. In the absence of nuclear staining, one should question the validity of results.

HMB-45: Unlike S100 protein, HMB-45 is a rather specific marker for malignant melanomas. Rare non-melanocytic lesions that may express HMB-45, eg, angiomyolipomas and pulmonary lymphangiomyomas, are not normally in the differential diagnosis of melanomas. On the other hand, HMB-45 is not a sensitive marker for malignant melanomas. Close to 50% of spindle cell melanomas and almost all desmoplastic variants are negative for this protein. Furthermore, a positive reaction for HMB-45 could be focal and hence, false-negative staining in small biopsies may create a problem. HMB-45 is not a marker of malignancy in melanocytic lesions as many nevi express this protein.

Miettinen 1993, McNutt 1998, Cochran 1993, Blessing 1998.

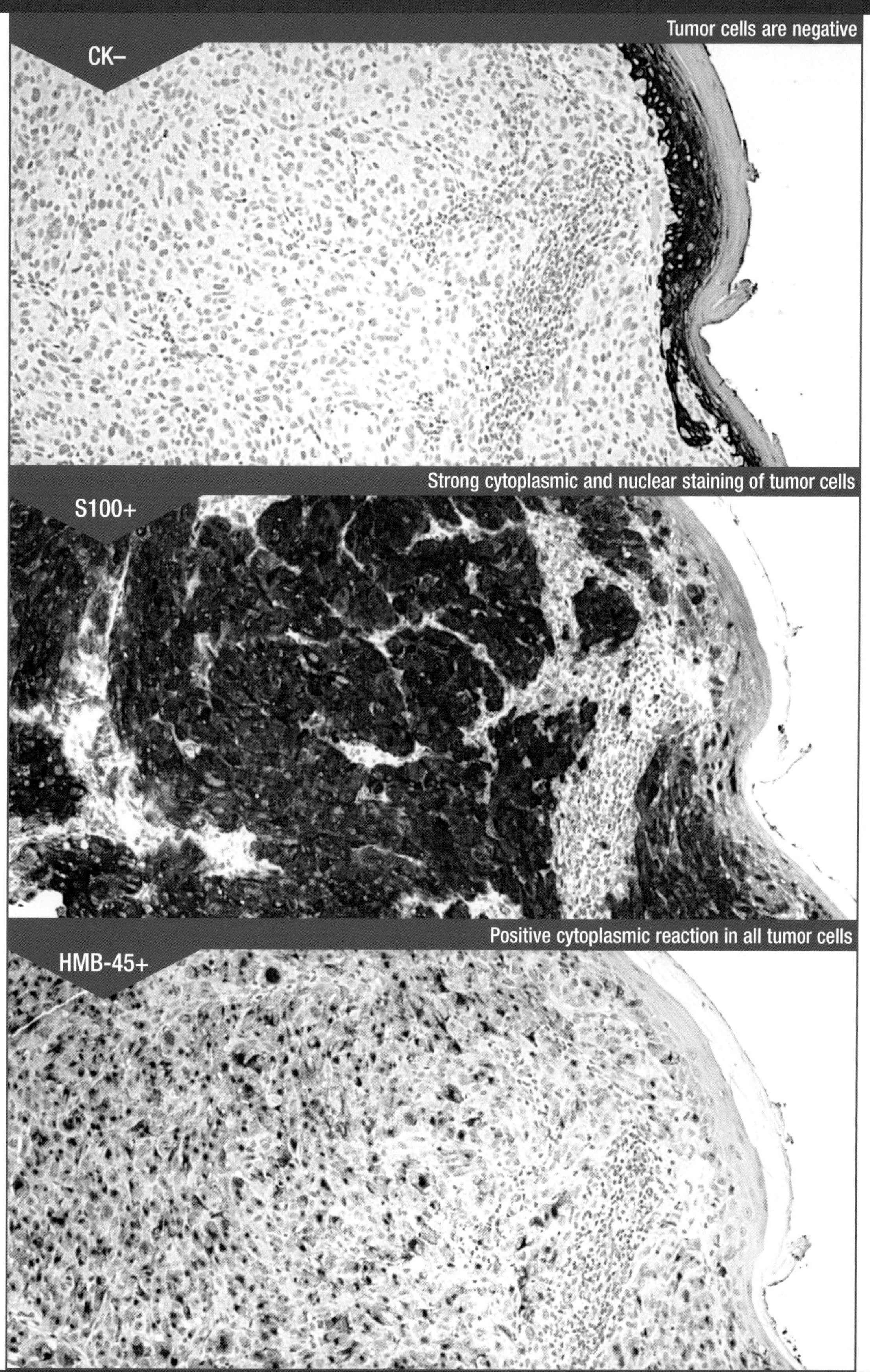

Diagnosis: Amelanotic Malignant Melanoma

Large Cell Carcinomas vs Malignant Large Cell Lymphoma

Biopsy of abdominal lymph node

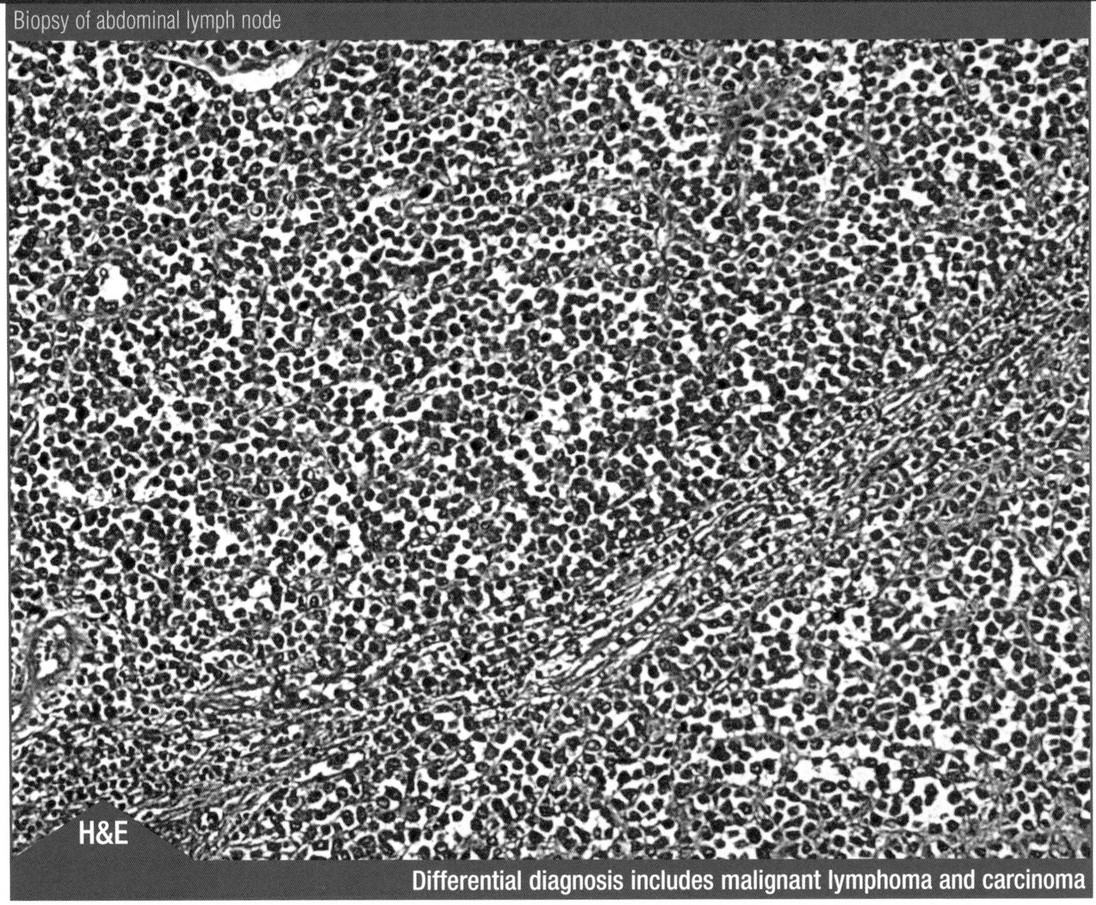

Differential diagnosis includes malignant lymphoma and carcinoma

Large Cell Carcinoma vs Malignant Large Cell Lymphoma			
	Cytokeratin (CK)	CD45	CD20
Carcinoma	+	–	–
Lymphoma	–	+	+

Helpful Hints

CD45 (leukocyte common antigen) is a specific and rather sensitive marker of malignant lymphomas. A few immunoblastic and anaplastic large cell lymphomas may be negative for CD45. The correct classification of these lesions can be aided by the use of immunoglobulin light chains and CD30 respectively. Since the majority of large cell lymphomas particularly in extranodal sites are B cell type, the addition of CD20 to the panel will improve the diagnostic sensitivity and specificity.

Poppema 1996, Riley 2000.

All tumor cells are positive for cytokeratin

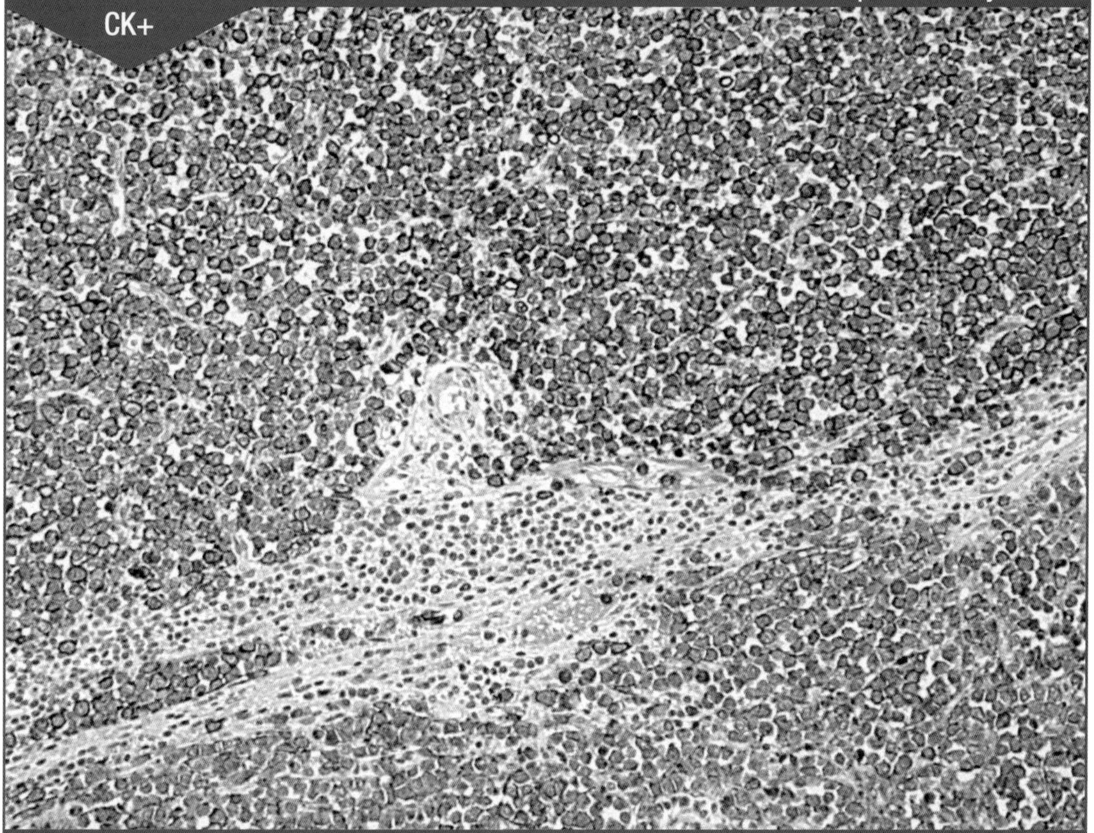

CK+

Tumor cells are negative while host lymphocytes react positively

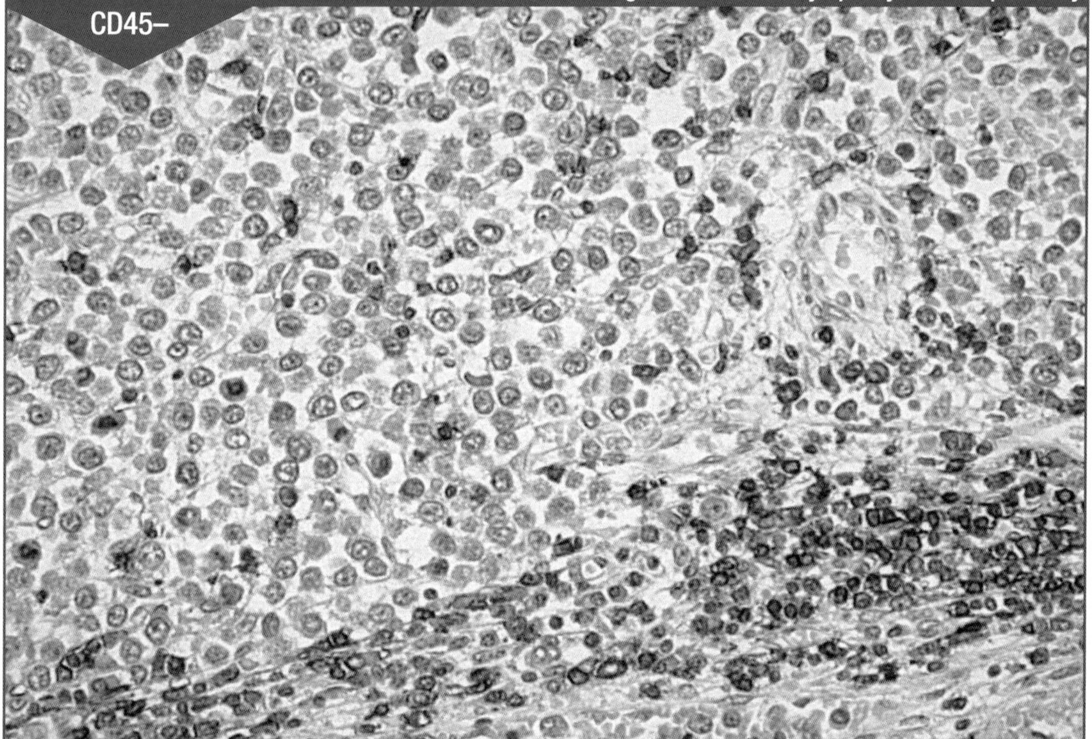

CD45–

Diagnosis: Metastatic Carcinoma

Tumor of small intestine

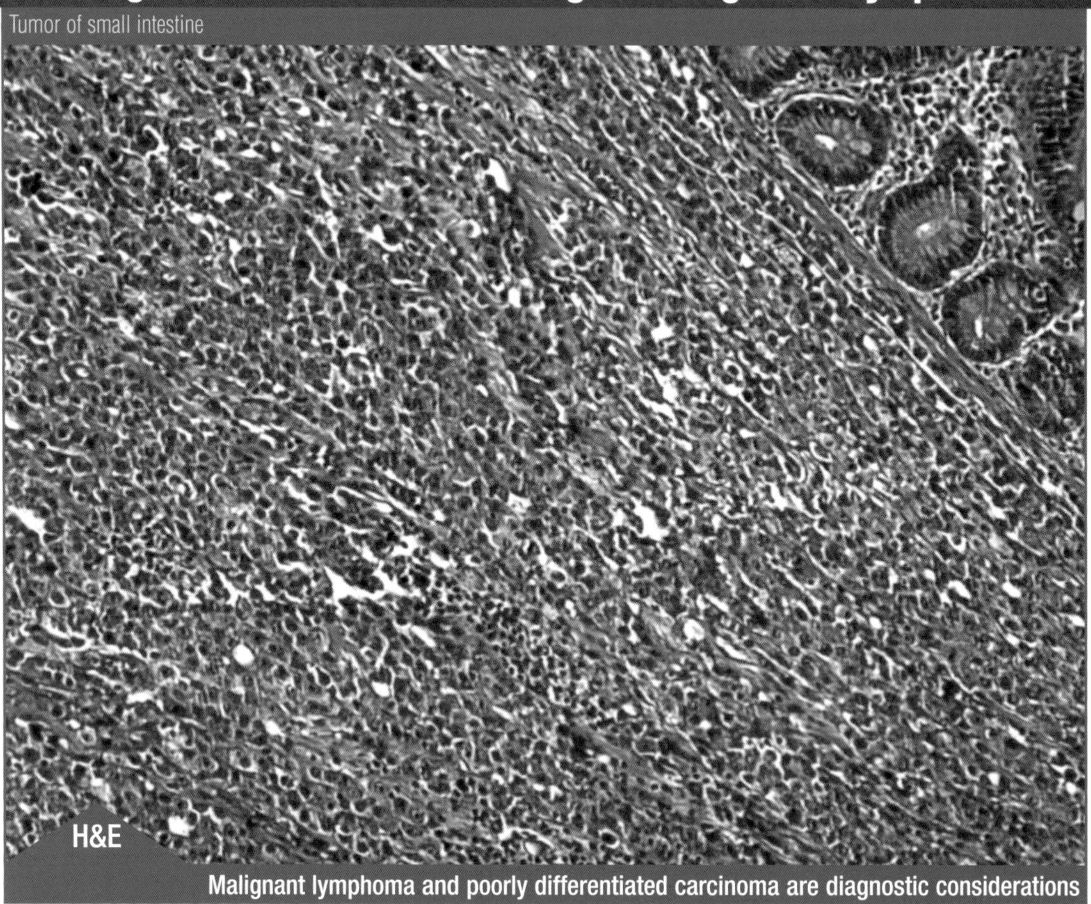

Malignant lymphoma and poorly differentiated carcinoma are diagnostic considerations

Large Cell Carcinoma vs Malignant Large Cell Lymphoma			
	Cytokeratin (CK)	CD45	CD20
Carcinoma	+	–	–
Lymphoma	–	+	+

Helpful Hints

CD45 (leukocyte common antigen) is a specific and rather sensitive marker of malignant lymphomas. A few immunoblastic and anaplastic large cell lymphomas may be negative for CD45. The correct classification of these lesions can be aided by the use of immunoglobulin light chains and CD30 respectively. Since the majority of large cell lymphomas particularly in extranodal sites are B cell type, the addition of CD20 to the panel will improve the diagnostic sensitivity and specificity.

Poppema 1996, Riley 2000.

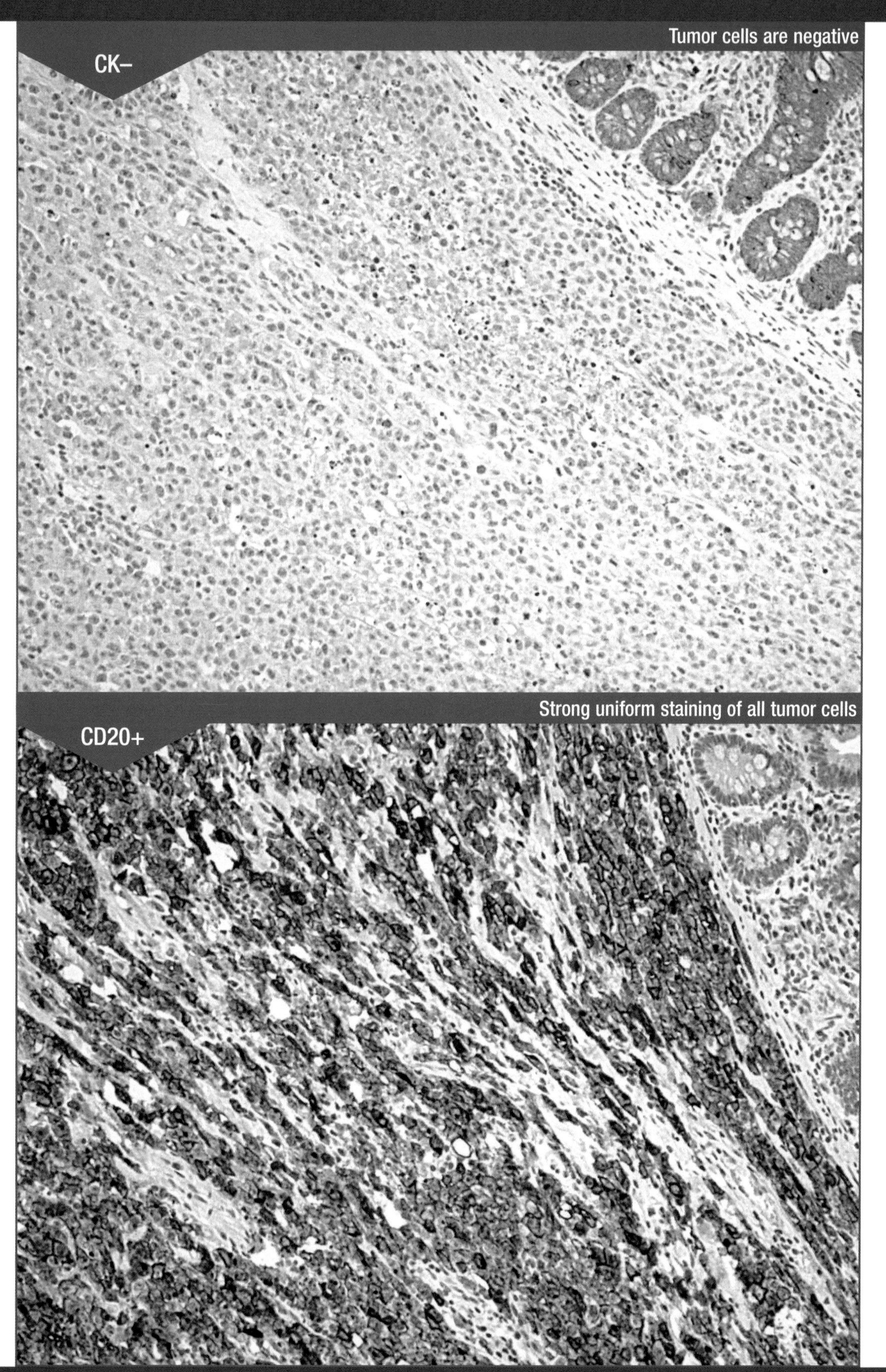

Diagnosis: Malignant Lymphoma, Large B Cell Type

Retroperitoneal lymph node in a patient with history of seminoma

H&E

Seminoma; but rule out large cell lymphoma

Large Cell Carcinomas vs Seminoma			
	Cytokeratin (CK)	PLAP	KIT (CD117)
Carcinoma	+	–	S
Seminoma	–	+	+

Helpful Hints

Cytokeratin: Focal, weak staining for cytokeratins may occasionally be seen in seminomas. The reaction, when present, however, is different than that of carcinoma in extent and intensity.

Placental Alkaline Phosphatase (PLAP): Although not completely specific, this antigen is expressed by the majority of germinomas (seminomas and dysgerminomas). The clinical information, especially the location of tumor (ie, mediastinum, retroperitoneum) should be taken into consideration before choosing PLAP as a diagnostic marker. Indiscriminate use of PLAP in antibody panels may lead to diagnostic errors.

Although not truly specific, **KIT (CD117)** is also a marker for seminomas. Similar to PLAP, this antigen is expressed by intratubal germ cell tumors as well.

Hamilton-Dutoit 1990, Koshida 1990, Cherville 2000.

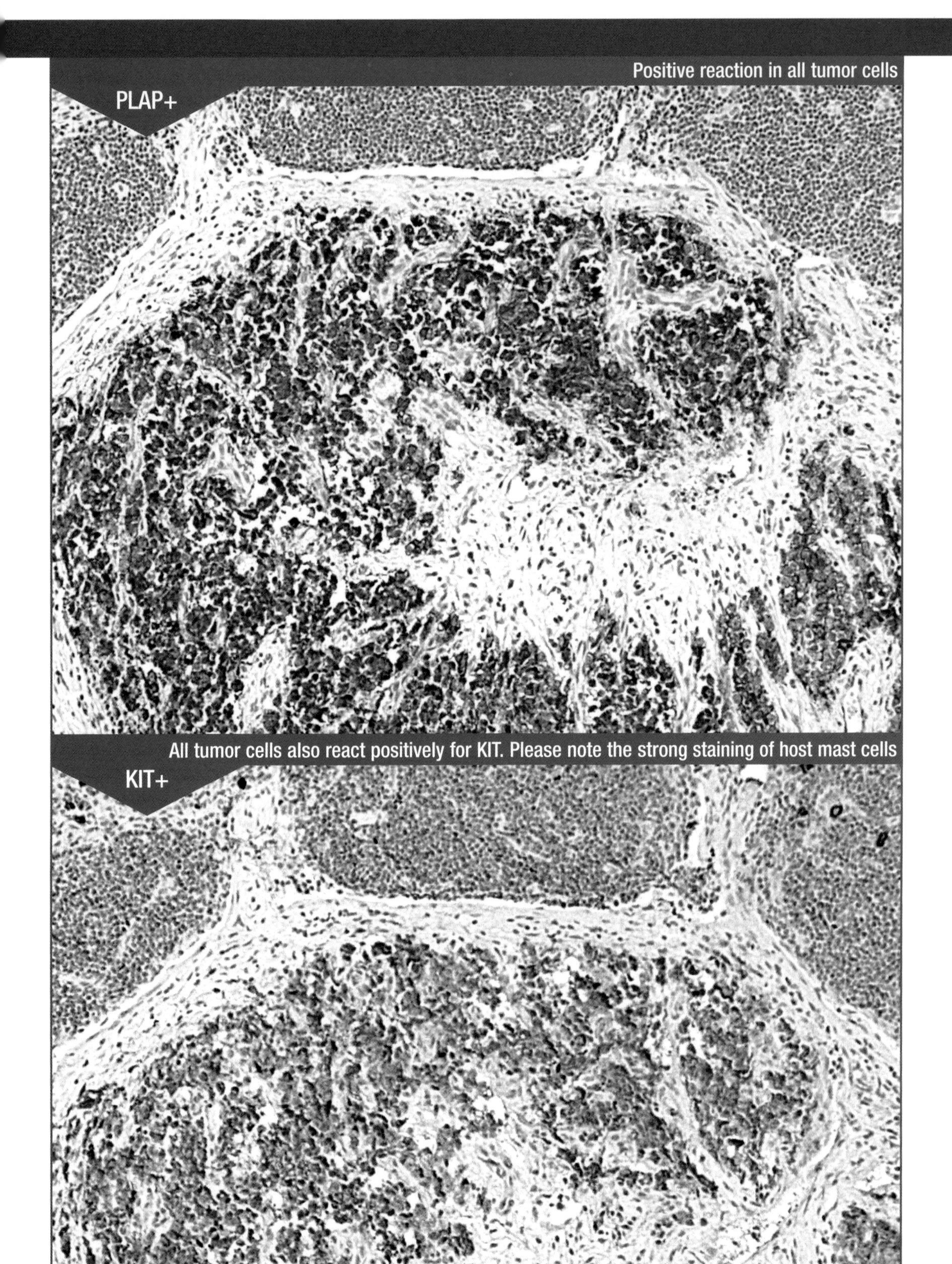

Diagnosis: Seminoma in Retroperitoneal Lymph Node

Inguinal lymph node biopsy; no prior history of malignancy

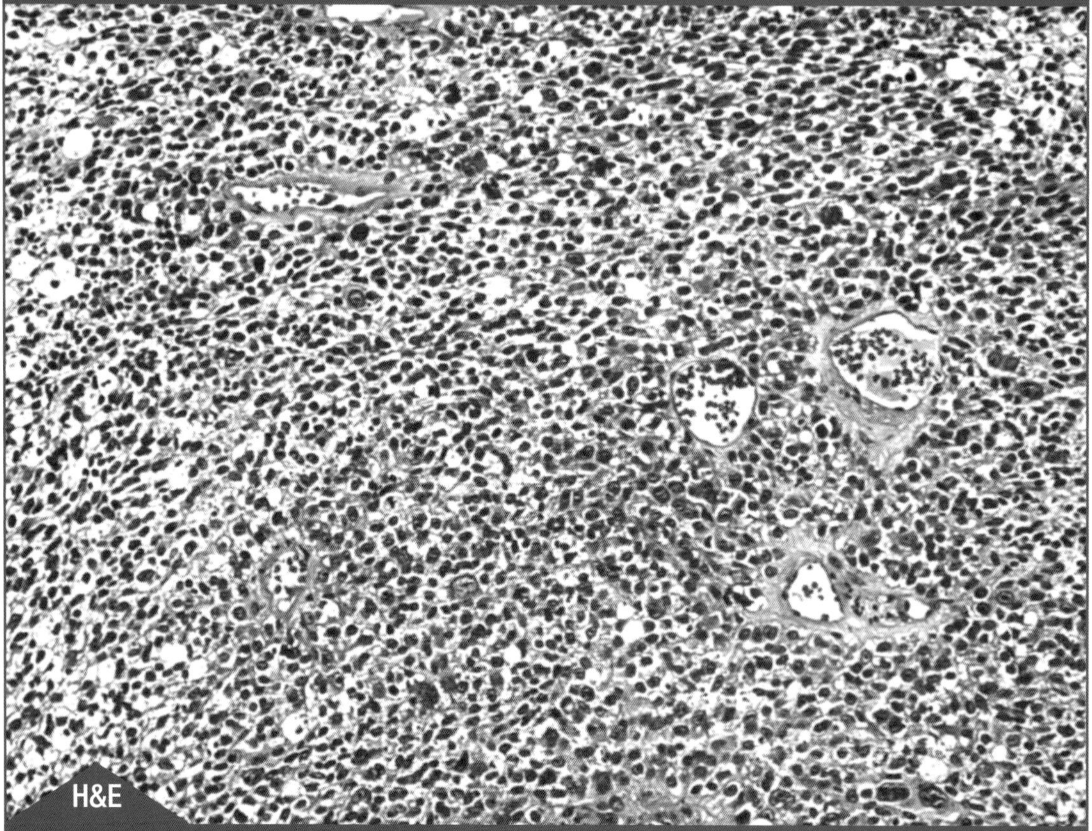

H&E

Anaplastic large cell malignant tumor

Malignant Melanoma vs Malignant Lymphoma		
	S100 Protein	CD45
Melanoma	+	–
Lymphoma	–	+

Helpful Hints

S100 protein: Although S100 protein is the most sensitive marker for malignant melanoma; it is by no means the most specific one. A number of non-melanocytic neoplasms could show a positive reaction for S100 protein. Positive staining of occasional carcinomas is usually focal, as opposed to malignant melanomas where the reaction is usually diffuse throughout the tumor. A true positive reaction for S100 protein is both cytoplasmic and nuclear. In the absence of nuclear staining, one should question the validity of results.

Melan-A: Please see p 32.

CD45 (leukocyte common antigen) is a specific and rather sensitive marker of malignant lymphomas. A few immunoblastic and anaplastic large cell lymphomas may be negative for CD45. In those instances, immunoglobulin light chains and CD30 could be used to resolve the above differential diagnoses respectively.

Poppema 1996, McNutt 1993, Cochran 1993.

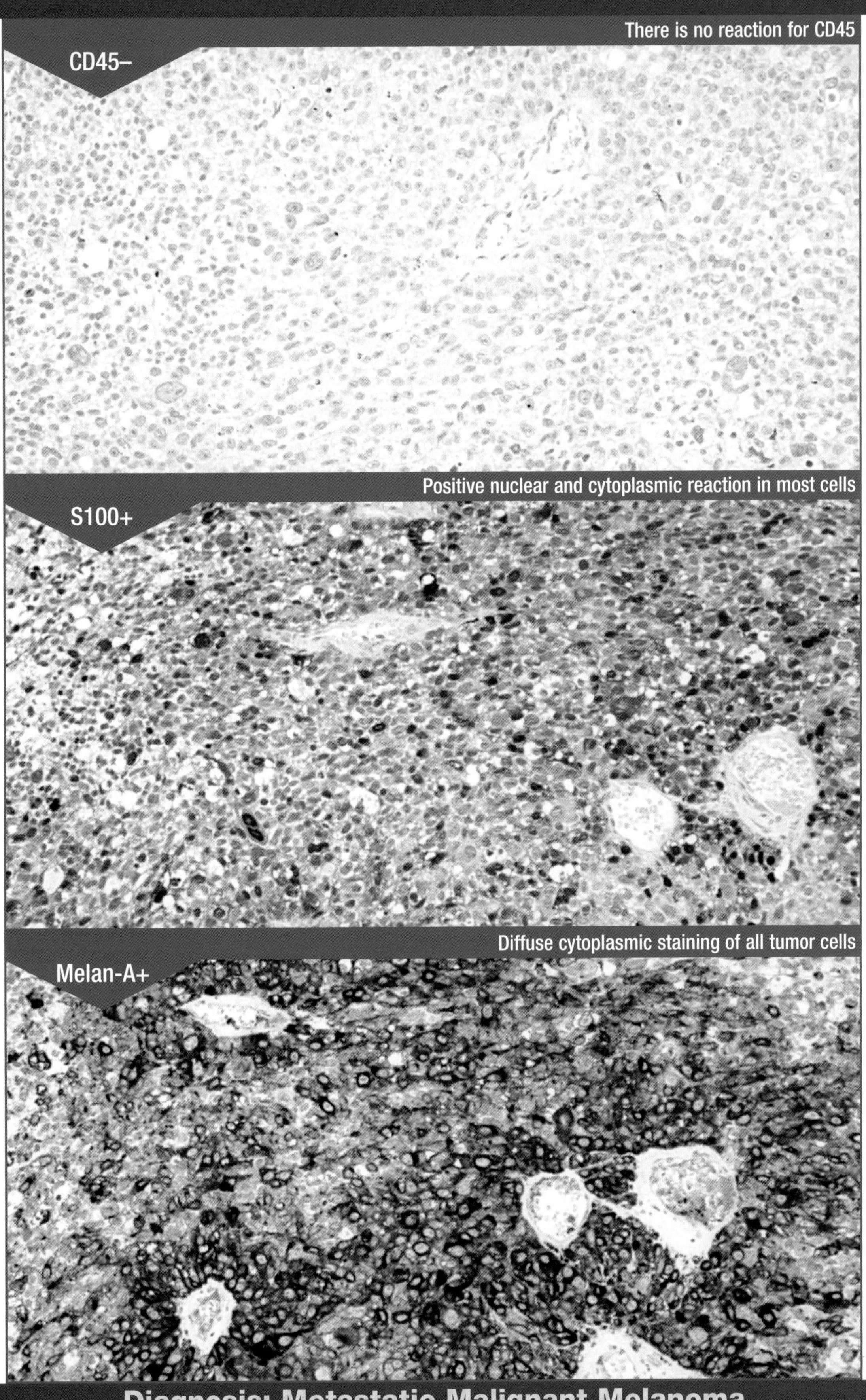

Diagnosis: Metastatic Malignant Melanoma

Malignant Melanoma vs Large Cell Malignant Lymphoma

Cervical lymph node

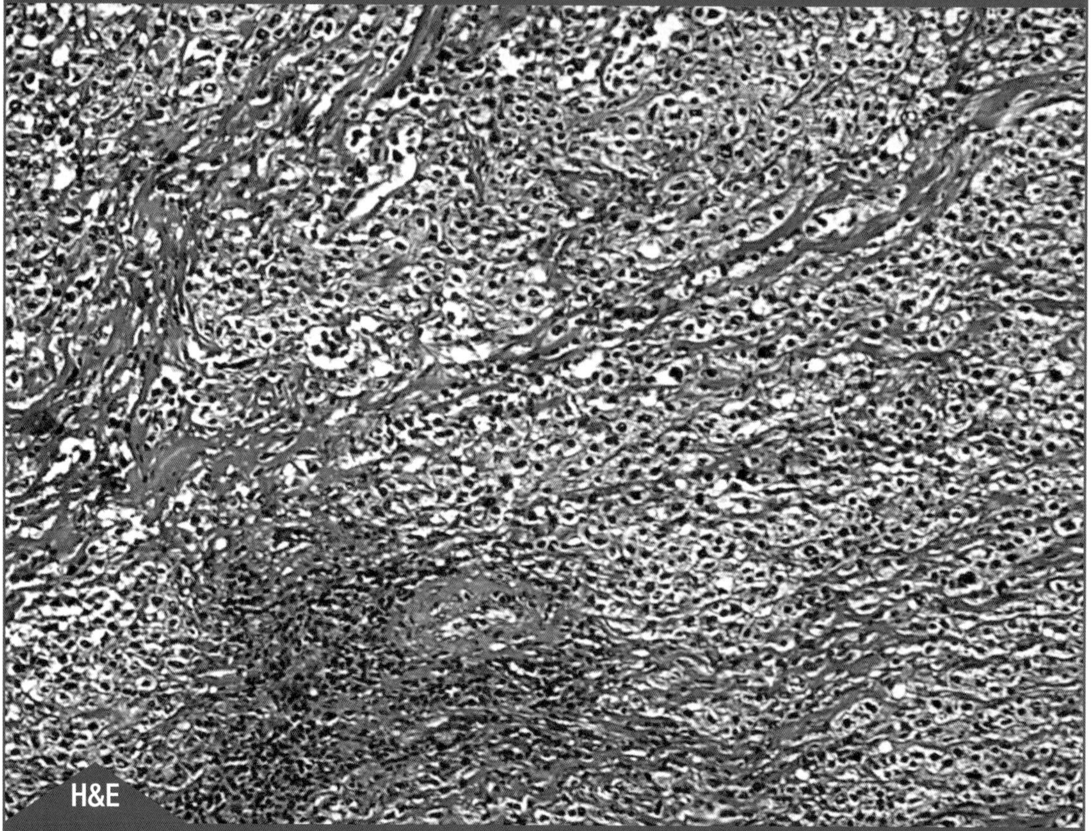

H&E

Anaplastic malignant neoplasm

Malignant Melanoma vs Malignant Lymphoma		
	S100 Protein	CD20
Melanoma	+	–
Lymphoma	–	+

Helpful Hints

S100 protein: Although S100 protein is the most sensitive marker for malignant melanoma; it is by no means the most specific one. A number of non-melanocytic neoplasms could show a positive reaction for S100 protein. Positive staining of occasional carcinomas is usually focal, as opposed to malignant melanomas where the reaction is usually diffuse throughout the tumor. A true positive reaction for S100 protein is both cytoplasmic and nuclear. In the absence of nuclear staining, one should question the validity of results.

CD20: The majority of large cell lymphomas, particularly at extranodal sites, are B cell type.

Poppema 1996, McNutt 1993.

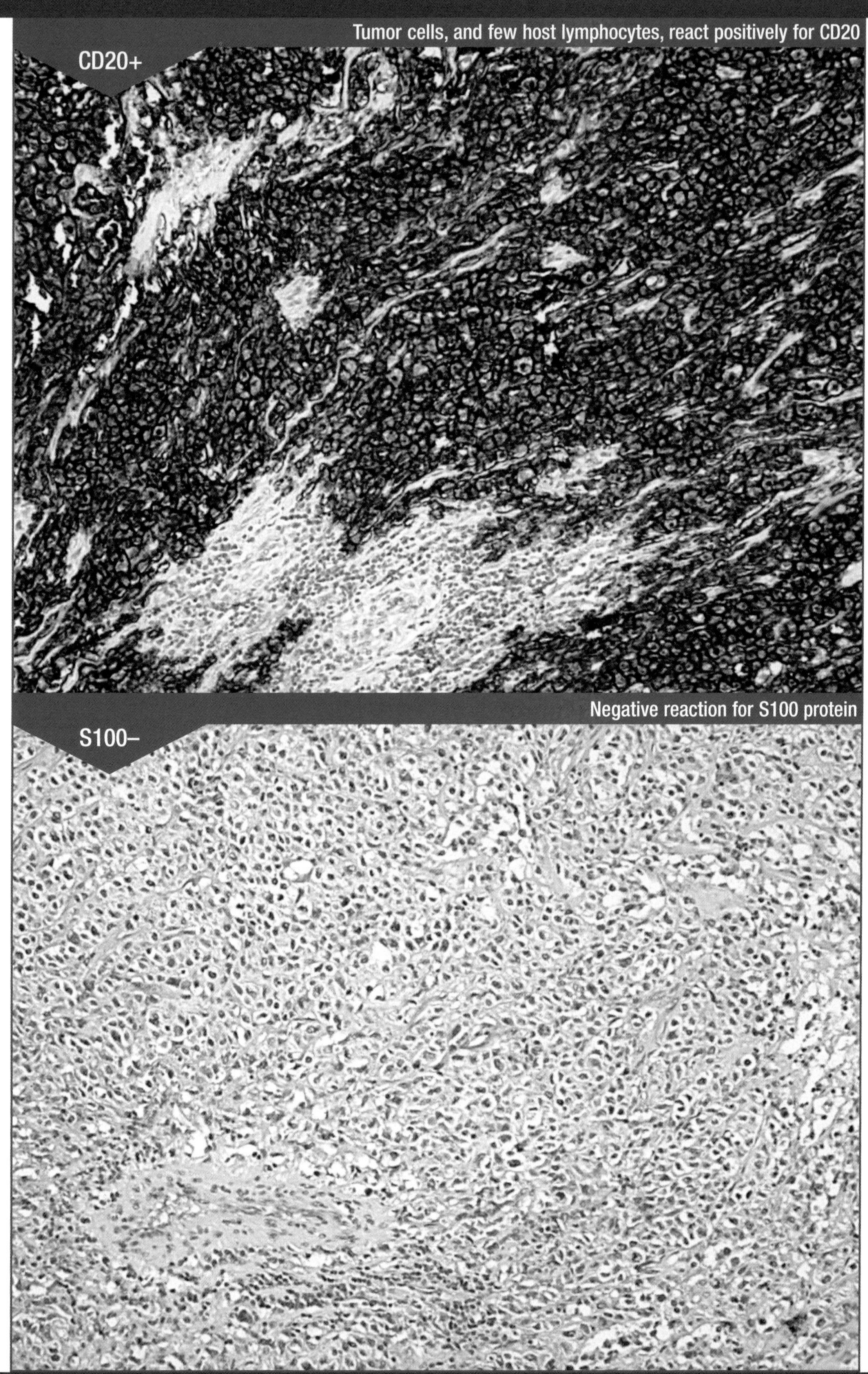

Diagnosis: Malignant Lymphoma, Large B Cell Type

Abdominal mass biopsy in a 51 year old male

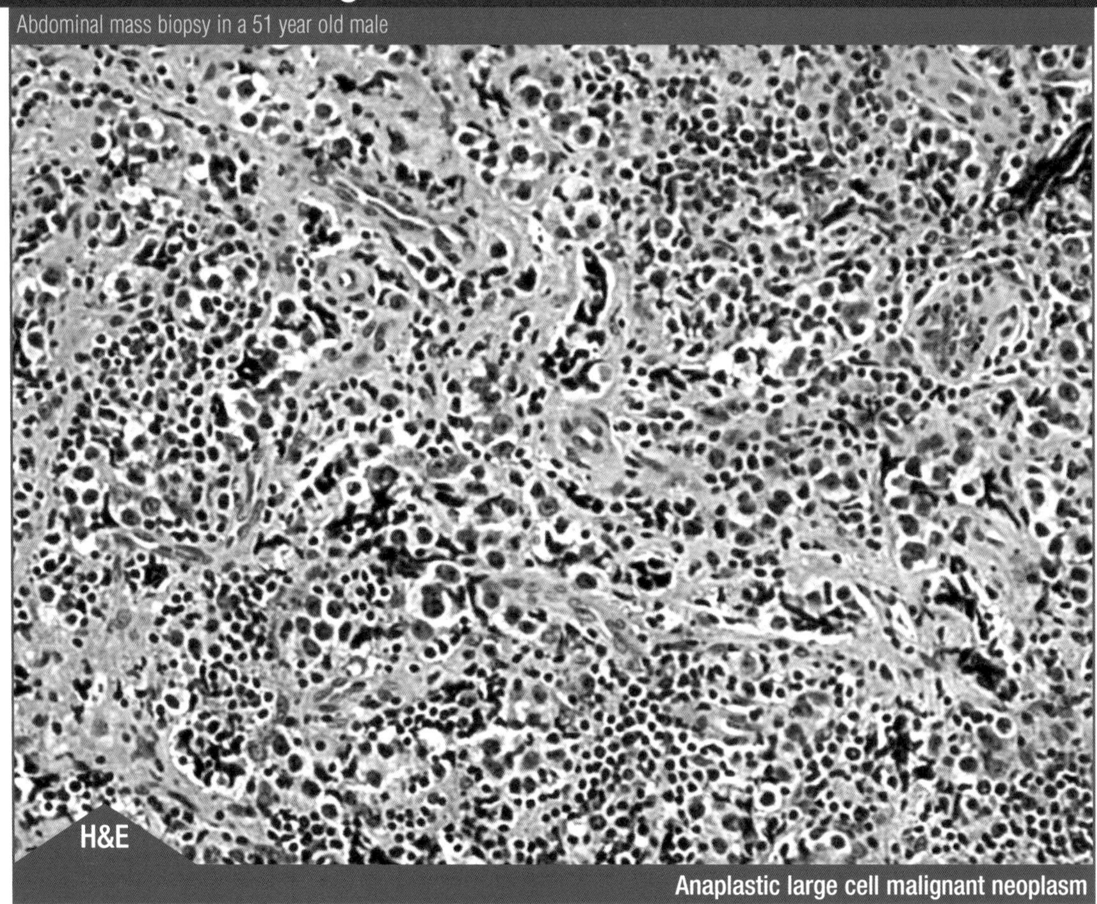

Anaplastic large cell malignant neoplasm

Malignant Melanoma vs Seminoma		
	S100 Protein	PLAP
Melanoma	+	−
Seminoma	−	+

Helpful Hints

S100 protein: Although S100 protein is the most sensitive marker for malignant melanoma; it is by no means the most specific one. A number of non-melanocytic neoplasms could show a positive reaction for S100 protein. Positive staining of occasional carcinomas is usually focal, as opposed to malignant melanomas where the reaction is usually diffuse throughout the tumor. A true positive reaction for S100 protein is both cytoplasmic and nuclear. In the absence of nuclear staining, one should question the validity of the results.

Placental Alkaline Phosphatase (PLAP): Although not completely specific, this antigen is expressed by the majority of germinomas (seminomas, dysgerminomas). The clinical information, especially the location of tumor (ie, mediastinum, retroperitoneum) should be taken into consideration before choosing PLAP as a diagnostic marker. Indiscriminate use of PLAP in antibody panels may lead to diagnostic errors.

Hamilton-Dutoit 1990, Koshida 1990, Cochran 1993.

*We later learned that it was a primary tumor that arose from an undescended testis.

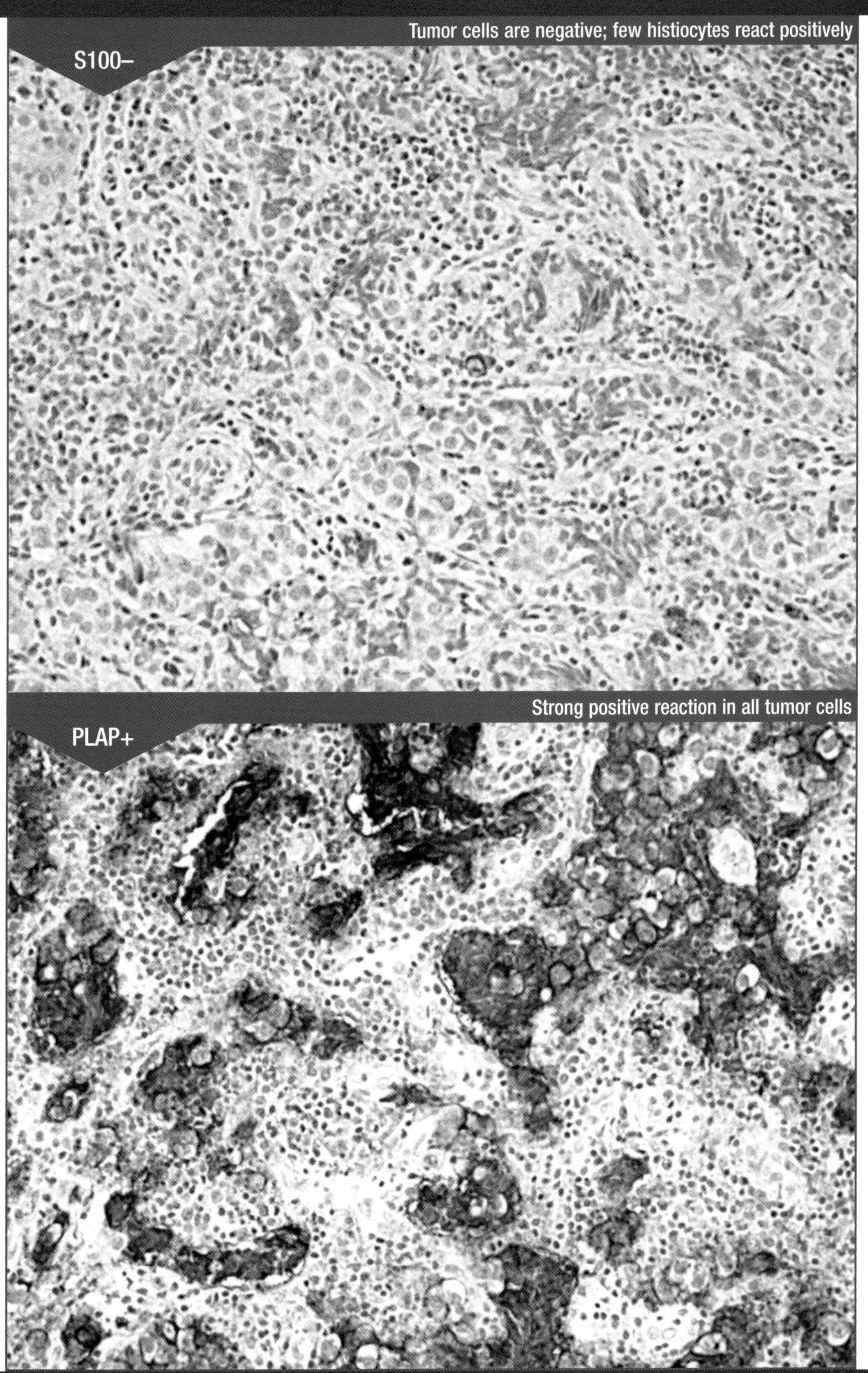

Diagnosis: "Metastatic" Seminoma*

Malignant Large Cell Lymphoma vs Seminoma

Mediastinal biopsy

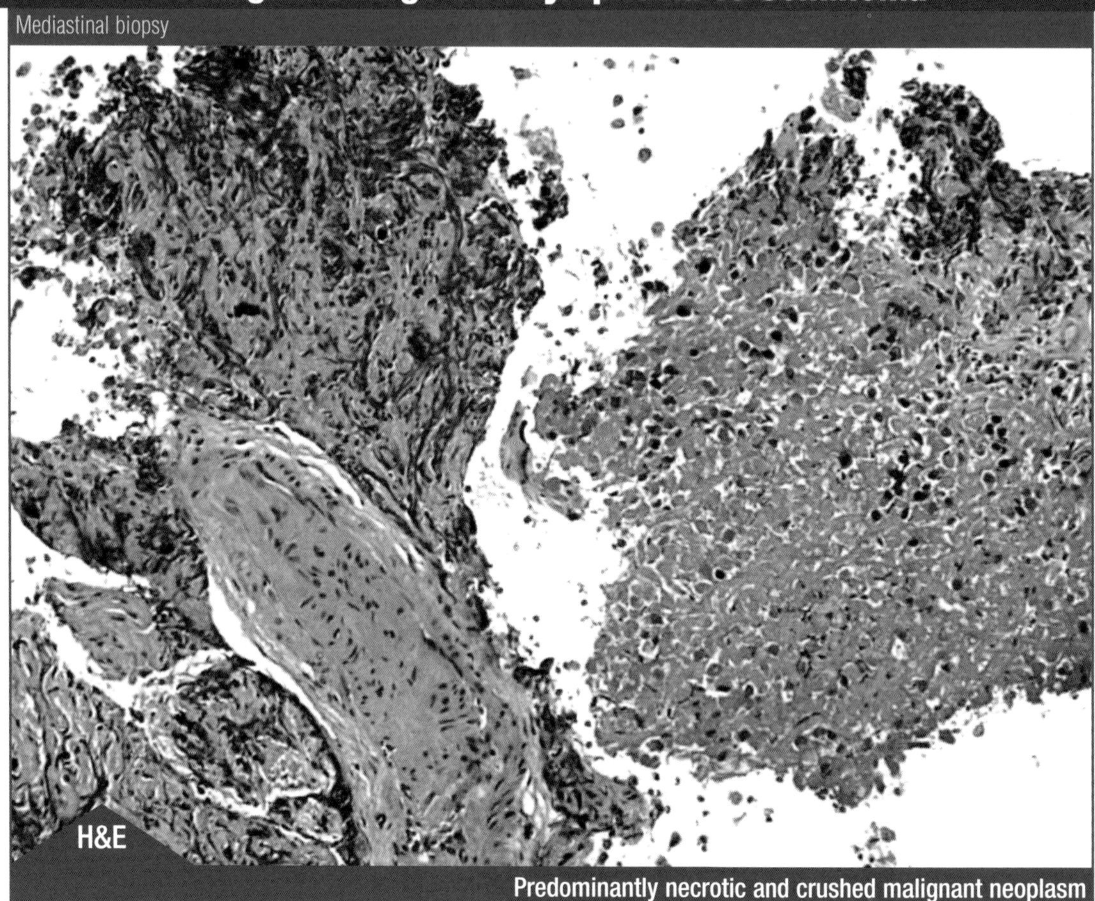

Predominantly necrotic and crushed malignant neoplasm

Malignant Lymphoma vs Seminoma		
	CD45	PLAP
Lymphoma	+	–
Seminoma	–	+

Helpful Hints

This differential diagnosis is not uncommon particularly in small biopsies from mediastinum and retroperitoneum. It is important to note that crushed or necrotic lymphoma cells still react positively for CD45 as do seminoma cell for PLAP.

Placental Alkaline Phosphatase (PLAP): Although not completely specific, this antigen is expressed by the majority of germinomas (seminomas, dysgerminomas). The clinical information, especially the location of tumor (ie, mediastinum, retroperitoneum) should be taken into consideration before choosing PLAP as a diagnostic marker. Indiscriminate use of PLAP in antibody panels may lead to diagnostic errors.

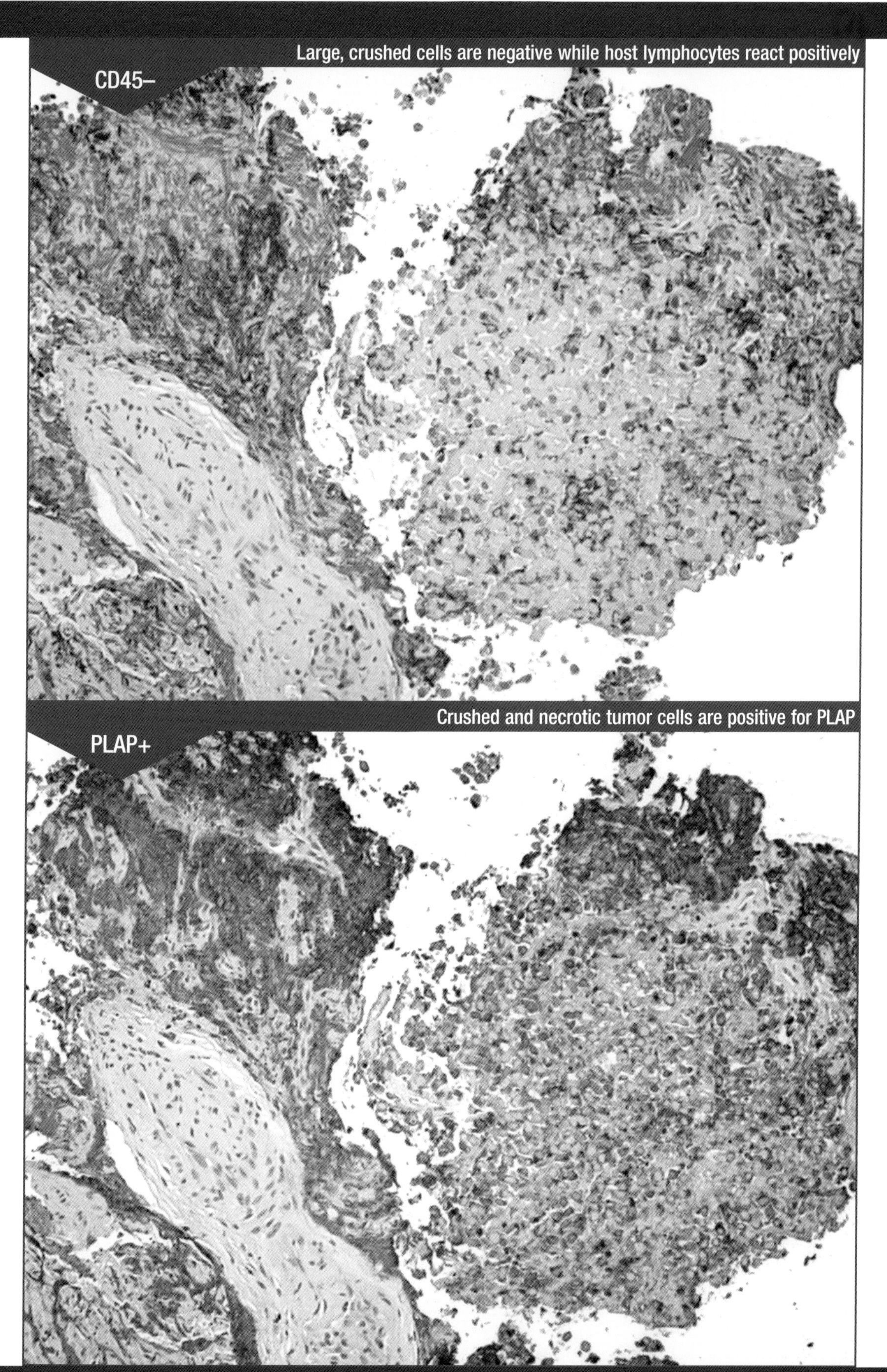

Diagnosis: Seminoma of Mediastinum

Orchiectomy specimen

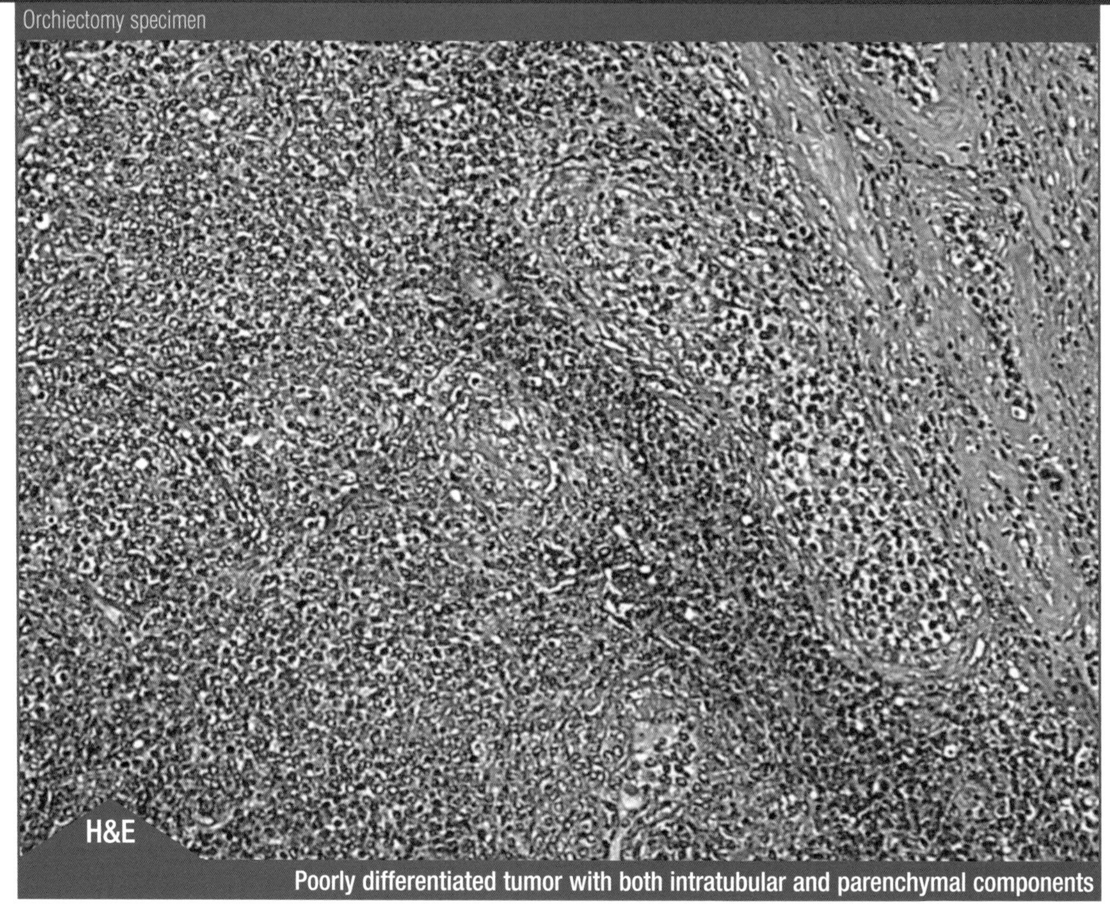

Poorly differentiated tumor with both intratubular and parenchymal components

Malignant Lymphoma vs Seminoma		
	CD45	PLAP
Lymphoma	+	–
Seminoma	–	+

Helpful Hints

This differential diagnosis is not uncommon particularly in small biopsies from mediastinum and retroperitoneum. It is important to note that crushed or necrotic lymphoma cells still react positively for CD45 as do seminoma cell for PLAP.

Placental Alkaline Phosphatase (PLAP): Although not completely specific, this antigen is expressed by the majority of germinomas (seminomas, dysgerminomas). The clinical information, especially the location of tumor (ie, mediastinum, retroperitoneum) should be taken into consideration before choosing PLAP as a diagnostic marker. Indiscriminate use of PLAP in antibody panels may lead to diagnostic errors.

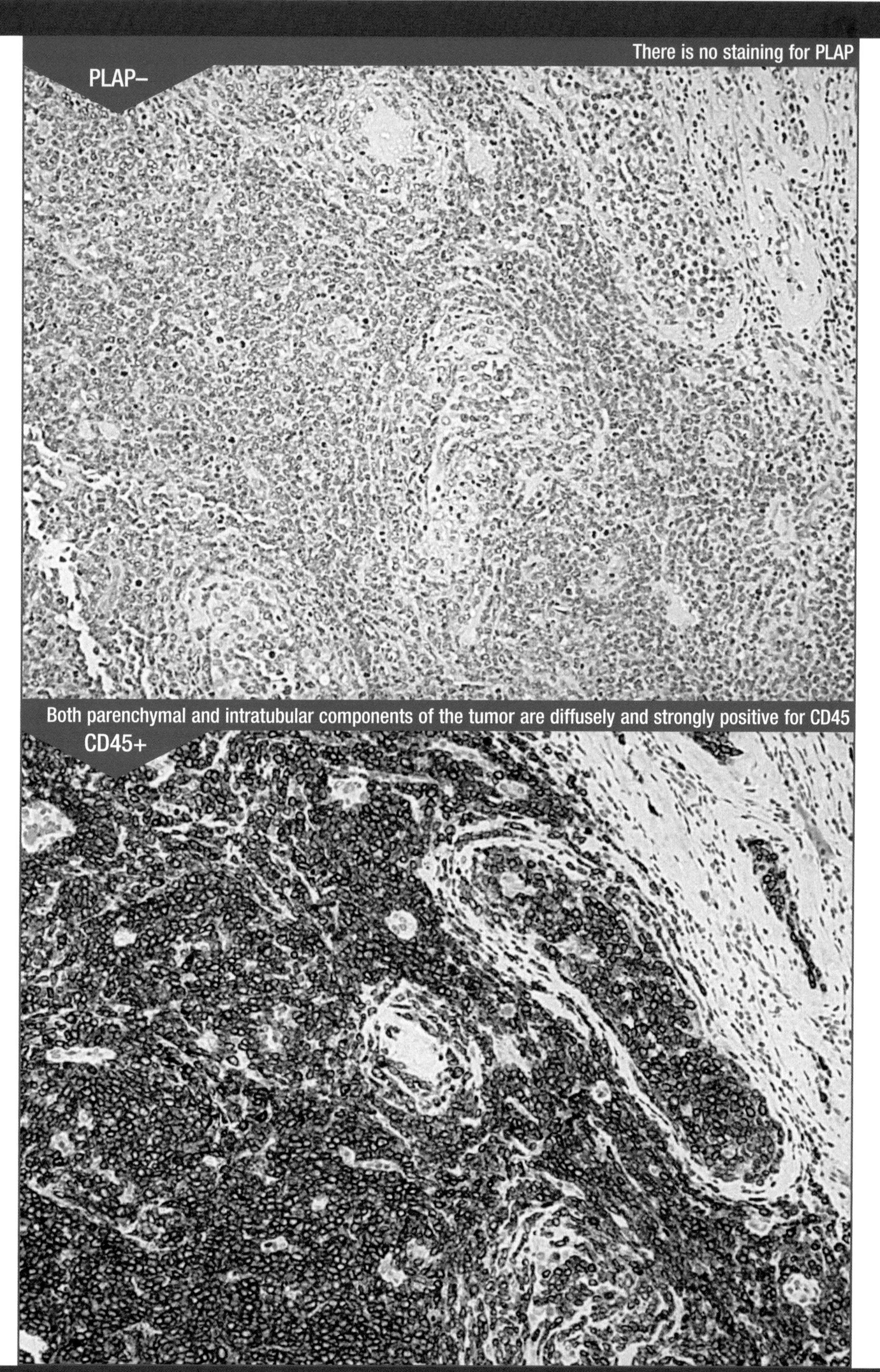

Diagnosis: Malignant Large Cell Lymphoma of Testis

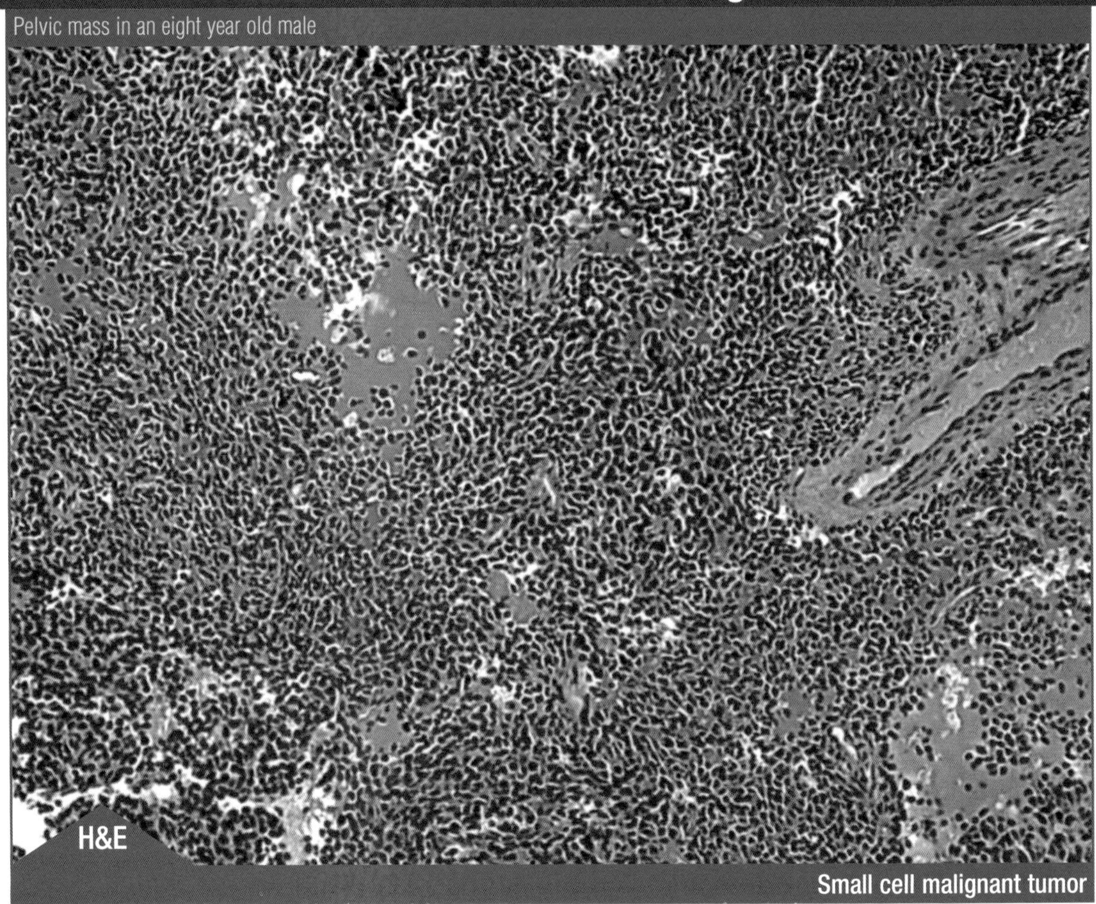

Small Cell Carcinoma vs Ewing/PNET*	Cytokeratin (CK)	CD99 (MIC2)
Small Cell Carcinoma	+	–
Ewing/PNET*	–	+

Helpful Hints

Cytokeratin: In most small cell carcinomas the reaction for cytokeratin is either perinuclear or in paranuclear punctate form. This staining pattern although helpful in distinguishing small cell carcinomas from non-small cell carcinomas is by no means by itself diagnostic.

CD99 (MIC2) is expressed by a number of tumors and as such is not diagnostic of any specific entity. It is however, helpful within a limited differential diagnostic possibility such as the above example. Reactivity for CD99 is usually diffuse in positive tumors and could occasionally be mistaken for non-specific background staining.

Amann 1999.

*PNET, Primitive neuroectodermal tumors

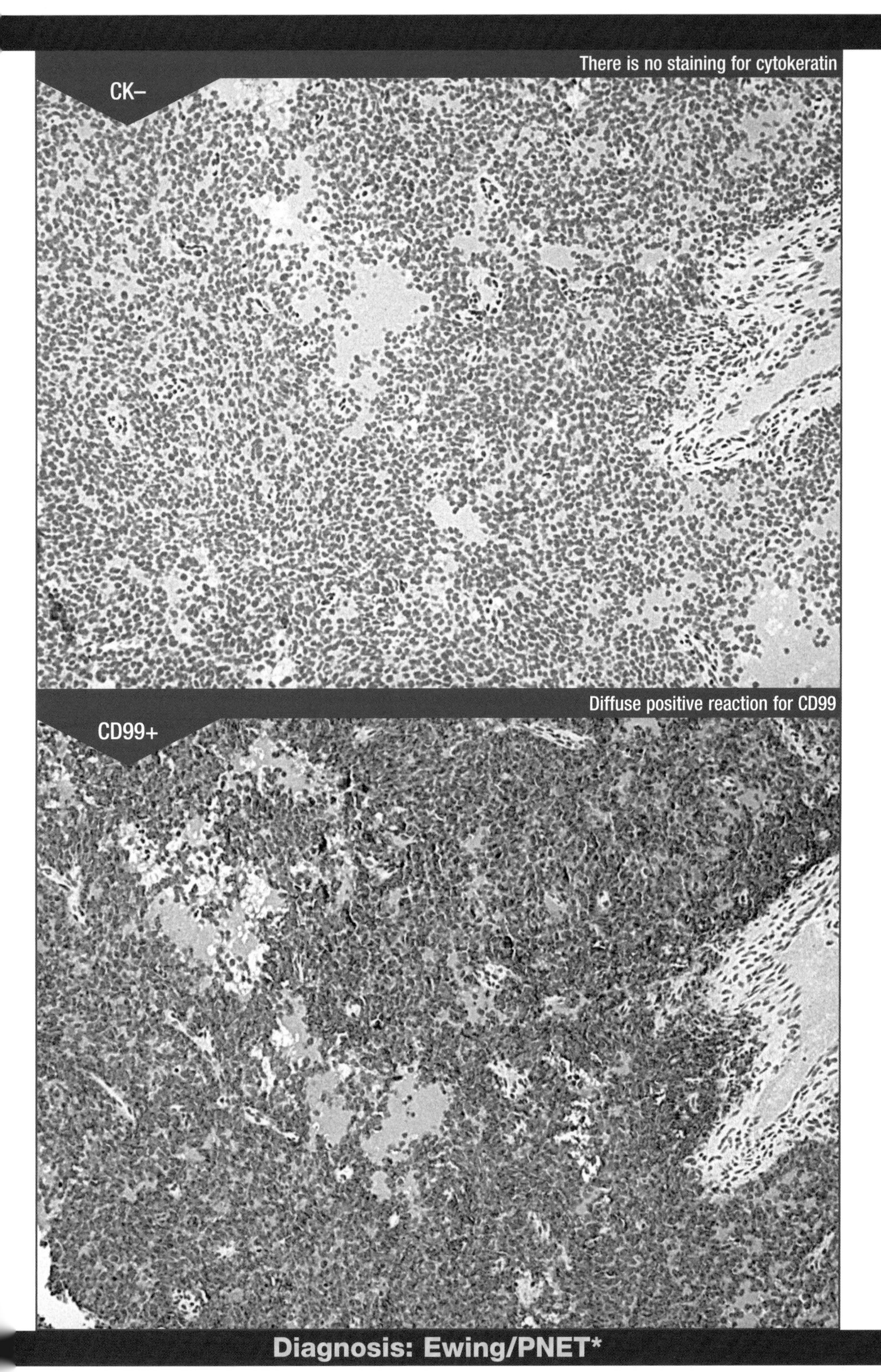

Diagnosis: Ewing/PNET*

Biopsy of nasal mucosa

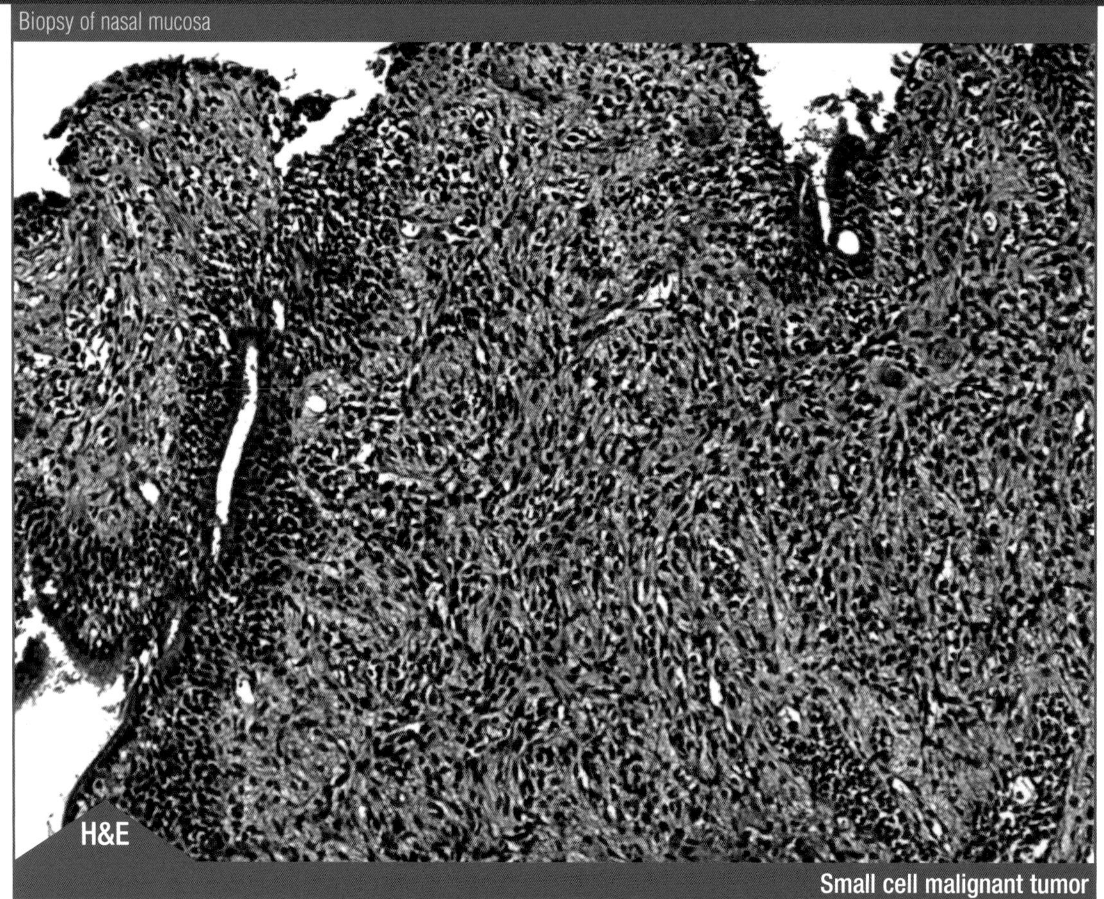

Small cell malignant tumor

Small Cell Carcinoma vs Rhabdomyosarcoma		
	Cytokeratin (CK)	Desmin
Small Cell Carcinoma	+	–
Rhabdomyosarcoma	–	+

Helpful Hints

In this differential diagnosis, positivity for **desmin** establishes the diagnosis of rhabdomyosarcoma. Since leiomyosarcoma ordinarily do not present as a small cell tumor, there is no need to further characterize a desmin-positive small cell tumor for rhabdomyoblastic differentiation. If needed, however, one could use a marker for rhabdomyoblast. *(See next case.)*

Truong 1990.

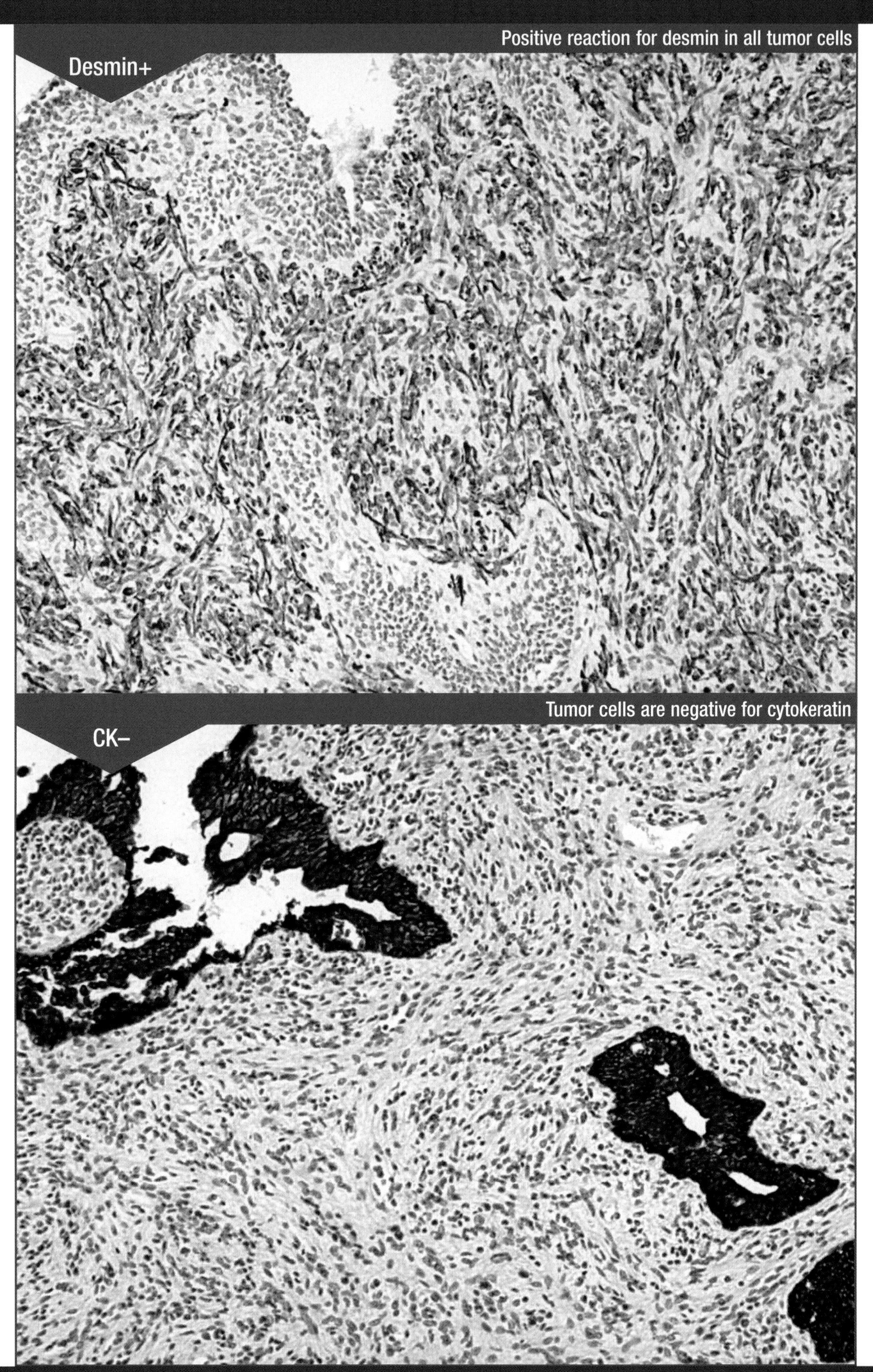

Diagnosis: Rhabdomyosarcoma, Embryonal Type

Biopsy of soft tissue mass in the neck of a young female

H&E

Small cell malignant tumor. There is a hint of cytoplasmic eosinophilia in some cells

Rhabdomyosarcoma vs Ewing/PNET*

	Desmin	Myogenin	CD99
Rhabdomyosarcoma	+	+	–
Ewing/PNET*	–	–	+

Helpful Hints

Desmin: The majority of rhabdomyosarcomas, regardless of histologic subtypes, are positive for desmin. Since leiomyosarcomas do not present with small cell morphology, a desmin-positive small round cell tumor is in all likelihood a rhabdomyosarcoma. To confirm that diagnosis one could use a skeletal muscle marker. Because of lack of sensitivity, myoglobin is practically useless for that purpose. The most sensitive and specific markers for skeletal muscle differentiation are myogenin and MyoD1; we prefer the former.

Myogenin: Both myogenin and MyoD1 are intranuclear transcription factors that are expressed exclusively in early rhabdomyoblastic differentiation. The majority of rhabdomyosarcomas are positive for those markers, although more differentiated tumors may be only focally positive or completely negative. Similarly, alveolar rhabdomyosarcomas may only show focal reaction for myogenin.

Cui 1999.

*PNET, Primitive neuroectodermal tumors

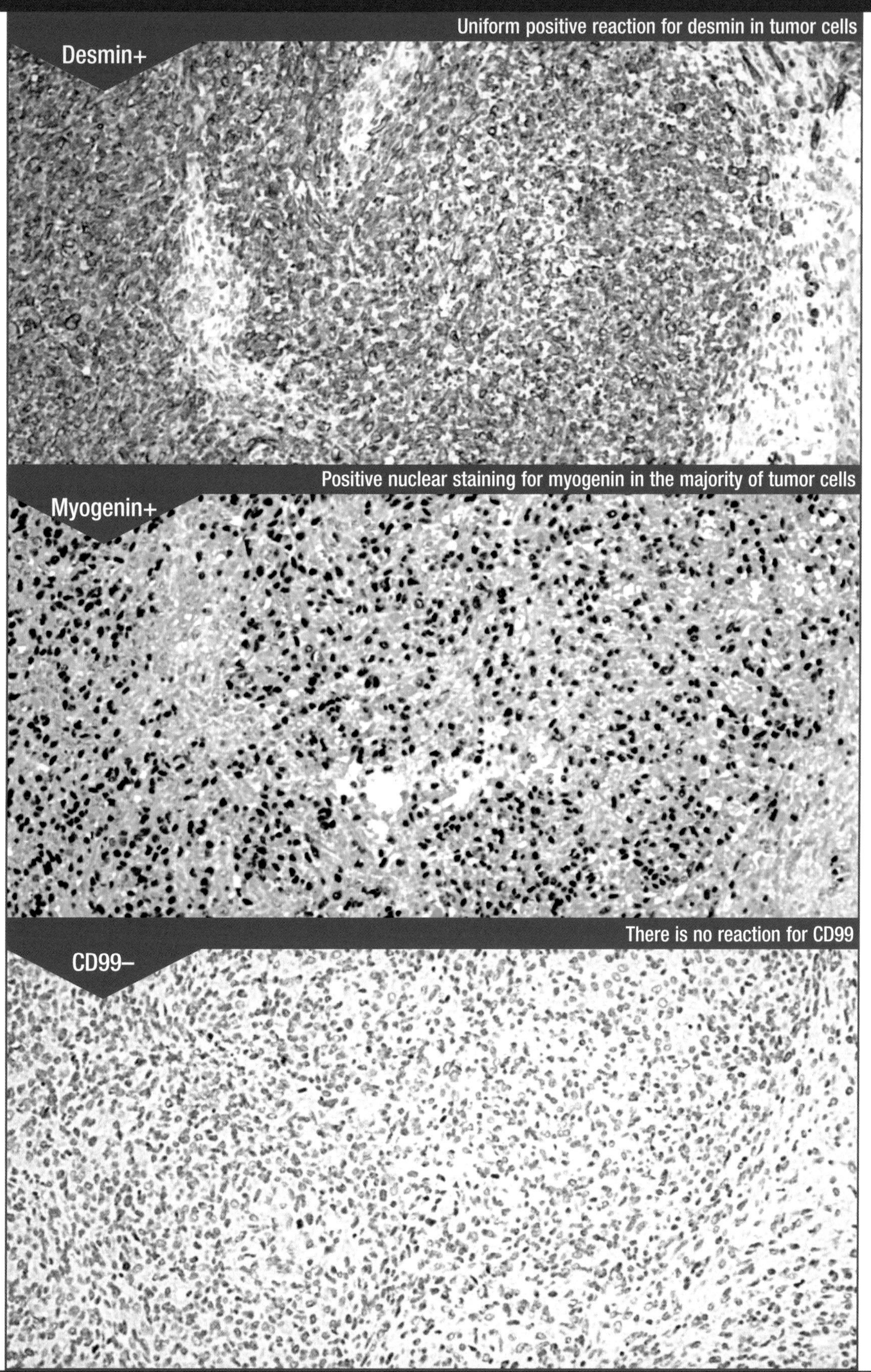
Uniform positive reaction for desmin in tumor cells
Desmin+
Positive nuclear staining for myogenin in the majority of tumor cells
Myogenin+
There is no reaction for CD99
CD99–
Diagnosis: Embryonal Rhabdomyosarcoma

Nasopharyngeal tumor

H&E

Alveolar rhabdomyosarcoma

Rhabdomyosarcoma vs Ewing/PNET*			
	Desmin	Myogenin	CD99
Rhabdomyosarcoma	+	+	–
Ewing/PNET*	–	–	+

Helpful Hints

Desmin: The majority of rhabdomyosarcomas, regardless of histologic subtypes, are positive for desmin. Since leiomyosarcomas do not present with small cell morphology, a desmin-positive small round cell tumor is in all likelihood a rhabdomyosarcoma. To confirm that diagnosis one could use a skeletal muscle marker. Because of lack of sensitivity, myoglobin is practically useless for that purpose. The most sensitive and specific markers for skeletal muscle differentiation are myogenin and MyoD1; we prefer the former.

Myogenin: Both myogenin and MyoD1 are intranuclear transcription factors that are expressed exclusively in early rhabdomyoblastic differentiation. The majority of rhabdomyosarcomas are positive for those markers, although more differentiated tumors may be only focally positive or completely negative. Similarly, alveolar rhabdomyosarcomas may only show focal reaction for myogenin.

Cui 1999.

*PNET, Primitive neuroectodermal tumors

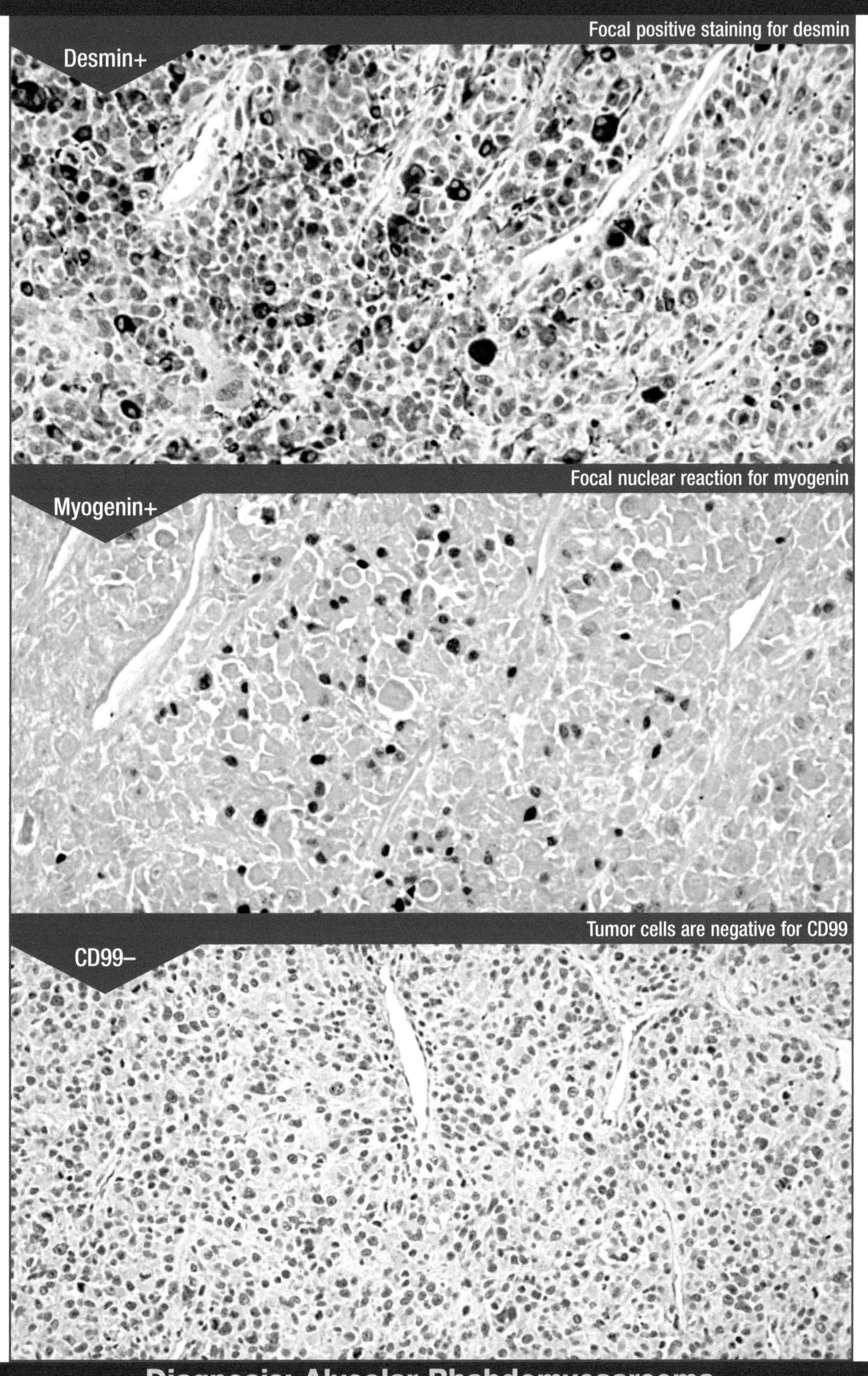

Diagnosis: Alveolar Rhabdomyosarcoma

Wedge biopsy of an ulcerated skin lesion

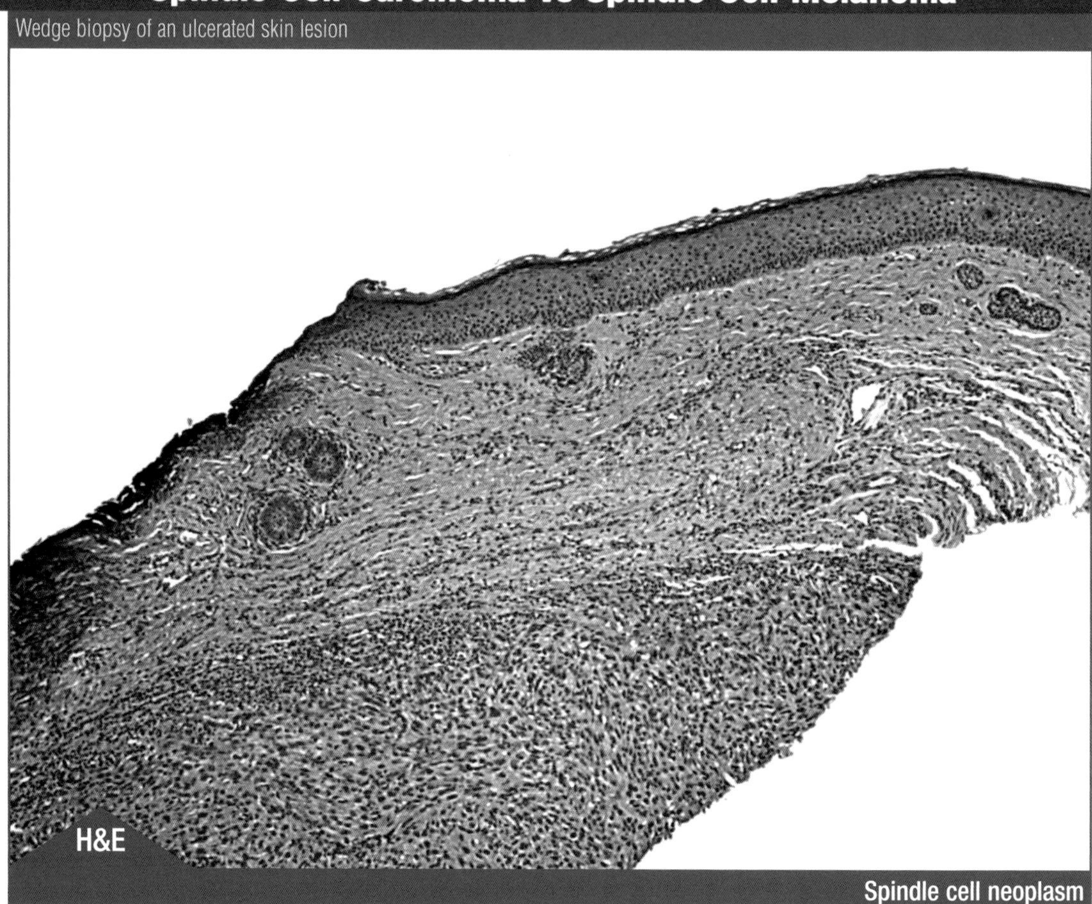

Spindle cell neoplasm

Spindle Cell Carcinoma vs Spindle Cell Melanoma		
	Cytokeratin	S100 Protein
Spindle Cell Carcinoma	+	–
Spindle Cell Melanoma	–	+

Helpful Hints

S100 protein: The great majority of spindle cell melanomas are positive for S100 protein, but only about 50% express HMB-45. Other melanocytic markers such as Melan-A and Tyrosinase may be helpful in this situation.

Miettinen 1993, Cochran 1993.

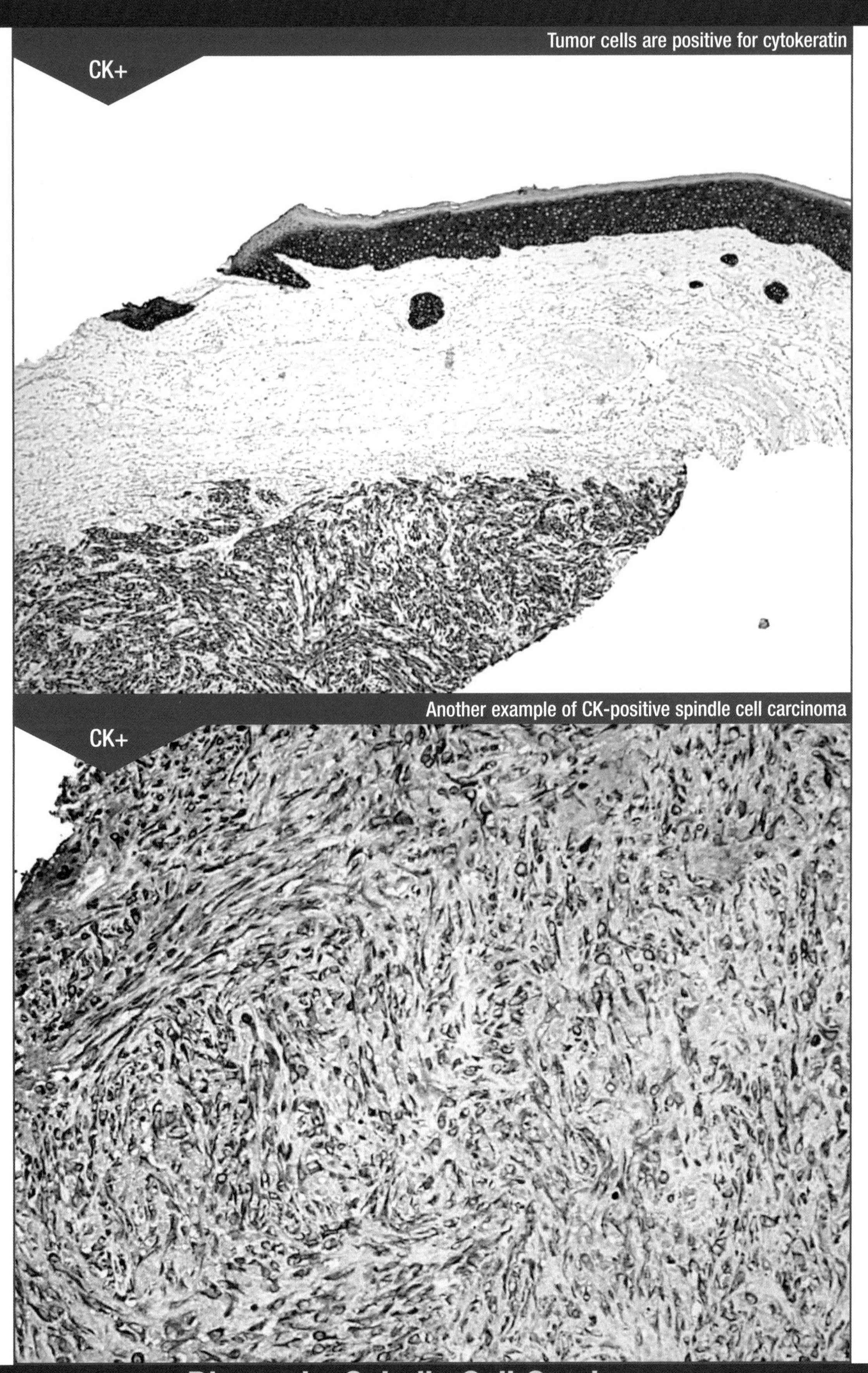

Diagnosis: Spindle Cell Carcinoma

Excision of a scalp tumor

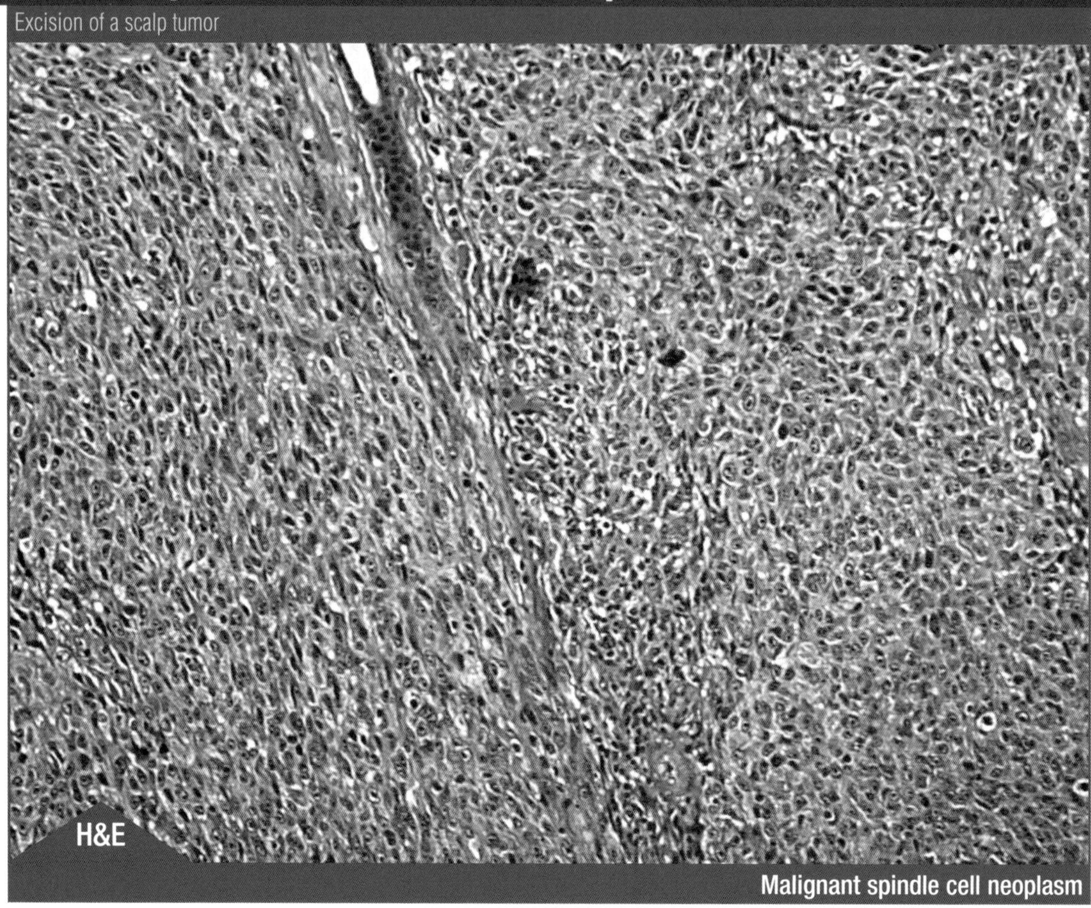

Malignant spindle cell neoplasm

Spindle Cell Carcinoma vs Spindle Cell Melanoma			
	Cytokeratin (CK)	S100	Melan-A
Spindle Cell Carcinoma	+	–	–
Spindle Cell Melanoma	–	+	+

Helpful Hints

S100 protein: The great majority of spindle cell melanomas are positive for S100 protein, but only about 50% express HMB-45. Other melanocytic markers such as Melan-A and Tyrosinase may be helpful in this situation.

Miettinen 1993, Cochran 1993.

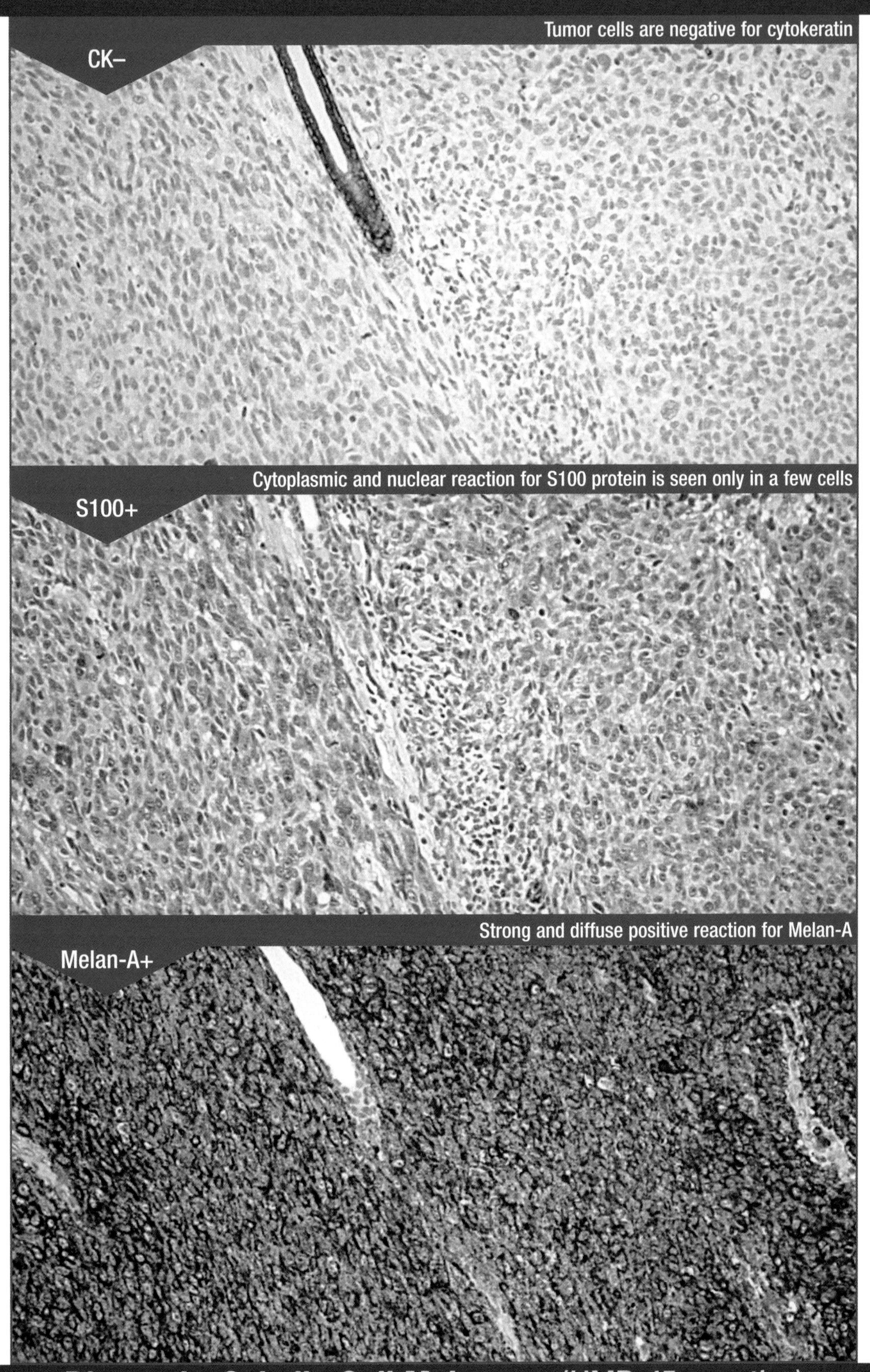

Diagnosis: Spindle Cell Melanoma (*HMB-45 negative*)

Biopsy of skin lesion from the shoulder area

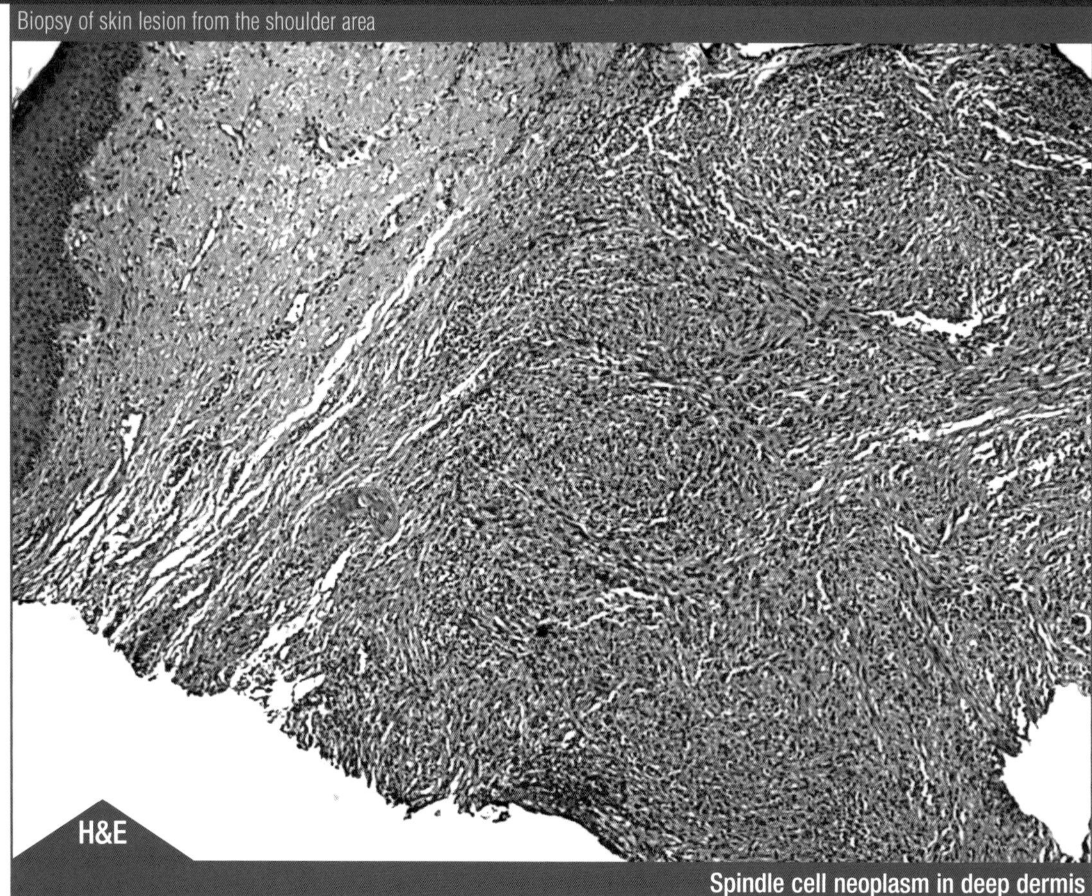

Spindle cell neoplasm in deep dermis

Spindle Cell Carcinoma vs Spindle Cell Melanoma			
	Cytokeratin (CK)	S100	HMB-45
Spindle Cell Carcinoma	+	–	–
Spindle Cell Melanoma	–	+	S

Helpful Hints

S100 protein: The great majority of spindle cell melanomas are positive for S100 protein, but only about 50% express HMB-45. Other melanocytic markers such as Melan-A and Tyrosinase may be helpful in this situation.

Miettinen 1993, Cochran 1993.

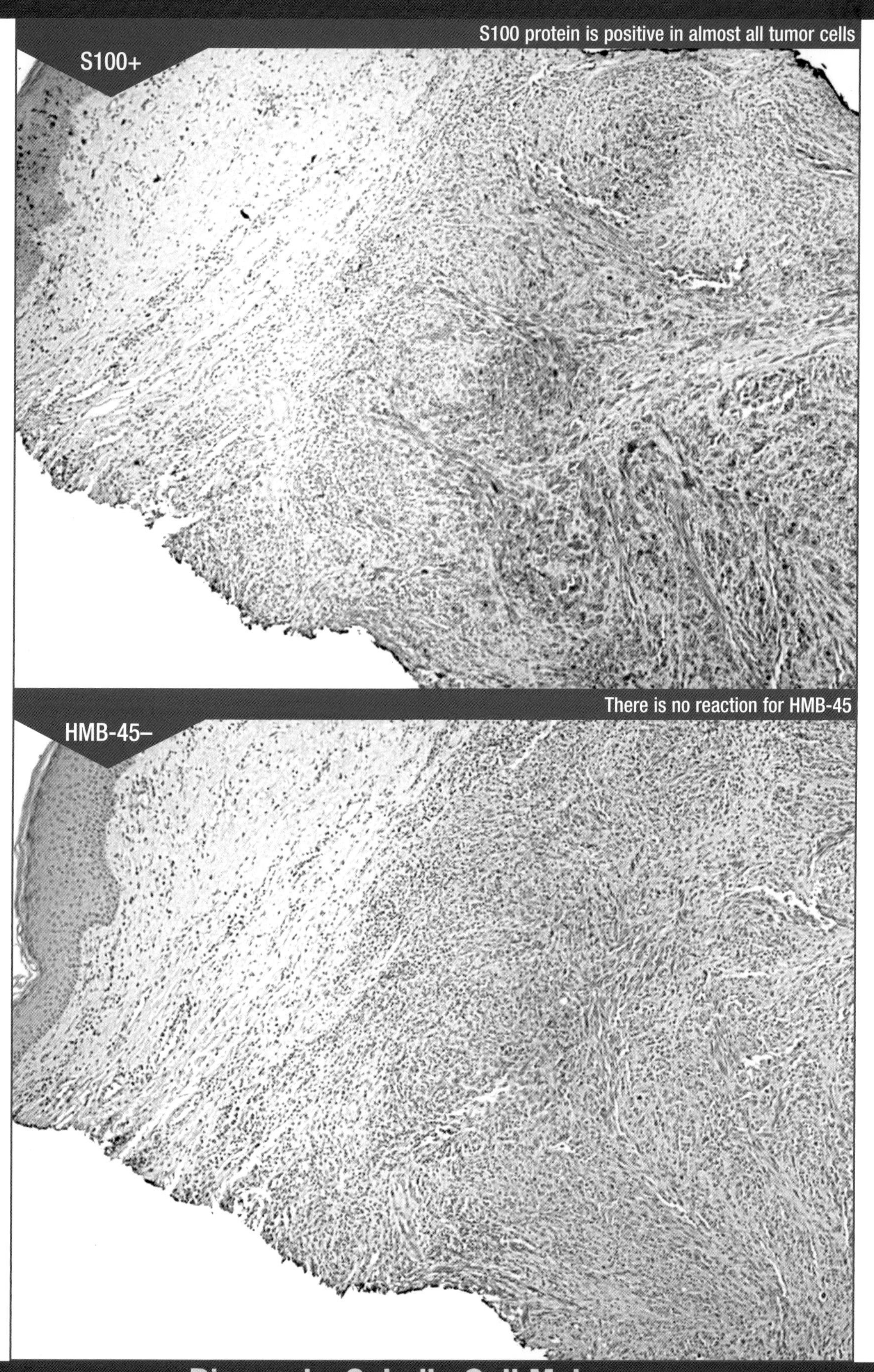

Diagnosis: Spindle Cell Melanoma

Biopsy of tumor in the dorsum of hand

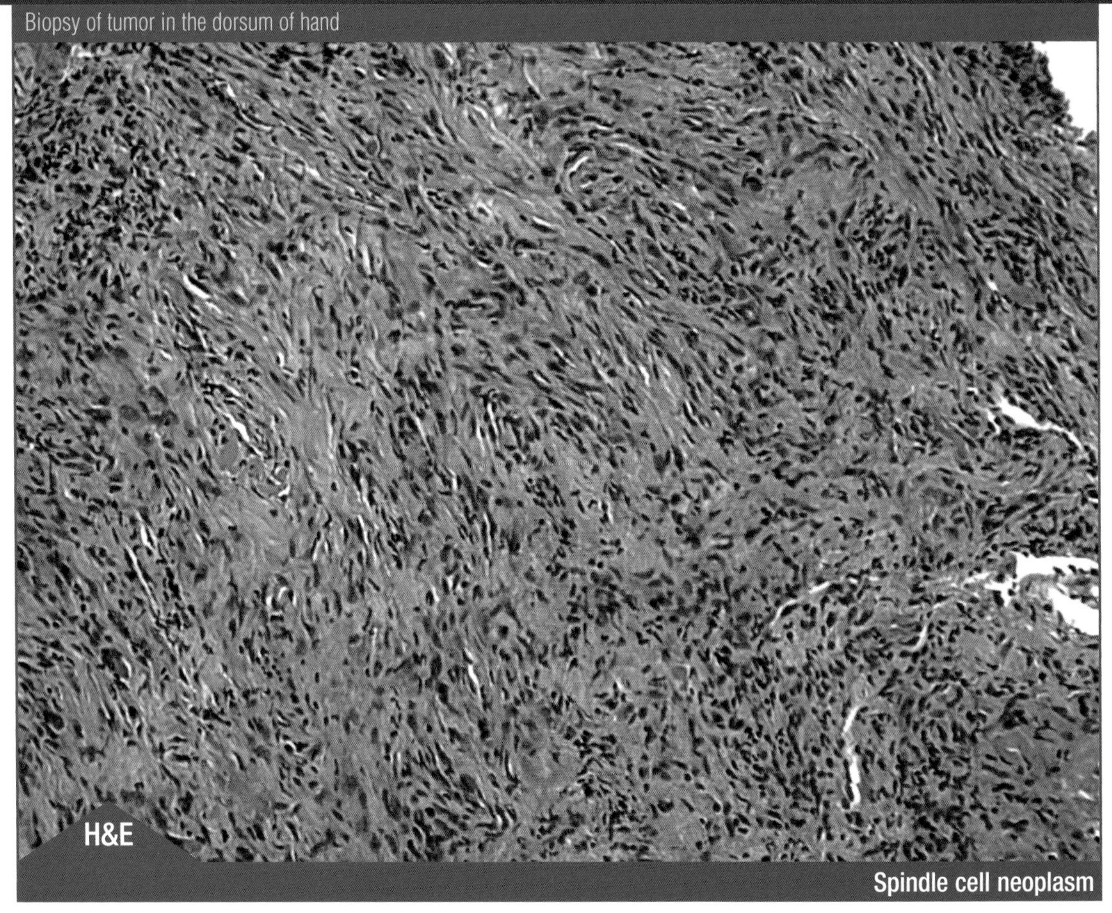

Spindle cell neoplasm

Spindle Cell Carcinoma vs Spindle Cell Sarcoma	
	Cytokeratin
Spindle Cell Carcinoma	+
Spindle Cell Sarcoma	–

Helpful Hints

Undifferentiated sarcomas are spindle cell malignant neoplasms that do not express any of the epithelial, melanocytic, muscle, or endothelial antigens.

Although focal cytokeratin expression has been reported in almost all types of sarcomas, this anomalous expression has very little practical diagnostic implications. Serious considerations nevertheless should be given to epithelioid hemangioendotheliomas and angiosarcomas (up to 25%) and synovial/epithelioid sarcomas (up to 100%) with regard to positive reaction for cytokeratins.

Miettinen 2000b, Meis-Kindblom 1998.

(See p 40 for the differential diagnosis with a synovial sarcoma).

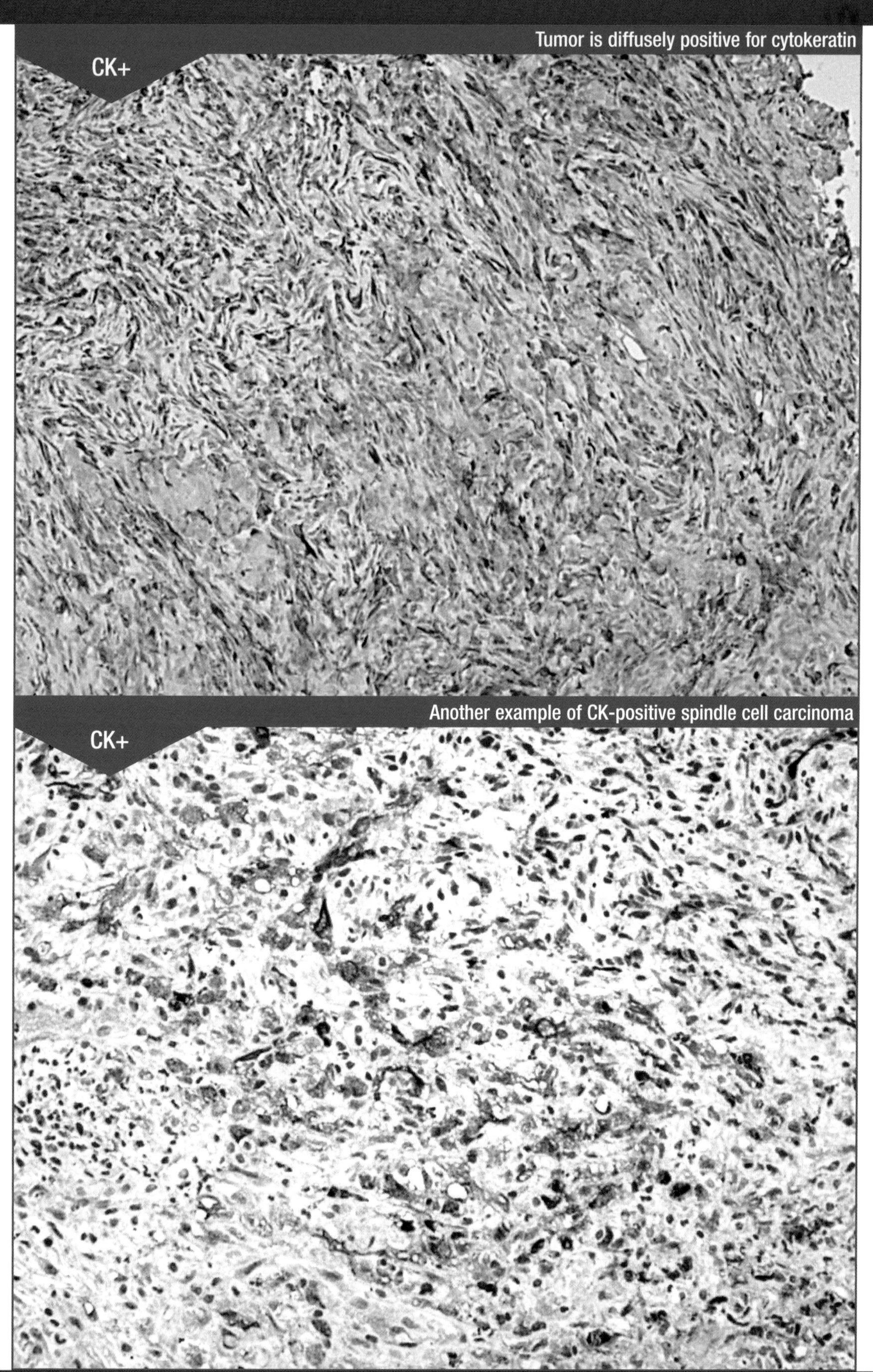

Diagnosis: Spindle Cell Carcinoma

Excision of a thigh mass

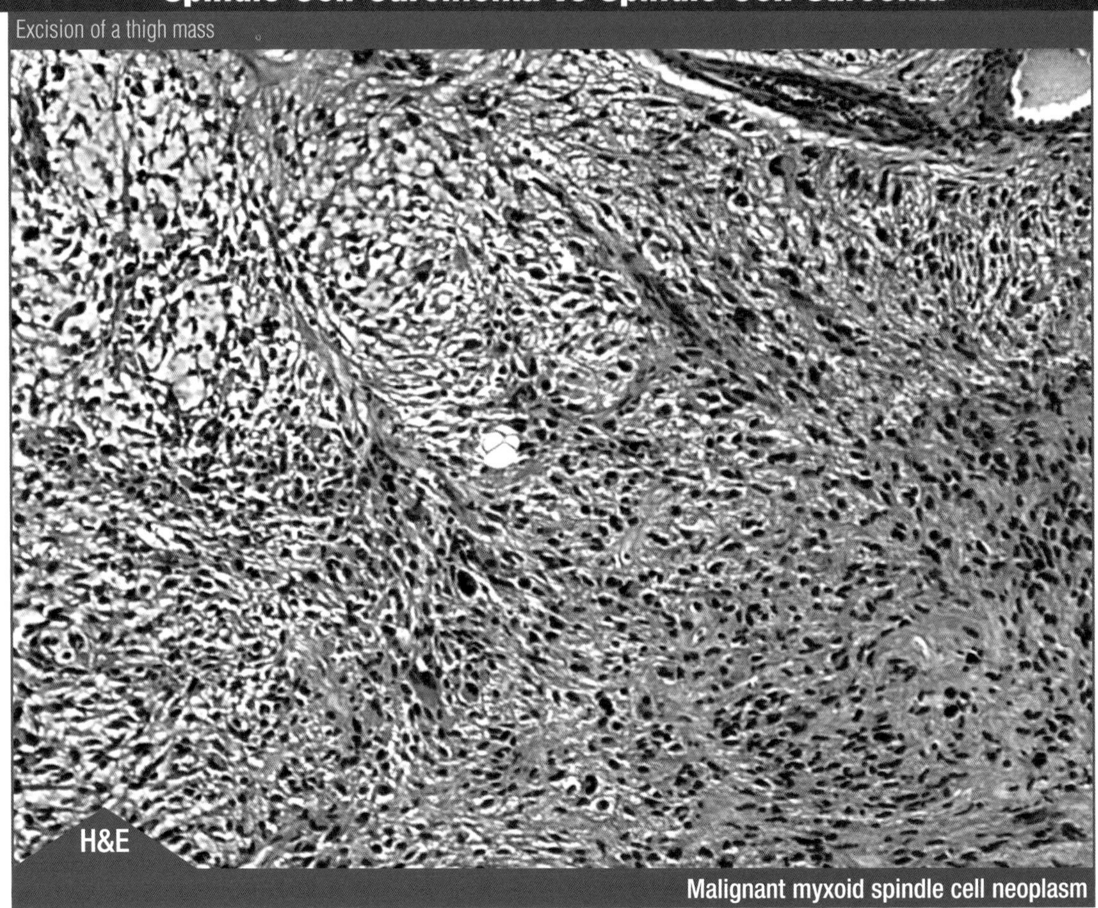

Malignant myxoid spindle cell neoplasm

Spindle Cell Carcinoma vs Spindle Cell Sarcoma	
	Cytokeratin
Spindle Cell Carcinoma	+
Spindle Cell Sarcoma	–

Helpful Hints

Undifferentiated sarcomas are spindle cell malignant neoplasms that do not express any of the epithelial, melanocytic, muscle, or endothelial antigens. We usually use **S100 protein** and **H-Caldesmon** in such cases.

Although focal cytokeratin expression has been reported in almost all types of sarcomas, this anomalous expression has very little practical diagnostic implications. Serious considerations nevertheless should be given to epithelioid hemangioendotheliomas and angiosarcomas (up to 25%) and synovial/epithelioid sarcomas (up to 100%) with regard to positive reaction for cytokeratins.

H-Caldesmon is demonstrable in the majority of smooth muscle neoplasms. We do not advocate the use of other so called muscle markers, such as smooth muscle actin and muscle specific actin simply because they are elaborated by a number of other unrelated soft tissue tumors.

Miettinen 2000b, Meis-Kindblom 1998.

*Probably Malignant Fibrous Histiocytoma.

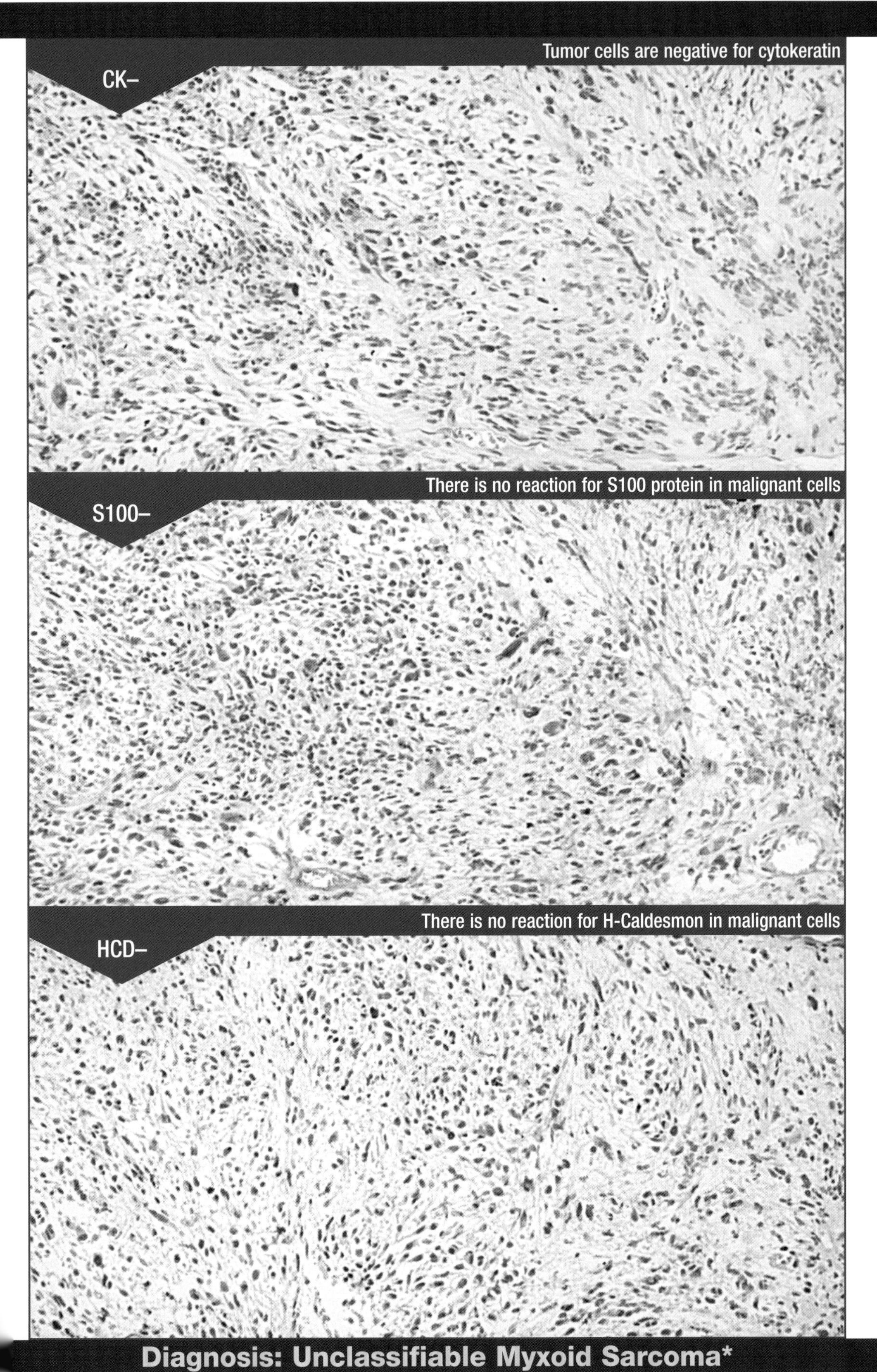
Tumor cells are negative for cytokeratin
CK–
There is no reaction for S100 protein in malignant cells
S100–
There is no reaction for H-Caldesmon in malignant cells
HCD–
Diagnosis: Unclassifiable Myxoid Sarcoma*

Synovial Sarcoma vs Spindle Cell Carcinoma

Biopsy of mass in the ankle of a young male

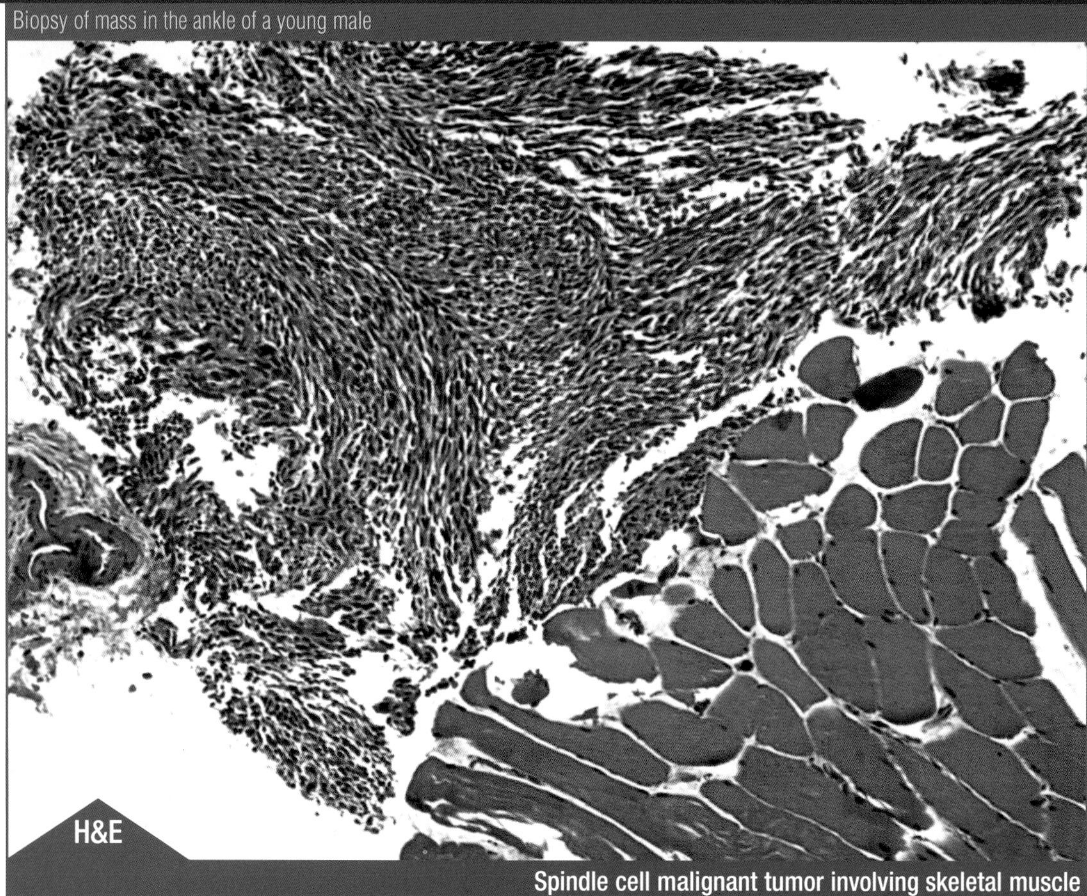

Spindle cell malignant tumor involving skeletal muscle

Synovial Sarcoma vs Spindle Cell Carcinoma		
	CD99	BCL-2
Synovial Sarcoma	+	+
Spindle Cell Carcinoma	–	–

Helpful Hints

Epithelial markers, such as cytokeratin and Epithelial Membrane Antigen (EMA) are expressed either focally or diffusely by both synovial sarcomas and spindle cell carcinomas. It is therefore, not possible to separate these lesions by the above markers. **CD99** and **BCL-2**, on the other hand, are expressed by the majority of synovial sarcomas but rarely by spindle cell carcinomas.

Fisher 1998, Folpe 1998, Dan'ura 2002.

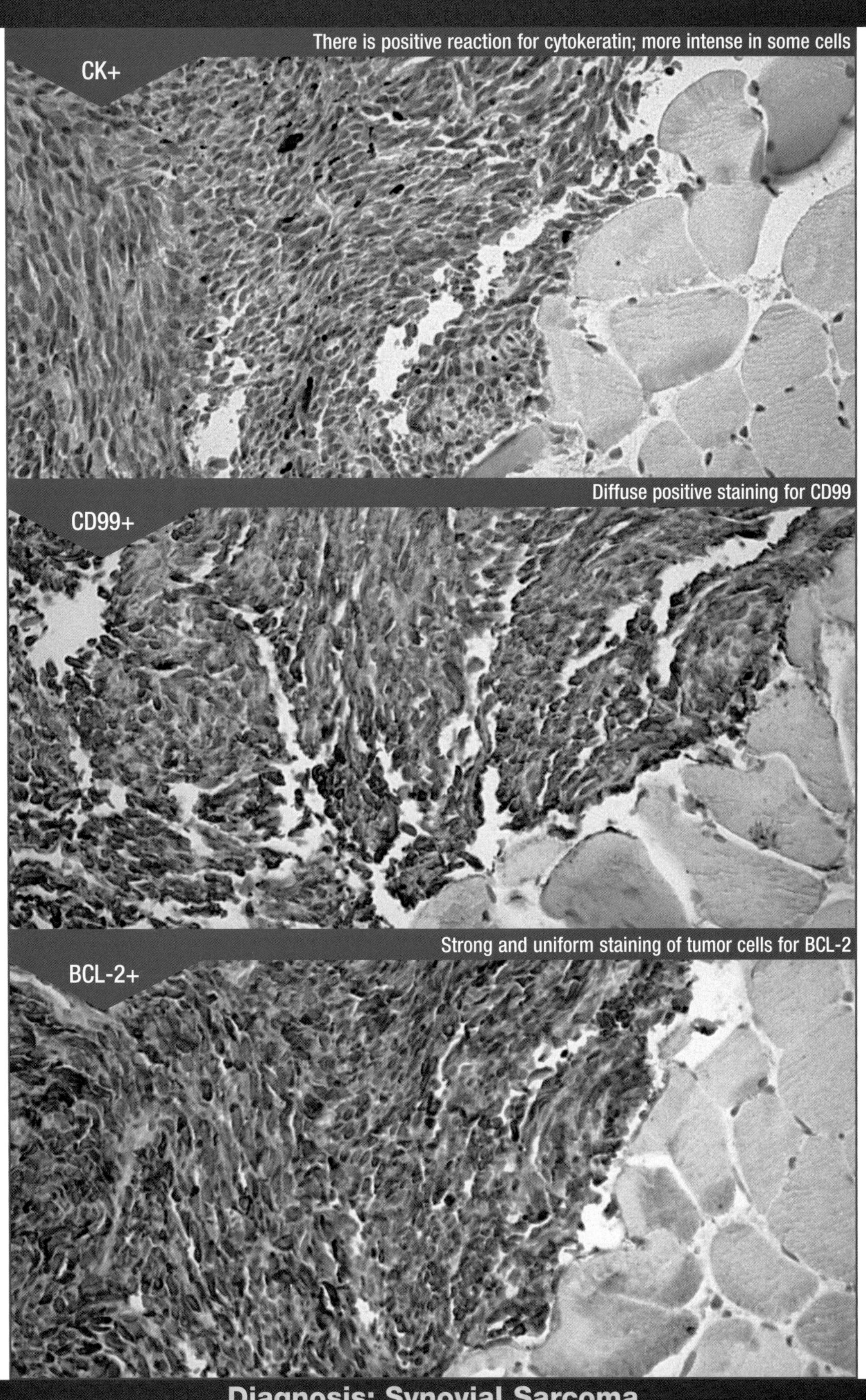

Diagnosis: Synovial Sarcoma

Tumor in the inguinal area

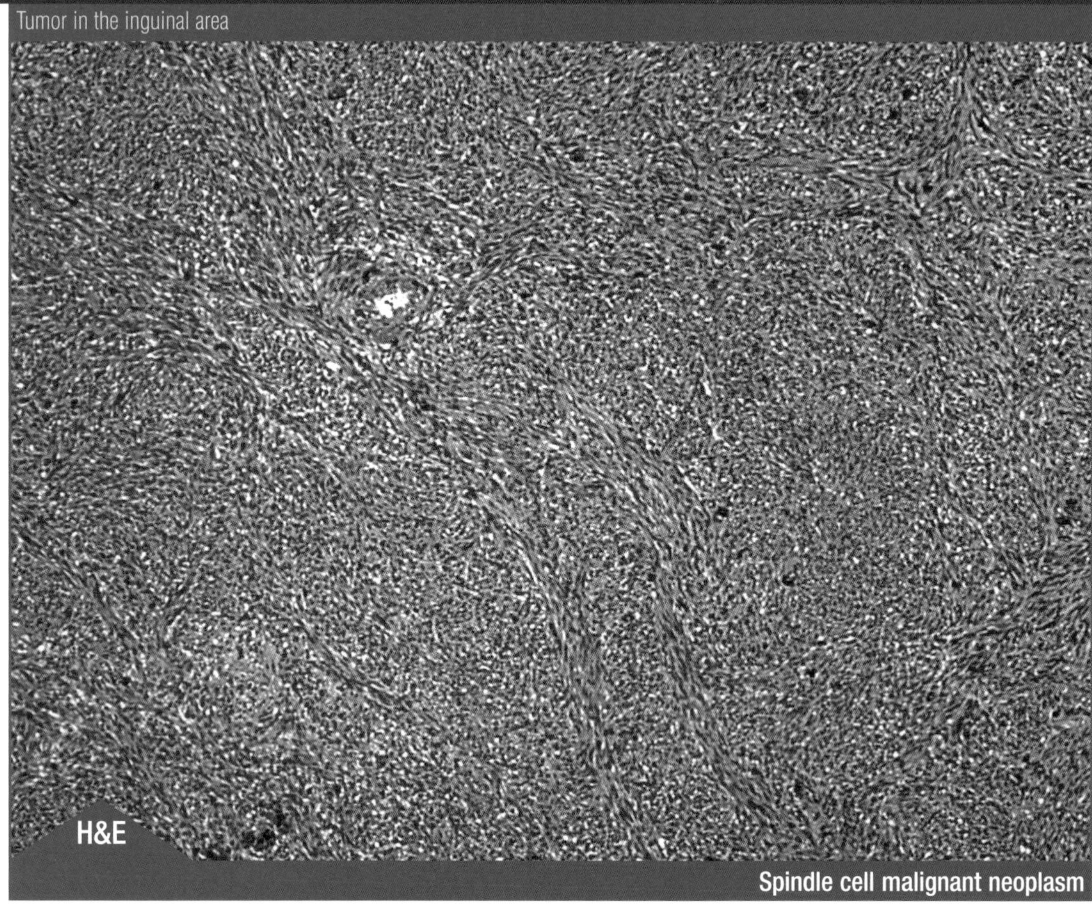

Spindle cell malignant neoplasm

Synovial Sarcoma vs Spindle Cell Carcinoma			
	Desmin	H-Caldesmon	S100 Protein
Neurogenic Sarcoma	–	–	S
Leiomyosarcoma	S	+	–

Helpful Hints

Desmin: Unlike those occurring in the uterus, only about 50% of extrauterine leiomyosarcomas express desmin.

H-Caldesmon, on the other hand, is demonstrable in the majority of smooth muscle neoplasms. We do not advocate the use of other so called muscle markers, such as smooth muscle actin and muscle specific actin simply because they are elaborated by a number of other unrelated soft tissue tumors.

S100: Not all neurogenic sarcomas are positive for S100 protein, and when positive, the expression is usually focal. This is in contrast to melanomas that are frequently diffusely positive for this antigen.

Hisaoka 2001.

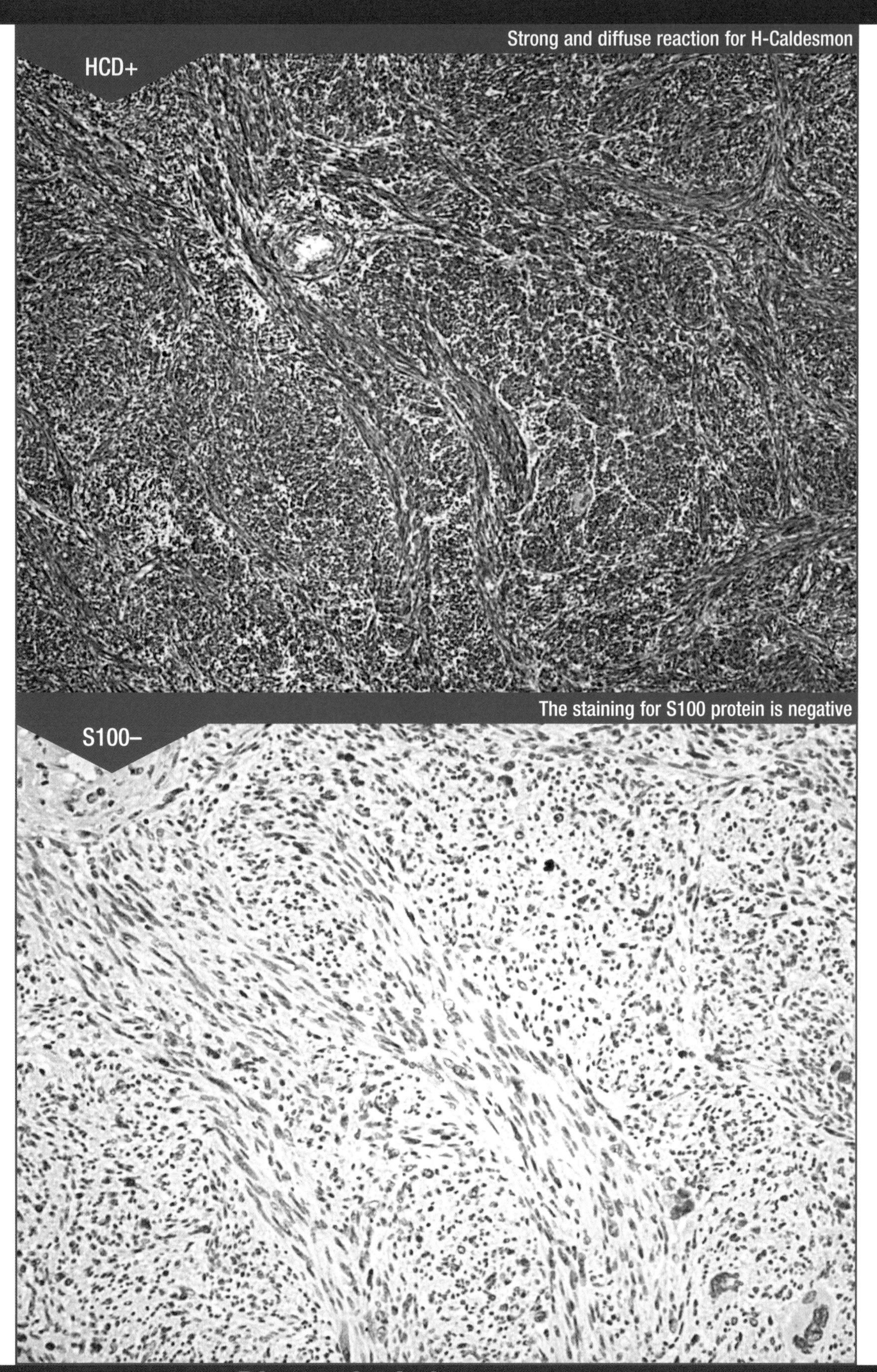
Strong and diffuse reaction for H-Caldesmon
HCD+
The staining for S100 protein is negative
S100–
Diagnosis: Leiomyosarcoma

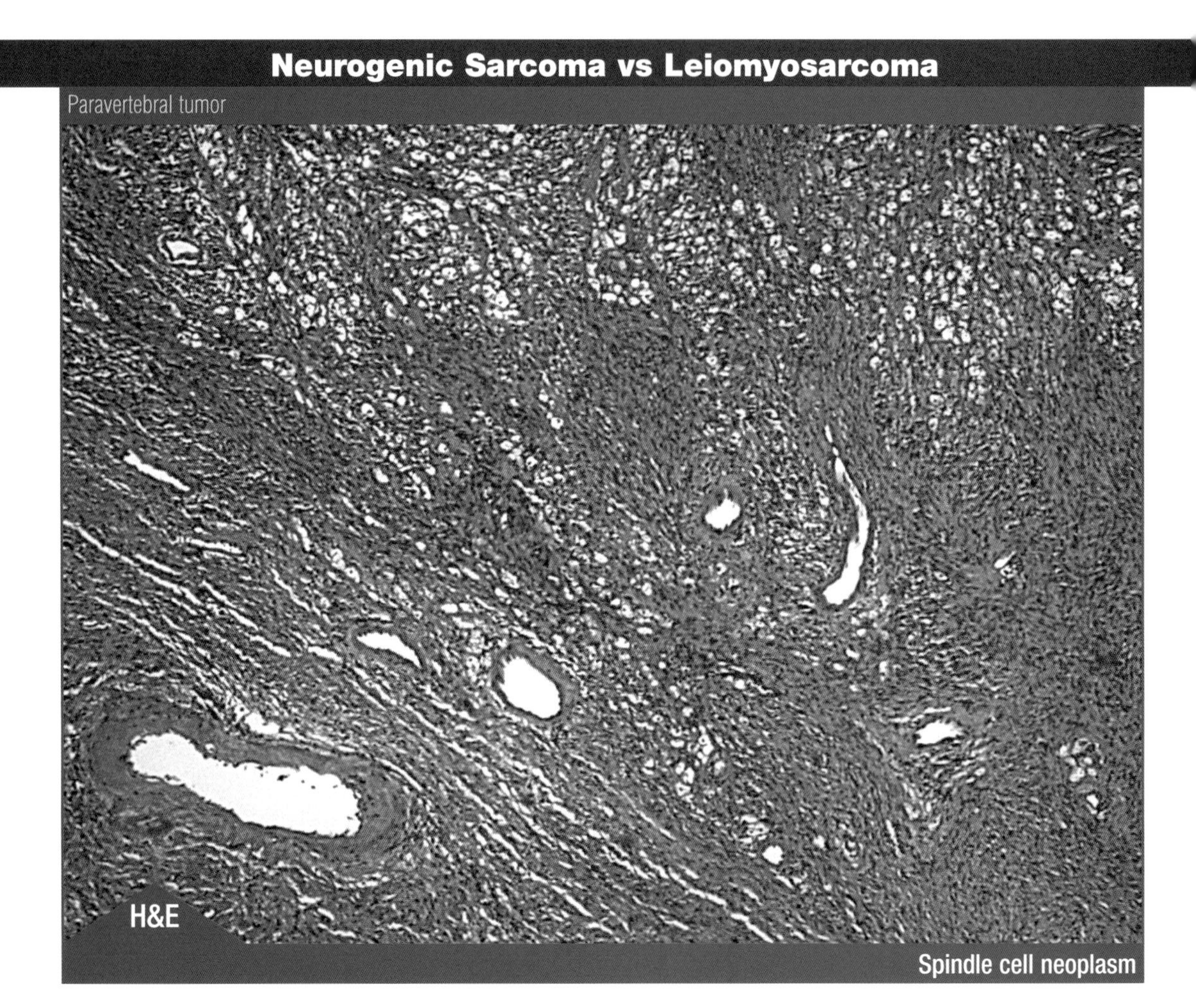

Neurogenic Neoplasm vs Leiomyosarcoma	Desmin	H-Caldesmon	S100 Protein
Neurogenic Neoplasm	–	–	S
Leiomyosarcoma	S	+	–

Helpful Hints

Desmin: Unlike those occurring in the uterus, only about 50% of extrauterine leiomyosarcomas express desmin.

H-Caldesmon, on the other hand, is demonstrable in the majority of smooth muscle neoplasms. We do not advocate the use of other so called muscle markers, such as smooth muscle actin and muscle specific actin simply because they are elaborated by a number of other unrelated soft tissue tumors.

S100: Not all neurogenic sarcomas are positive for S100 protein, and when positive, the expression is usually focal. This is in contrast to melanomas that are frequently diffusely positive for this antigen.

Hisaoka 2001.

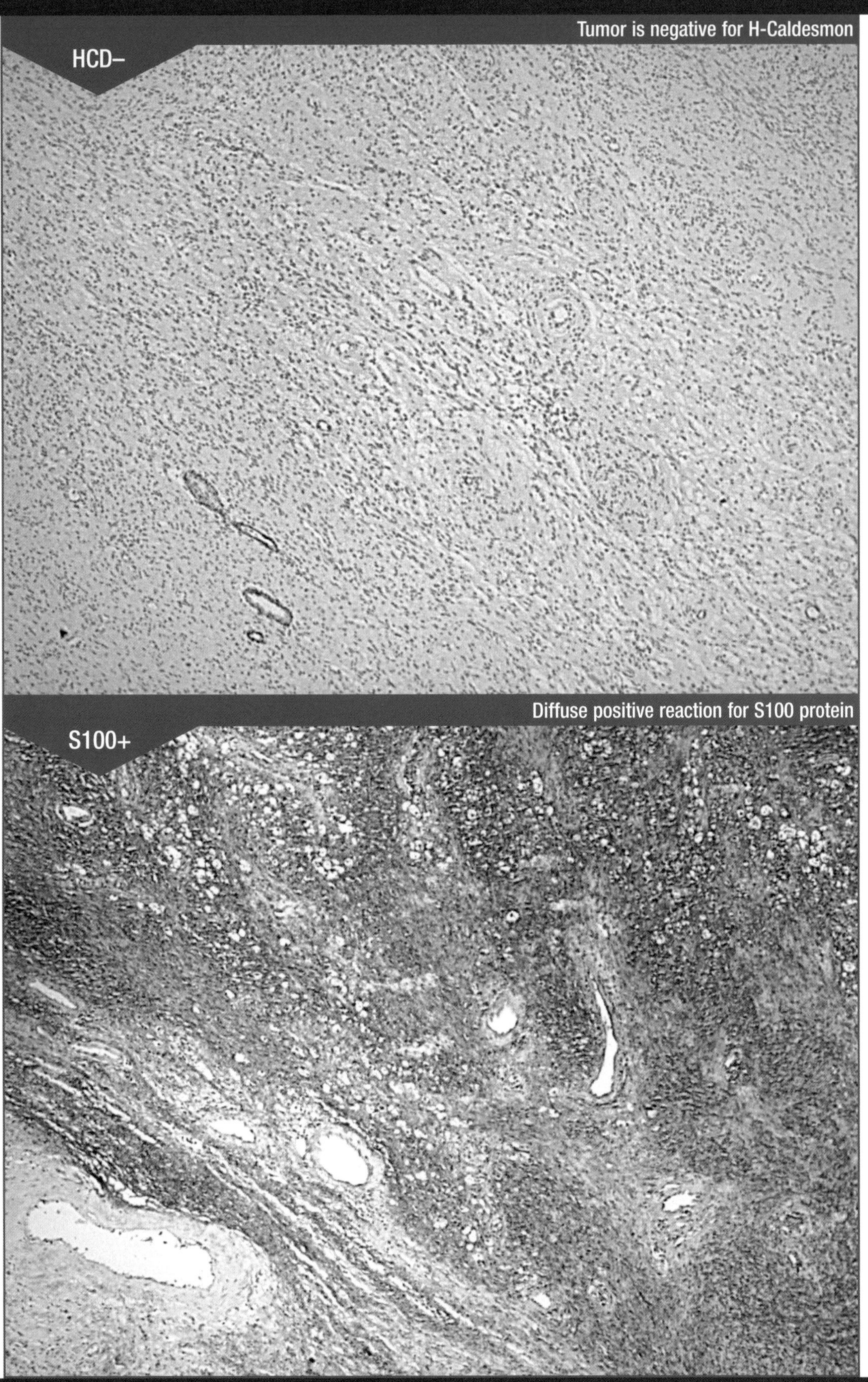

Diagnosis: Nerve Sheath Neoplasm *(Benign by H&E)*

Axillary lesion of a patient with history of radiation therapy for breast cancer

H&E

Changes suggestive of lymphangiosarcoma

Angiosarcoma vs Lymphangiosarcoma			
	CD31	vWF	D2-40
Angiosarcoma	+	+	–
Lymphangiosarcoma	+	S	+

Helpful Hints

Factor VIII-related antigen (**vWF**) and **CD31** are both expressed by endothelial cells and megakaryocytes. CD31 is also expressed by some hematolymphoid cells. In the proper histologic settings, positivity for one or both markers denotes the endothelial differentiation of the neoplasm. Both epithelioid hemangioendotheliomas and angiosarcomas are usually positive for vWF and CD31 but lymphangiosarcomas may be negative for vWF.

D2-40: This is a newly described marker expressed by the lymphatic endothelium but not by vascular endothelium. D2-40 is also expressed by a wide range of other normal and neoplastic cells.

DeYoung 1995, McComb1982, Kahn 2002.

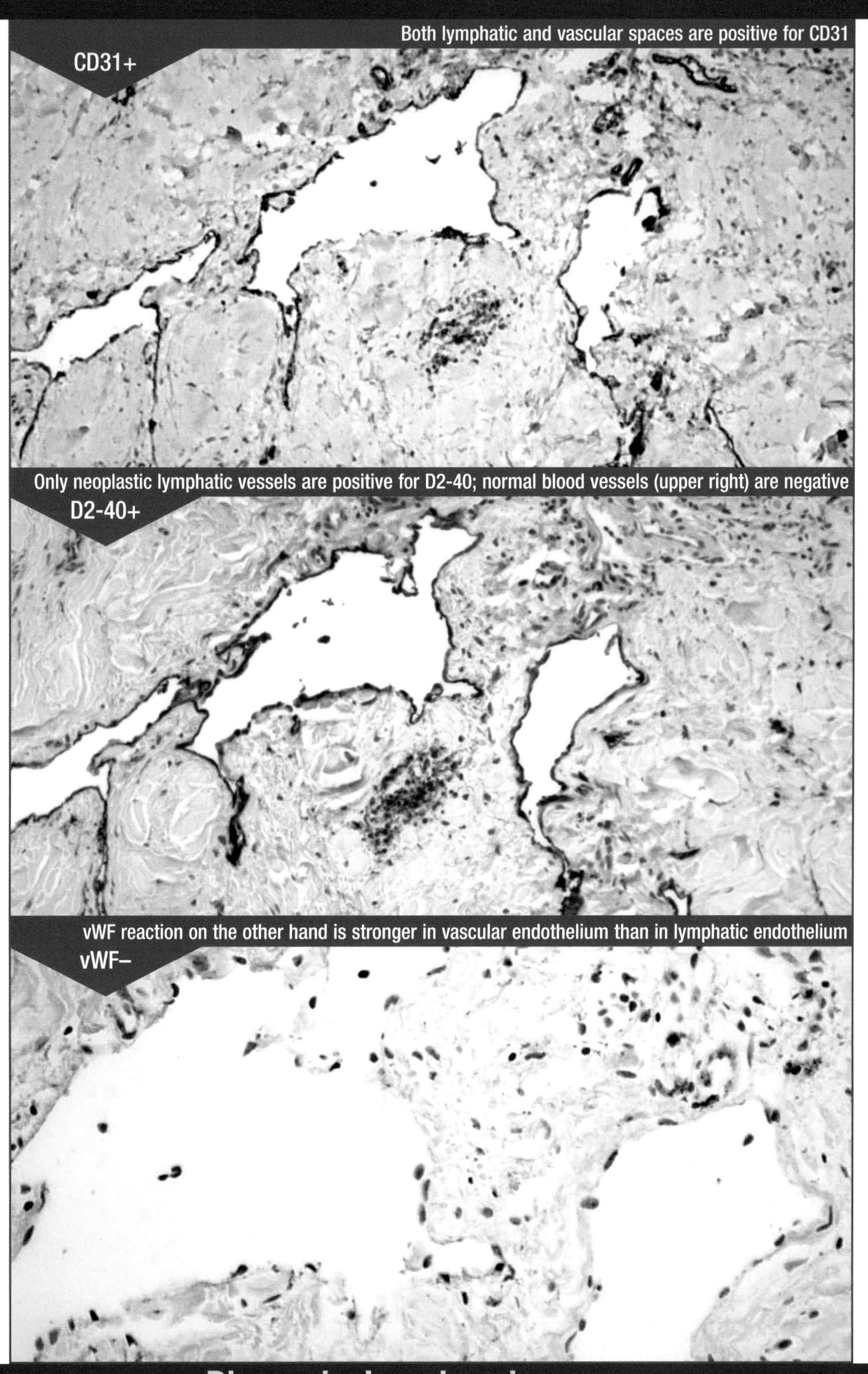
Both lymphatic and vascular spaces are positive for CD31
CD31+
Only neoplastic lymphatic vessels are positive for D2-40; normal blood vessels (upper right) are negative
D2-40+
vWF reaction on the other hand is stronger in vascular endothelium than in lymphatic endothelium
vWF–
Diagnosis: Lymphangiosarcoma

Large, pedunculated tumor of the arm

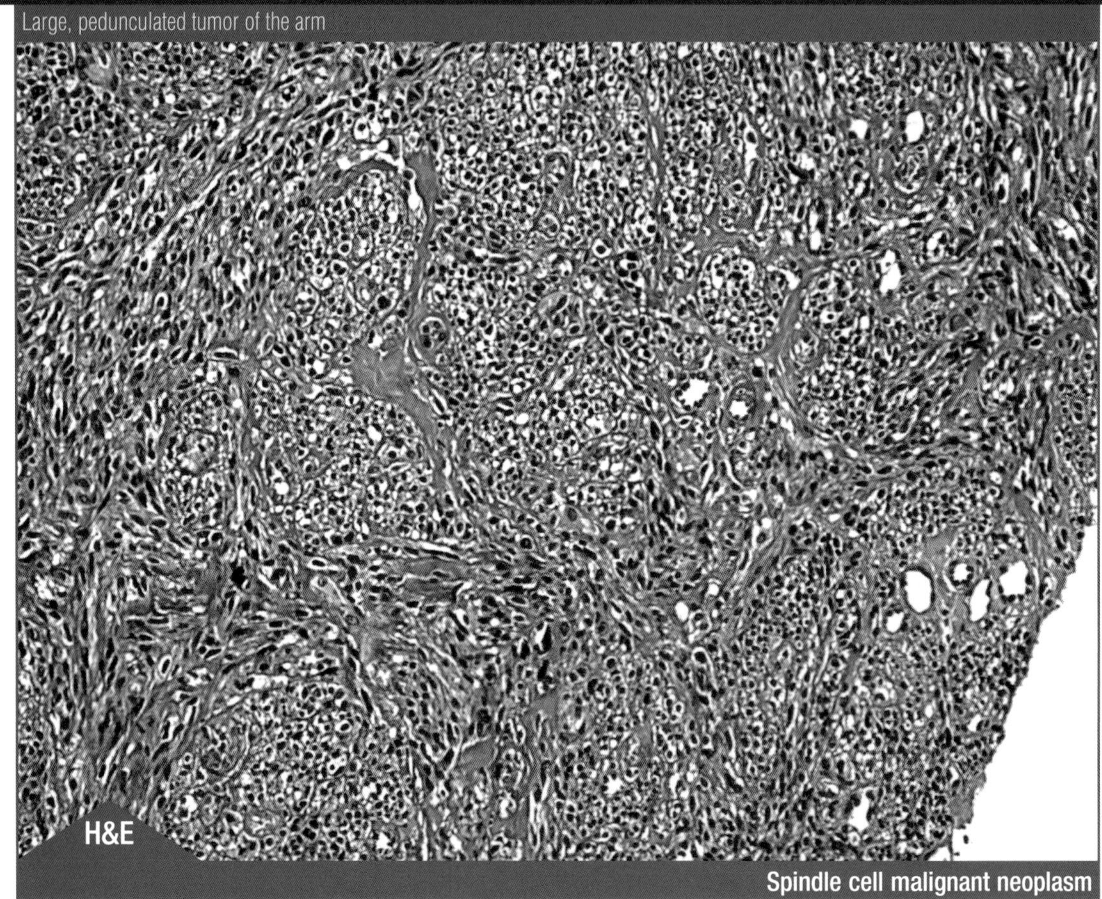

Spindle cell malignant neoplasm

Neurogenic Sarcoma vs Spindle Cell Melanoma		
	Melan-A	Tyrosinase
Neurogenic Sarcoma	–	–
Spindle Cell Melanoma	+	+

Helpful Hints

Although neither Melan-A or Tyrosinase are specific for melanomas, positivity for one or both in the above situation is strongly in favor of a malignant melanoma.

Busam 1999, Hofbauer 1998.

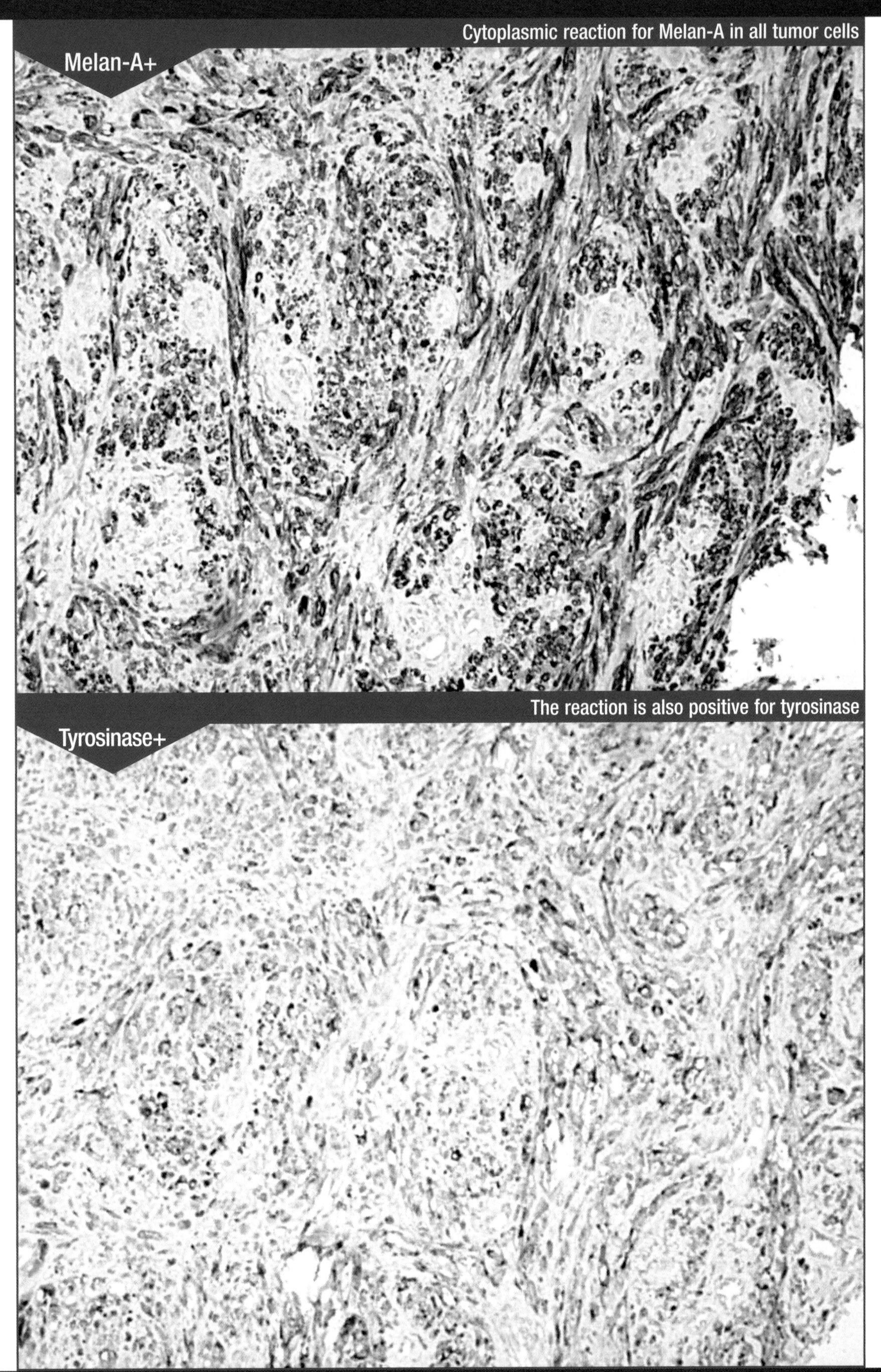

Cytoplasmic reaction for Melan-A in all tumor cells

The reaction is also positive for tyrosinase

Diagnosis: Spindle Cell Malignant Melanoma

Posterior pharyngeal mass

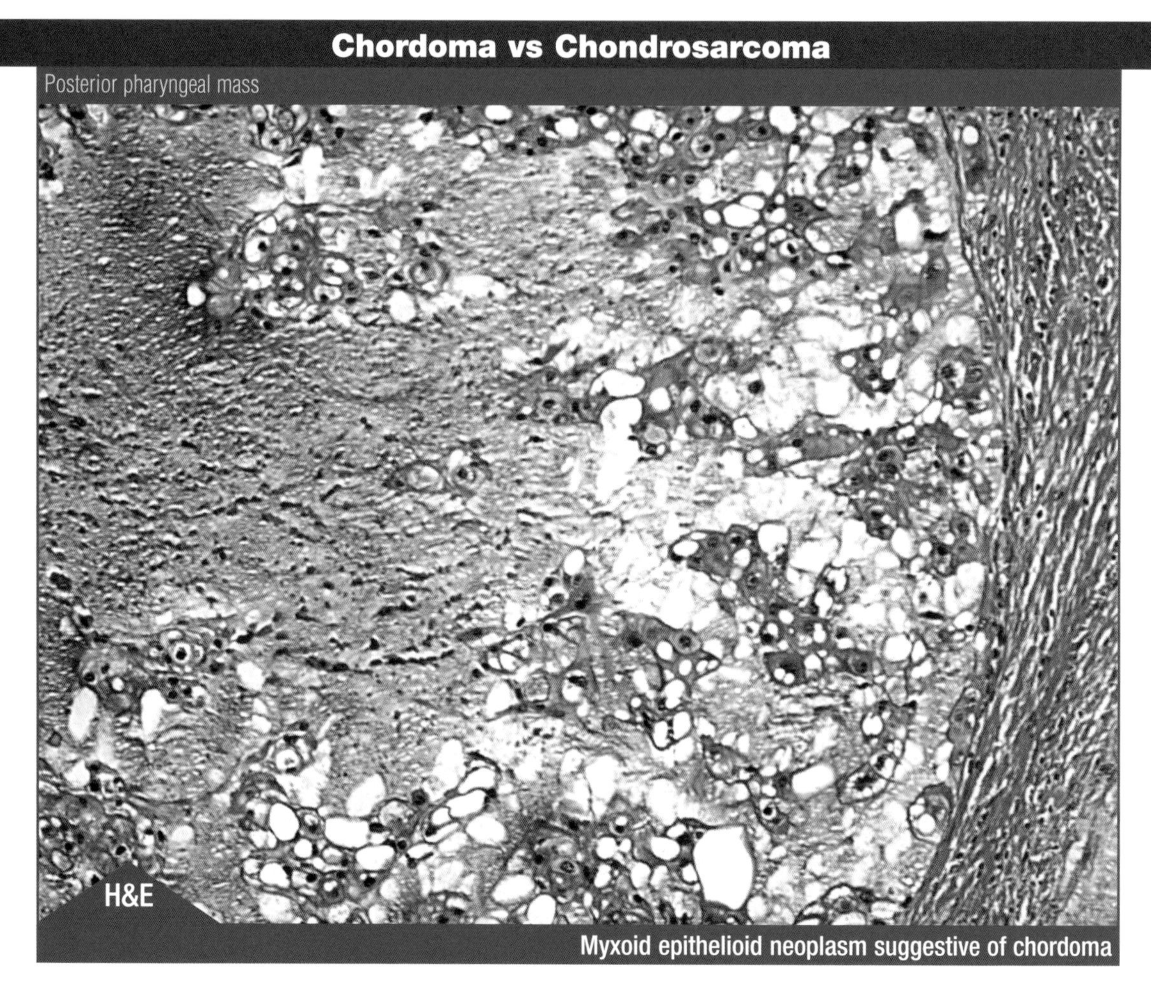

Myxoid epithelioid neoplasm suggestive of chordoma

Chordoma vs Chondrosarcoma		
	Cytokeratin (CK)	Epithelial Membrane Antigen (EMA)
Chordoma	+	+
Chondrosarcoma	–	–

Helpful Hints

Both chordomas and chondrosarcomas are positive for S100 protein, therefore, there appears to be no practical reason to use S100 in their differential diagnosis. Cytokeratin and EMA are on the other hand expressed by chordomas and not chondrosarcomas.

O'Hara 1998.

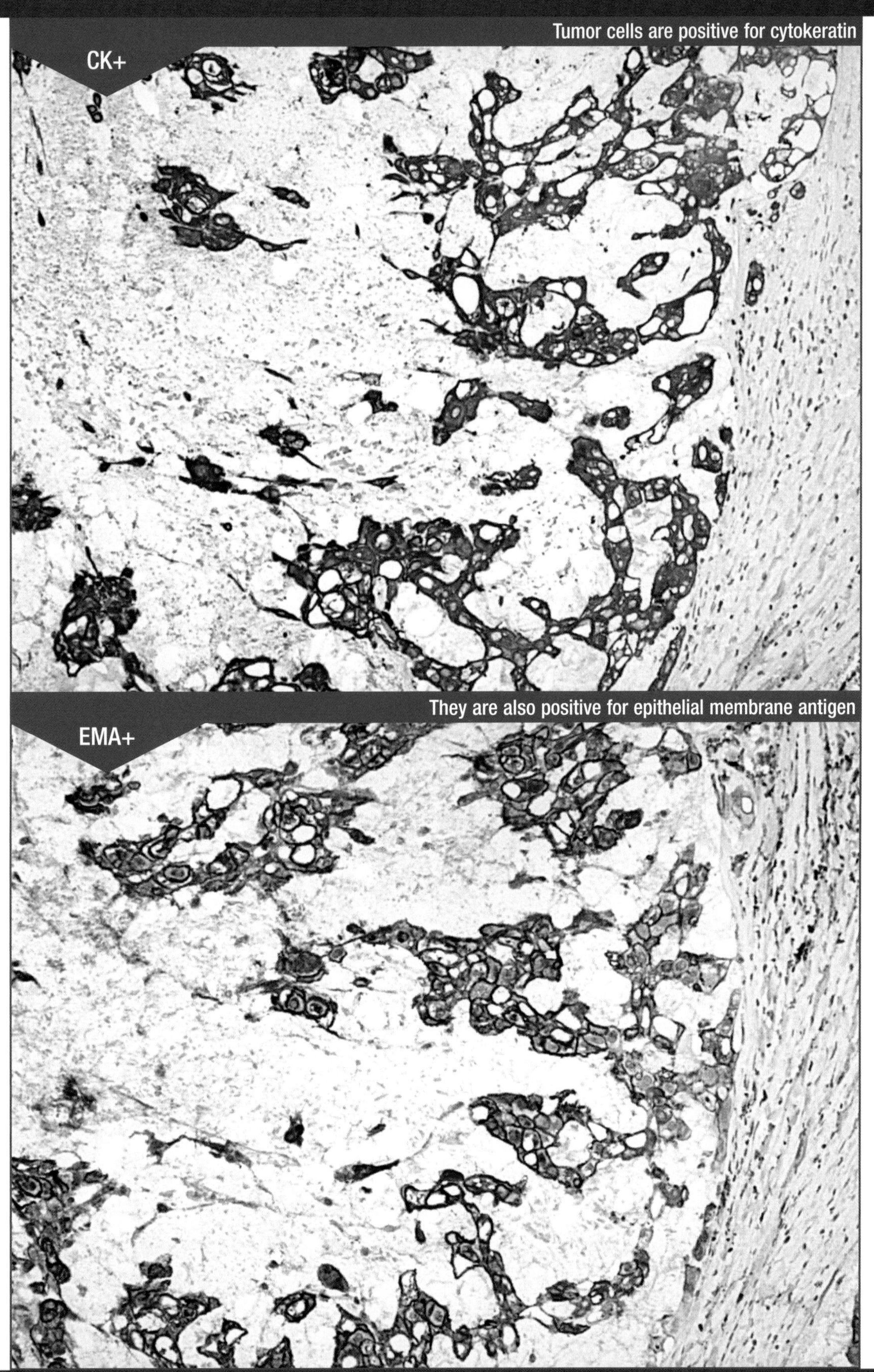

Diagnosis: Chordoma

Epithelioid Hemangioendothelioma vs Poorly Differentiated Carcinoma

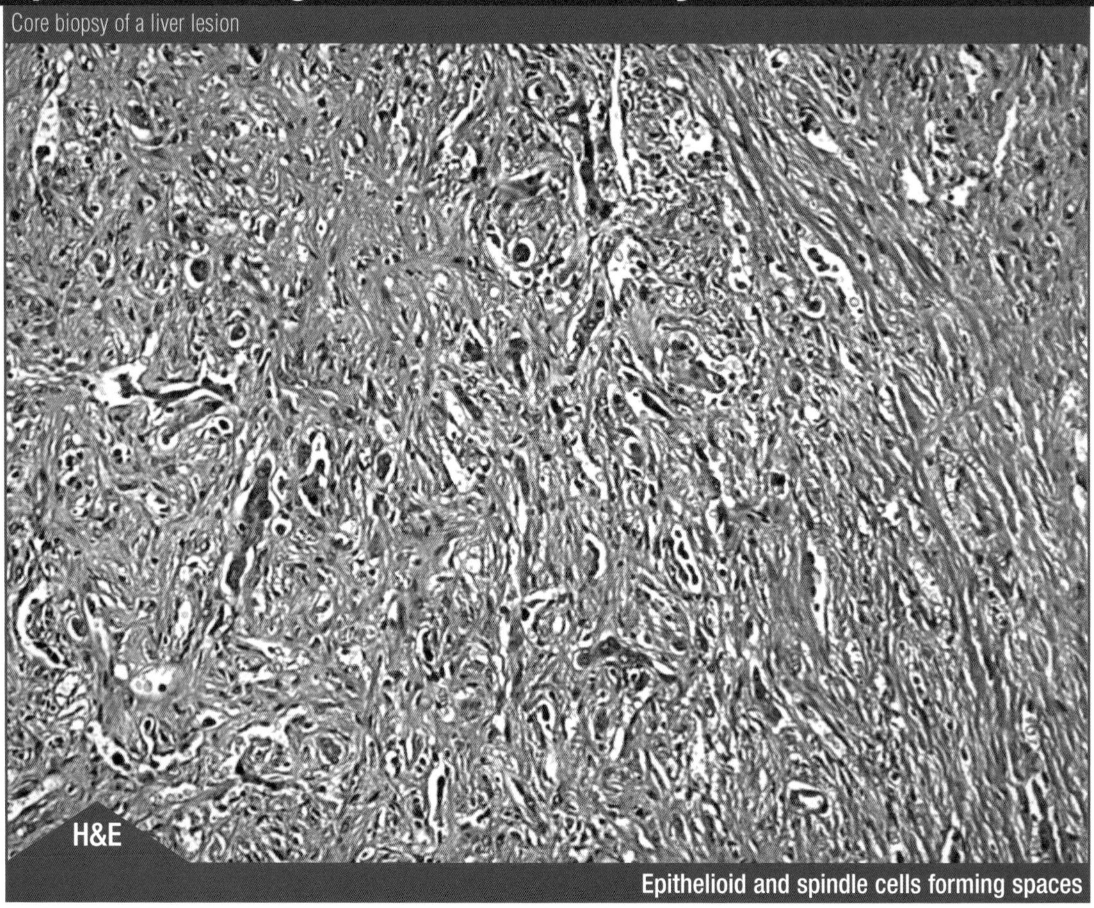

Core biopsy of a liver lesion

Epithelioid and spindle cells forming spaces

Epithelioid Angiosarcoma/EHE vs Poorly Differentiated Carcinoma

	Cytokeratin (CK)	CD31	vWF
Epithelioid Angiosarcoma/EHE	S	+	+
Poorly Differentiated Carcinoma	+	–	–

Helpful Hints

Factor VIII-related antigen (**vWF**) and **CD31** are both expressed by endothelial cells and megakaryocytes. CD31 is also expressed by some hematolymphoid cells. In the proper histologic settings, positivity for one or both markers denotes the endothelial differentiation of the neoplasm. Both epithelioid hemangioendotheliomas and angiosarcomas are usually positive for vWF and CD31.

Cytokeratin is included here to remind us that epithelioid hemangioendotheliomas and epithelioid angiosarcomas can express cytokeratin in up to 25% of cases. It is therefore, the positivity for vWF and CD31 that helps most in establishing the diagnosis of these entities.

CD34: Because of its expression by a wide range of different cells and tumors, we do not recommend CD34 as an endothelial cell marker. Furthermore, CD34 may not be positive in some angiosarcomas.

D2-40: This is a newly described marker expressed by the lymphatic endothelium but not vascular endothelium. D2-40 is also expressed by a wide range of other neoplasms.

DeYoung 1995, McComb 1982, Kahn 2002, Miettinen 2000a.

EHE, epithelioid hemangioendothelioma; vWF, von Willebrand factor

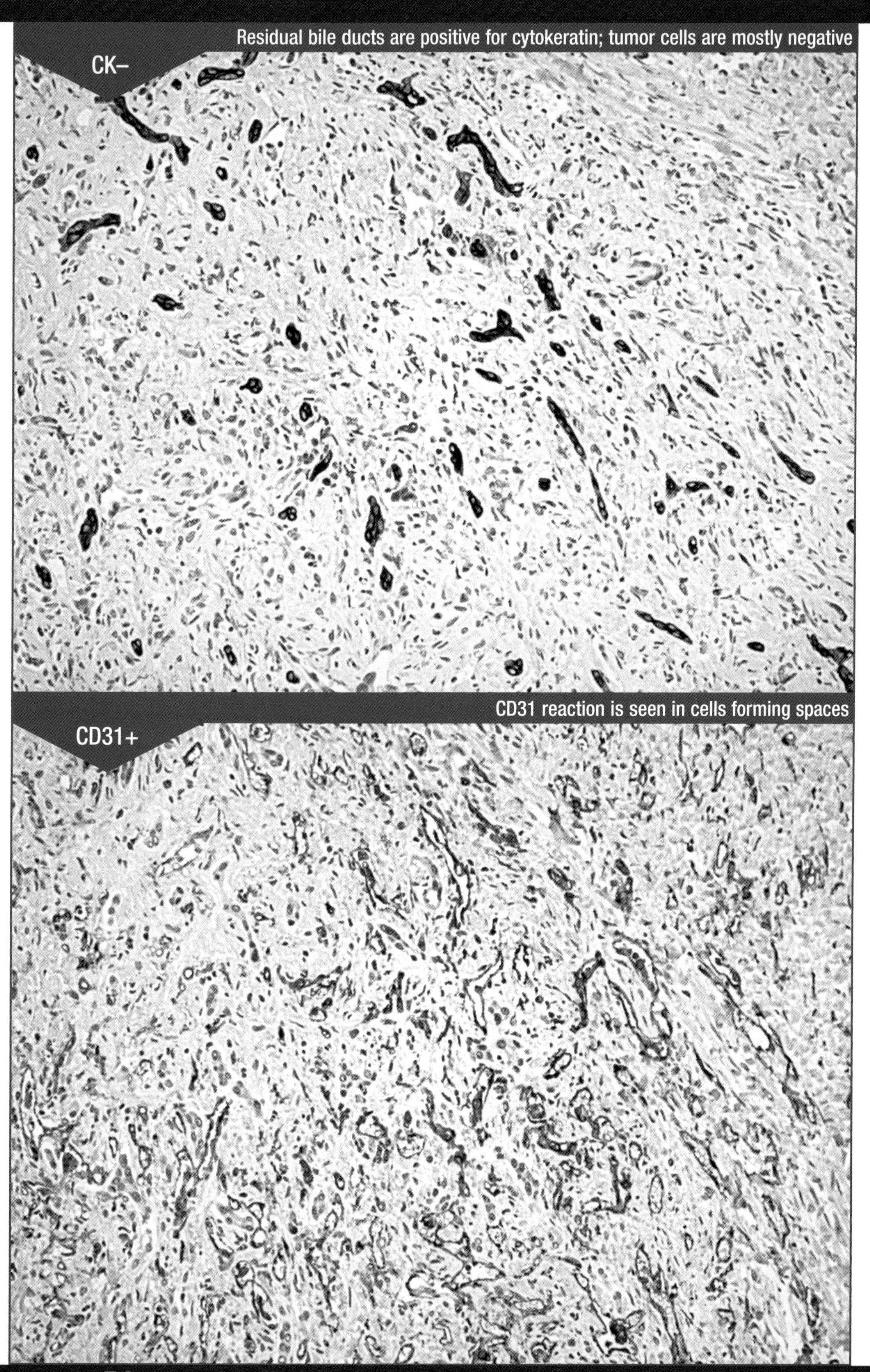

Diagnosis: Epithelioid Hemangioendothelioma

Biopsy of a breast mass

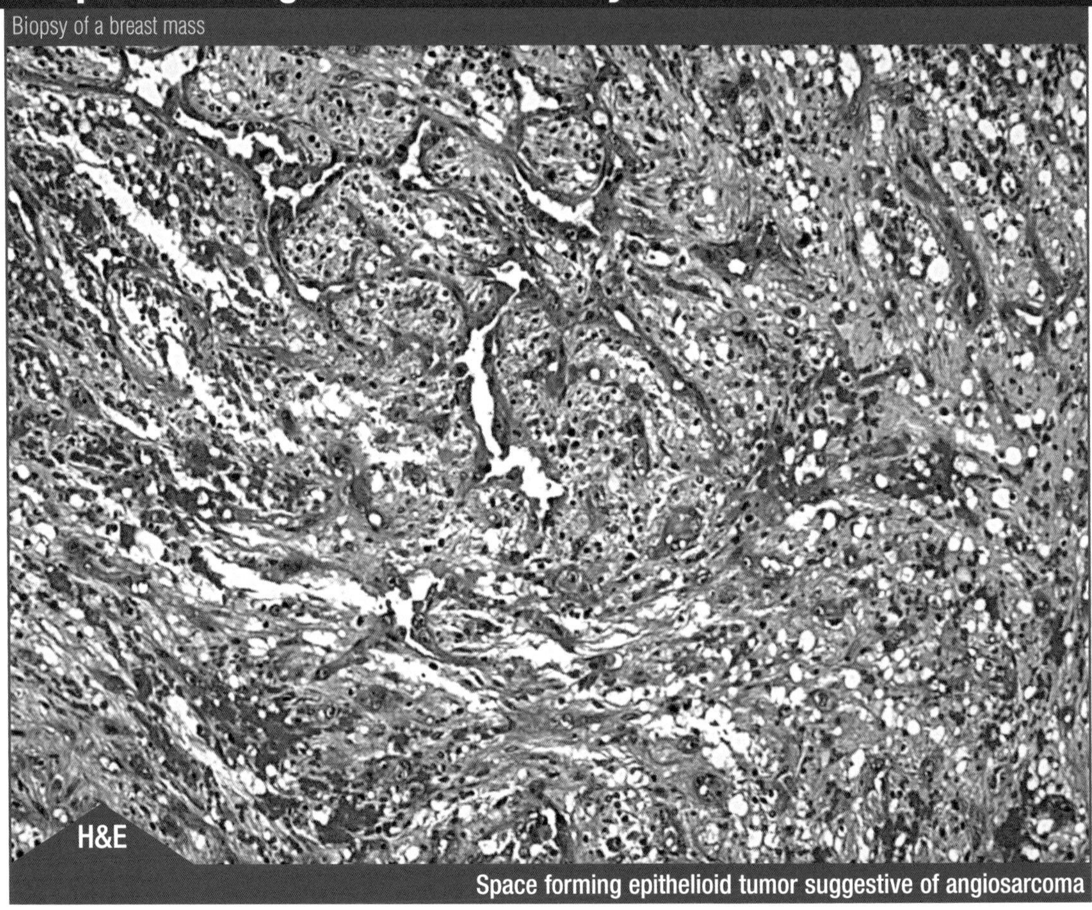

Space forming epithelioid tumor suggestive of angiosarcoma

Epithelioid Angiosarcoma/EHE vs Poorly Differentiated Carcinoma			
	Cytokeratin (CK)	CD31	vWF
Epithelioid Angiosarcoma/EHE	S	+	+
Poorly Differentiated Carcinoma	+	–	–

Helpful Hints

Factor VIII-related antigen (**vWF**) and **CD31** are both expressed by endothelial cells and megakaryocytes. CD31 is also expressed by some hematolymphoid cells. In the proper histologic settings, positivity for one or both markers denotes the endothelial differentiation of the neoplasm. Both epithelioid hemangio-endotheliomas and angiosarcomas are usually positive for vWF and CD31.

Cytokeratin is included here to remind us that epithelioid hemangioendotheliomas and epithelioid angiosarcomas can express cytokeratin in up to 25% of cases. It is therefore, the positivity for vWF and CD31 that helps most in establishing the diagnosis of these entities.

CD34: Because of its expression by a wide range of different cells and tumors, we do not recommend CD34 as an endothelial cell marker. Furthermore, CD34 may not be positive in some angiosarcomas.

D2-40: This is a newly described marker expressed by the lymphatic endothelium but not vascular endothelium. D2-40 is also expressed by a wide range of other neoplasms.

DeYoung 1995, McComb 1982, Kahn 2002, Miettinen 2000a.

EHE, epithelioid hemangioendothelioma; vWF, von Willebrand factor

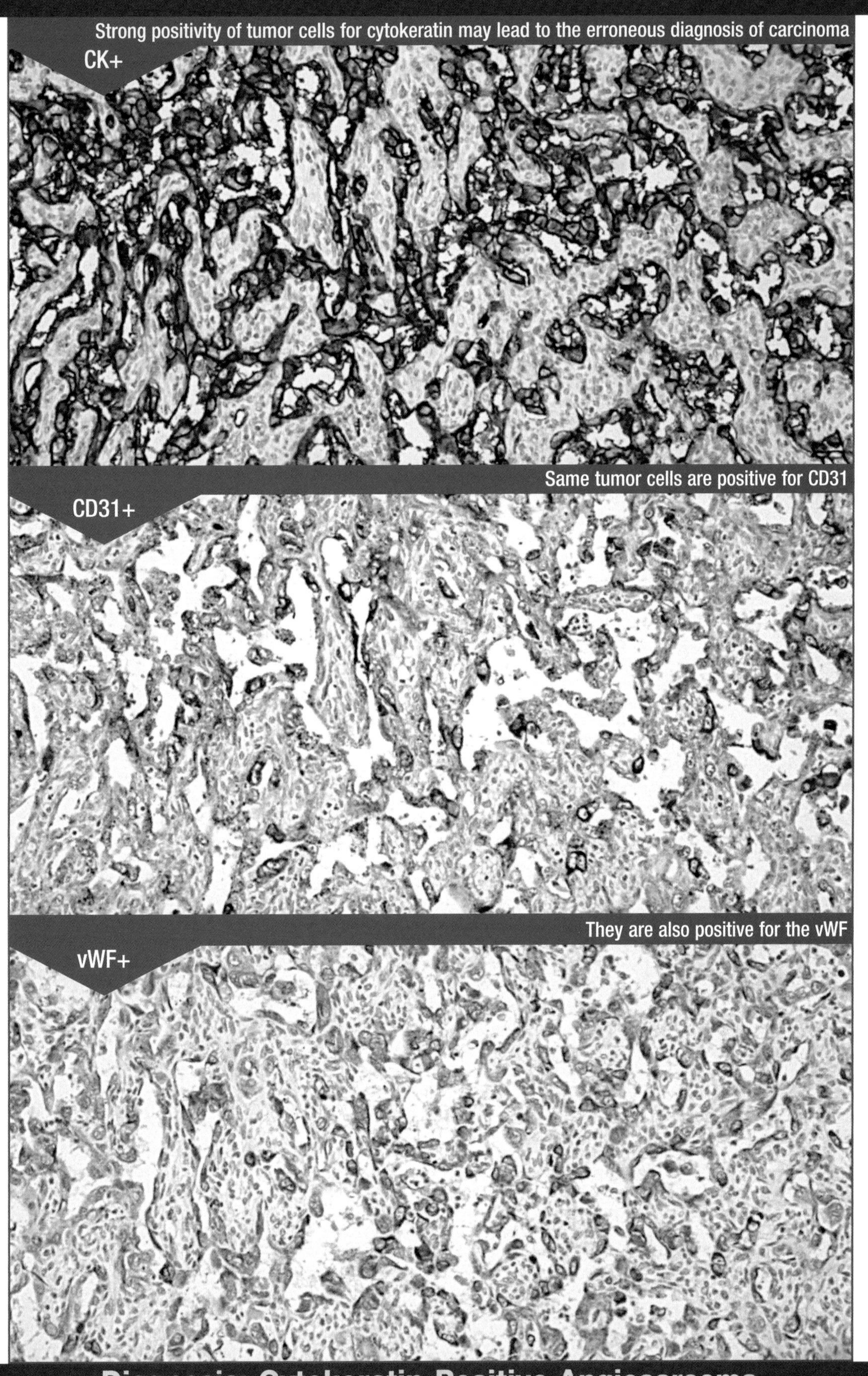

Diagnosis: Cytokeratin-Positive Angiosarcoma

Tumor of scalp in an elderly male

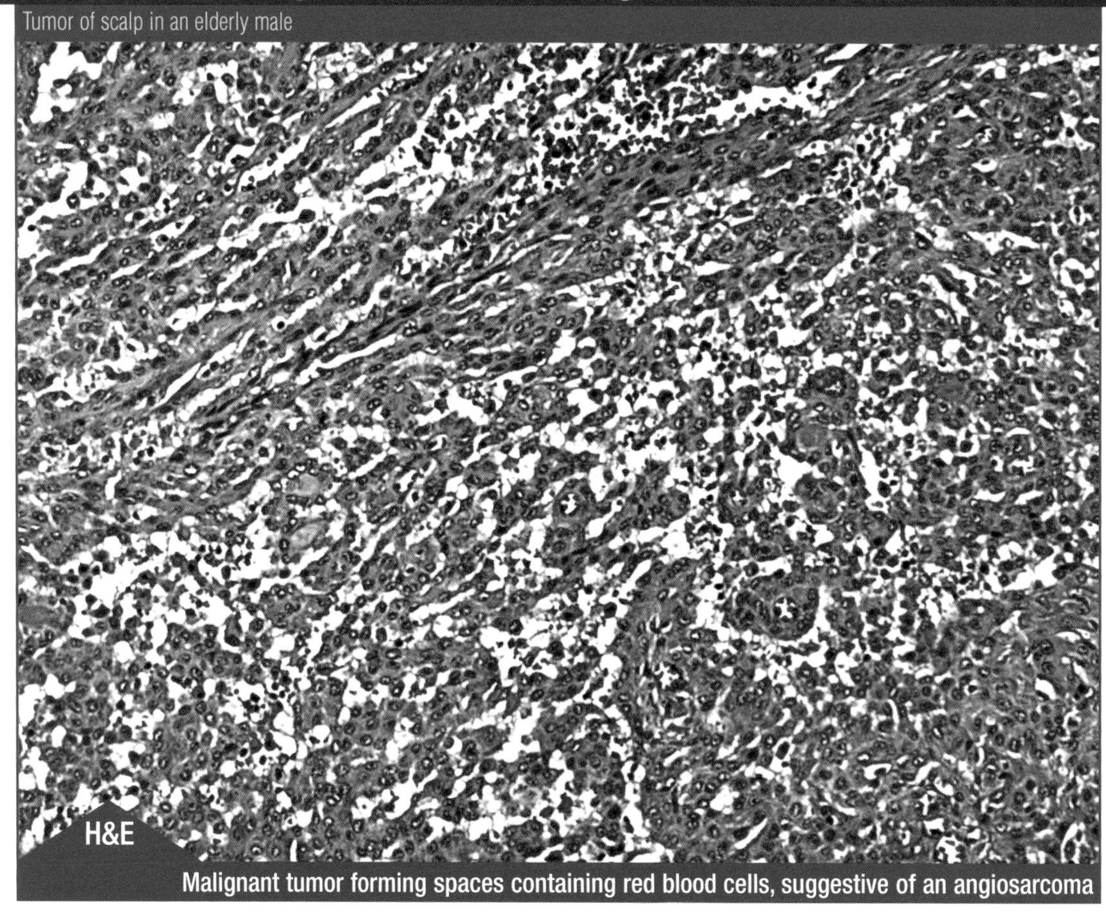

Malignant tumor forming spaces containing red blood cells, suggestive of an angiosarcoma

Epithelioid Angiosarcoma vs Poorly Differentiated Carcinoma			
	Cytokeratin (CK)	CD31	vWF
Epithelioid Angiosarcoma	S	+	+
Poorly Differentiated Carcinoma	+	–	–

Helpful Hints

Factor VIII-related antigen (**vWF**) and **CD31** are both expressed by endothelial cells and megakaryocytes. CD31 is also expressed by some hematolymphoid cells. In the proper histologic settings, positivity for one or both markers denotes the endothelial differentiation of the neoplasm. Both epithelioid hemangioendotheliomas and angiosarcomas are usually positive for vWF and CD31.

Cytokeratin is included here to remind us that epithelioid hemangioendotheliomas and epithelioid angiosarcomas can express cytokeratin in up to 25% of cases. It is therefore, the positivity for vWF and CD31 that helps most in establishing the diagnosis of these entities.

CD34: Because of its expression by a wide range of different cells and tumors, we do not recommend CD34 as an endothelial cell marker. Furthermore, CD34 may not be positive in some angiosarcomas.

DeYoung 1995, McComb 1982, Kahn 2002, Miettinen 2000a.

vWF, von Willebrand factor

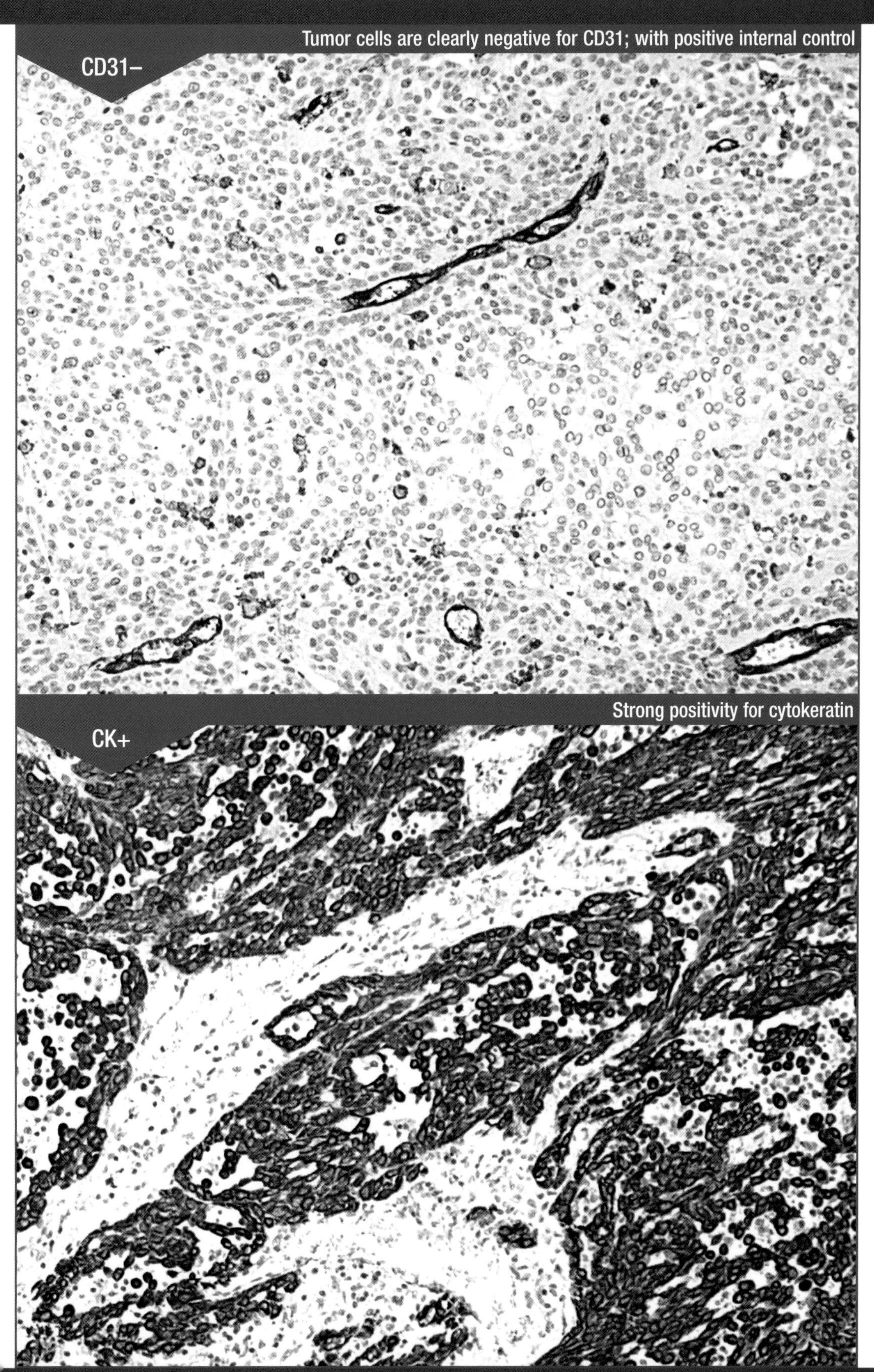

Diagnosis: Acantholytic Squamous Cell Carcinoma

Gastric biopsy

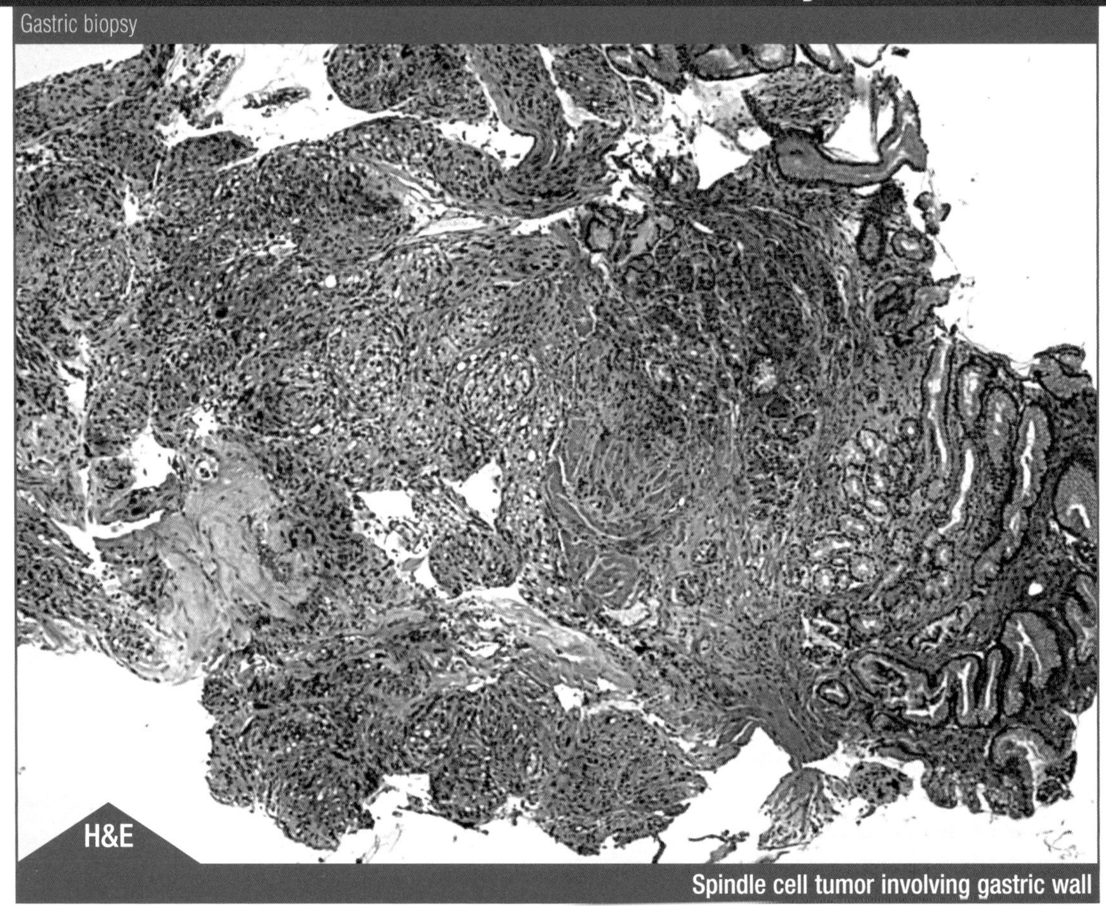

Spindle cell tumor involving gastric wall

Gastrointestinal Stromal Tumor vs Leiomyosarcoma		
	KIT	Desmin
GI Stromal Tumor	+	–
Leiomyosarcoma	–	S

Helpful Hints

KIT: This protein is expressed by more than 85% of gastrointestinal stromal tumors (GIST), whereas it is usually negative in leiomyosarcomas. True positivity for KIT in GISTs is usually strong and diffuse. This is important because focal weak reaction for KIT could be seen in wide range of soft tissue tumors.

CD34: the majority of GISTs also express this marker. Unlike KIT, however, CD34 may be positive in morphologically similar tumors and hence, its diagnostic utility is relatively limited.

Desmin is positive in more than 50% of extrauterine leiomyosarcomas. Most GISTs are negative for this antigen. We do not recommend the use of H-Caldesmon in this situation as it may also be positive in GISTs.

About one-third of KIT-negative GISTs harbor a mutation in platelet-derived growth factor receptor alpha (PDGFR). These tumors also show positivity for PDGFR by immunohistochemistry.

Miettinen 2001, Yi 2005.

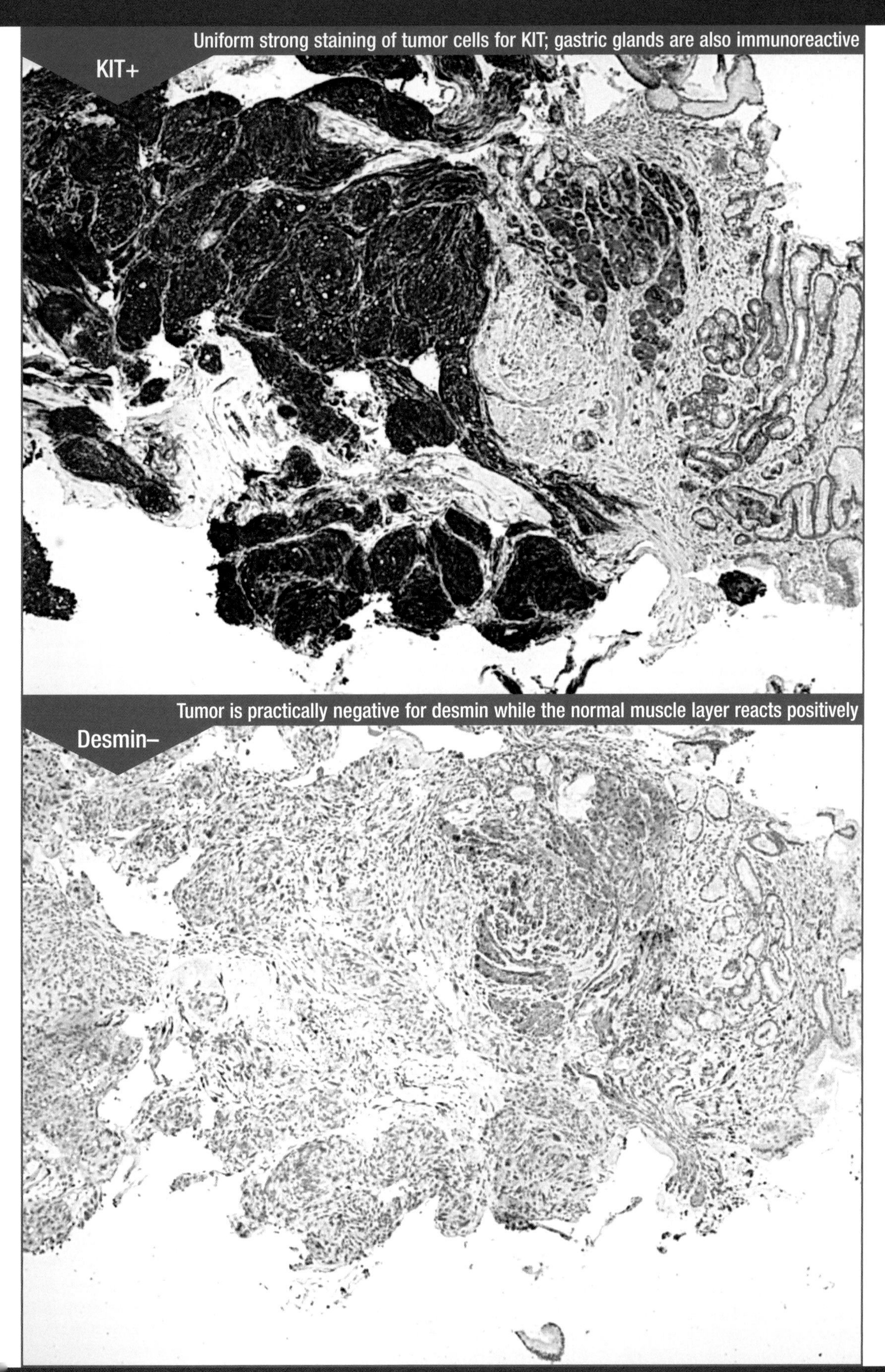

Diagnosis: Gastrointestinal Stromal Tumor

Gastric Biopsy

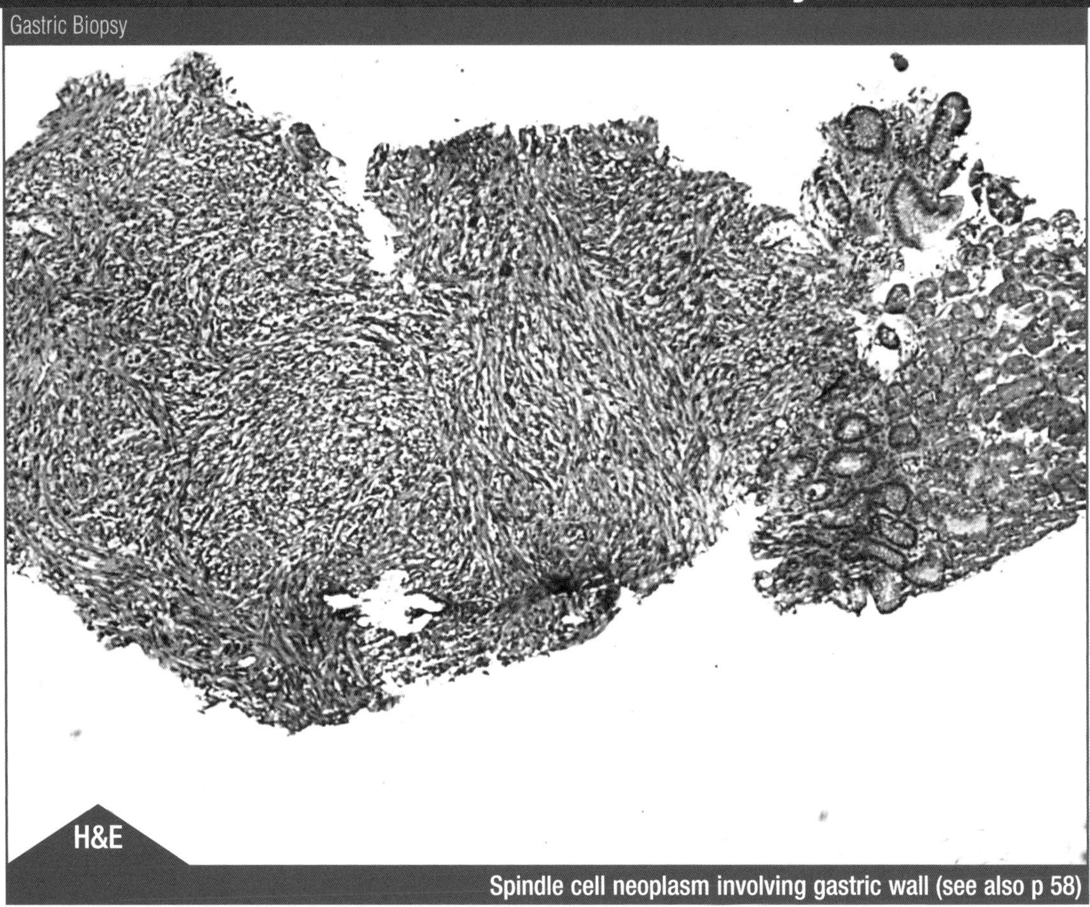

Spindle cell neoplasm involving gastric wall (see also p 58)

Gastrointestinal Stromal Tumor vs Leiomyosarcoma		
	KIT	Desmin
GI Stromal Tumor	+	–
Leiomyosarcoma	–	S

Helpful Hints

KIT: This protein is expressed by more than 85% of gastrointestinal stromal tumors (GIST), whereas it is usually negative in leiomyosarcomas. True positivity for KIT in GISTs is usually strong and diffuse. This is important because focal weak reaction for KIT could be seen in wide range of soft tissue tumors.

CD34: the majority of GISTs also express this marker. Unlike KIT, however, CD34 may be positive in morphologically similar tumors and hence, its diagnostic utility is relatively limited.

Desmin is positive in more than 50% of extrauterine leiomyosarcomas. Most GISTs are negative for this antigen. We do not recommend the use of H-Caldesmon in this situation as it may also be positive in GISTs.

About one-third of KIT-negative GISTs harbor a mutation in platelet-derived growth factor receptor alpha (PDGFR). These tumors also show positivity for PDGFR by immunohistochemistry.

Miettinen 2001, Yi 2005.

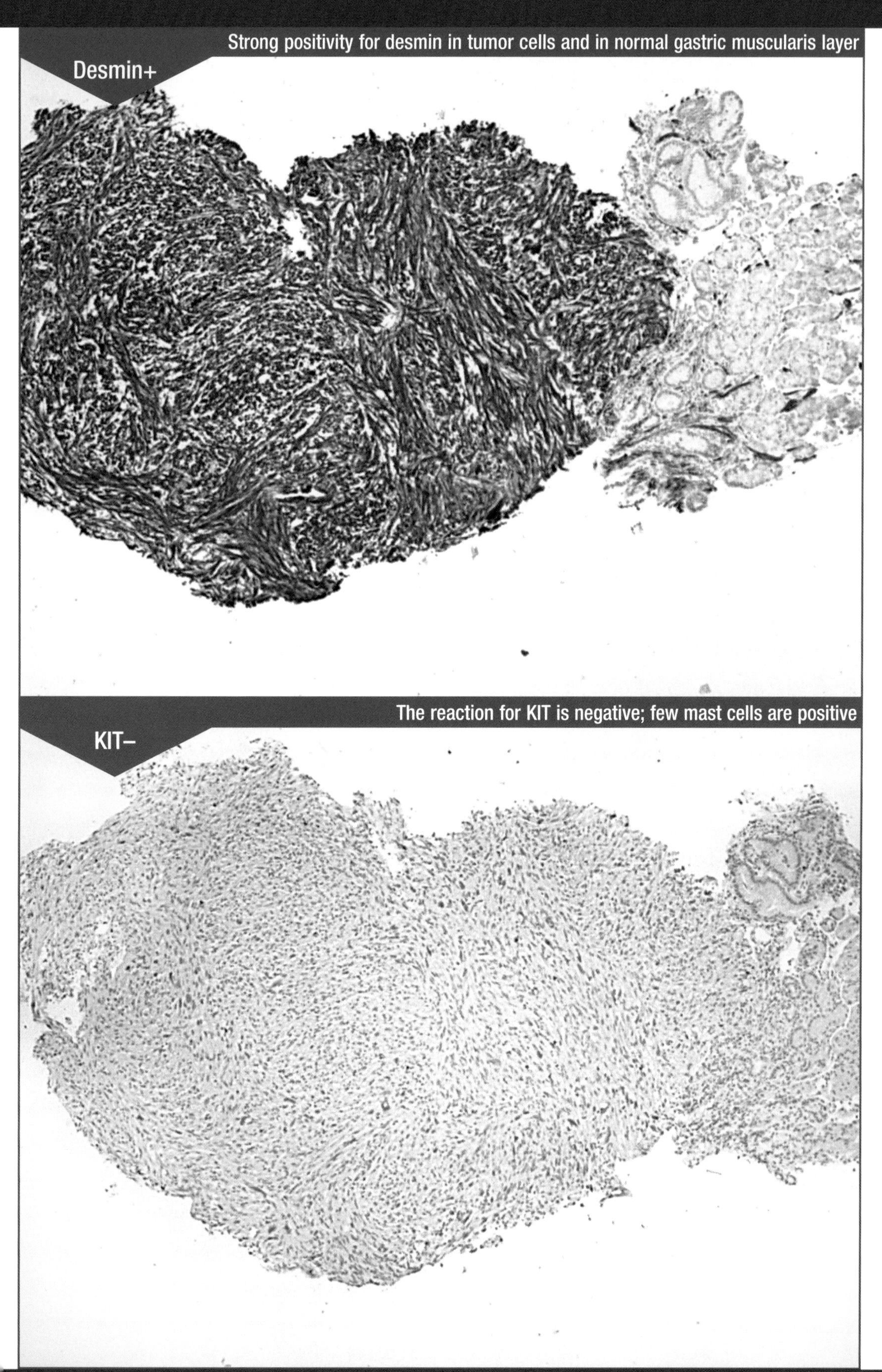

Diagnosis: Leiomyosarcoma

Biopsy of an abdominal tumor

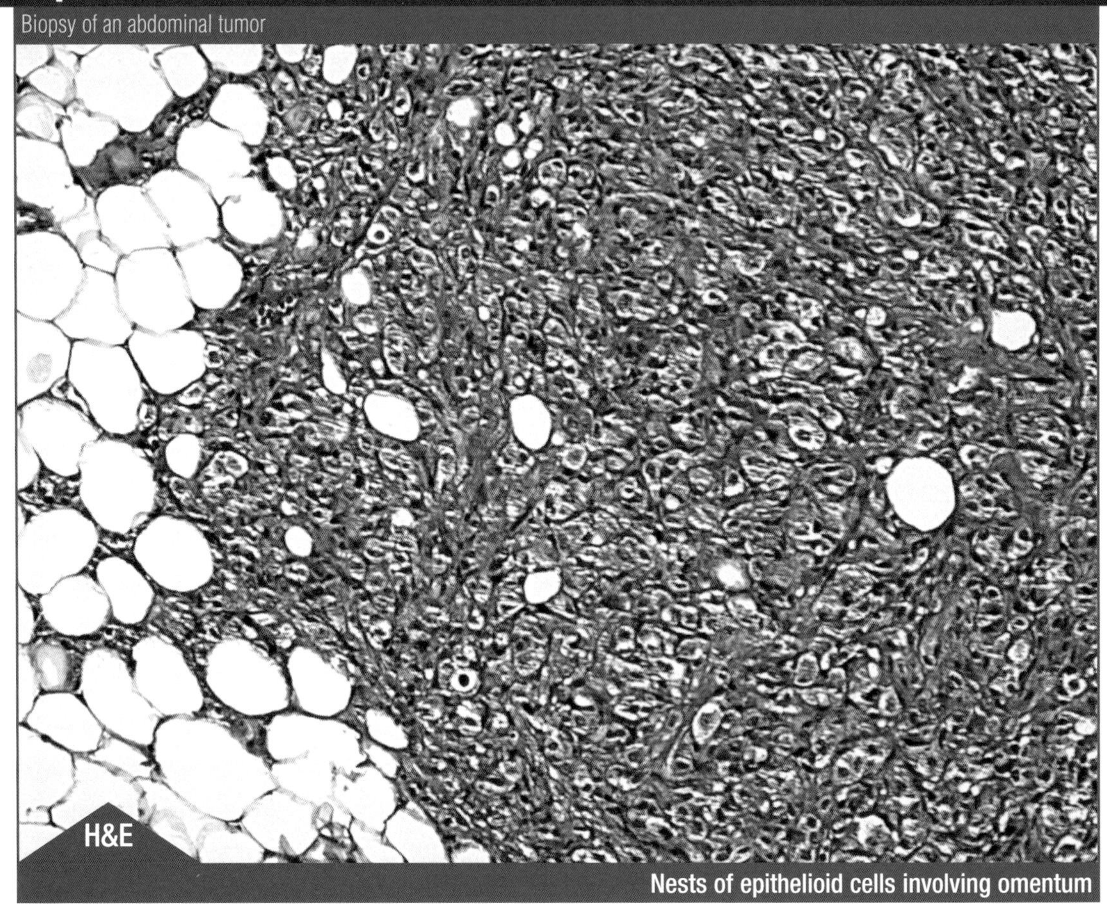

Nests of epithelioid cells involving omentum

Epithelioid Gastrointestinal Stromal Tumor vs Metastatic Carcinoma		
	KIT	Cytokeratin (CK)
Epithelioid GIST	+	–
Metastatic Carcinoma	–	+

Helpful Hints

KIT: This protein is expressed by the majority of gastrointestinal stromal tumors, whereas it is usually negative in leiomyosarcomas. True positivity for KIT in GISTs is usually strong and diffuse.

About one-third of KIT-negative GISTs harbor a mutation in platelet-derived growth factor receptor alpha (PDGFR). These tumors also show positivity for **PDGFR** by immunohistochemistry.

Miettinen 2001, Yi 2005.

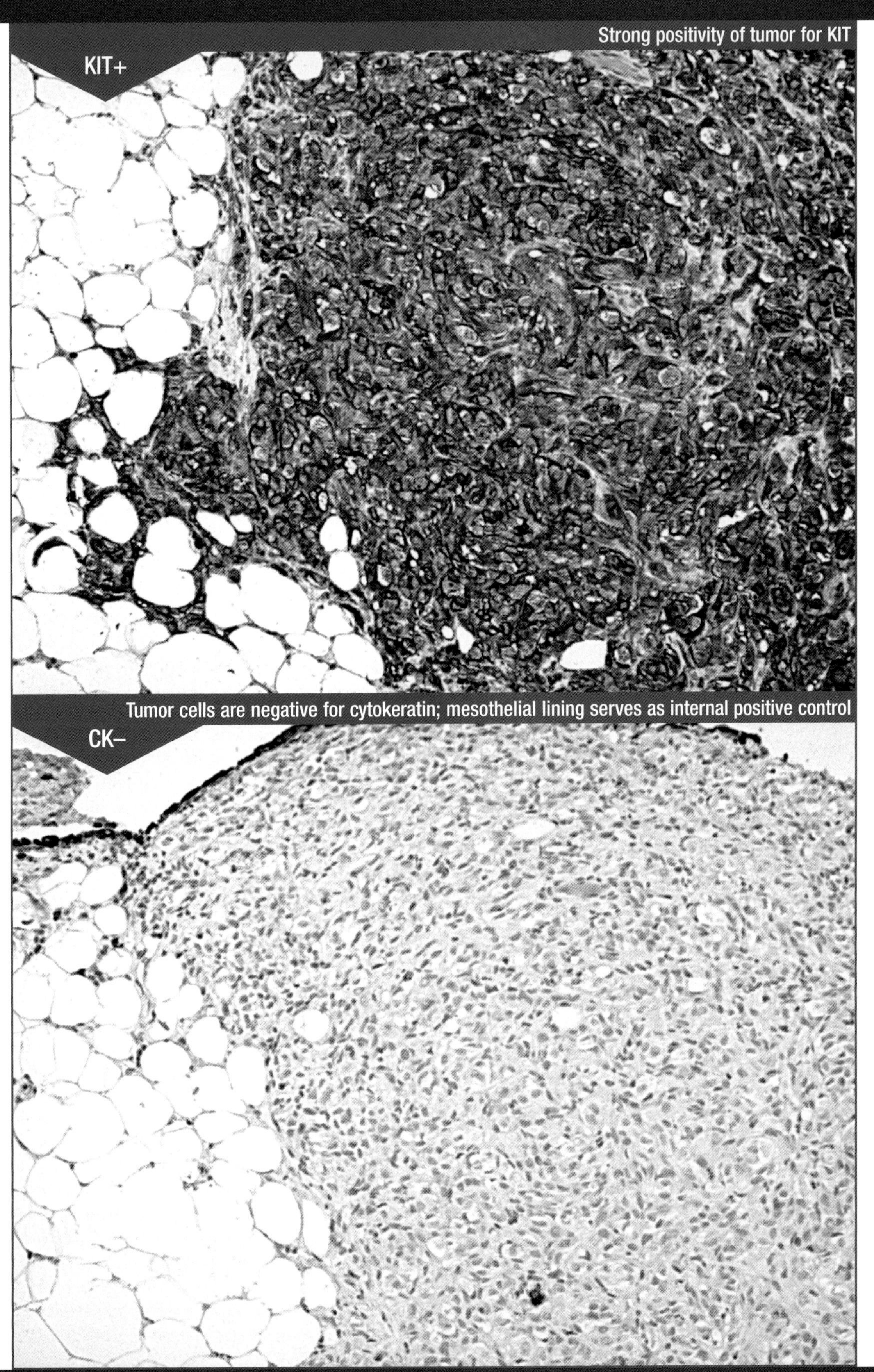

Diagnosis: Epithelioid Gastrointestinal Stromal Tumor

Gastrointestinal Tract Lymphoma vs Poorly Differentiated Carcinoma

Gastric biopsy

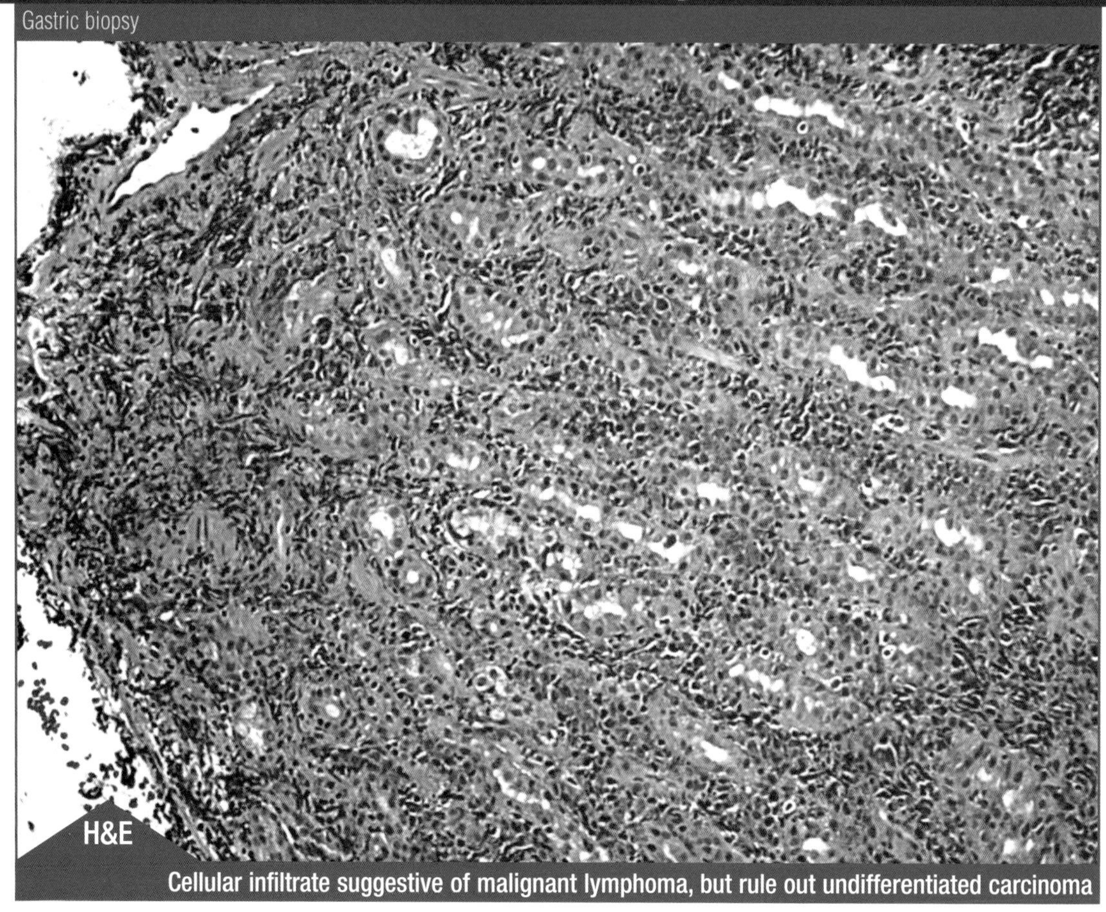

Cellular infiltrate suggestive of malignant lymphoma, but rule out undifferentiated carcinoma

Gastrointestinal Tract Lymphoma vs Poorly Differentiated Carcinoma		
	Cytokeratin (CK)	CD45, CD 20
GI Tract Lymphoma	–	+
Poorly Differentiated Ca	+	–

Helpful Hints

This is a relatively common differential diagnostic problem. The first thing one has to establish is morphological evidence of malignancy. The next step is to identify the phenotype of the malignant cells by the above small panel. Since the great majority of GI tract lymphomas are large B cell type, one could use **CD20** instead of, or in addition to **CD45**.

When the cells are small and the differential diagnosis is between a benign lymphoid infiltrate and a small cell lymphoma, immunohistochemistry is seldom useful. In these instances gene rearrangement studies are indicated.

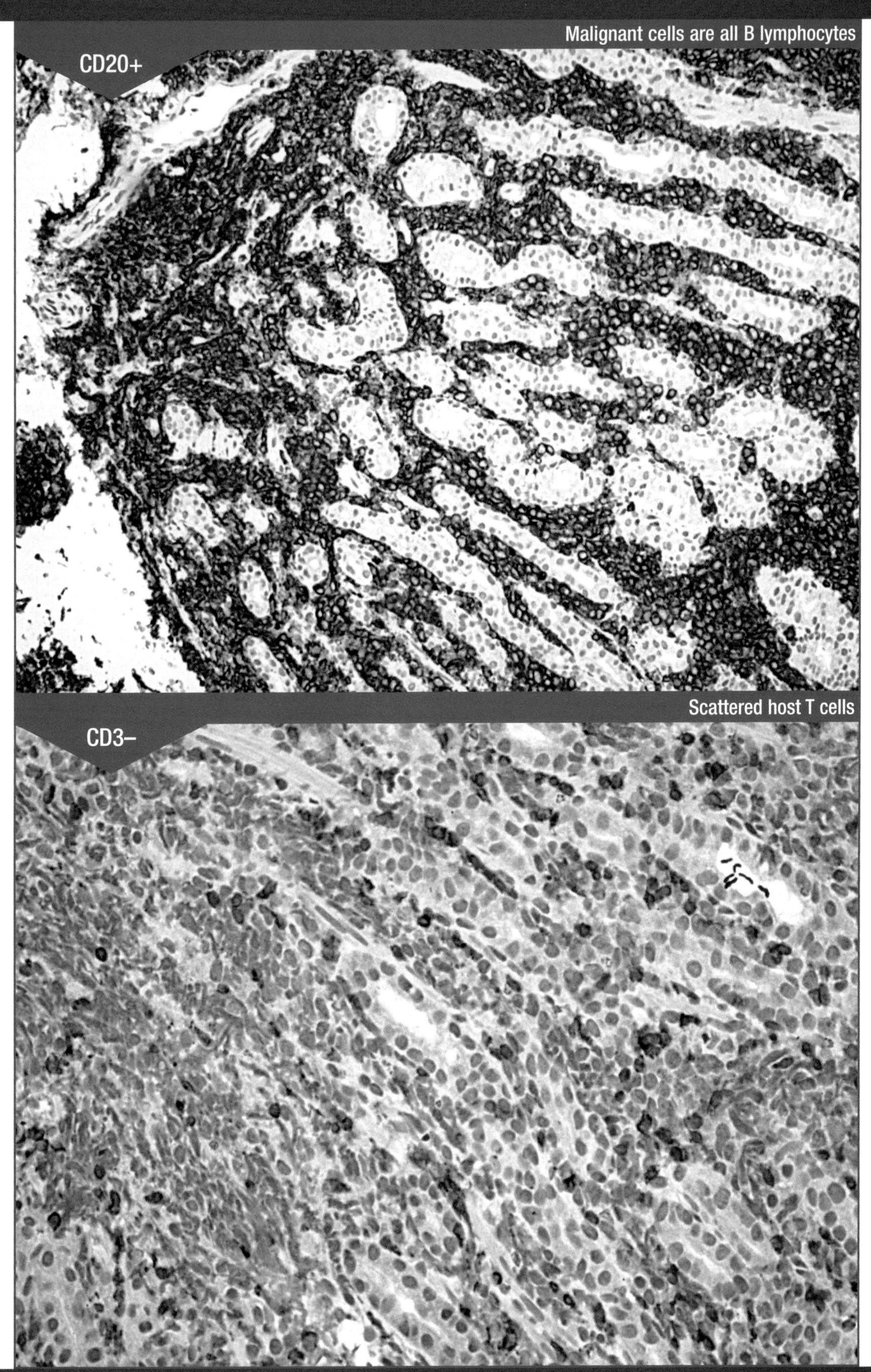

Diagnosis: Malignant Lymphoma, Large B Cell Type

Gastric biopsy

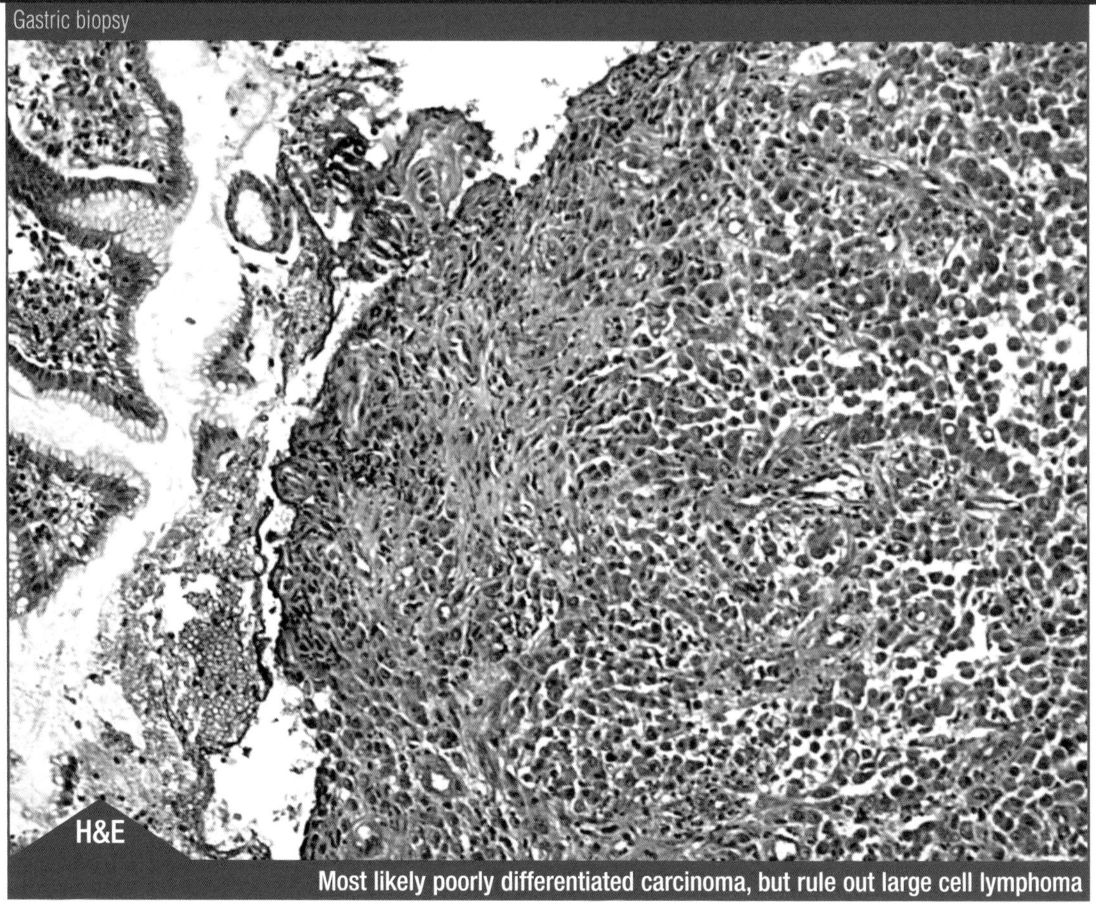

Most likely poorly differentiated carcinoma, but rule out large cell lymphoma

Gastrointestinal Tract Lymphoma vs Poorly Differentiated Carcinoma		
	Cytokeratin (CK)	CD45, CD20
GI Tract Lymphoma	–	+
Poorly Differentiated Ca	+	–

Helpful Hints

This is a relatively common differential diagnostic problem. The first thing one has to establish is morphological evidence of malignancy. The next step is to identify the phenotype of the malignant cells by the above small panel. Since the great majority of GI tract lymphomas are large B cell type, one could use **CD20** instead of, or in addition to **CD45**.

When the cells are small and the differential diagnosis is between a benign lymphoid infiltrate and a small cell lymphoma, immunohistochemistry is seldom useful. In these instances gene rearrangement studies are indicated.

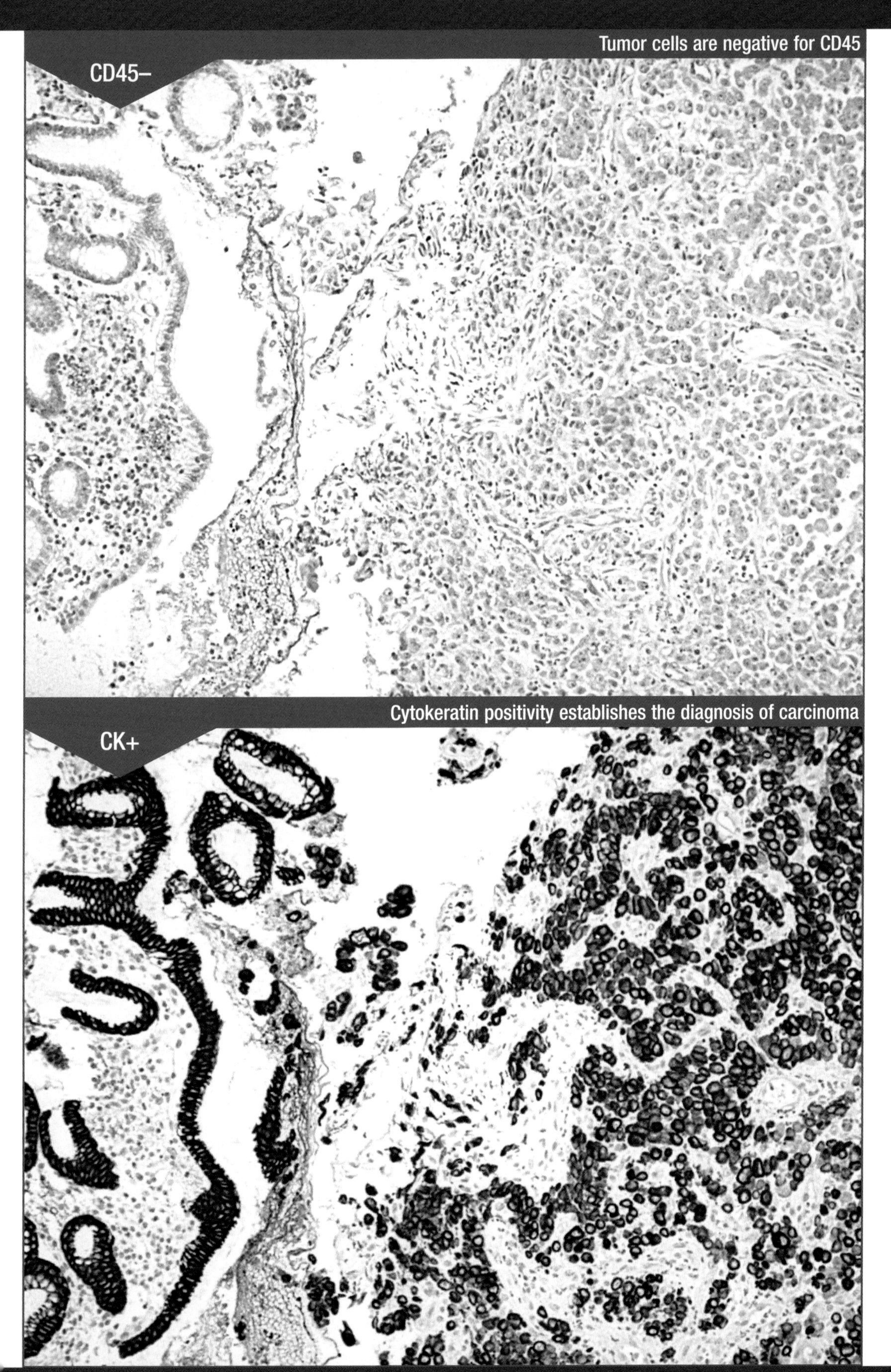

Diagnosis: Poorly Differentiated Carcinoma

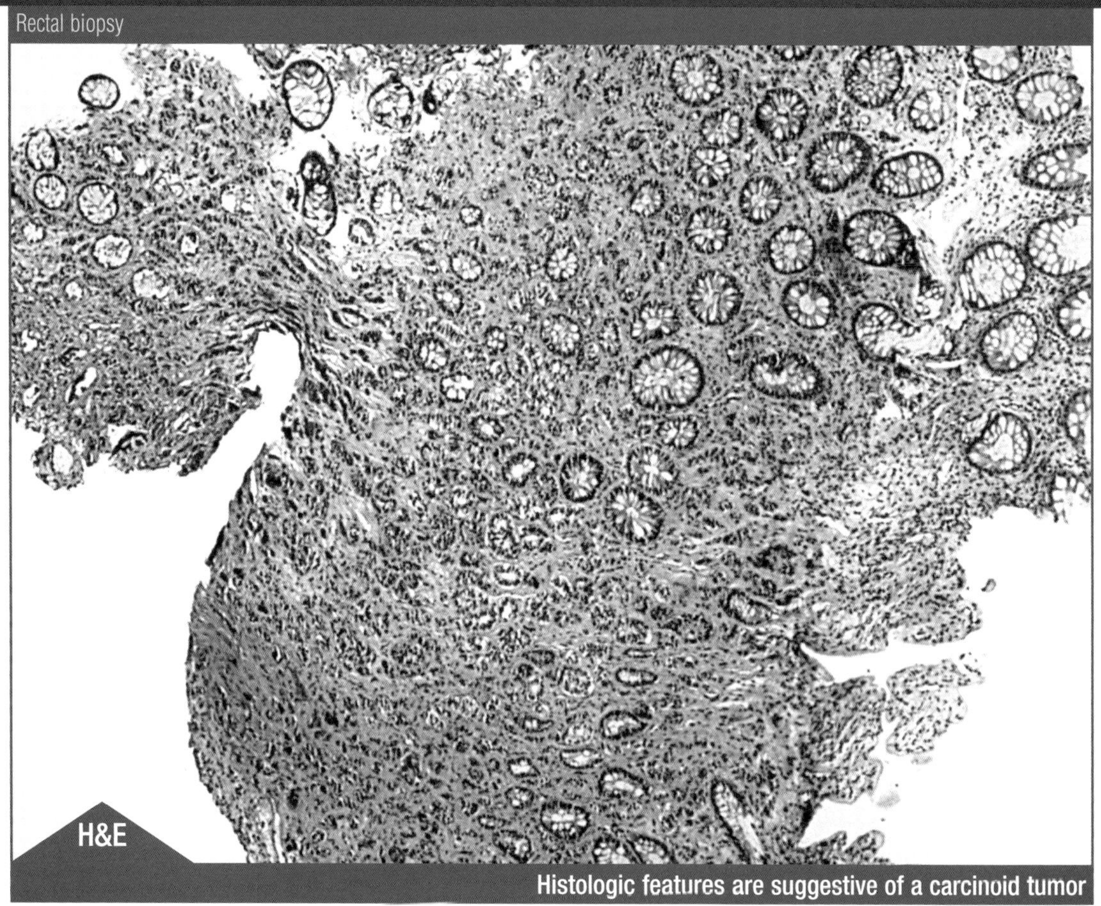

Histologic features are suggestive of a carcinoid tumor

Gastrointestinal Tract Carcinoid vs Gastrointestinal Tract Carcinoma			
	Chromogranin (Chrg)	Synaptophysin (SP)	CEA
GI Tract Carcinoid	+	+	–
GI Tract Carcinoma	–	–	+

Helpful Hints

Chromogranin: Most carcinoids of the GI tract are positive for chromogranin A. Occasional gastric and most colorectal carcinoids may be negative for chromogranin. In such cases, one may use **synaptophysin** with the understanding that some non-endocrine carcinomas can also be positive for synaptophysin.

When the endocrine nature of a tumor is established the expression of individual hormones may be detected; the most prevalent is **serotonin (5HT)**.

CEA: Polyclonal antibodies to CEA react with the majority of GI tract adenocarcinomas; monoclonal varieties are less sensitive. True carcinoids of the GI tract are seldom positive for CEA.

Wilander 1989.

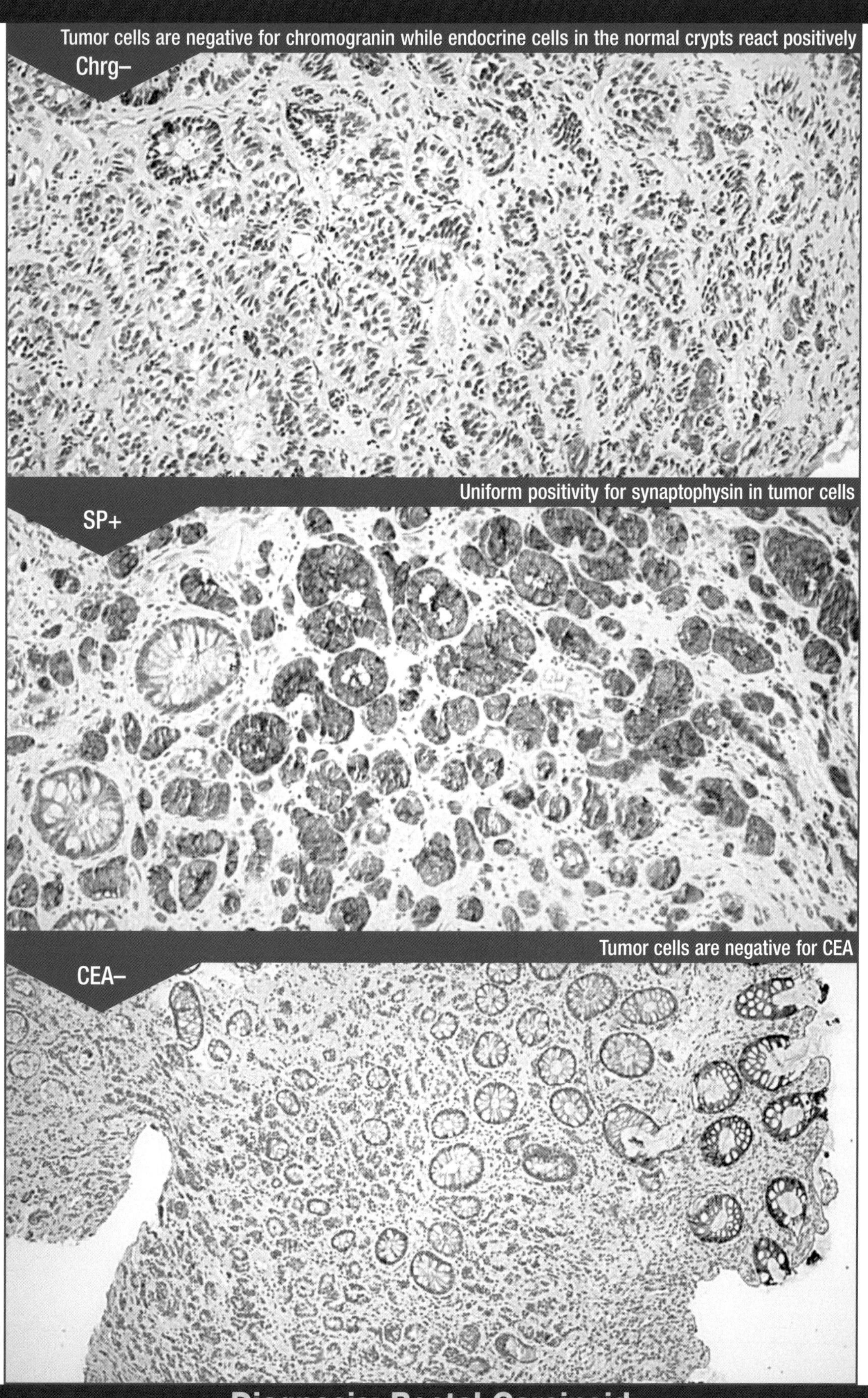

Diagnosis: Rectal Carcinoid

Laparoscopic biopsy of the colonic wall

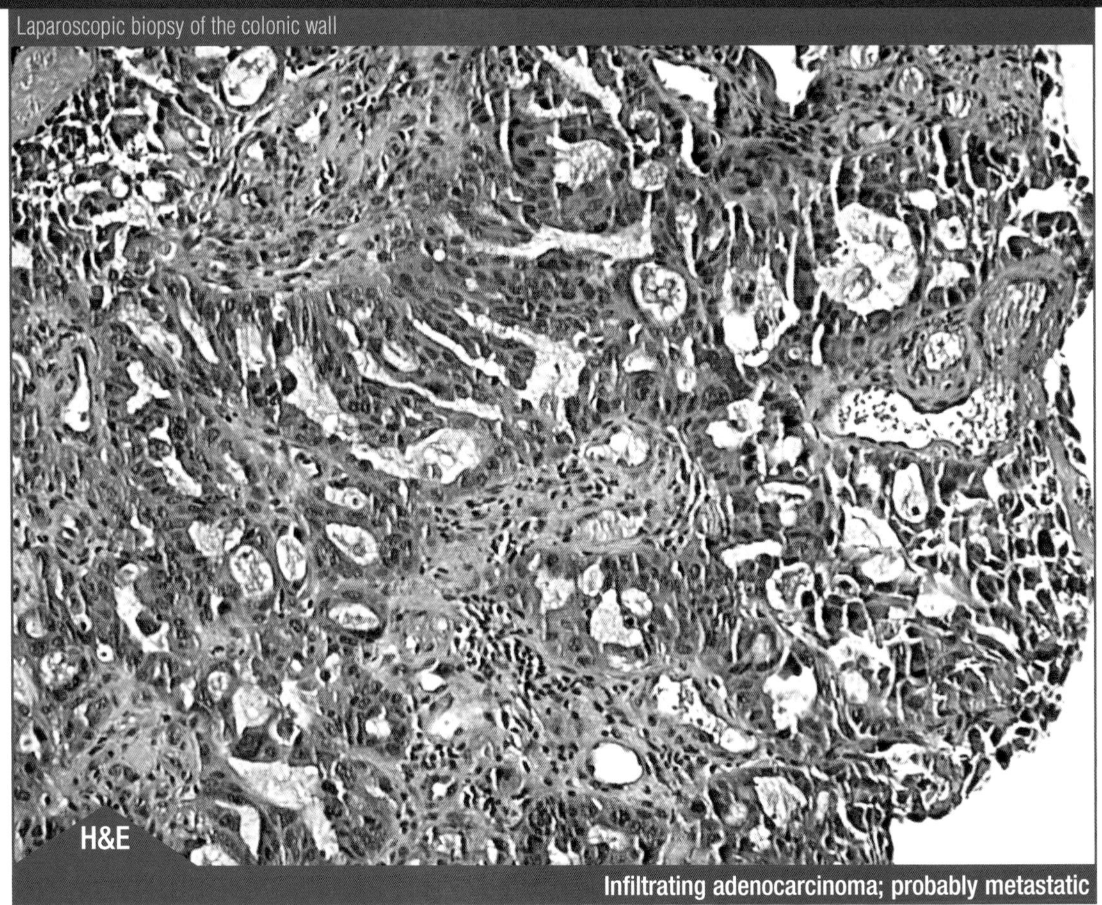

Infiltrating adenocarcinoma; probably metastatic

Colonic Adenocarcinoma vs Metastatic Ovarian Carcinoma		
	CK20	Estrogen Receptor (ER)
Colonic Adenocarcinoma	+	–
Metastatic Ovarian Ca	–	+

Helpful Hints

Metastatic ovarian carcinomas in the colon usually involve the wall externally. The majority are either serous or endometrioid type and usually express **estrogen receptor** (**ER**). Unlike breast carcinomas that either uniformly express ER in all tumor cells, or are clearly negative, gynecologic tumors may stain focally for ER (when ER antibody 1D5 is used). The phenotypic profile of mucinous ovarian carcinomas could be identical to that of colonic carcinomas and at times it is impossible to distinguish them from each other. With the exception of pseudomyxoma peritoneii, mucinous ovarian neoplasms seldom spread in abdominal peritoneum or intestinal serosa. Mucinous carcinomas of the ovary are usually negative for ER. Other helpful markers to distinguish metastatic nonmucinous carcinoma of the ovary from primary colonic adenocarcinomas are **CK20**, **CK7** and **CA-125**. The latter two are expressed by ovarian but not colonic carcinomas. CA-125 is not specific for ovarian carcinomas because a number of other carcinomas as well as mesotheliomas may also be positive for this marker.

In adequately fixed tissue a focal reaction for ER is usually seen in gynecologic tumors. Breast cancers are either completely negative or diffusely positive.

Loy 1996, Koelma1987, Nadji 2005.

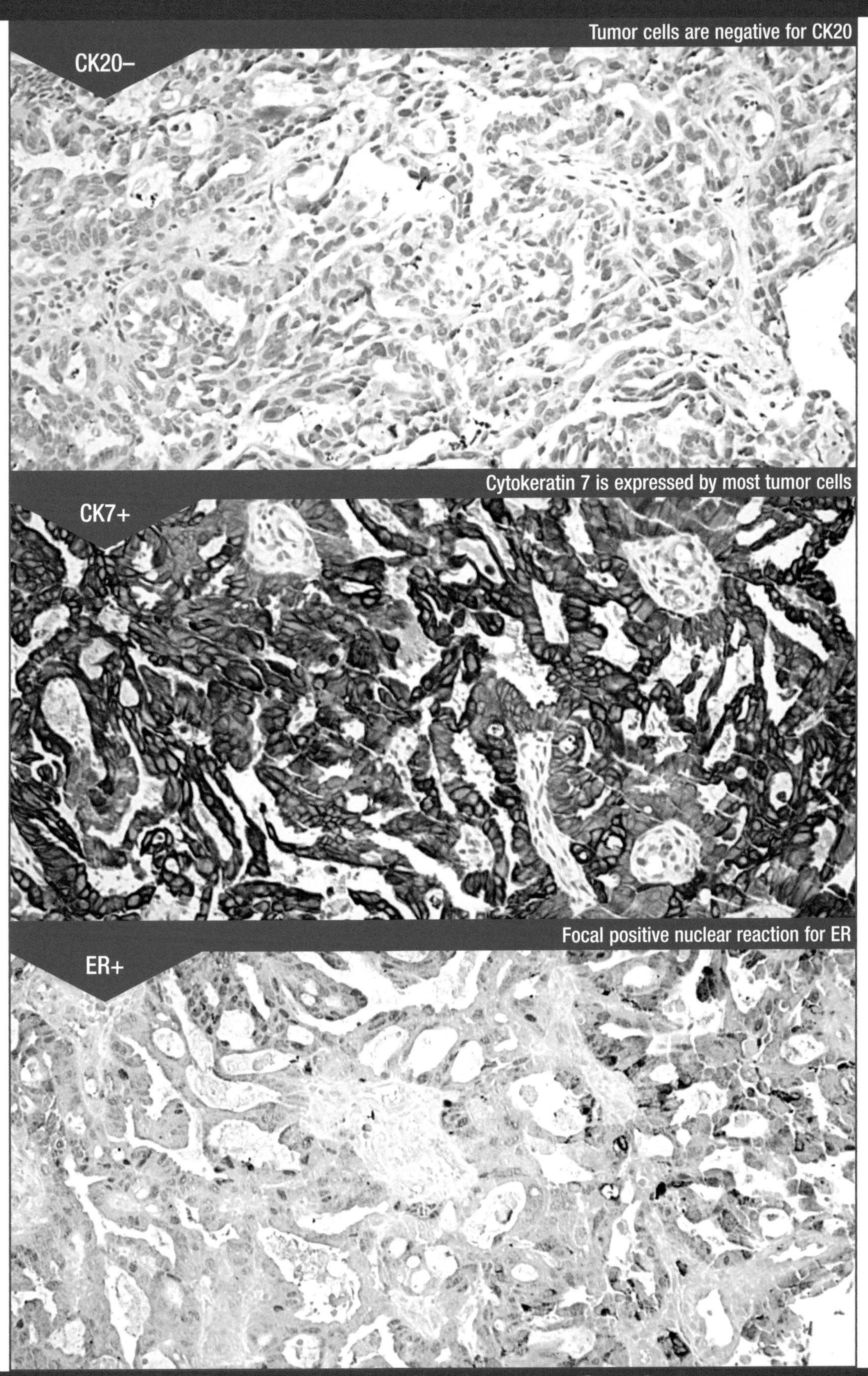
Tumor cells are negative for CK20
CK20–
Cytokeratin 7 is expressed by most tumor cells
CK7+
Focal positive nuclear reaction for ER
ER+
Diagnosis: Metastatic Ovarian Carcinoma

Appendectomy specimen

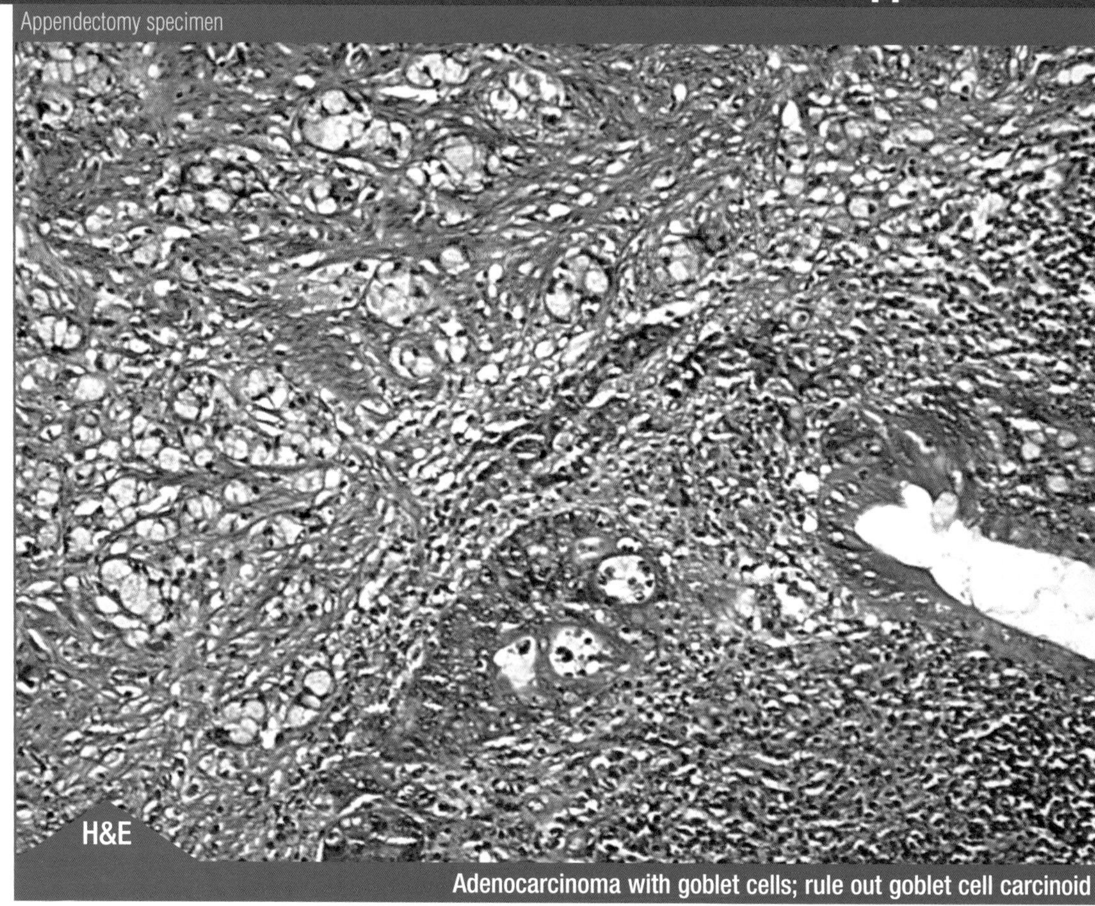

Adenocarcinoma with goblet cells; rule out goblet cell carcinoid

Goblet Cell Carcinoid vs Adenocarcinoma of Appendix			
	Chromogranin (Chrg)	5-HT	CK20
Goblet Cell Carcinoid	+	+	S
Adenocarcinoma of Appendix	–	–	+

Helpful Hints

Goblet cell carcinoids of appendix are morphologically similar to adenocarcinomas but immunohistochemically express endocrine markers. These tumors are positive for both **chromogranin** and **serotonin** (**5-HT**). Similar to adenocarcinomas of colon, adenocarcinomas of appendix are usually diffusely positive for **CK20** while goblet cell carcinoids are either negative or focally positive.

Wilander 1989.

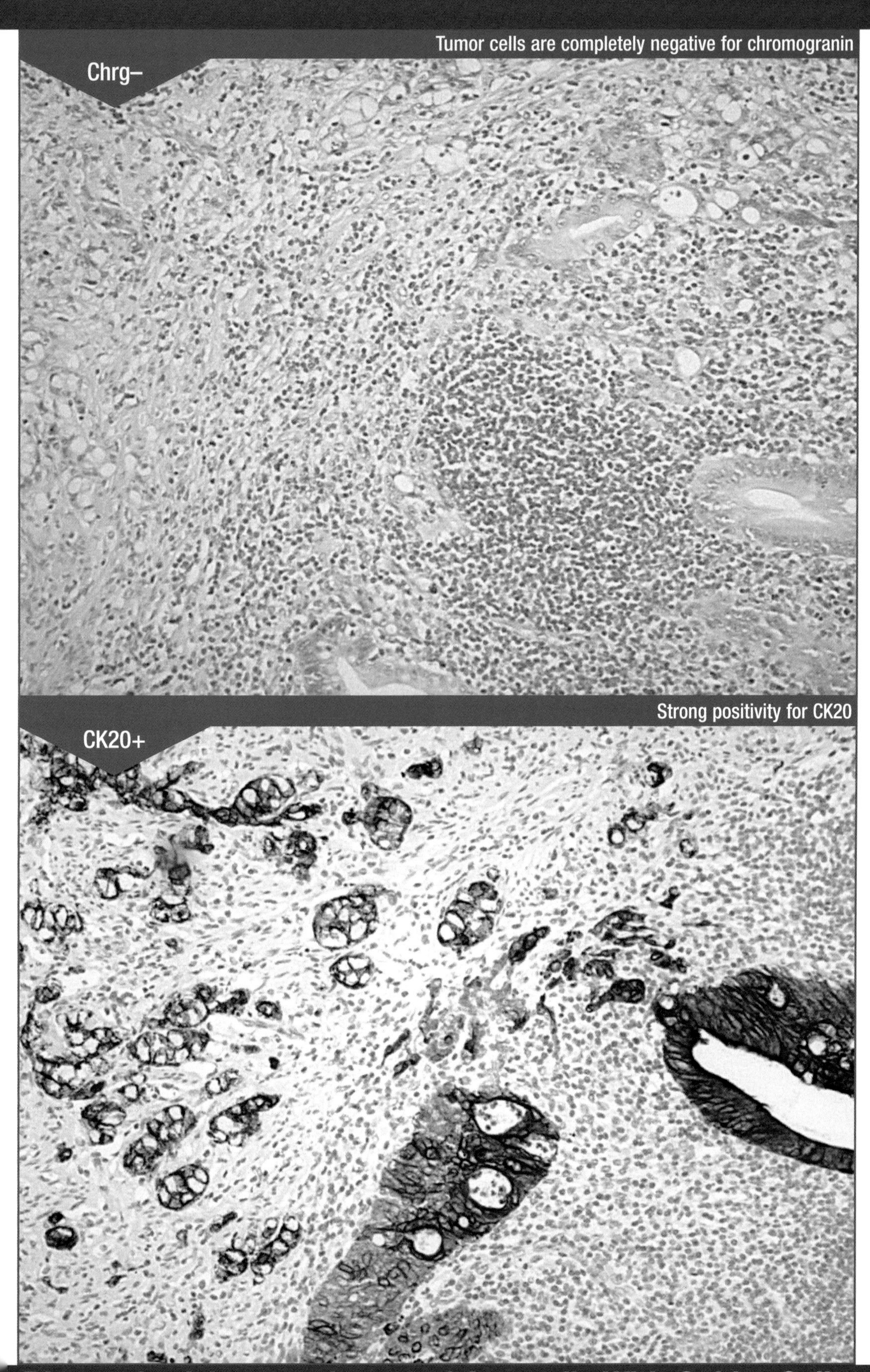

Diagnosis: Adenocarcinoma of Appendix With Goblet Cells

Gastric biopsy

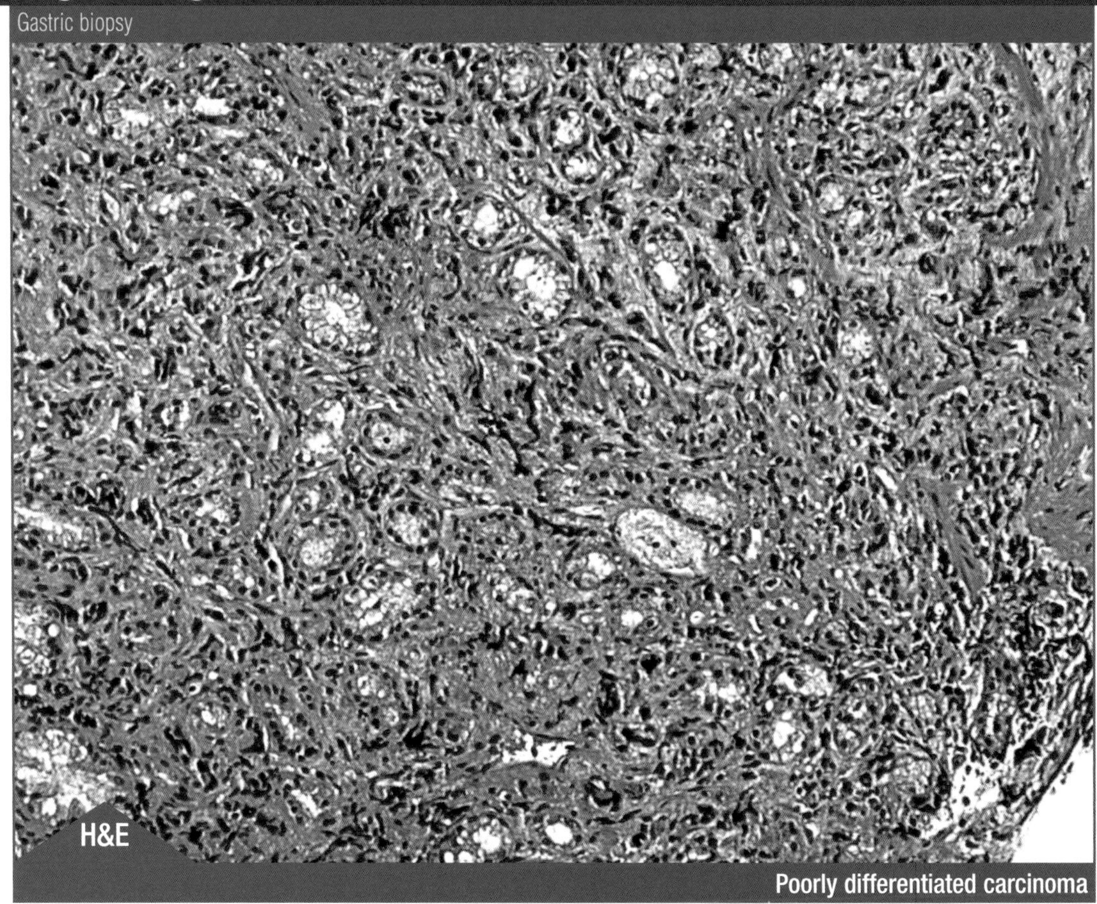

Poorly differentiated carcinoma

Signet Ring Cell Carcinoma of Stomach vs Metastatic Lobular Carcinoma of Breast		
	Cytokeratin (CK)	Estrogen Receptor (ER)
Signet Ring Cell Carcinoma of Stomach	+	–
Metastatic Lobular Carcinoma of Breast	+	+

Helpful Hints

Both primary signet ring cell carcinoma of stomach and metastatic lobular carcinomas of breast are positive for cytokeratin and EMA. The only distinguishing marker for these two entities is ER. With the exception of rare pleomorphic variants, all lobular carcinomas of the breast are positive for estrogen receptor. ER is not expressed by gastrointestinal tract carcinomas when antibody 1D5 is used.

Nadji 2005.

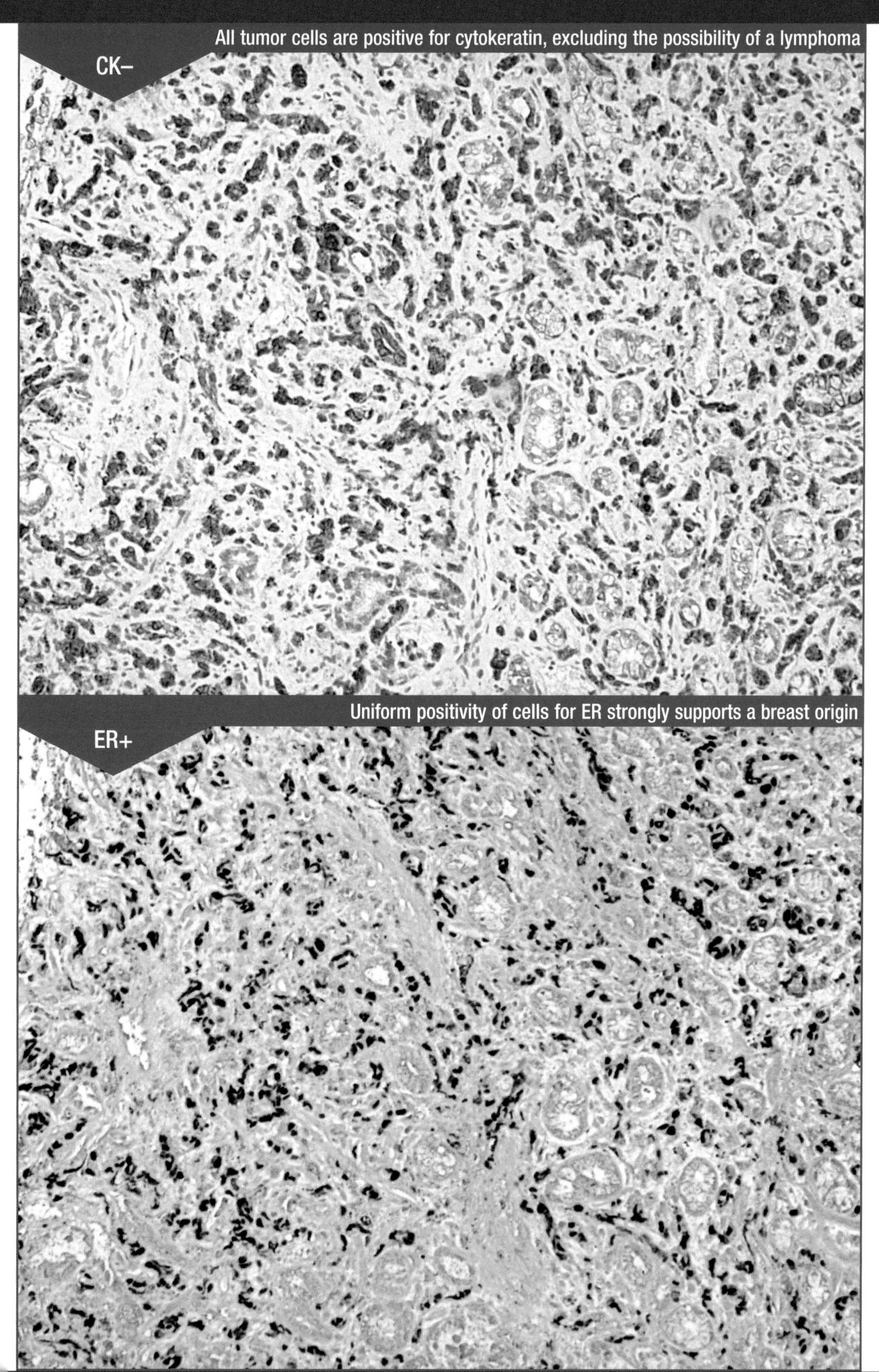

Diagnosis: Metastatic Carcinoma of Breast

Tumor in the body of pancreas

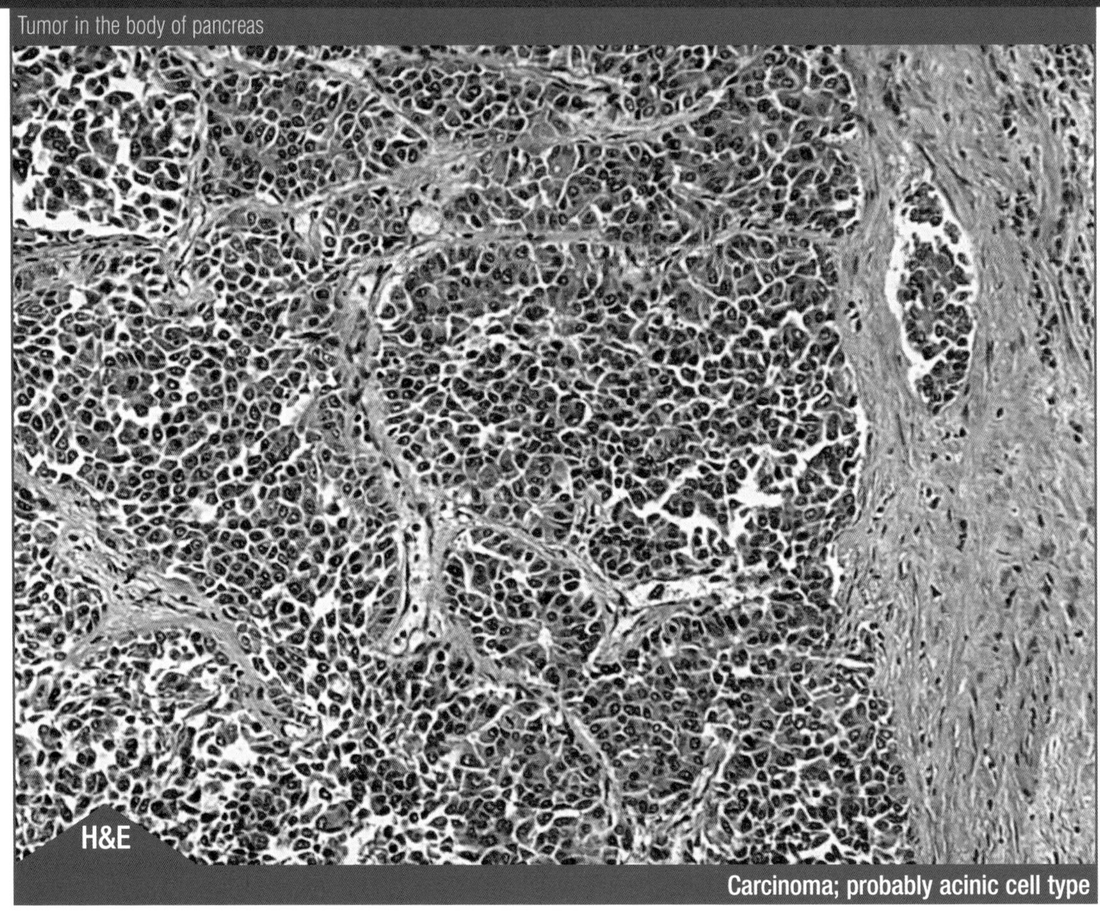

Carcinoma; probably acinic cell type

Ductal Adenocarcinoma vs Acinic Cell Carcinoma		
	CEA	Amylase/Lipase/Trypsin
Pancreatic Ductal Carcinoma	+	–
Acinic Cell Carcinoma	–	+

Helpful Hints

CEA: The majority of pancreatic ductal carcinomas are positive for CEA particularly when polyclonal anti-CEA antibody is used. Conversely, acinic cell carcinomas of the pancreas are usually negative for CEA.

Acinic cell carcinomas are likely to express one or more antigens elaborated by normal pancreatic acini. These include **pancreatic amylase**, **lipase**, and **trypsin**. These markers are normally not expressed by ductal carcinomas. One should note that antibodies to salivary gland amylase do not cross-react with pancreatic amylase and vice versa.

Klimstra 1992.

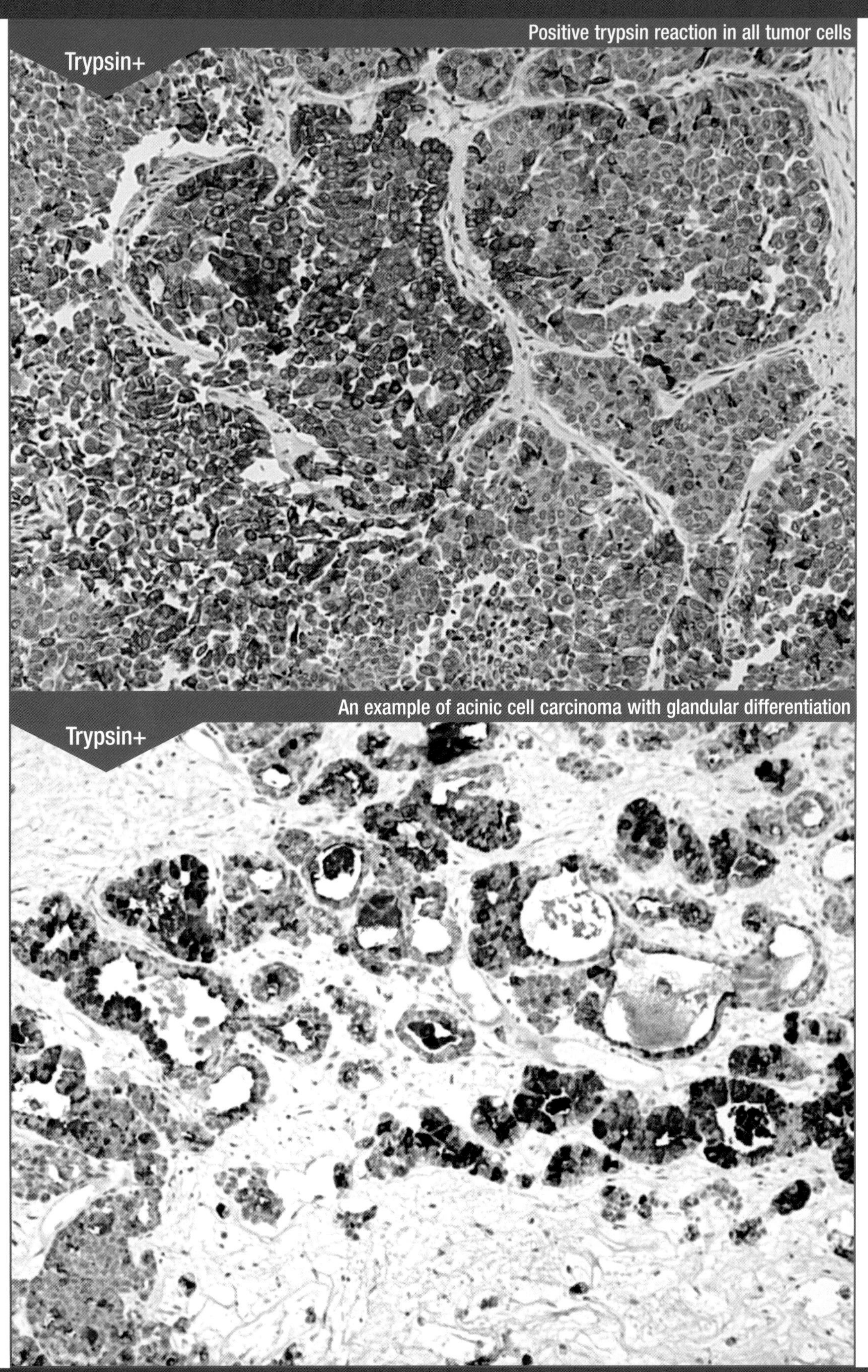

Positive trypsin reaction in all tumor cells

An example of acinic cell carcinoma with glandular differentiation

Diagnosis: Acinic Cell Carcinoma of Pancreas

Tumor in the body of pancreas

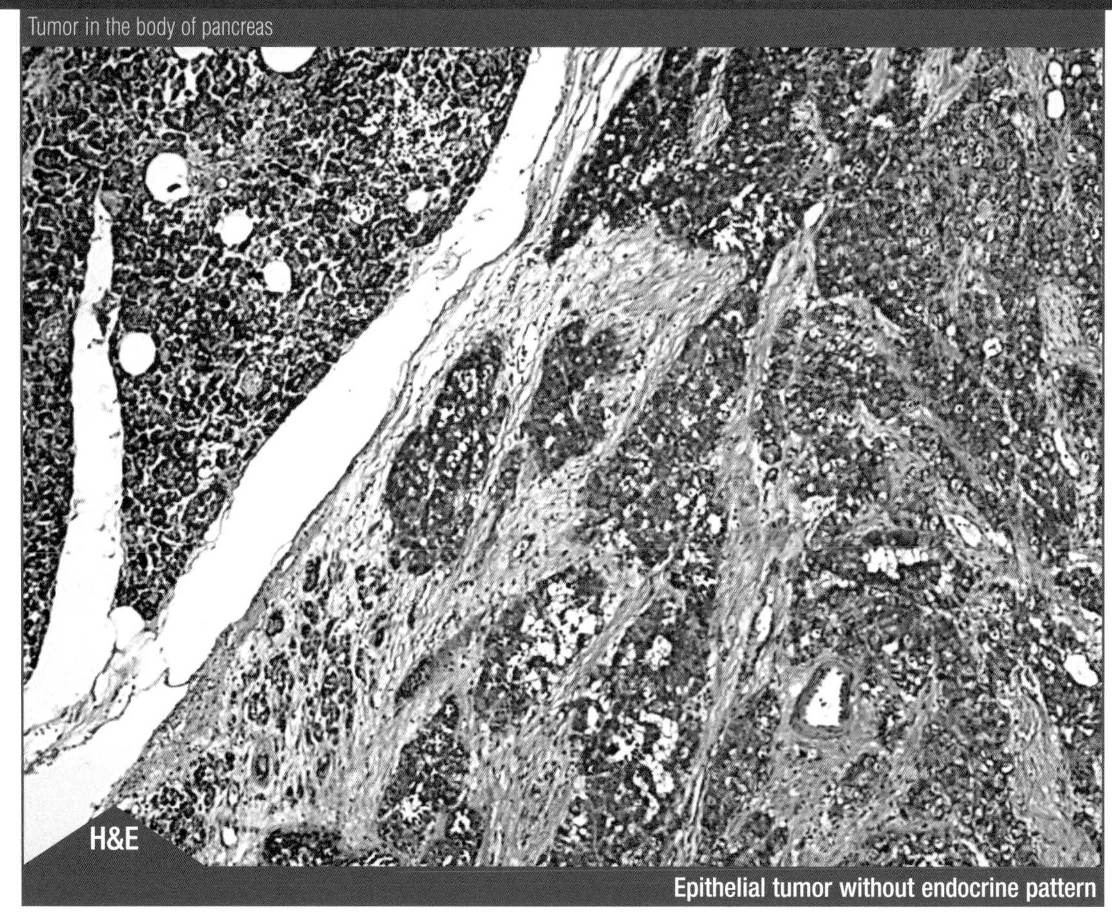

Epithelial tumor without endocrine pattern

Islet Cell Tumor vs Acinic Cell Carcinoma		
	Chromogranin (Chrg)	Amylase/Lipase/Trypsin
Islet Cell Tumor	+	–
Acinic Cell Carcinoma	–	+

Helpful Hints

Pancreatic islet cell tumors and acinic cell carcinomas may show similar morphologic features. The combination of **chromogranin** and **acinar cell markers** usually solves this problem. Rare cases of mixed acinic-islet cell tumors of pancreas are reported; presumably they express both endocrine and acinar cell antigens.

Tobita 2001.

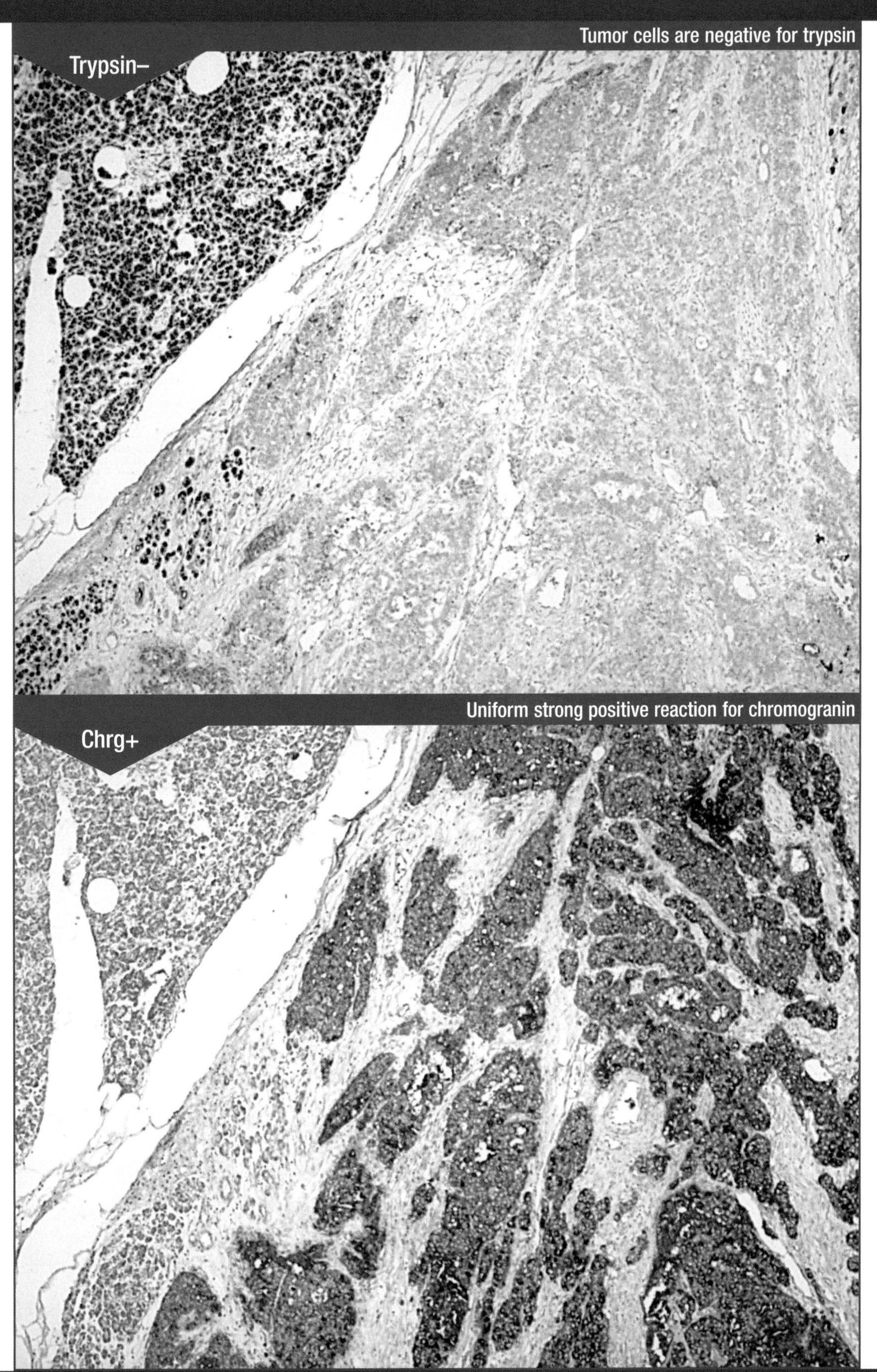

Diagnosis: Islet Cell Tumor

Pancreatic tumor

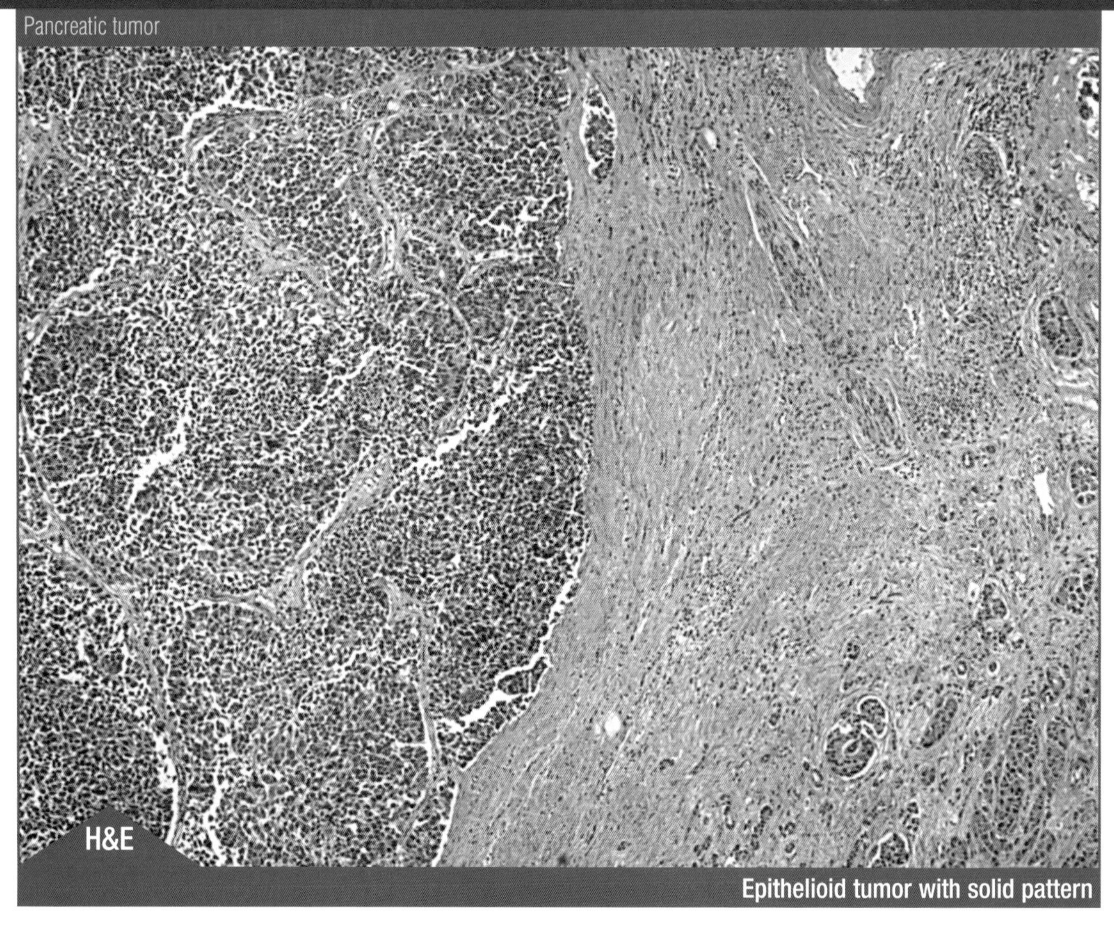

Epithelioid tumor with solid pattern

Islet Cell Tumor vs Acinic Cell Carcinoma		
	Chromogranin (Chrg)	Amylase/Lipase/Trypsin
Islet Cell Tumor	+	–
Acinic Cell Carcinoma	–	+

Helpful Hints

Pancreatic islet cell tumors and acinic cell carcinomas may show similar morphologic features. The combination of **chromogranin** and **acinar cell markers** usually solves this problem. Rare cases of mixed acinic-islet cell tumors of pancreas are reported; presumably they express both endocrine and acinar cell antigens.

Tobita 2001.

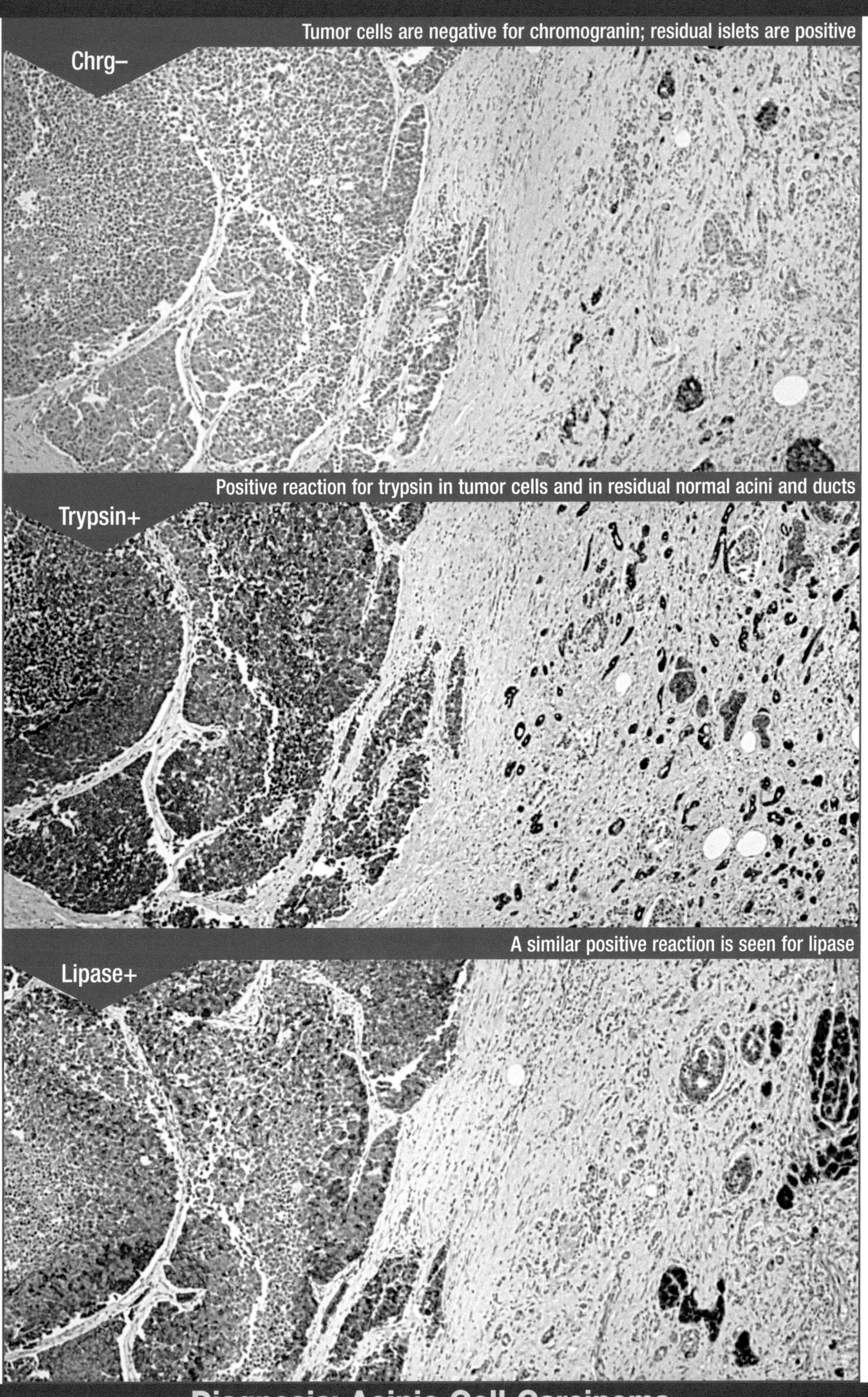

Diagnosis: Acinic Cell Carcinoma

Tumor of the body of pancreas

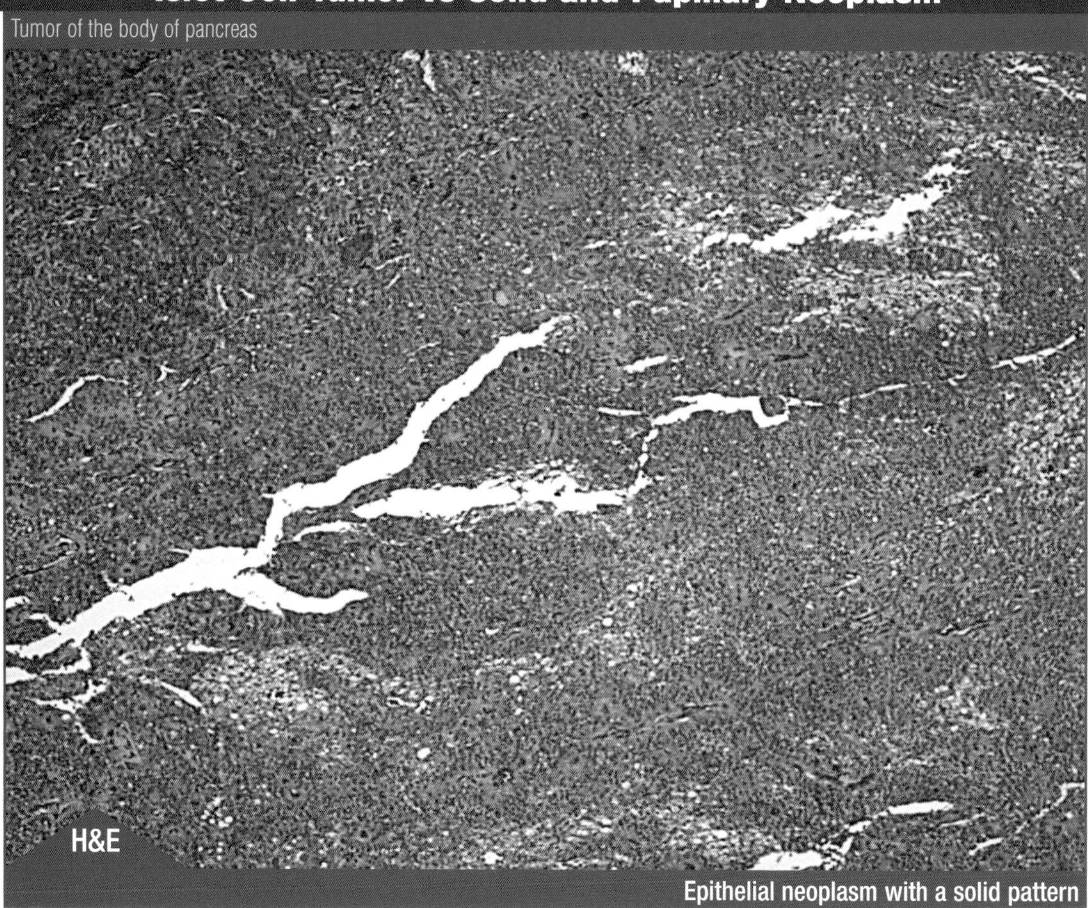

Epithelial neoplasm with a solid pattern

Islet Cell Tumor vs Solid and Papillary Neoplasm	
	Chromogranin (Chrg)
Islet Cell Tumor	+
Solid and Papillary Neoplasm	–

Helpful Hints

Pancreatic islet cell tumors and solid and papillary tumors share overlapping morphologic features and hence, immunohistochemistry is always necessary for their proper classification. The best marker for this purpose is **chromogranin** because it is expressed by the majority of islet cell tumors but not by solid and papillary neoplasms. Other neuroendocrine markers, such as **Neuronal Enolase** (**NSE**) maybe expressed by both tumors.

Wick 2001, Choi 2002.

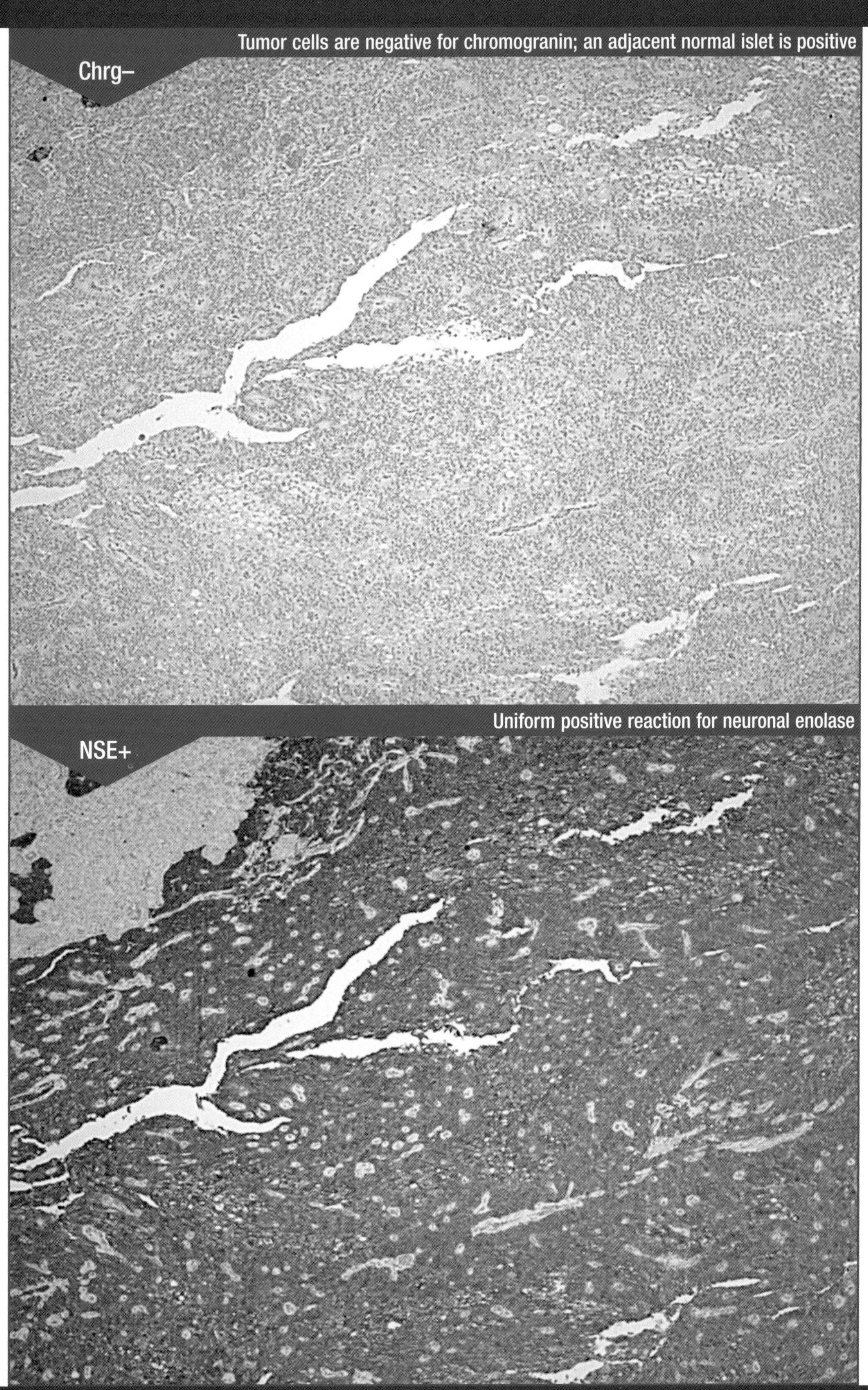

Diagnosis: Solid and Papillary Neoplasm

Resected primary tumor of the liver

H&E

Hepatocellular carcinoma and cholangiocarcinoma are possibilities

Hepatocellular Carcinoma vs Cholangiocarcinoma		
	Cytokeratin 7 (CK7)	Hepatocellular Antigen (HCA)
Hepatocellular Carcinoma	–	+
Cholangiocarcinoma	+	–

Helpful Hints

CK7: In normal liver, CK7 decorates normal bile ducts but not hepatocytes. This marker is ideal for identification of ductules in biopsies from transplant liver and in cases of bile duct atresia. While cholangiocarcinomas stain strongly for CK7, hepatocellular carcinomas do not. The exceptions are those rare cases of combined hepatocellular-cholangiocarcinoma in which the cholangio component reacts positively for CK7. It should be noted that CK7 does not separate cholangiocarcinoma from metastatic carcinomas of upper GI tract, lung, and pancreatobiliary system.

Hepatocellular antigen (**HEP PAR1 or HCA**) is an undefined cytoplasmic antigen that is present in normal liver and in the majority of hepatocellular carcinomas. This marker is also expressed, albeit less commonly, by foregut-derived adenocarcinomas, such as lung and upper GI tract. Unlike hepatocellular carcinomas, these tumors always express CK7.

We do not use alpha-fetoprotein (AFP) for the diagnosis of hepatocellular carcinoma. Less than 20% of hepatocellular carcinomas are positive for this antigen. Furthermore, up to 10% of carcinomas of upper gastrointestinal tract and pancreatobiliary system may also express AFP.

Duval 2000, Lau 2002c.

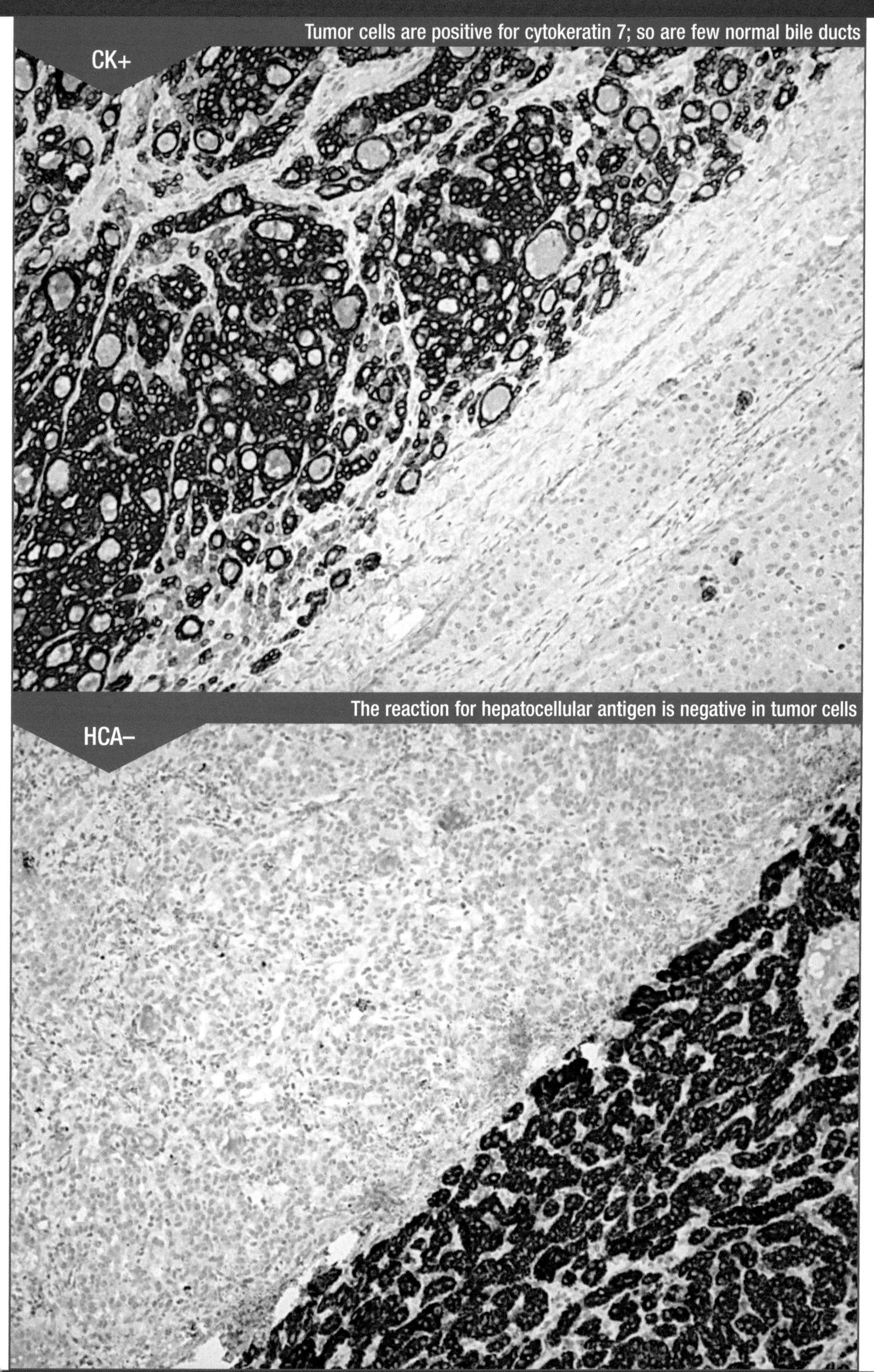

Diagnosis: Cholangiocarcinoma

Core biopsy of liver

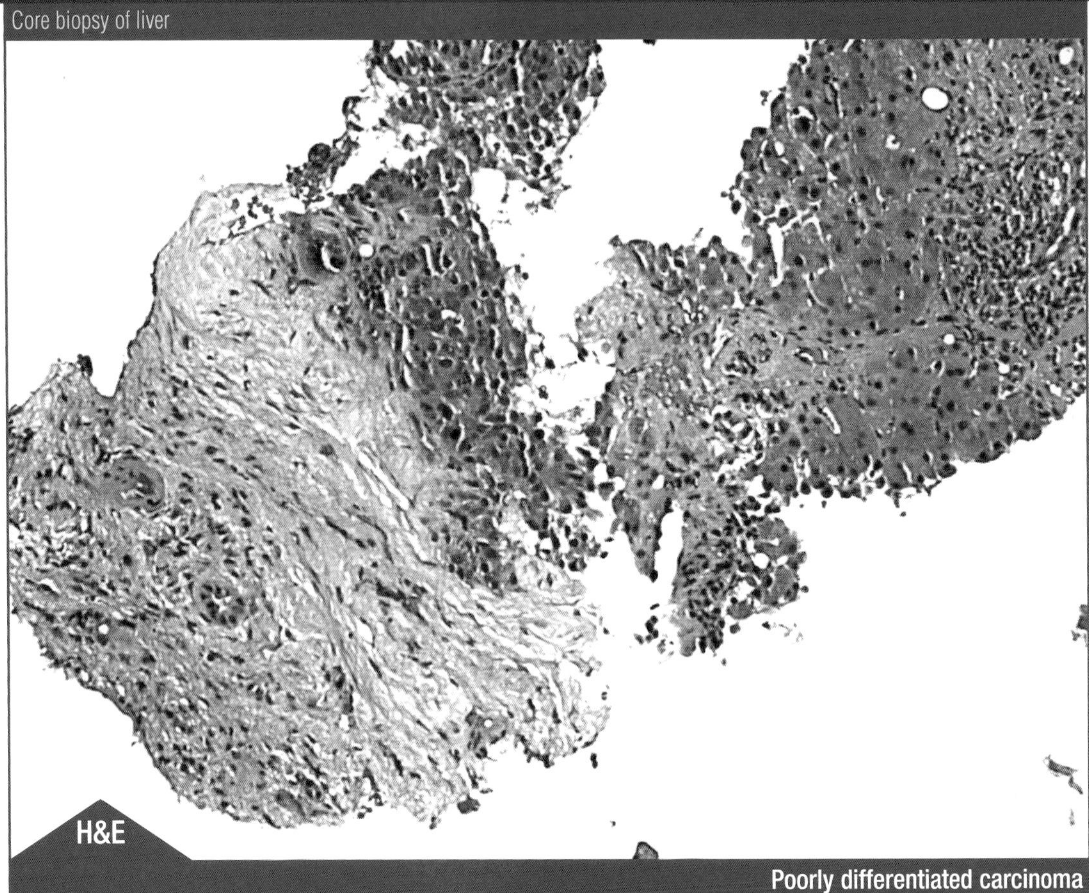

Poorly differentiated carcinoma

Hepatocellular Carcinoma vs Cholangiocarcinoma		
	Cytokeratin 7 (CK7)	Hepatocellular Antigen (HCA)
Hepatocellular Carcinoma	–	+
Cholangiocarcinoma	+	–

Helpful Hints

CK7: In normal liver, CK7 decorates normal bile ducts but not hepatocytes. This marker is ideal for identification of ductules in biopsies from transplant liver and in cases of bile duct atresia. While cholangiocarcinomas stain strongly for CK7, hepatocellular carcinomas do not. The exceptions are those rare cases of combined hepatocellular-cholangiocarcinoma in which the cholangio component reacts positively for CK7. It should be noted that CK7 does not separate cholangiocarcinoma from metastatic carcinomas of upper GI tract, lung, and pancreatobiliary system.

Hepatocellular antigen (**HEP PAR1 or HCA**) is an undefined cytoplasmic antigen that is present in normal liver and in the majority of hepatocellular carcinomas. This marker is also expressed, albeit less commonly, by foregut-derived adenocarcinomas, such as lung and upper GI tract. Unlike hepatocellular carcinomas, these tumors always express CK7.

We do not use alpha-fetoprotein (AFP) for the diagnosis of hepatocellular carcinoma. Less than 20% of hepatocellular carcinomas are positive for this antigen. Furthermore, up to 10% of carcinomas of upper gastrointestinal tract and pancreatobiliary system may also express AFP.

Duval 2000, Lau 2002c.

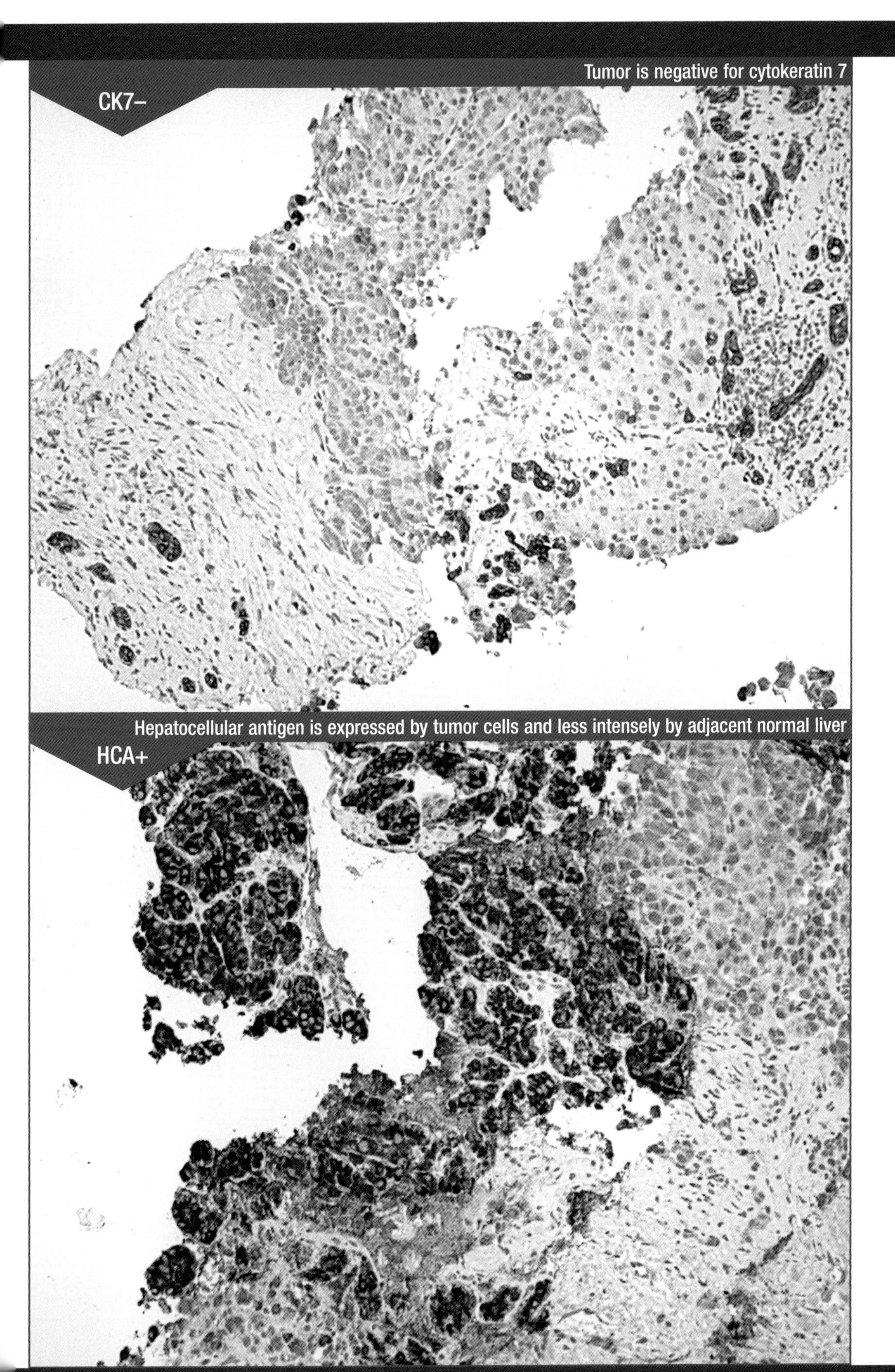

Diagnosis: Hepatocellular Carcinoma

Resected tumor of the liver

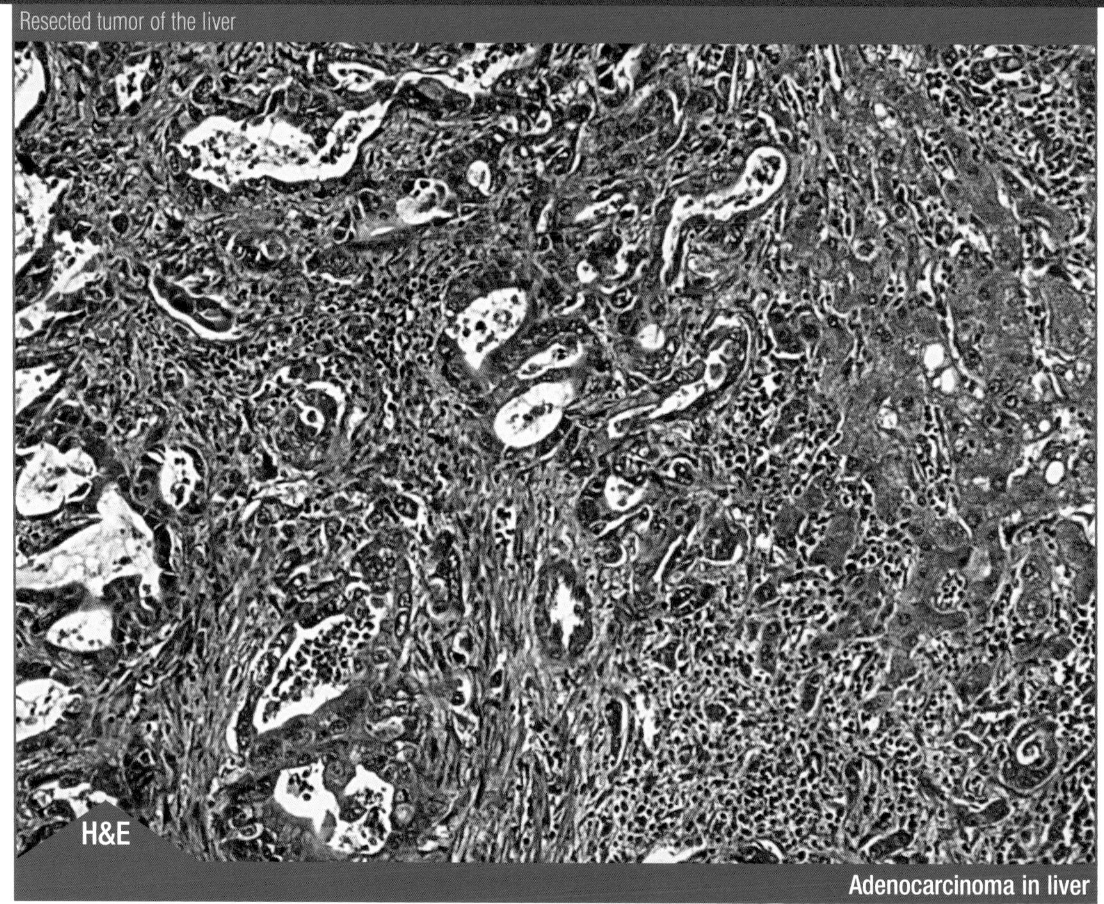

Adenocarcinoma in liver

Hepatocellular Carcinoma vs Metastatic Adenocarcinoma		
	Cytokeratin 7 (CK7)	Hepatocellular Antigen (HCA)
Hepatocellular Carcinoma	–	+
Metastatic Adenocarcinoma	+	–

Helpful Hints

Similar to cholangiocarcinomas, most metastatic adenocarcinomas to liver react positively for **CK7** (colonic adenocarcinoma is an exception). Hepatocellular carcinomas, on the other hand, are usually negative. As was discussed before, **HCA** may rarely be expressed by upper GI tract and lung carcinomas. These tumors, however, are always positive for CK7.

Duval 2000, Lau 2002.

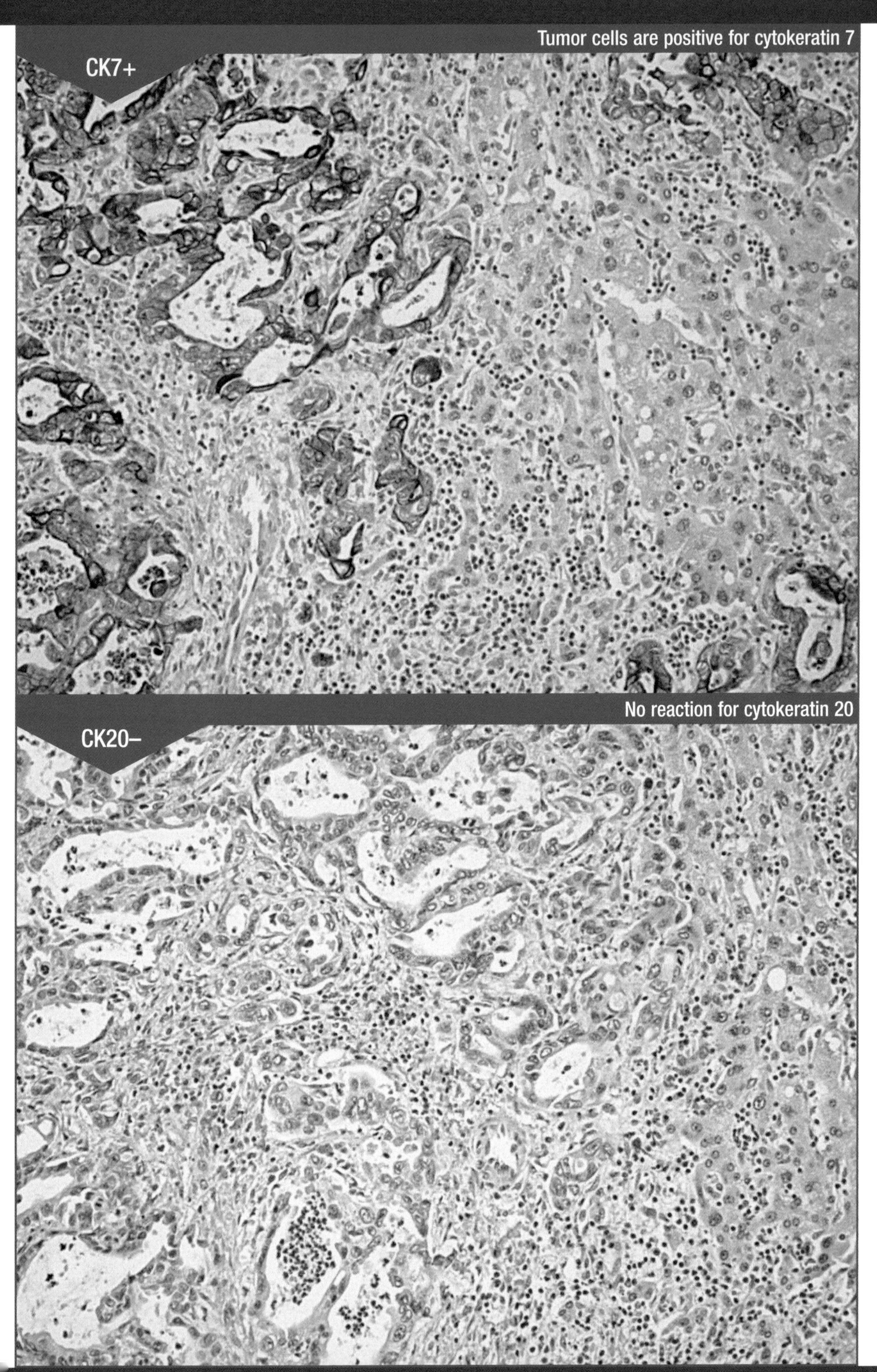

Diagnosis: Metastatic Adenocarcinoma *(pancreas by history)*

Hepatocellular Carcinoma vs Metastatic Colonic Adenocarcinoma

Resection of single liver nodule in a patient with history of colonic carcinoma

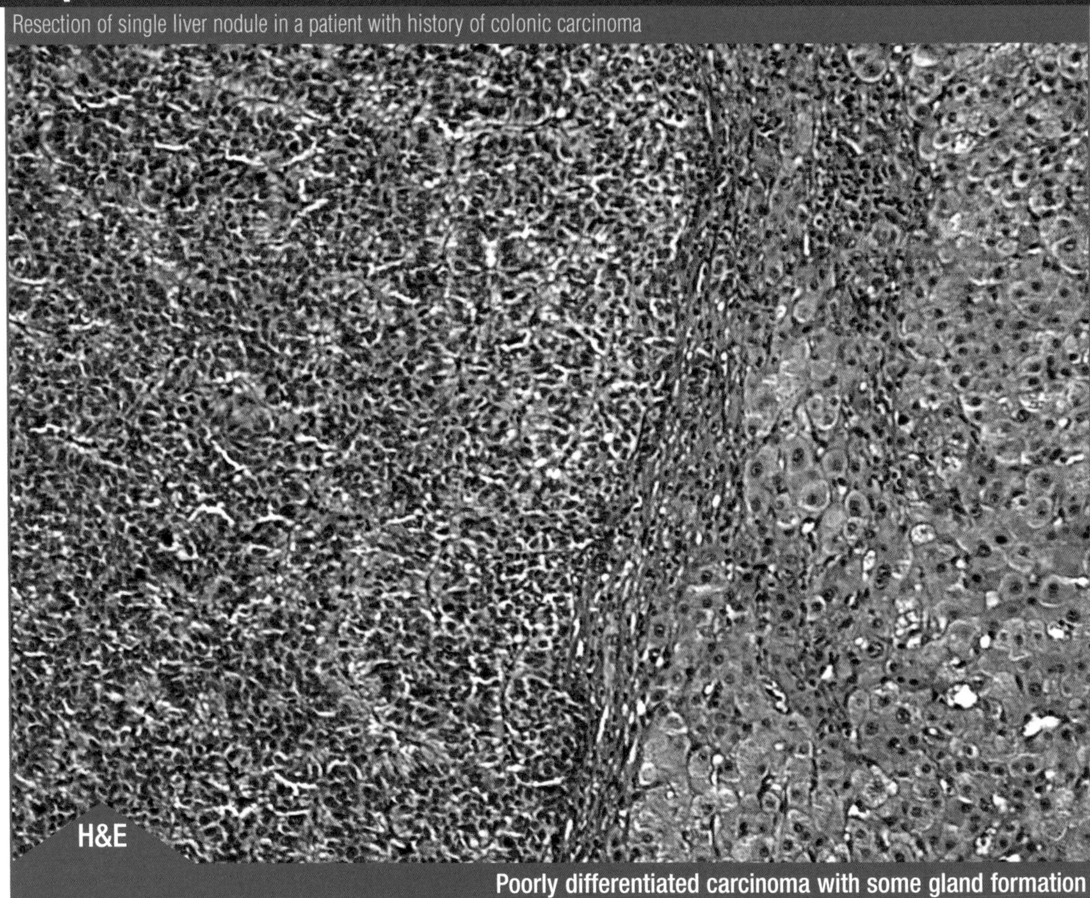

Poorly differentiated carcinoma with some gland formation

Hepatocellular Carcinoma vs Metastatic Colonic Adenocarcinoma		
	Cytokeratin 20 (CK20)	Hepatocellular Antigen (HCA)
Hepatocellular Carcinoma	–	+
Metastatic Colonic Carcinoma	+	–

Helpful Hints

Most metastatic colonic carcinomas could be distinguished from hepatocellular carcinomas by histomorphology alone. Occasionally less differentiated colonic carcinomas may create a diagnostic problem. **CK20** is expressed by the majority of colonic carcinomas regardless of their degree of differentiation. Hepatocellular carcinomas are always negative for CK20. On the other hand, **HCA** is practically never present in colonic adenocarcinomas.

Duval 2000, Lau 2002.

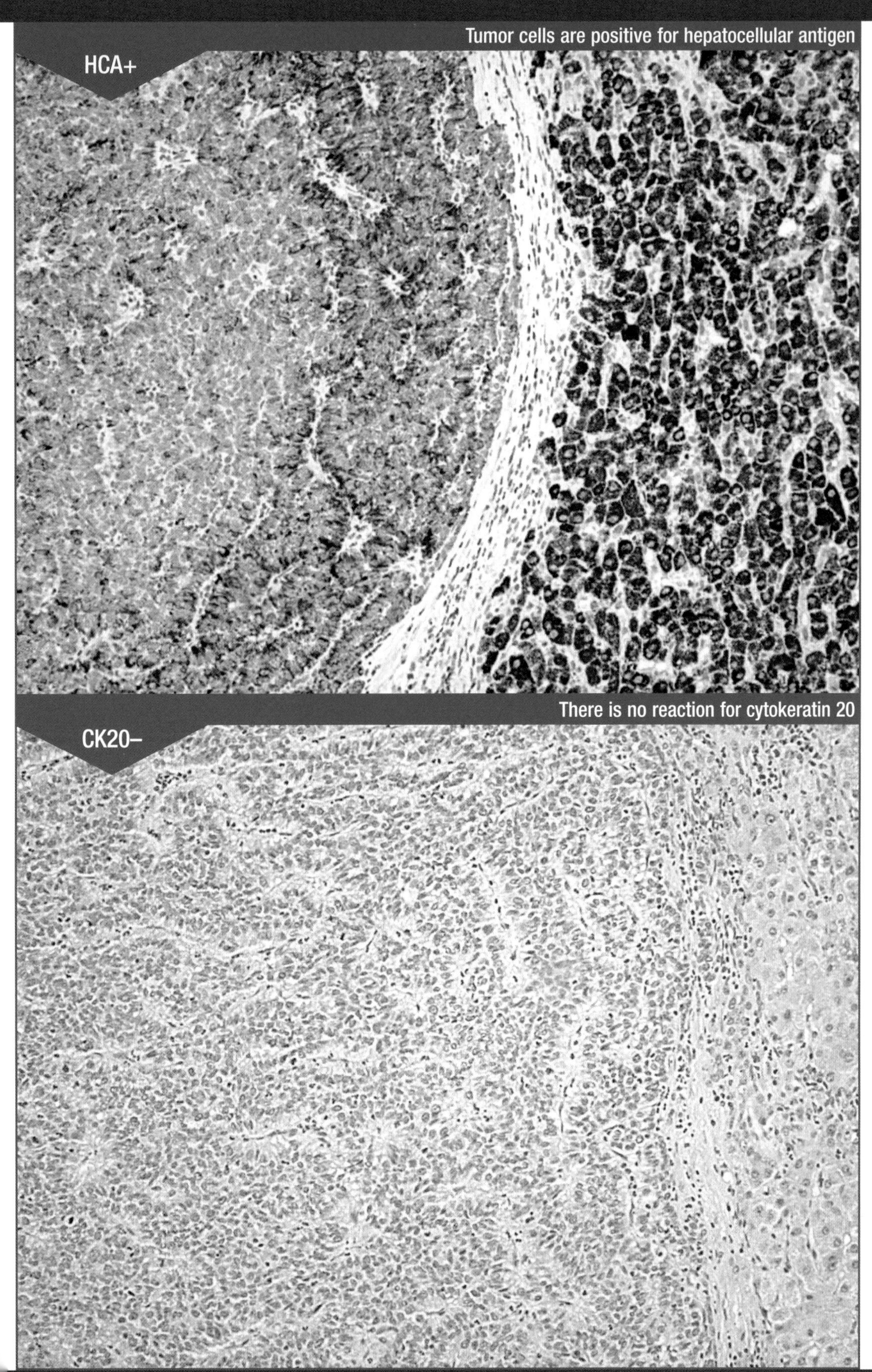

Diagnosis: Hepatocellular Carcinoma; Poorly Differentiated

Segmental resection of liver

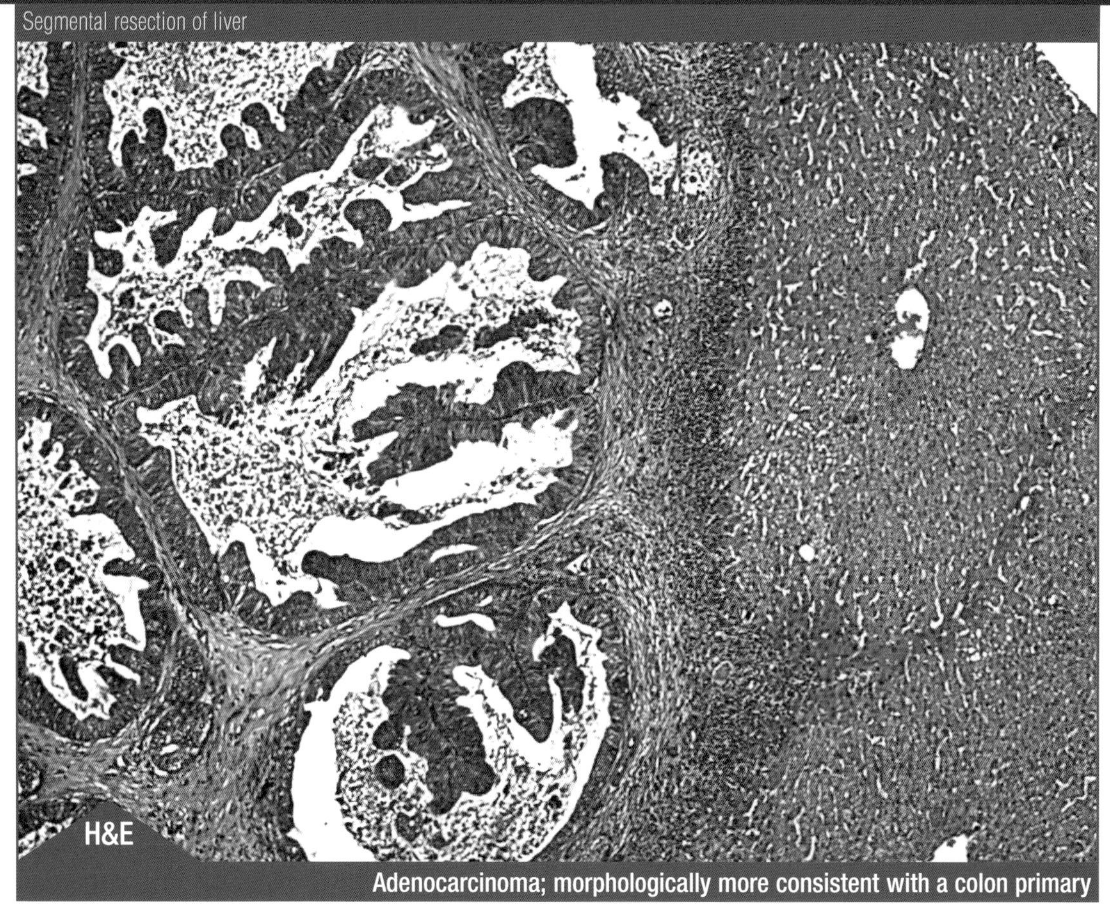

Adenocarcinoma; morphologically more consistent with a colon primary

Cholangiocarcinoma vs Metastatic Colonic Adenocarcinoma		
	Cytokeratin 7 (CK7)	Cytokeratin 20 (CK20)
Cholangiocarcinoma	+	–
Metastatic Colonic Adeno Ca	–	+

Helpful Hints

A combination of **CK7** and **CK20** will separate most cholangiocarcinomas from metastatic colonic carcinomas in liver. It should be noted that occasionally few CK20-positive cells may be seen in cholangiocarcinomas, but the overwhelming cellular reactivity is for CK7.

CDX-2 also suggested to be used in this situation but this marker is not totally specific for colon cancer as it is expressed by a number of other adenocarcinomas.

Li 2004.

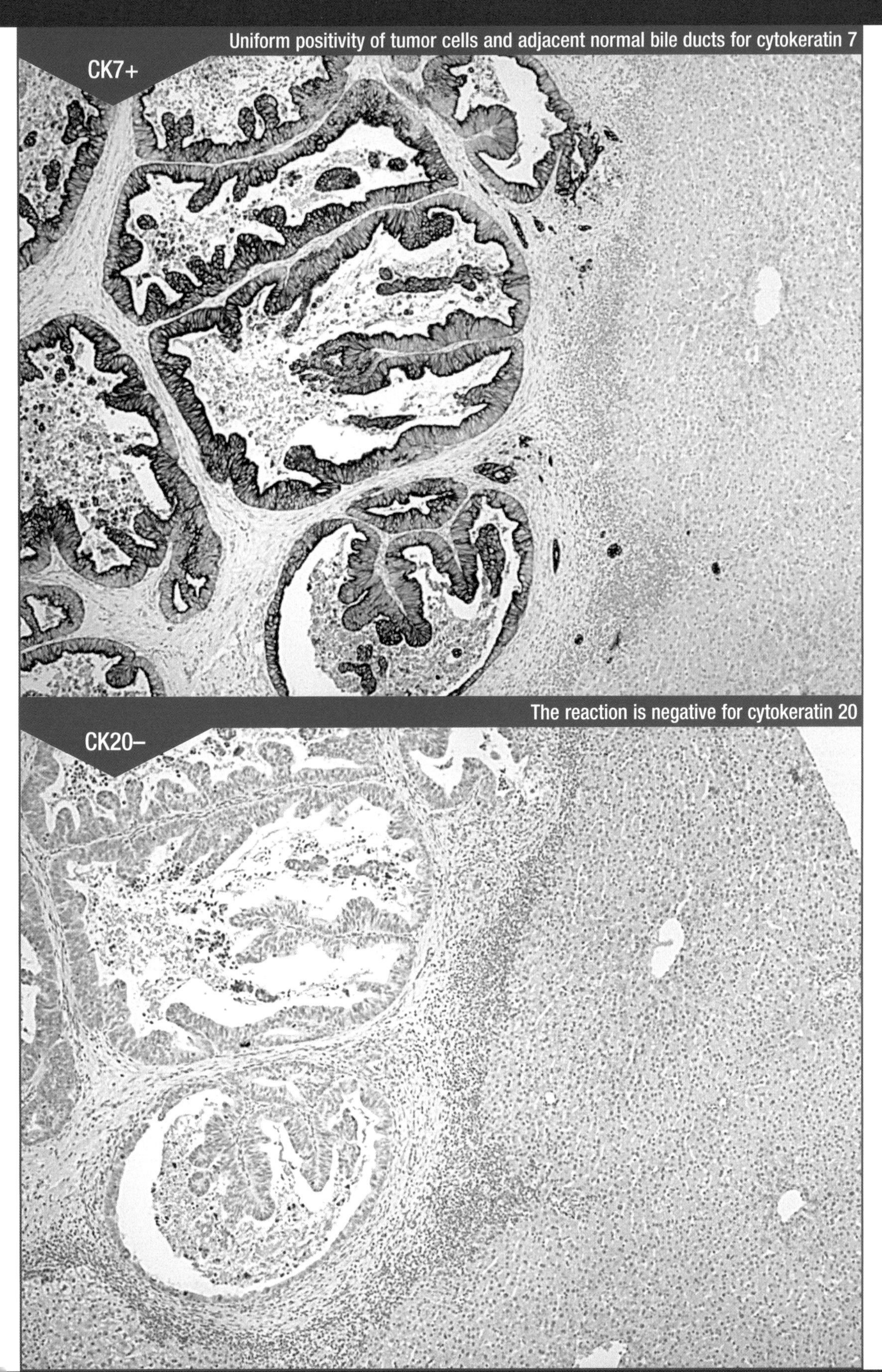

agnosis: Cholangiocarcinoma *(no evidence of a primary elsewhere)*

Core biopsy of a solitary nodule in liver; patient had a renal mass by x-ray

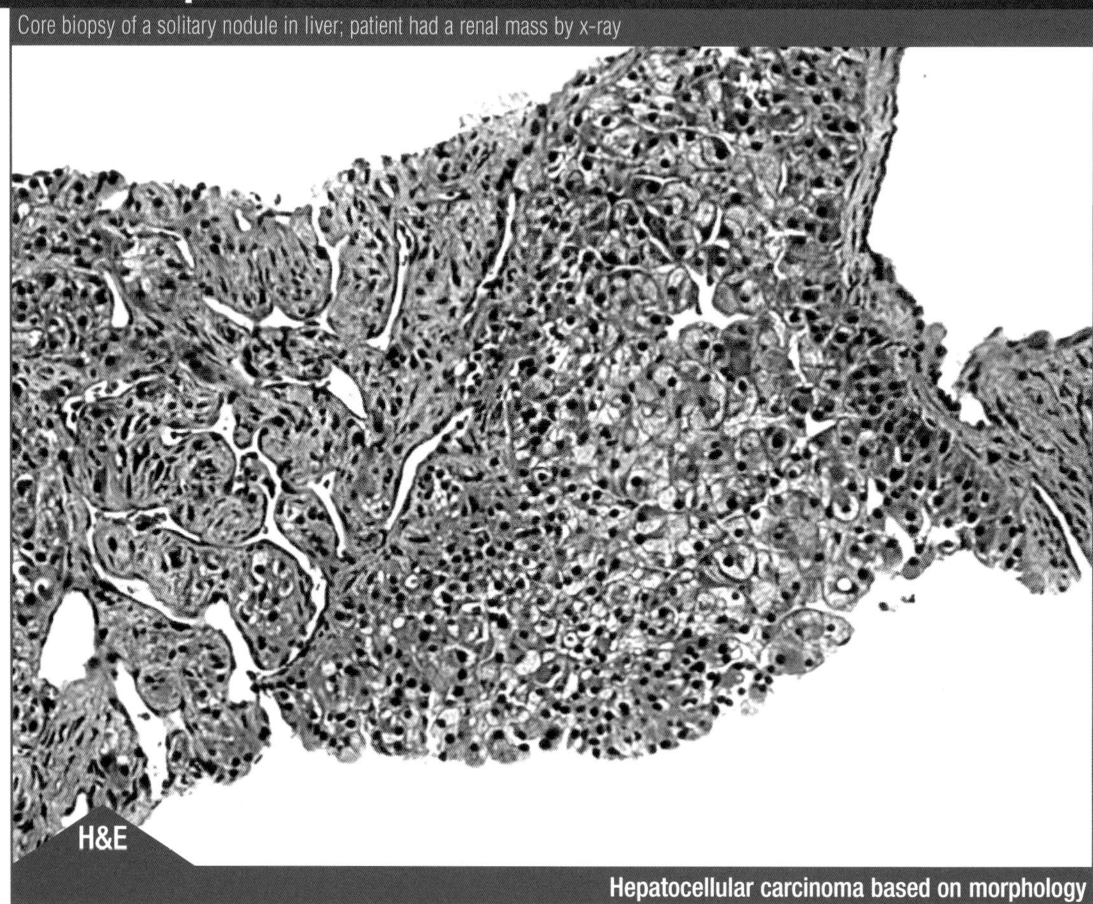

Hepatocellular carcinoma based on morphology

Hepatocellular Carcinoma vs Renal Cell Carcinoma			
	HCA	RCA	EMA
Hepatocellular Ca	+	–	–
Renal Cell Ca	–	+	+

Helpful Hints

Renal cell carcinoma antigen (**RCC or RCA**) is normally found in renal proximal tubules and the majority of clear cell renal cell carcinomas. The expression of RCA is less common by chromophobe subtypes. Sarcomatoid renal cell carcinomas practically never react for RCA.

EMA may also be useful for the above differential diagnosis because it is expressed by most renal cell carcinomas but rarely by hepatocellular neoplasms. RCA is not completely specific for renal cell carcinomas; other tumors, such as yolk sac carcinomas may also express this marker.

Mulders 2003.

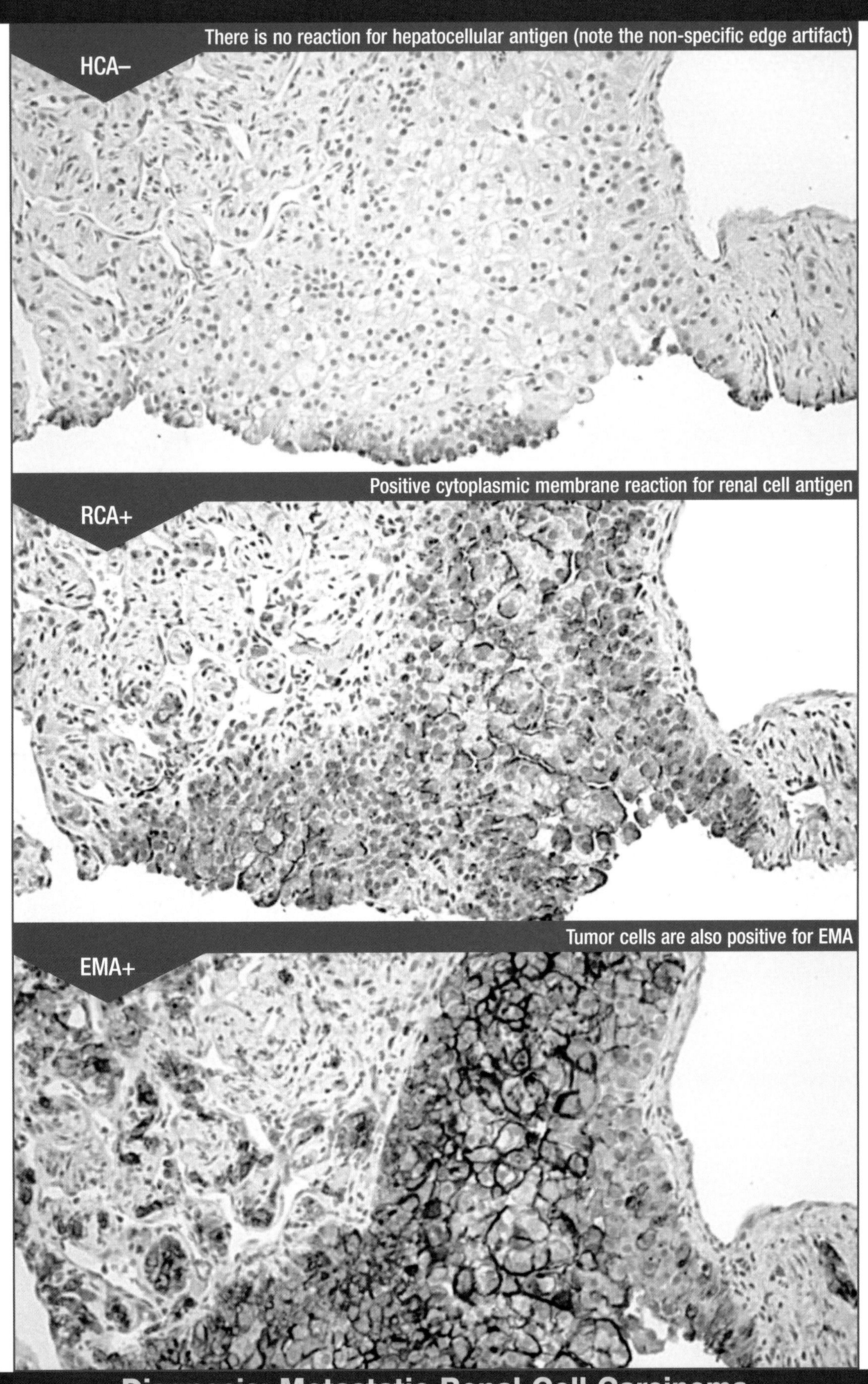

Diagnosis: Metastatic Renal Cell Carcinoma

Core biopsy of a solitary nodule in the liver

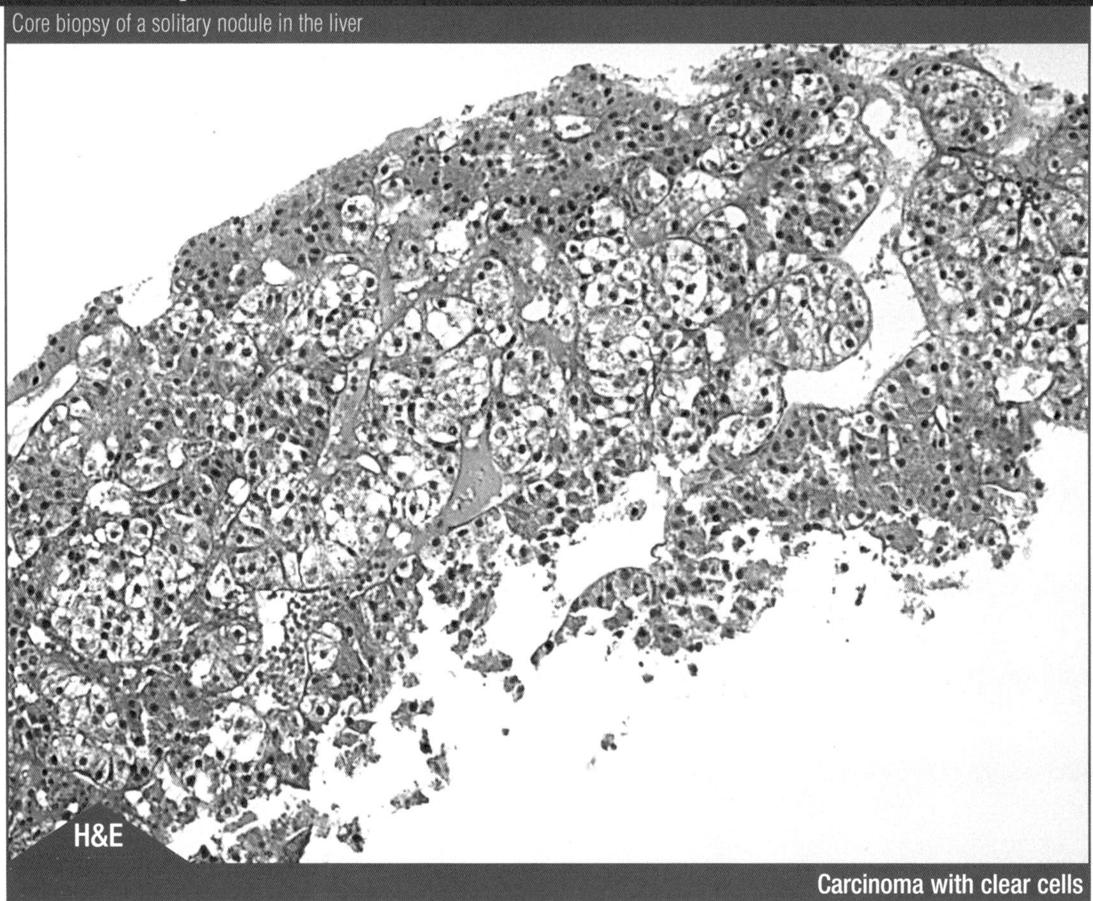

Carcinoma with clear cells

Hepatocellular Carcinoma vs Renal Cell Carcinoma	HCA	RCA	EMA
Hepatocellular Ca	+	–	–
Renal Cell Ca	–	+	+

Helpful Hints

Renal cell carcinoma antigen (**RCC or RCA**) is normally found in renal proximal tubules and the majority of clear cell renal cell carcinomas. The expression of RCA is less common by chromophobe subtypes. Sarcomatoid renal cell carcinomas practically never react for RCA.

EMA may also be useful for the above differential diagnosis because it is expressed by most renal cell carcinomas but rarely by hepatocellular neoplasms. RCA is not completely specific for renal cell carcinomas; other tumors, such as yolk sac carcinomas may also express this marker.

Mulders 2003.

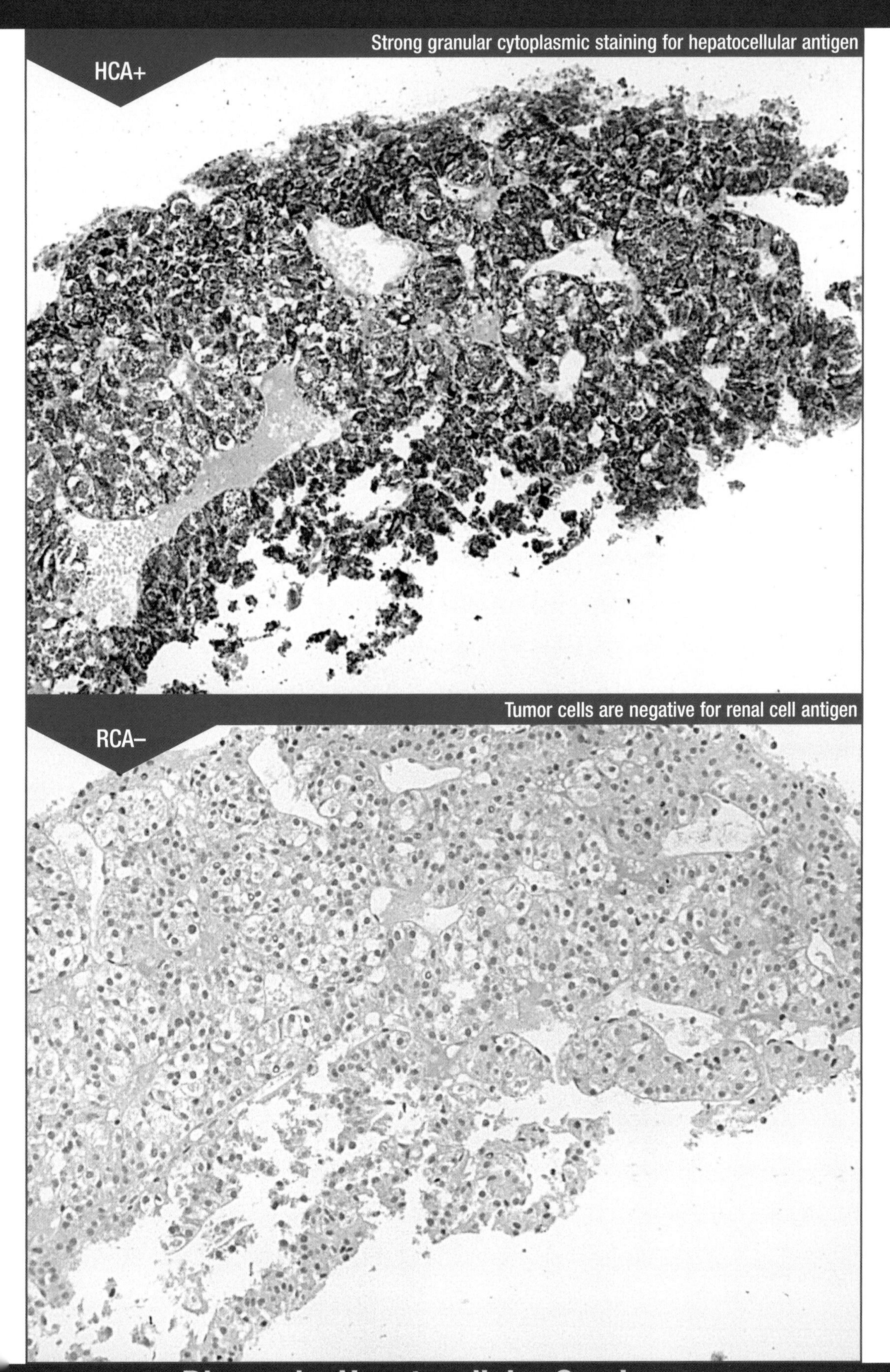

Diagnosis: Hepatocellular Carcinoma

Abdominal tumor in the region of adrenal gland

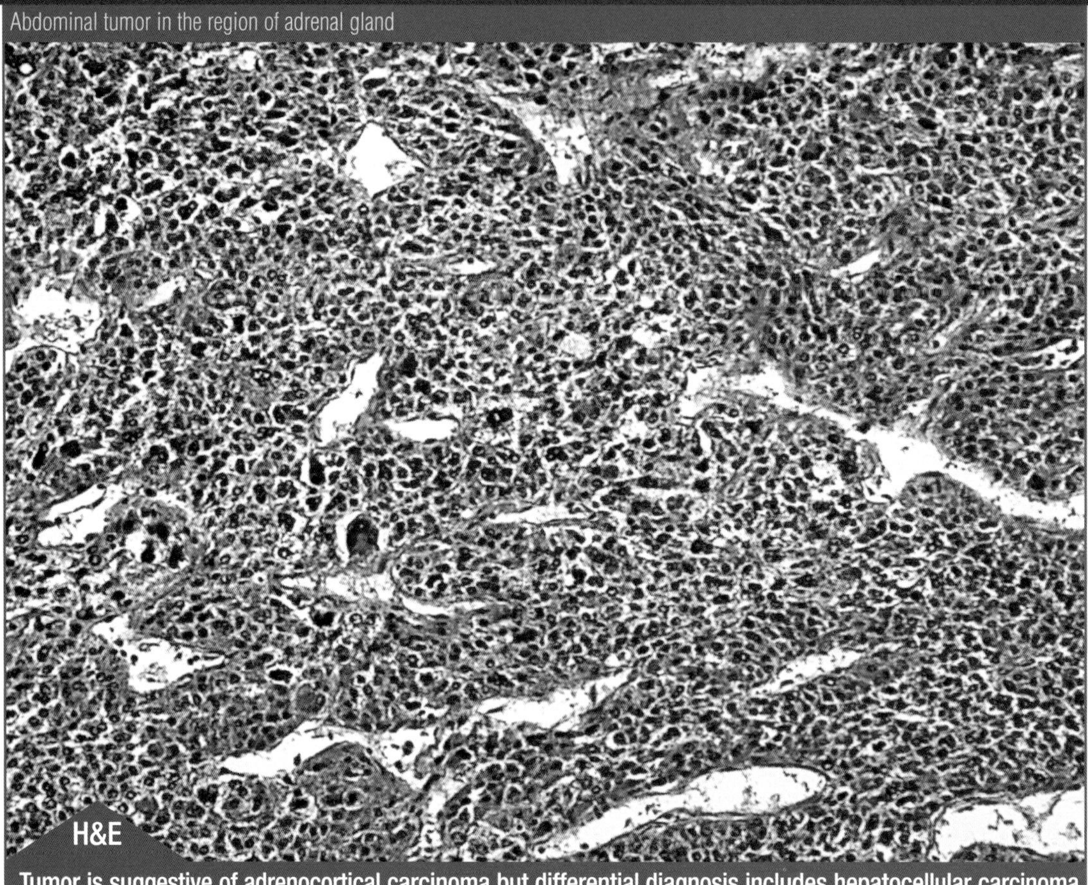

Tumor is suggestive of adrenocortical carcinoma but differential diagnosis includes hepatocellular carcinoma

Hepatocellular Carcinoma vs Adrenocortical Carcinoma		
	Hepatocellular Antigen (HCA)	Inhibin
Hepatocellular Carcinoma	+	–
Adrenocortical Carcinoma	–	+

Helpful Hints

Inhibin: Alpha inhibin is a marker for steroid producing cells including those in adrenal cortex and ovary. Most adrenocortical tumors, whether benign or malignant, at least focally express inhibin whereas adrenal medulla and pheochromocytomas are usually negative. Other inhibin-positive tumors include ovarian sex cord stromal neoplasms and steroid cell tumor. Inhibin is not present in hepatocellular carcinomas. Adrenocortical tumors and hepatocellular carcinomas share some morphologic features and hence, immunohistochemistry is needed for their correct classification.

Jorda 2002.

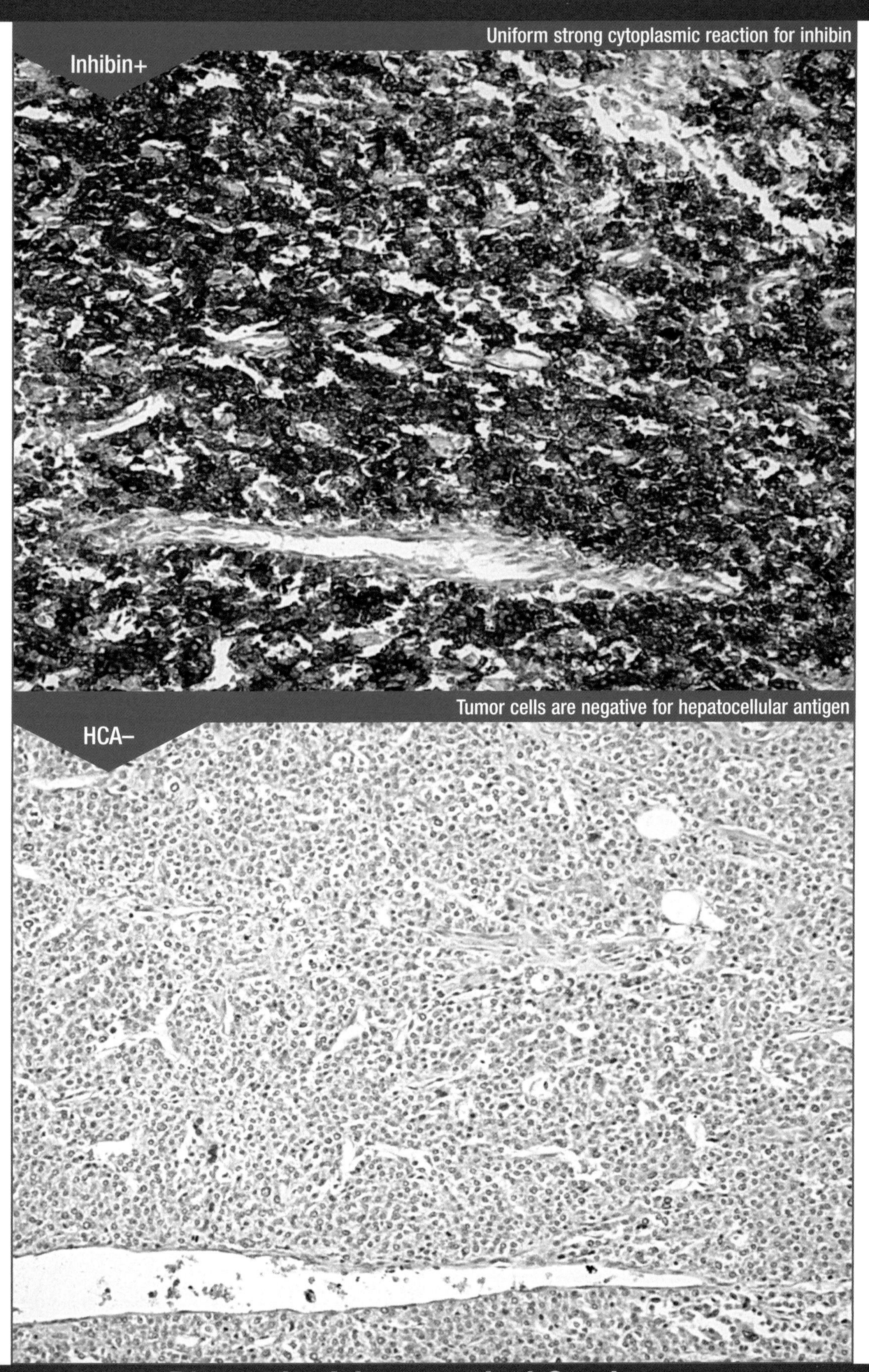

Diagnosis: Adrenocortical Carcinoma

Core biopsy of liver

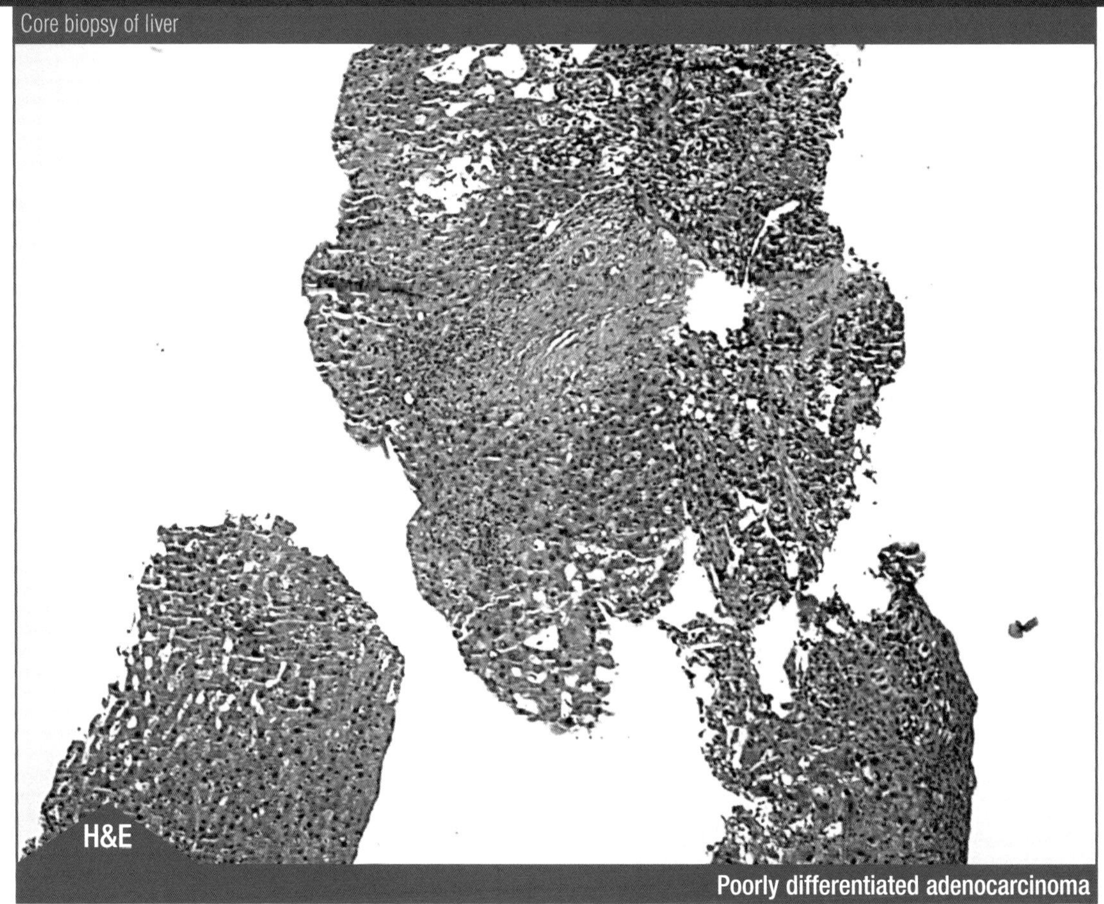

Poorly differentiated adenocarcinoma

Helpful Hints

Depending on the clinical history, histomorphology and availability of specific markers the site of origin of a number of metastatic tumors in the liver can be determined by using two or three antibodies. Here are some examples.

1. Metastatic adenocarcinoma of lung	TTF-1
2. Metastatic small cell carcinoma of lung	TTF-1
3. Metastatic neuroendocrine carcinoma	Chromogranin (Chrg) Synaptophysin (SP)
4. Metastatic prostatic carcinoma	PSA
5. Metastatic gastrointestinal stromal tumor	KIT
6. Metastatic malignant melanoma	S100, HMB-45

Positive nuclear reaction for TTF-1

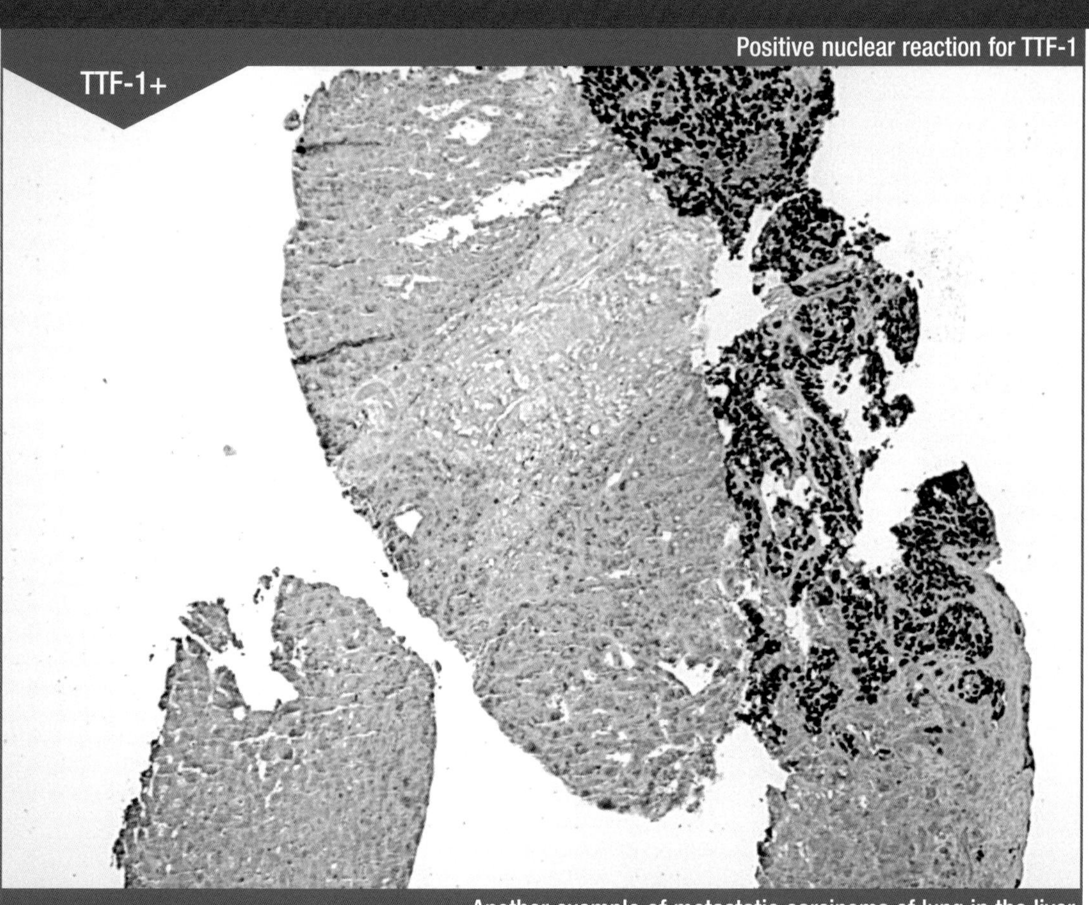

Another example of metastatic carcinoma of lung in the liver

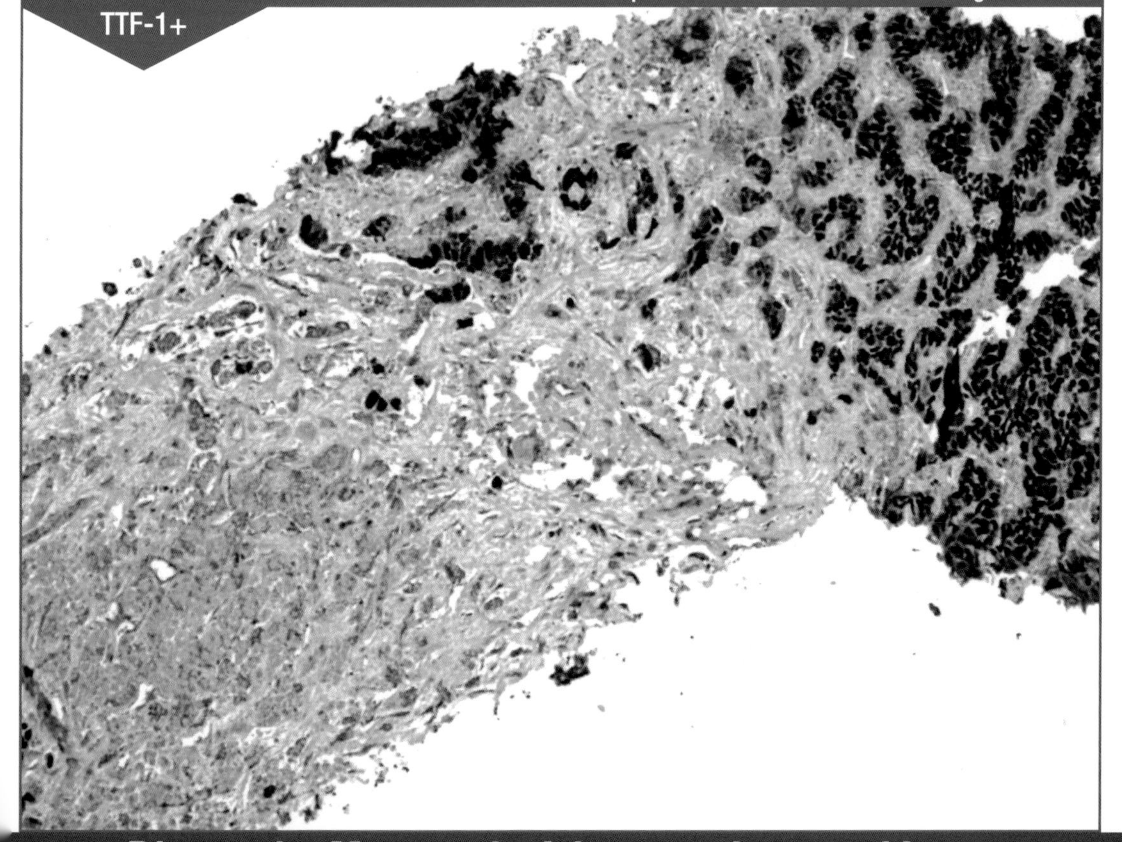

Diagnosis: Metastatic Adenocarcinoma of Lung

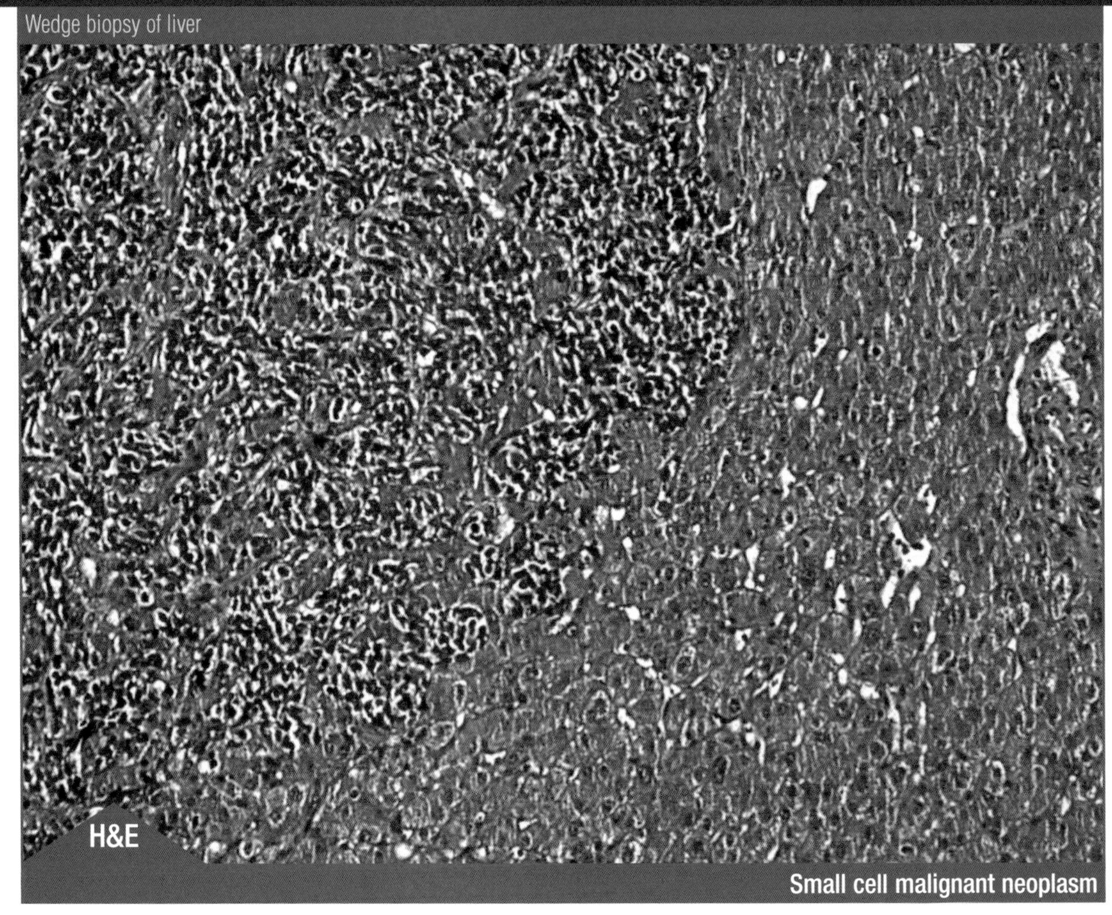

Small cell malignant neoplasm

Helpful Hints

Depending on the clinical history, histomorphology and availability of specific markers the site of origin of a number of metastatic tumors in the liver can be determined by using two or three antibodies. Here are some examples.

1. Metastatic adenocarcinoma of lung	TTF-1
2. Metastatic small cell carcinoma of lung	TTF-1
3. Metastatic neuroendocrine carcinoma	Chromogranin (Chrg) Synaptophysin (SP)
4. Metastatic prostatic carcinoma	PSA
5. Metastatic gastrointestinal stromal tumor	KIT
6. Metastatic malignant melanoma	S100, HMB-45

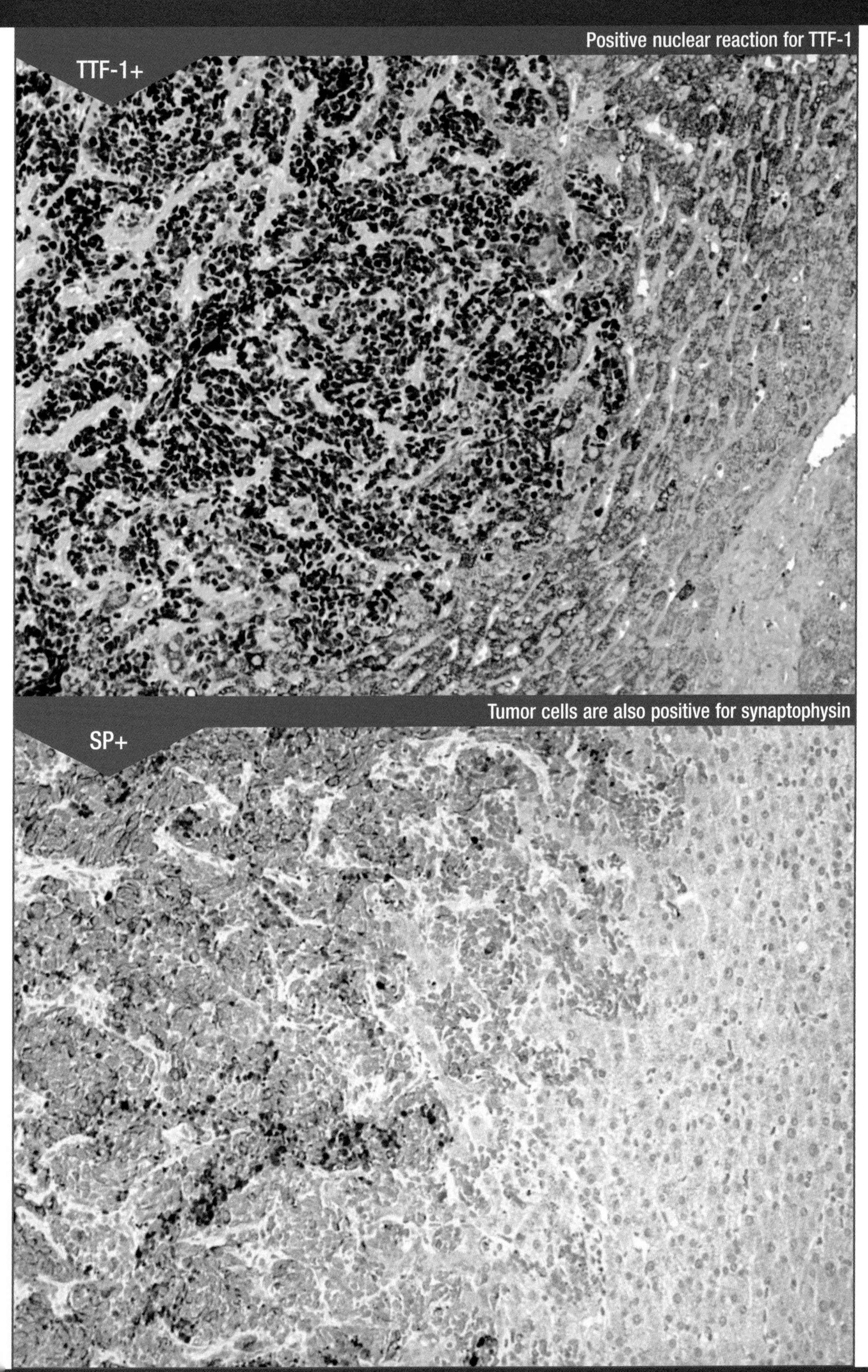

Diagnosis: Metastatic Small Cell Carcinoma of Lung

Core biopsy of liver

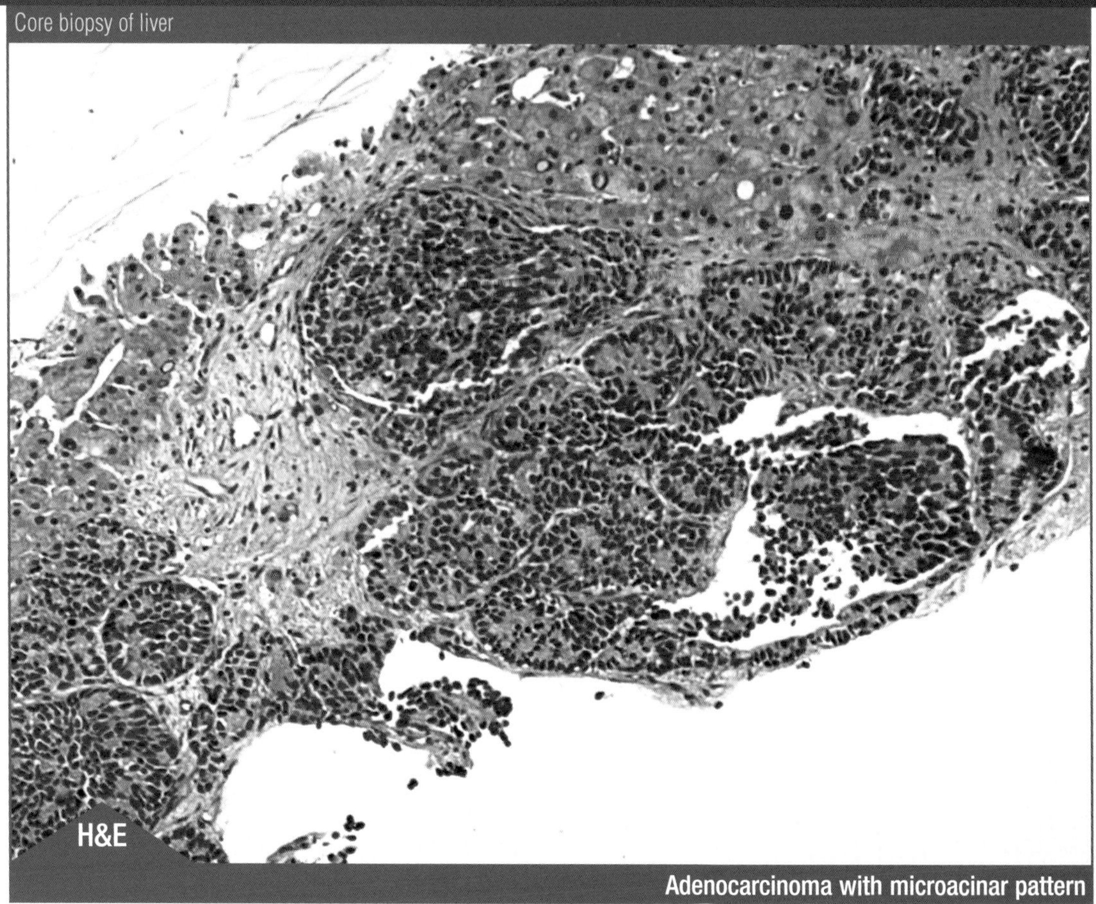

Adenocarcinoma with microacinar pattern

Helpful Hints

Depending on the clinical history, histomorphology and availability of specific markers the site of origin of a number of metastatic tumors in the liver can be determined by using two or three antibodies. Here are some examples.

1. Metastatic adenocarcinoma of lung	TTF-1
2. Metastatic small cell carcinoma of lung	TTF-1
3. Metastatic neuroendocrine carcinoma	Chromogranin (Chrg) Synaptophysin (SP)
4. Metastatic prostatic carcinoma	PSA
5. Metastatic gastrointestinal stromal tumor	KIT
6. Metastatic malignant melanoma	S100, HMB-45

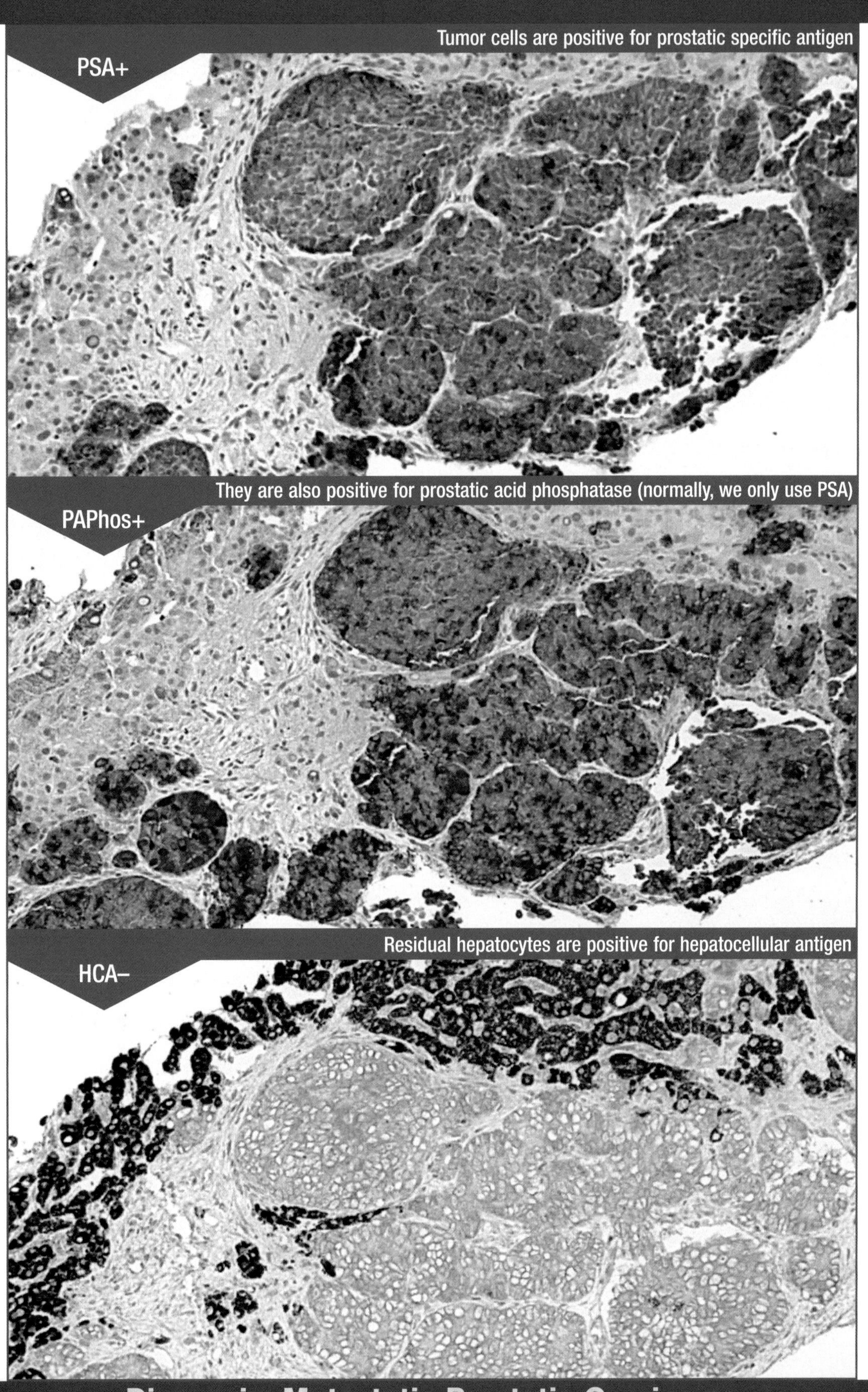

Diagnosis: Metastatic Prostatic Carcinoma

Core biopsy of liver

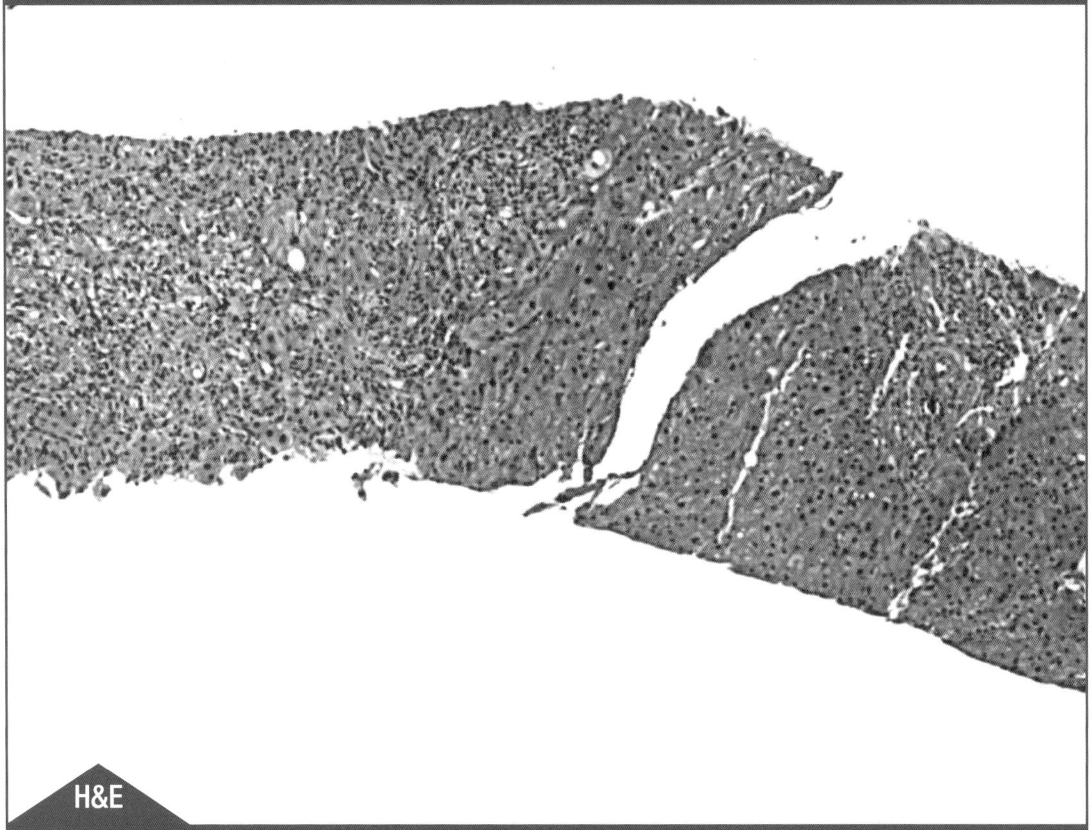

H&E

Poorly differentiated tumor with spindle cells

Helpful Hints

Depending on the clinical history, histomorphology and availability of specific markers the site of origin of a number of metastatic tumors in the liver can be determined by using two or three antibodies. Here are some examples.

1. Metastatic adenocarcinoma of lung	TTF-1
2. Metastatic small cell carcinoma of lung	TTF-1
3. Metastatic neuroendocrine carcinoma	Chromogranin (Chrg) Synaptophysin (SP)
4. Metastatic prostatic carcinoma	PSA
5. Metastatic gastrointestinal stromal tumor	KIT
6. Metastatic malignant melanoma	S100, HMB-45

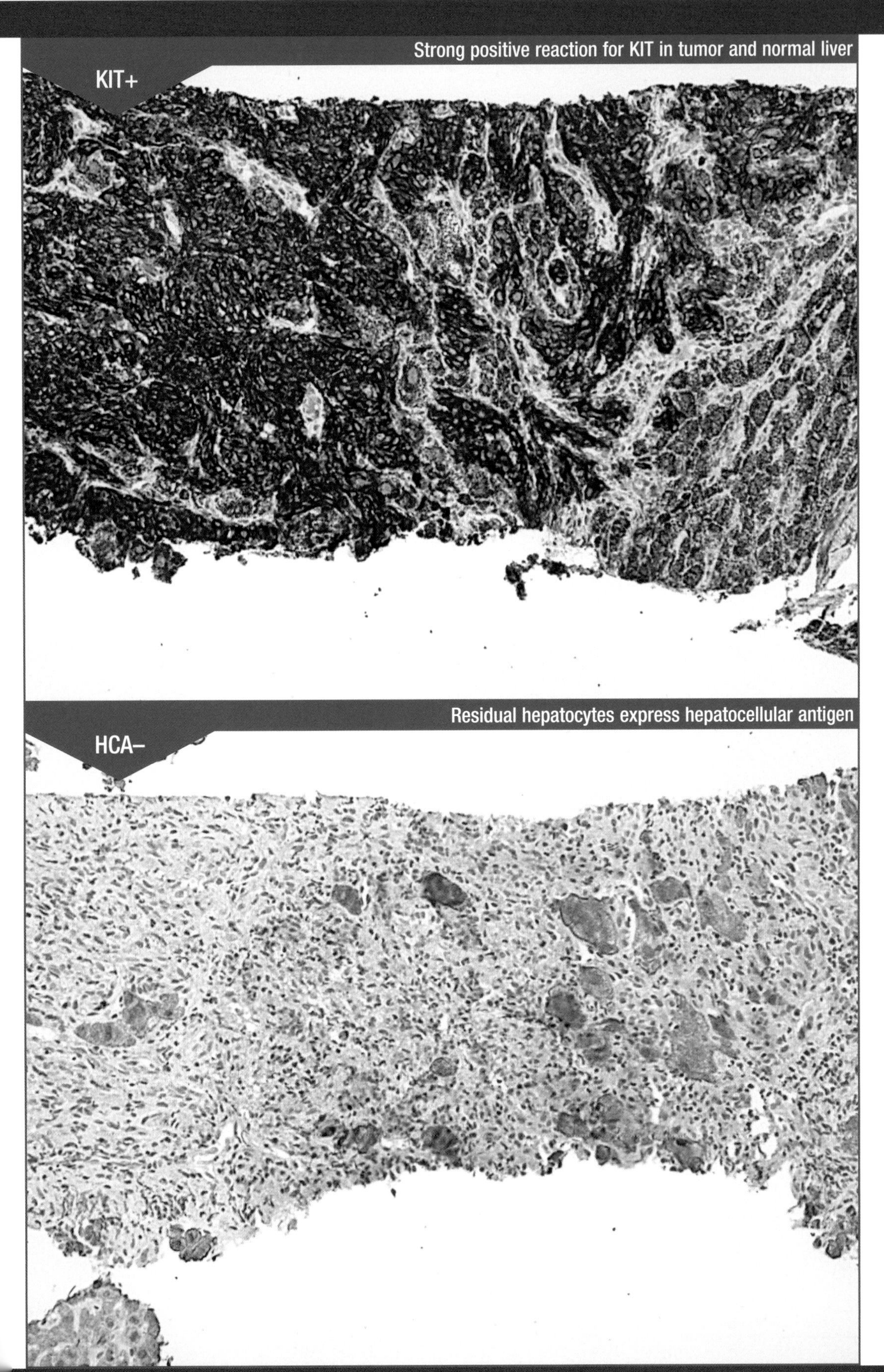

Strong positive reaction for KIT in tumor and normal liver

Residual hepatocytes express hepatocellular antigen

Diagnosis: Metastatic Gastrointestinal Stromal Tumor

Liver core biopsy in patient with history of malignant melanoma

H&E

Morphologically this tumor resembles hepatocellular carcinoma

Helpful Hints

Depending on the clinical history, histomorphology and availability of specific markers the site of origin of a number of metastatic tumors in the liver can be determined by using two or three antibodies. Here are some examples.

1. Metastatic adenocarcinoma of lung	TTF-1
2. Metastatic small cell carcinoma of lung	TTF-1
3. Metastatic neuroendocrine carcinoma	Chromogranin (Chrg) Synaptophysin (SP)
4. Metastatic prostatic carcinoma	PSA
5. Metastatic gastrointestinal stromal tumor	KIT
6. Metastatic malignant melanoma	S100, HMB-45

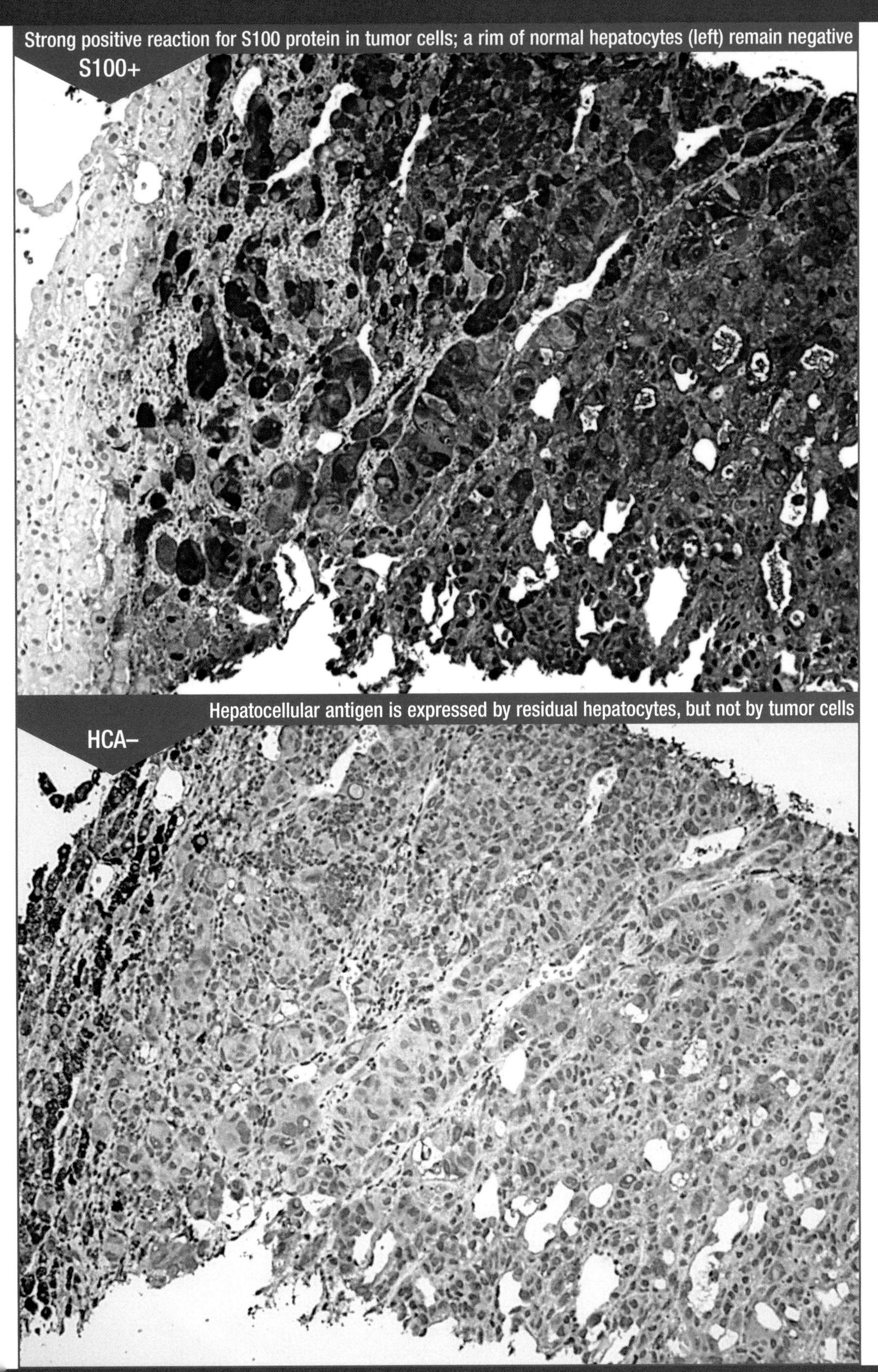

Diagnosis: Metastatic Malignant Melanoma

Bone biopsy in a patient with clinical evidence of a renal mass

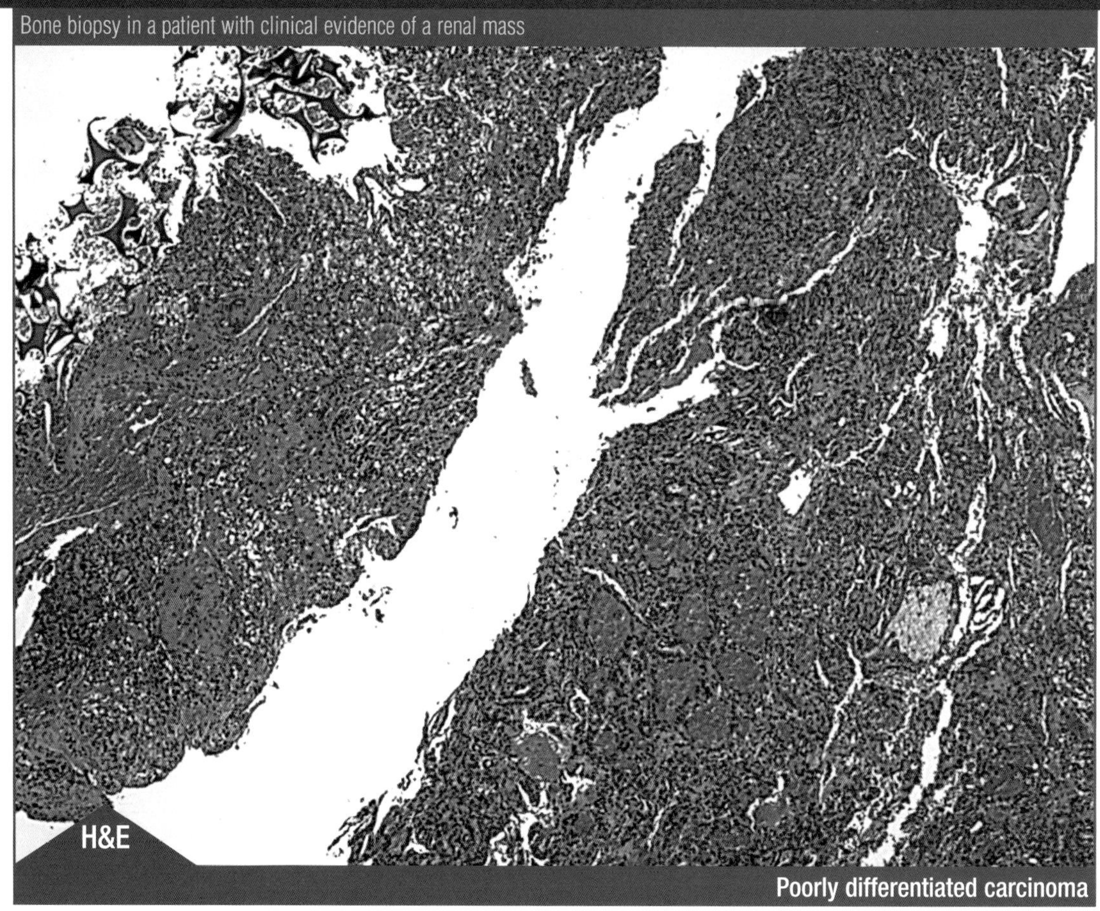

Poorly differentiated carcinoma

Renal Cell Carcinoma vs Urothelial Carcinoma			
	RCA	CEA	P63
Renal Cell Carcinoma	+	–	–
Urothelial Carcinoma	–	+	+

Helpful Hints

In some instances urothelial carcinomas of the renal pelvis may be difficult to differentiate from high-grade renal cell carcinomas, particularly in small biopsies. **RCA** is usually present in renal cell carcinomas but these tumors are always negative for **CEA**. Transitional cell carcinomas on the other hand do not express RCA but are usually positive for CEA, particularly when a polyclonal anti-CEA antibody is used. Most transitional cell carcinomas also express **P63**. This marker is not found in renal cell carcinomas. Other purported urothelial markers such as uroplakin and CK20 are less helpful.

Sim 1999.

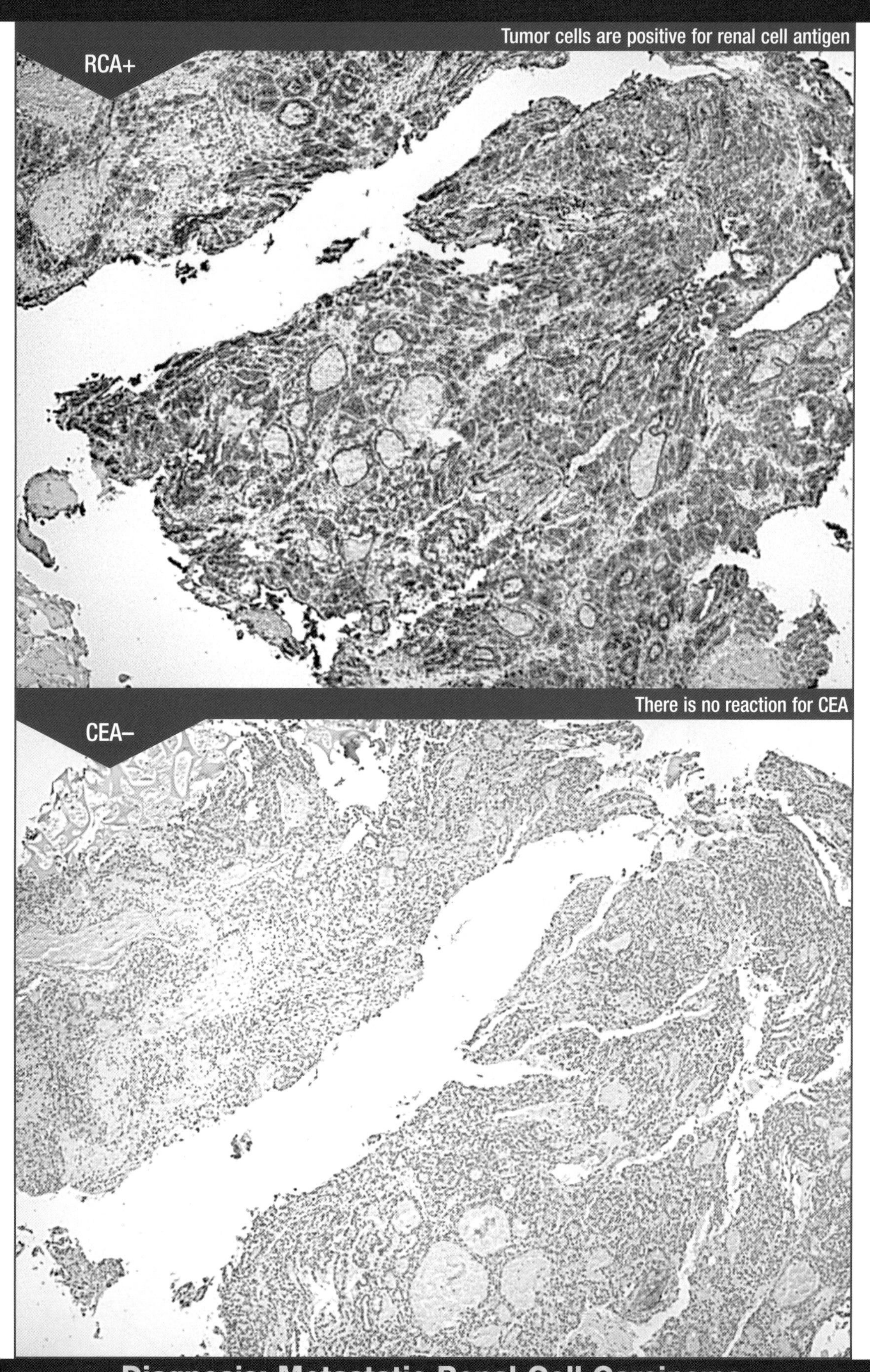

Diagnosis: Metastatic Renal Cell Carcinoma

Core biopsy of the kidney

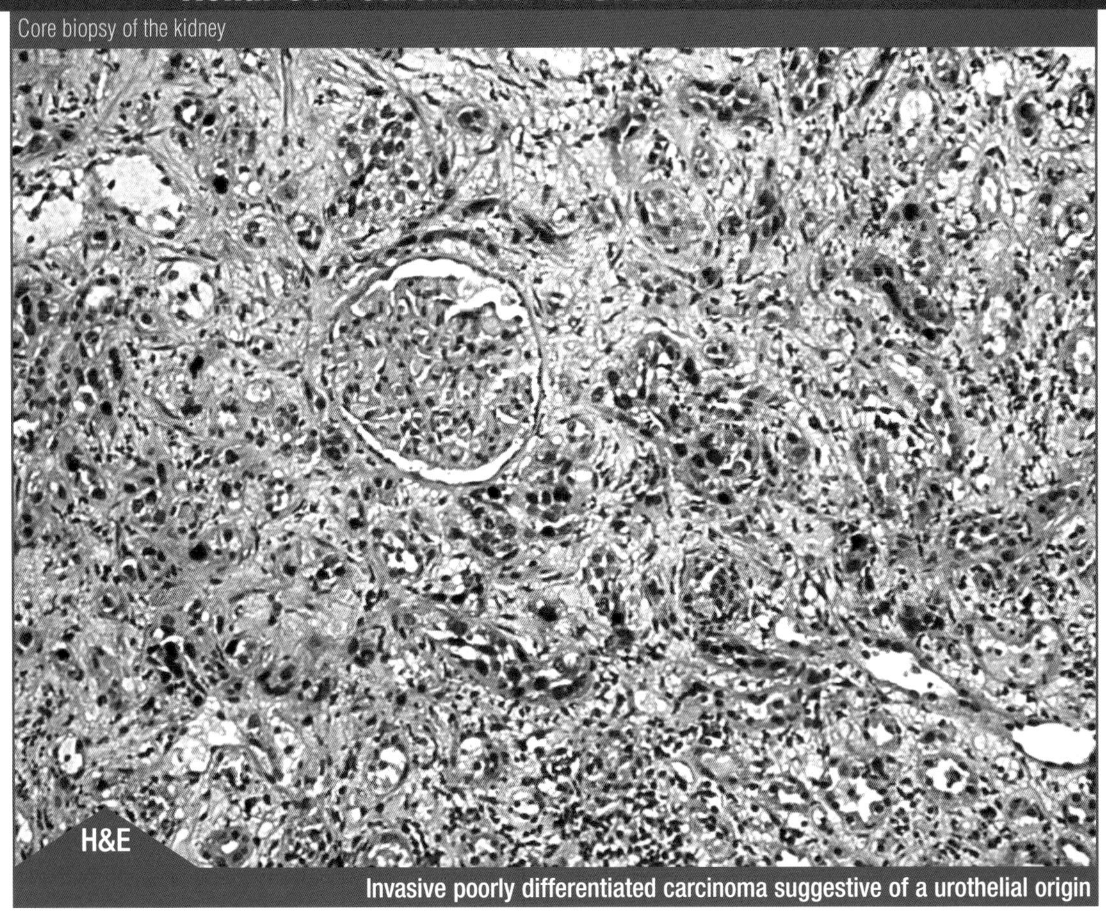

Invasive poorly differentiated carcinoma suggestive of a urothelial origin

Renal Cell Carcinoma vs Urothelial Carcinoma			
	RCA	CEA	P63
Renal Cell Carcinoma	+	–	–
Urothelial Carcinoma	–	+	+

Helpful Hints

In some instances urothelial carcinomas of the renal pelvis may be difficult to differentiate from high-grade renal cell carcinomas, particularly in small biopsies. **RCA** is usually present in renal cell carcinomas but these tumors are always negative for **CEA**. Transitional cell carcinomas on the other hand do not express RCA but are usually positive for CEA, particularly when a polyclonal anti-CEA antibody is used. Most transitional cell carcinomas also express **P63**. This marker is not found in renal cell carcinomas. Other purported urothelial markers such as uroplakin and CK20 are less helpful.

Sim 1999.

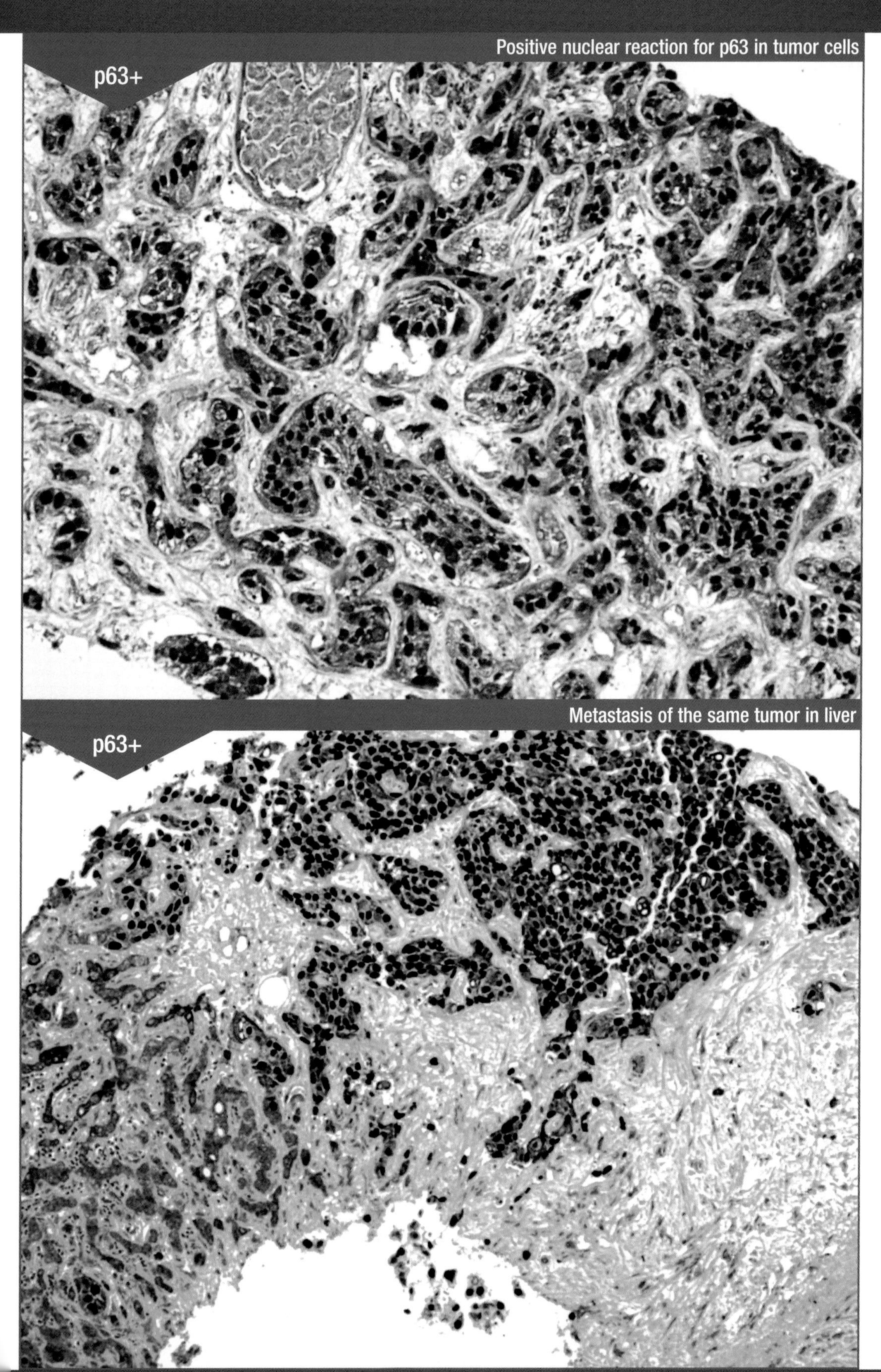

Diagnosis: Urothelial Carcinoma

Needle biopsies of kidney in a patient with renal and lung nodules

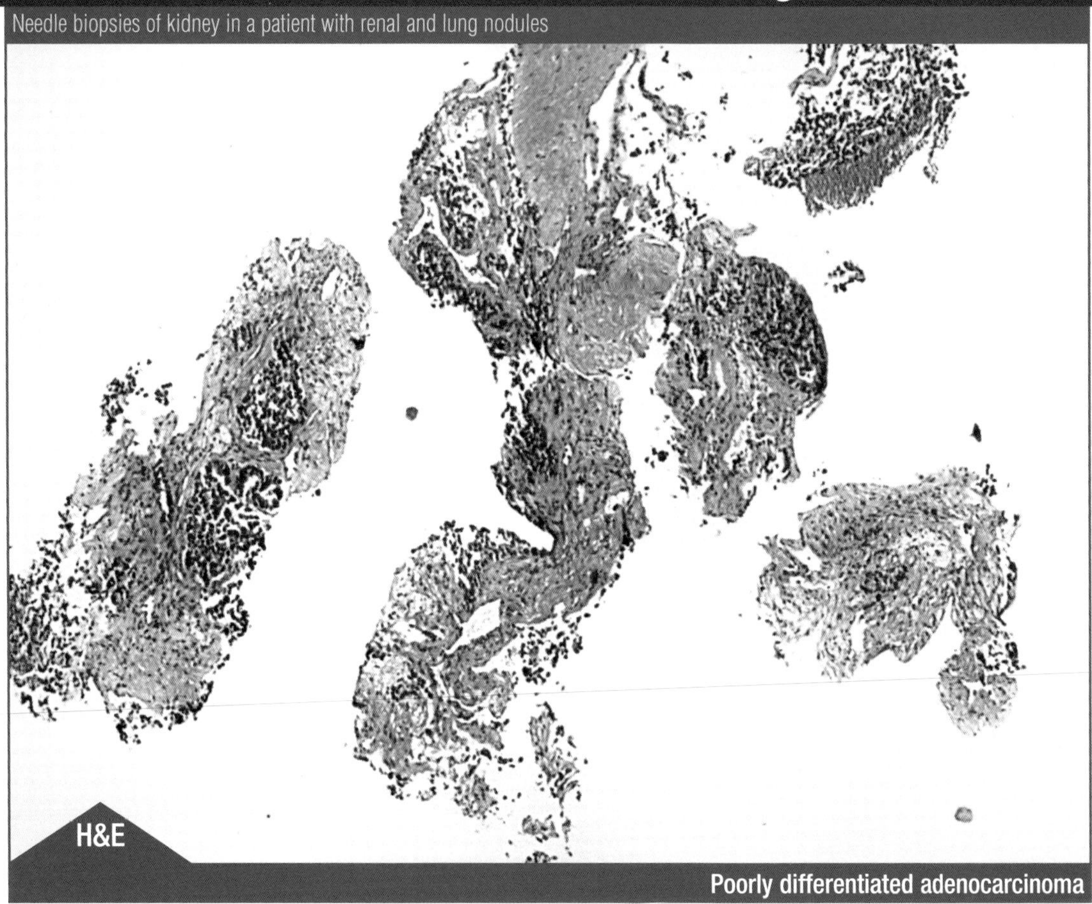

Poorly differentiated adenocarcinoma

Renal Cell Carcinoma vs Metastatic Lung Carcinoma			
	RCA	CEA	TTF-1
Renal Cell Carcinoma	+	–	–
Metastatic Lung Carcinoma	–	+	+

Helpful Hints

Thyroid transcription factor (**TTF-1**) is expressed by normal thyroid and lung. The majority of adenocarcinomas and small cell carcinomas of the lung are positive for TTF-1, while most squamous cell carcinomas are negative.

Most adenocarcinomas of the lung are **CEA** positive whereas renal cell carcinomas are always negative.

Renal cell antigen (**RCA**) is not expressed by carcinomas of the lung.

Lau 2002b.

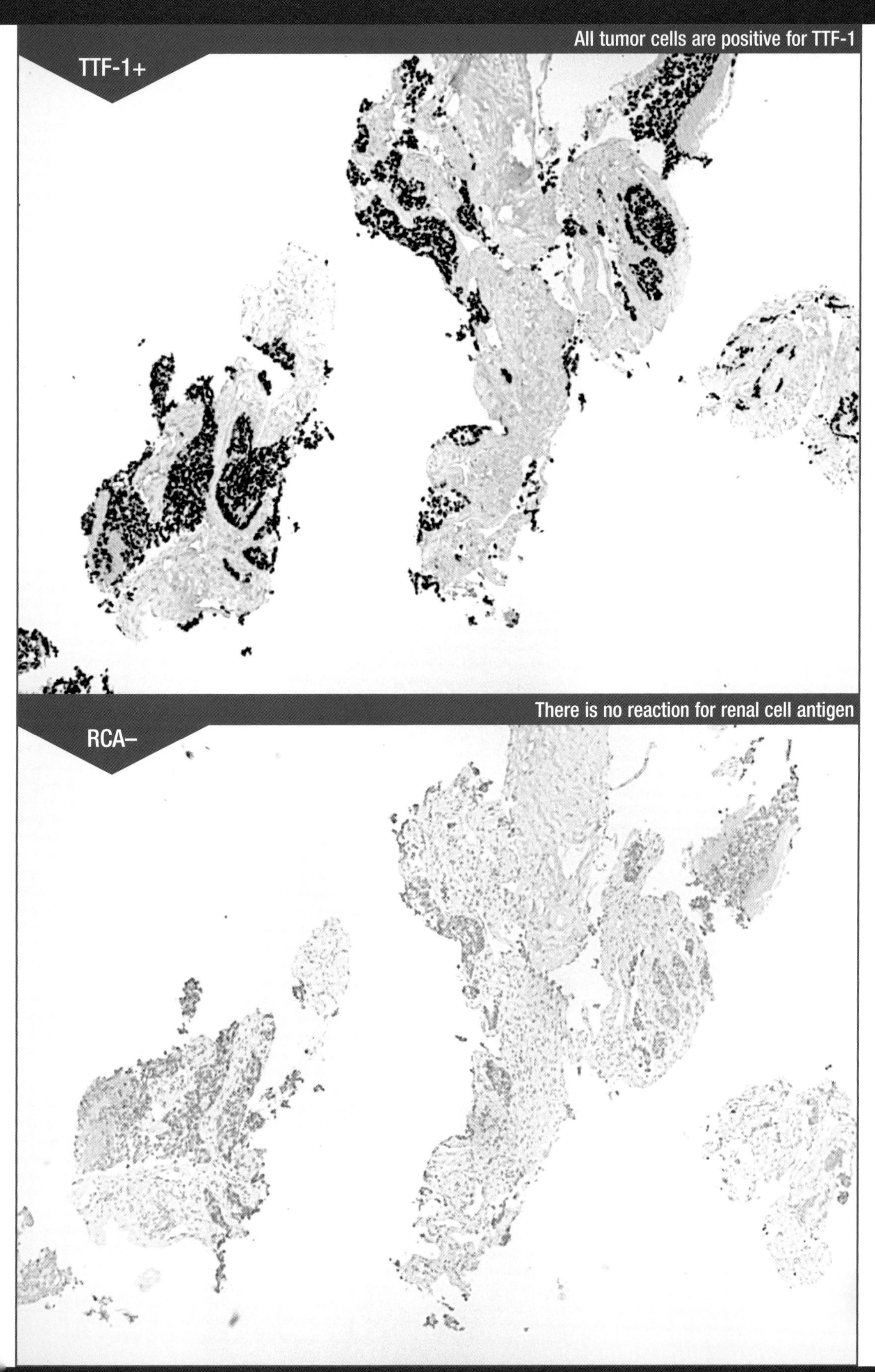

Diagnosis: Metastatic Adenocarcinoma of Lung

Cell block preparation from aspiration of a renal/adrenal mass

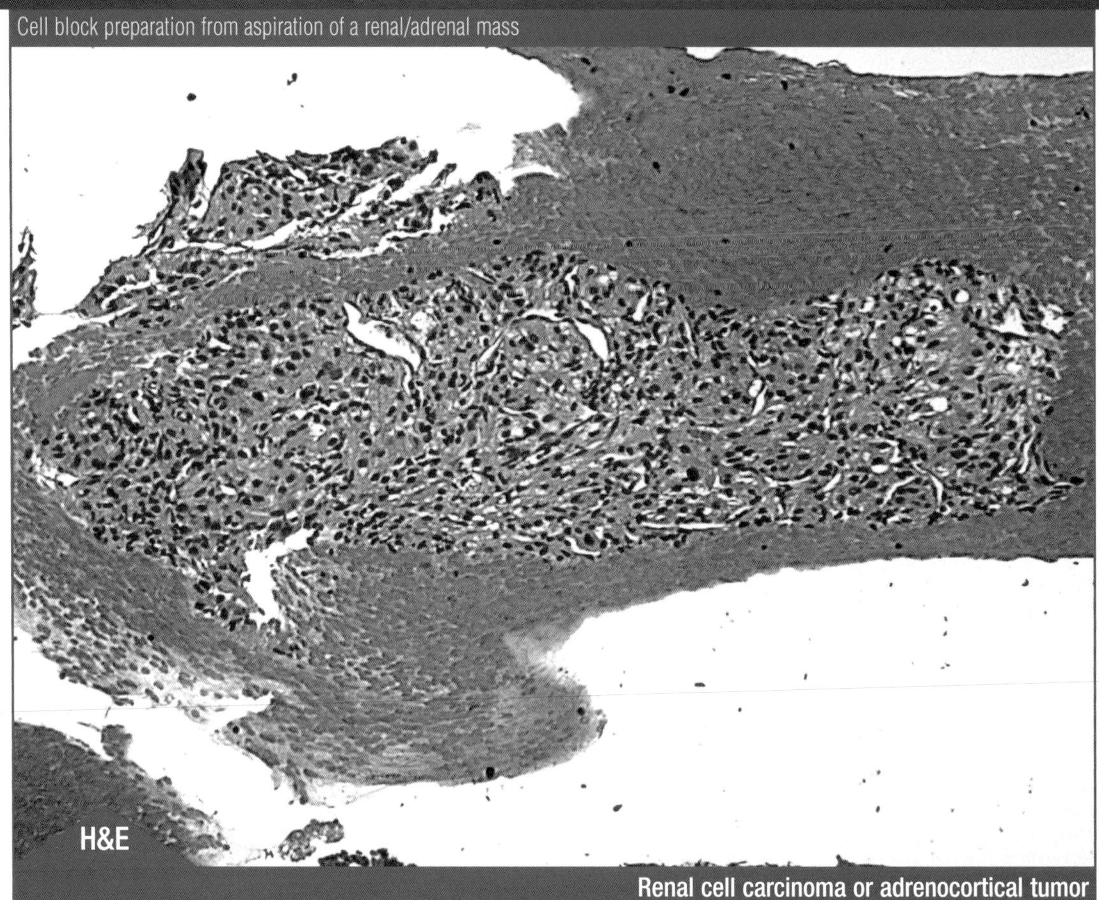

Renal cell carcinoma or adrenocortical tumor

Renal Cell Carcinoma vs Adrenocortical Tumor			
	Cytokeratin (CK)	EMA	Inhibin
Renal Cell Carcinoma	+	+	–
Adrenocortical Tumor	–	–	+

Helpful Hints

This differential diagnosis can usually be solved by demonstration of epithelial markers (**EMA and cytokeratin**) in renal cell carcinomas. Adrenocortical carcinomas do not react positively for EMA although occasional cytokeratin positivity is reported in these tumors. Furthermore, renal cell carcinomas are usually negative for **inhibin**.

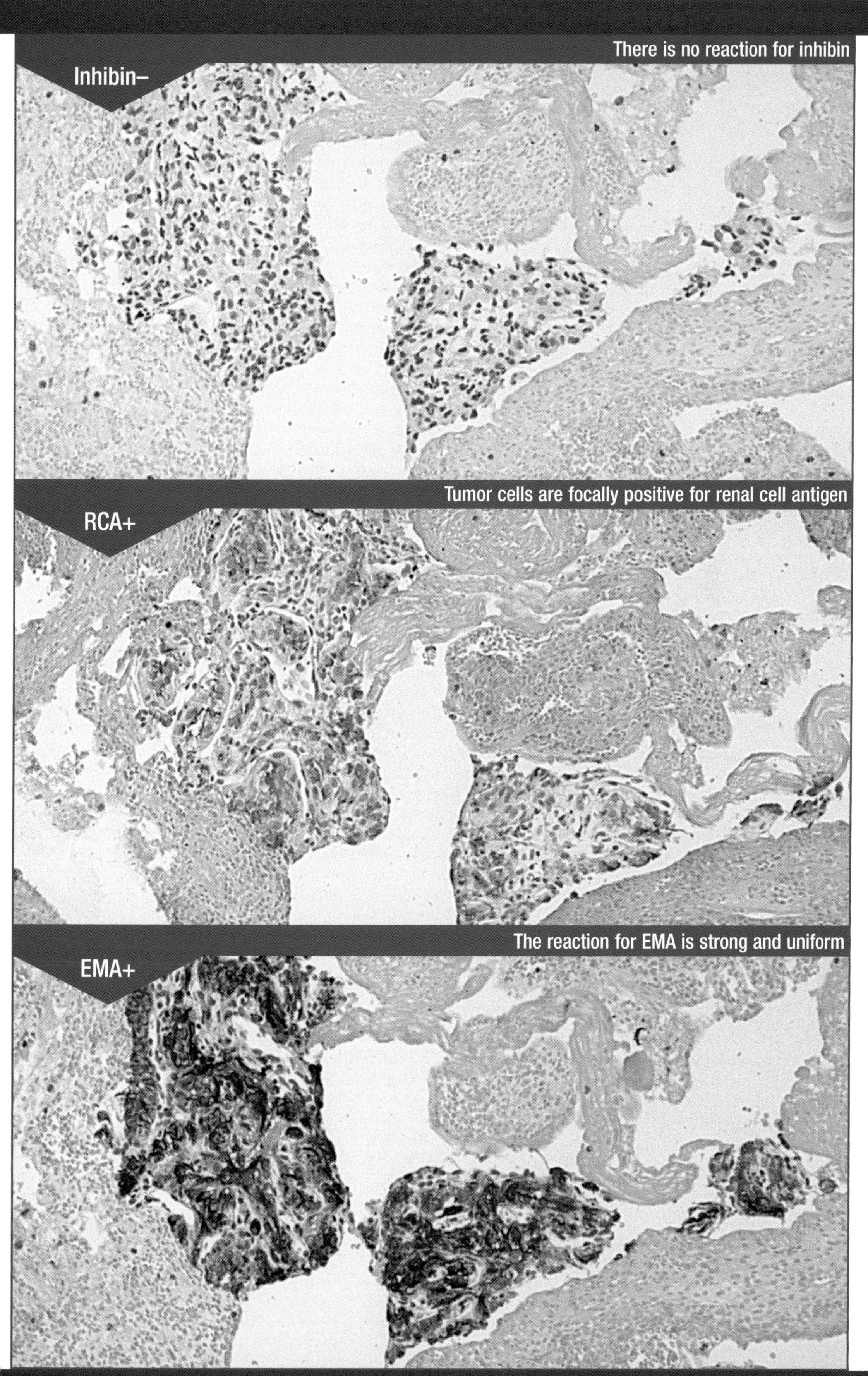
There is no reaction for inhibin
Inhibin–
Tumor cells are focally positive for renal cell antigen
RCA+
The reaction for EMA is strong and uniform
EMA+
Diagnosis: Renal Cell Carcinoma

Biopsy of a tumor in the renal/adrenal area

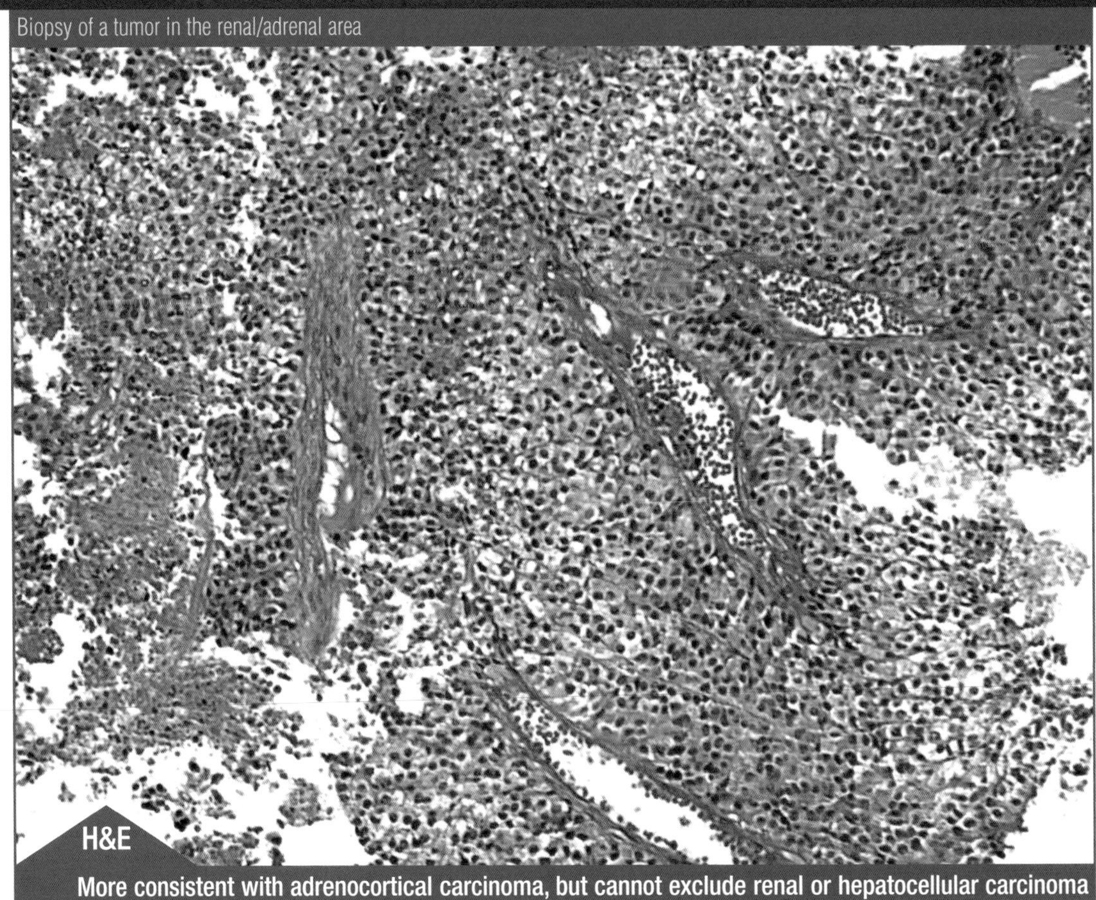

More consistent with adrenocortical carcinoma, but cannot exclude renal or hepatocellular carcinoma

Renal Cell Carcinoma vs Adrenocortical Tumor			
	Cytokeratin (CK)	EMA	Inhibin
Renal Cell Carcinoma	+	+	–
Adrenocortical Tumor	–	–	+

Helpful Hints

This differential diagnosis can usually be solved by demonstration of epithelial markers (**EMA** and **cytokeratin**) in renal cell carcinomas. Adrenocortical carcinomas do not react positively for EMA although occasional cytokeratin positivity is reported in these tumors. Furthermore, renal cell carcinomas are usually negative for **inhibin**.

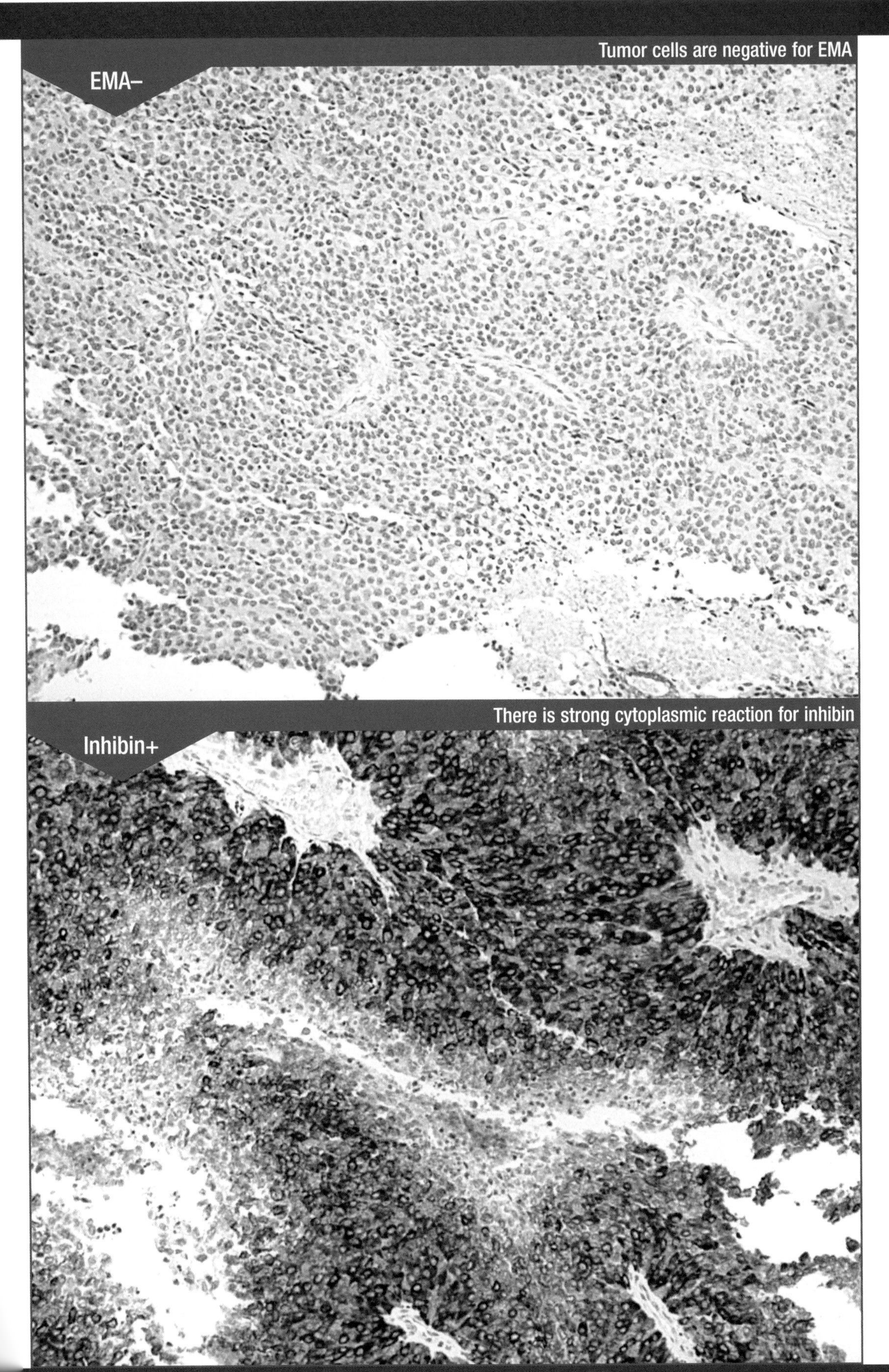
Tumor cells are negative for EMA
EMA–
There is strong cytoplasmic reaction for inhibin
Inhibin+
Diagnosis: Adrenocortical Tumor

Excision of a renal mass

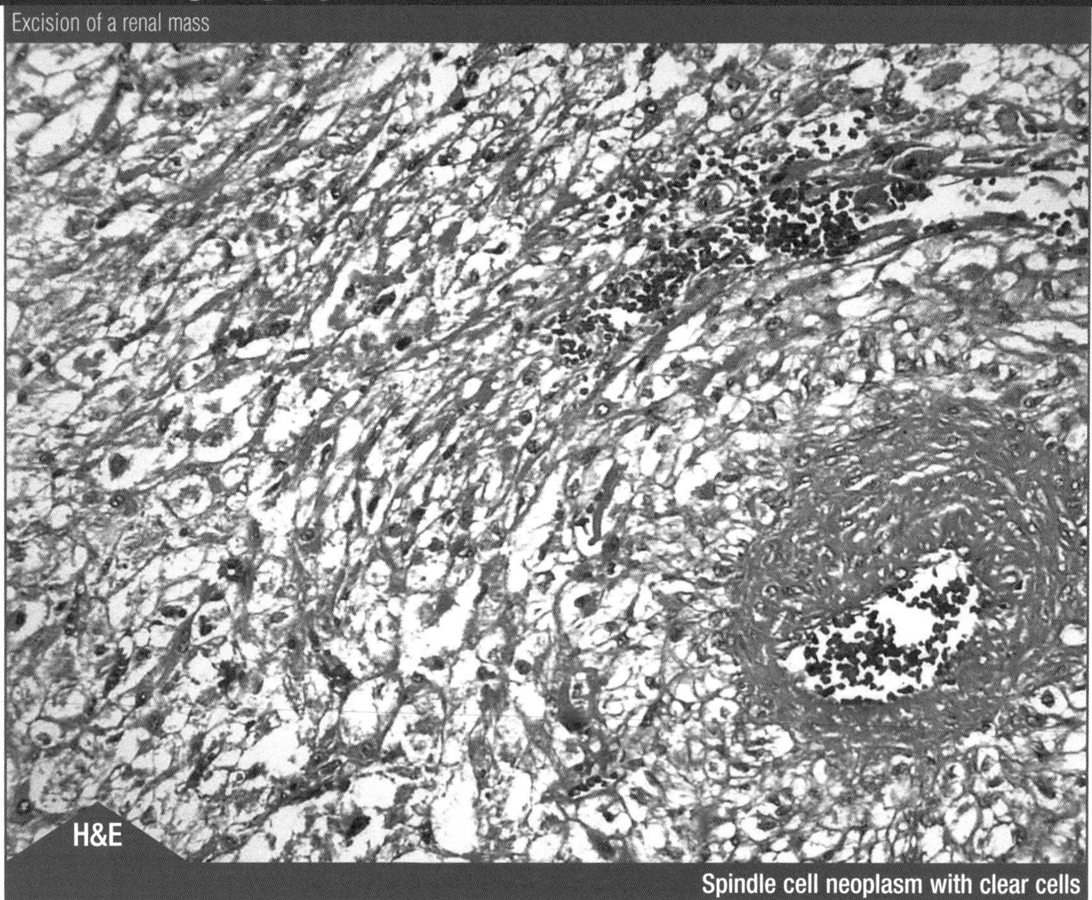

Spindle cell neoplasm with clear cells

Angiomyolipoma vs Sarcomatoid Renal Carcinoma			
	Cytokeratin (CK)	H-Caldesmon (HCD)	HMB-45
Angiomyolipoma	–	+	+
Sarcomatoid Renal Ca	+	–	–

Helpful Hints

Classic angiomyolipomas are easy to diagnose but the epithelioid and spindle cell varieties do not contain fat and may create a diagnostic problem with renal cell carcinomas. This differential diagnosis can usually be solved by demonstration of epithelial markers (**EMA** and **cytokeratin**) in renal cell carcinomas and **H-Caldesmon** and **HMB-45** in angiomyolipoma. The use of renal cell antigen in this situation is not warranted as it is usually negative in sarcomatoid renal cell carcinomas.

Sturtz 1994.

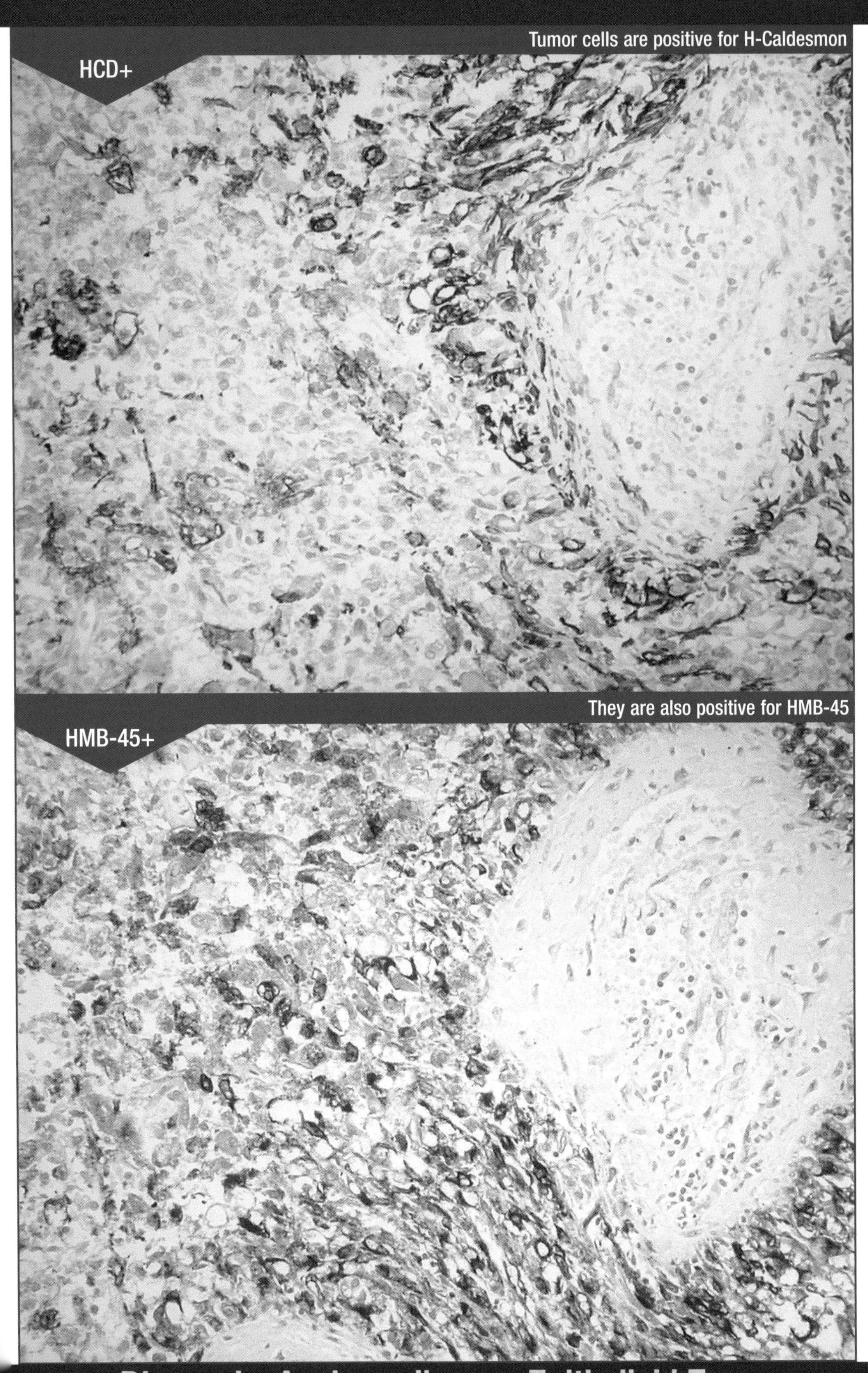

Diagnosis: Angiomyolipoma, Epithelioid Type

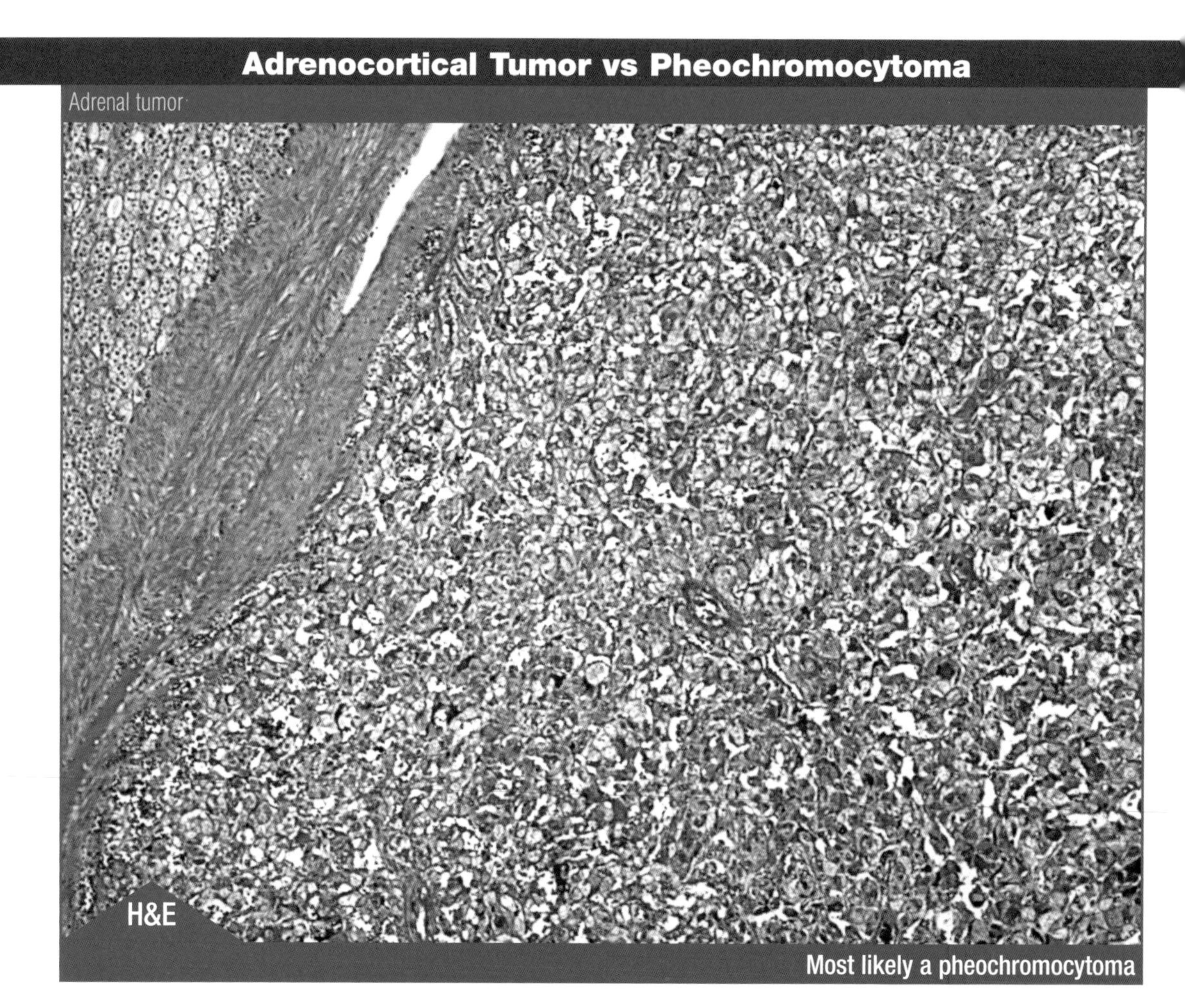

Most likely a pheochromocytoma

Adrenocortical Tumor vs Pheochromocytoma			
	Inhibin	Chromogranin (Chrg)	Synaptophysin
Adrenocortical Tumor	+	–	S
Pheochromocytoma	–	+	+

Helpful Hints

Pheochromocytomas are generally diffusely positive for **chromogranin** while adrenocortical tumors are always negative. **Synaptophysin** staining is not helpful because both tumors could be positive for this marker.

Schroder 1992.

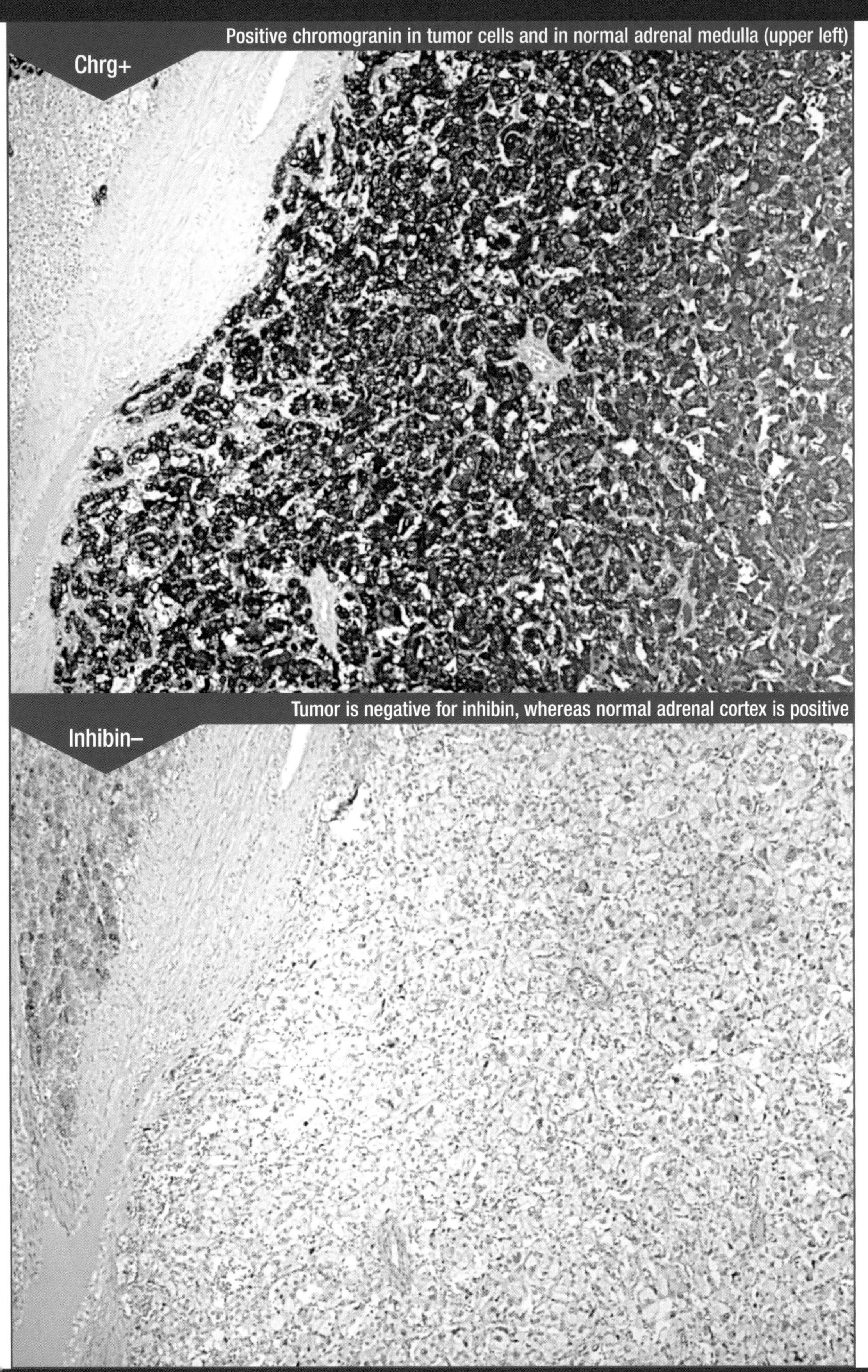

Diagnosis: Pheochromocytoma

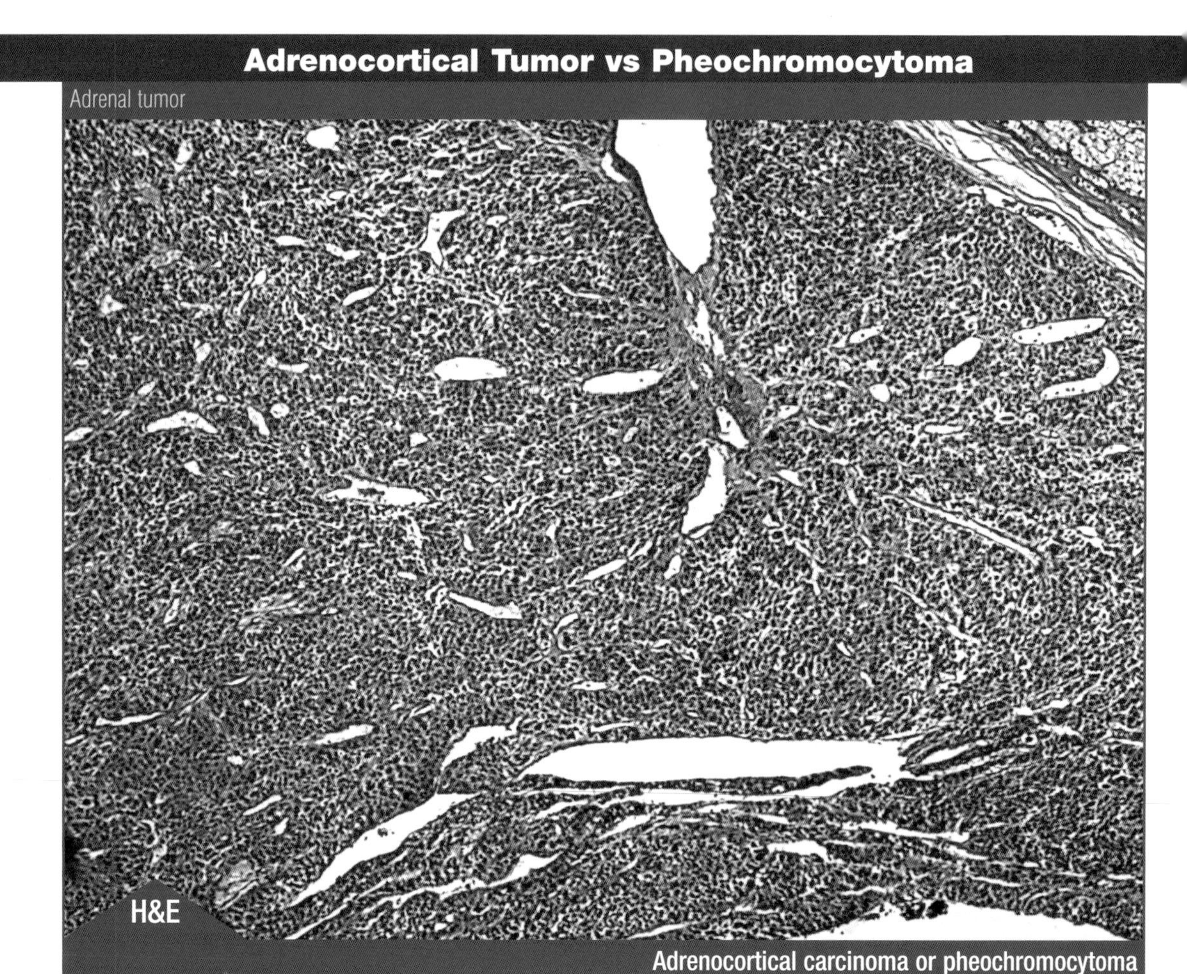

Adrenocortical carcinoma or pheochromocytoma

Adrenocortical Tumor vs Pheochromocytoma			
	Inhibin	Chromogranin (Chrg)	Synaptophysin (SP)
Adrenocortical Tumor	+	–	S
Pheochromocytoma	–	+	+

Helpful Hints

Pheochromocytomas are generally diffusely positive for **chromogranin** while adrenocortical tumors are always negative. **Synaptophysin** staining is not helpful because both tumors could be positive for this marker.

Schroder 1992.

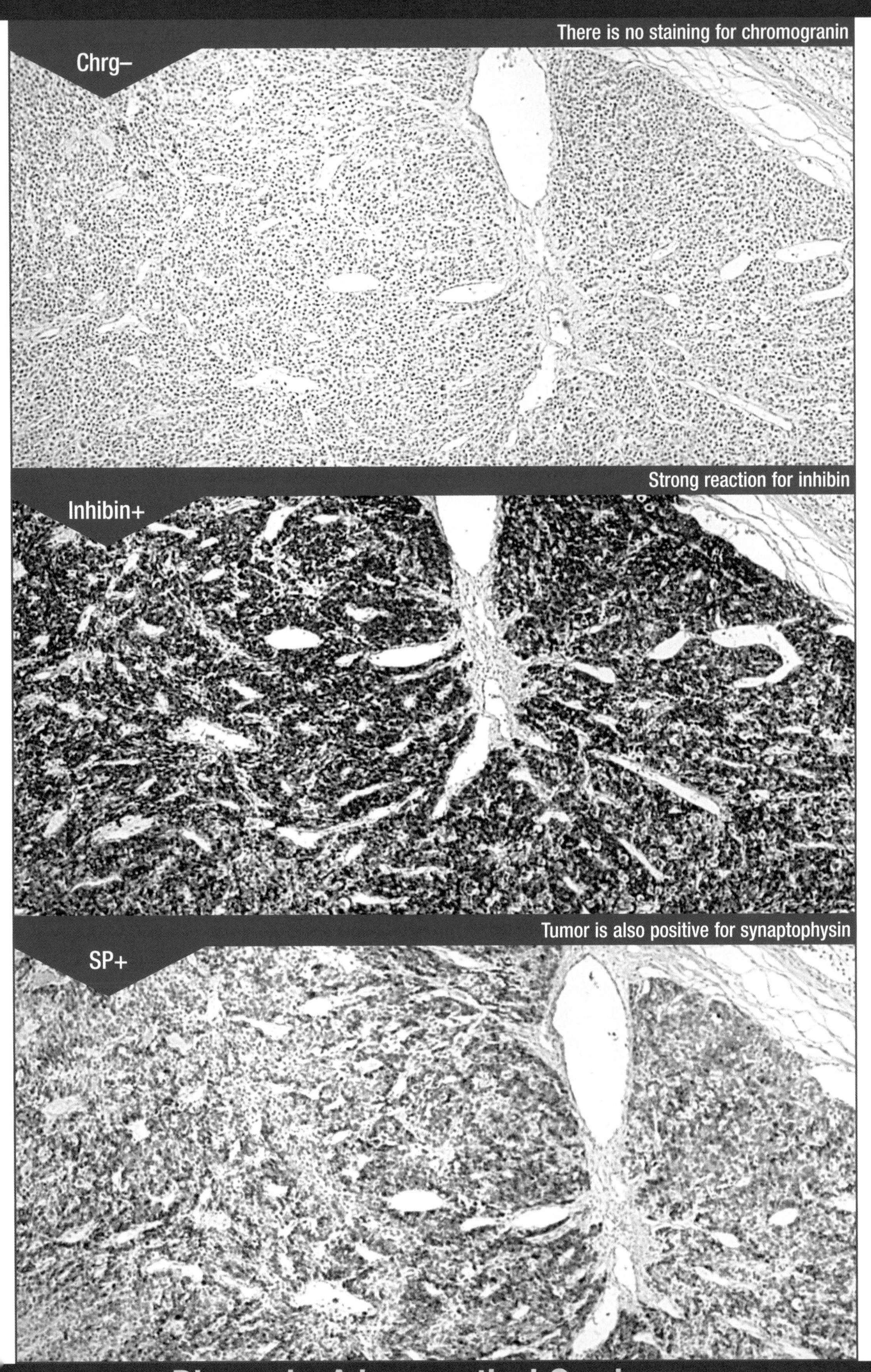

Diagnosis: Adrenocortical Carcinoma

Adrenal tumor

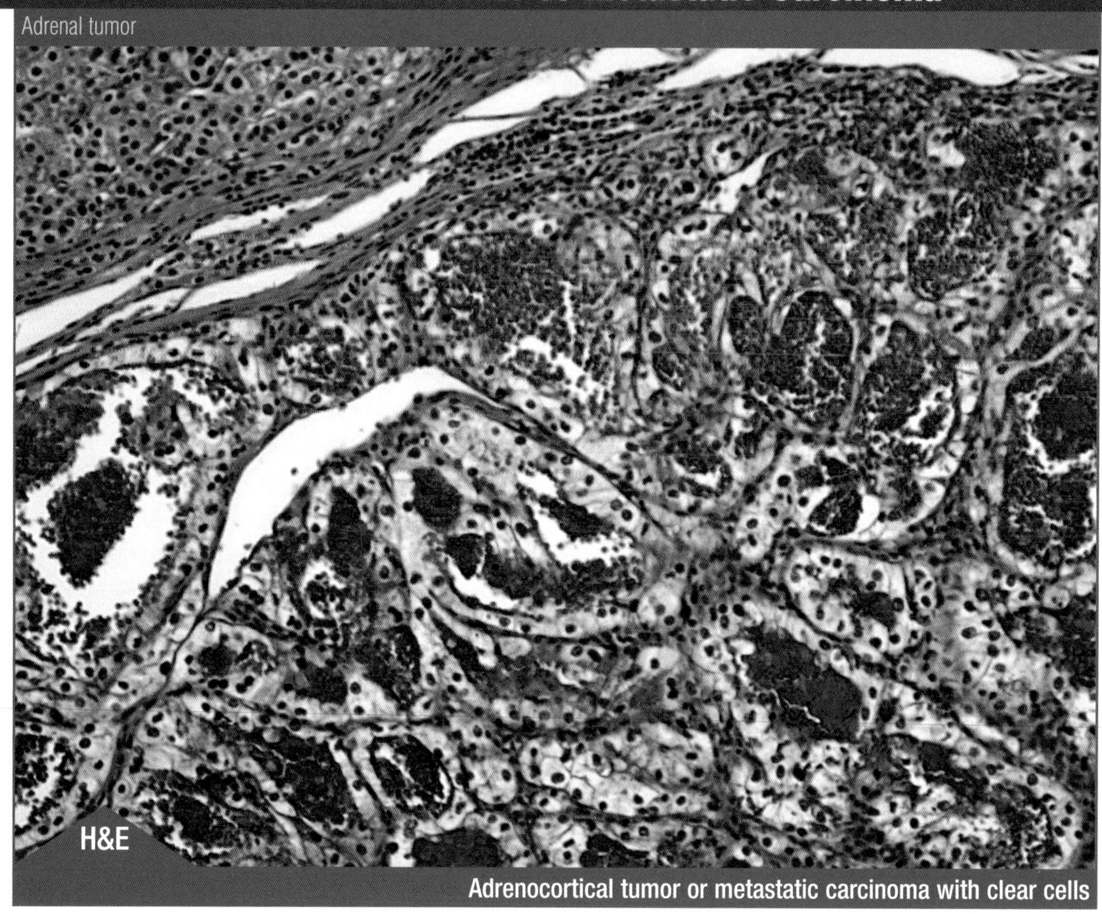

Adrenocortical tumor or metastatic carcinoma with clear cells

Adrenocortical Tumor vs Metastatic Carcinoma			
	Inhibin	Cytokeratin (CK)	EMA
Adrenocortical Tumor	+	–	–
Metastatic Carcinoma	–	+	+

Helpful Hints

A wide-spectrum **cytokeratin** antibody and **EMA** label most metastatic carcinomas to the adrenal. Adrenocortical tumors are rarely positive for cytokeratin or EMA.

Metastatic carcinomas to the adrenal are usually from the lung or kidney and are negative for **inhibin**. If a specific site for carcinoma is suspected, appropriate markers for that primary could be used.

Wieneke 2003, Fetsch 1999.

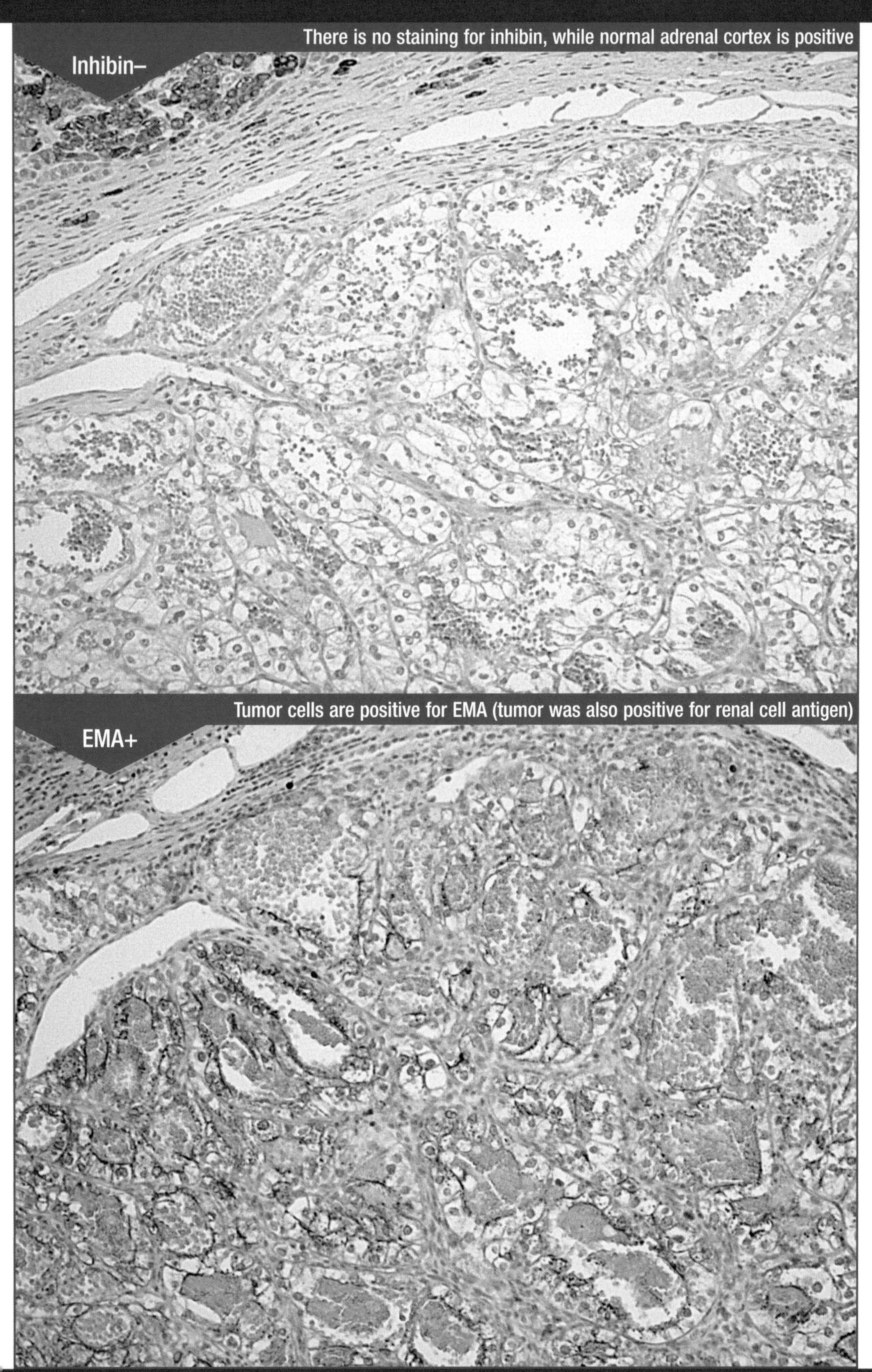

Diagnosis: Metastatic Renal Cell Carcinoma

Adrenal tumor

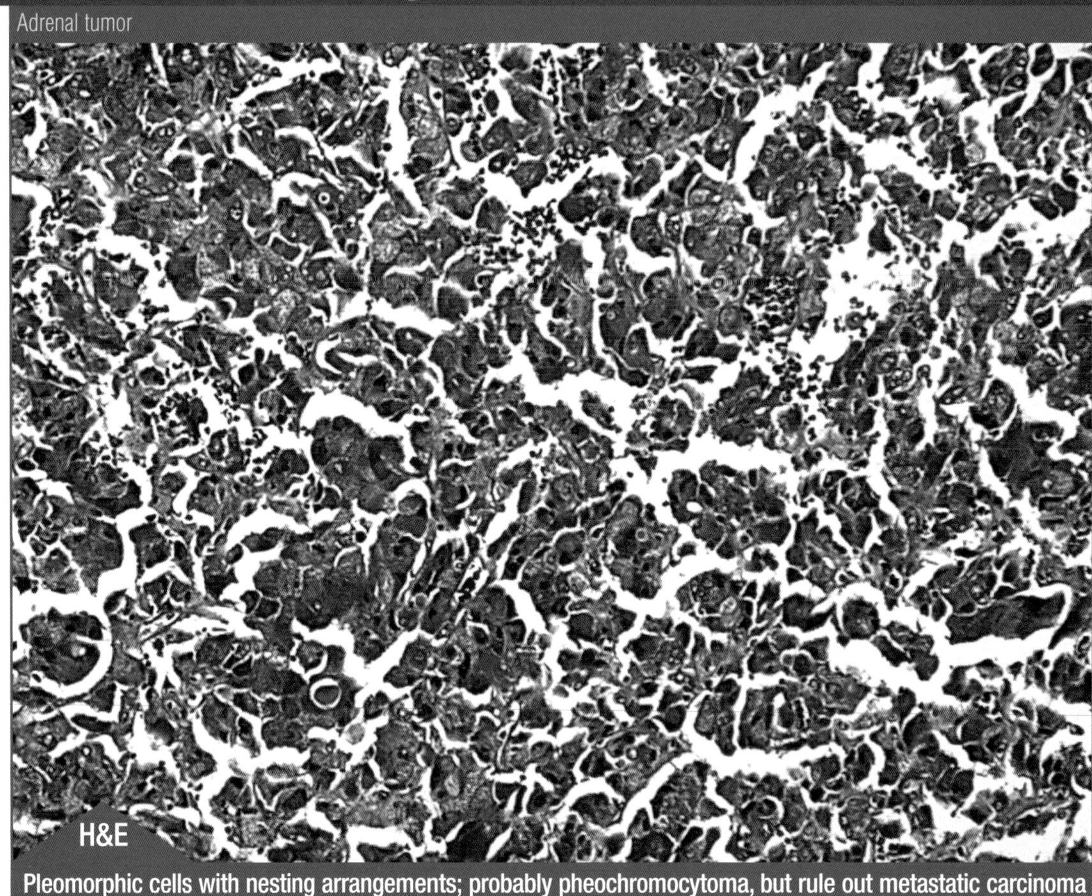

Pleomorphic cells with nesting arrangements; probably pheochromocytoma, but rule out metastatic carcinoma

Pheochromocytoma vs Metastatic Carcinoma		
	Chromogranin (Chrg)	Cytokerain (CK)
Pheochromocytoma	+	–
Metastatic Carcinoma	–	+

Helpful Hints

The majority of metastic carcinomas to the adrenal are from the lung. These tumors are uniformly positive for **cytokeratin** and usually negative for **chromogranin**. Conversely, pheochromocytomas are always positive for chromogranin and negative for cytokeratin.

Metastatic carcinomas to the adrenal from organs other than lung are also positive for cytokeratin. Furthermore, they may express their respective immunohistochemical markers, eg, RCA, ER.

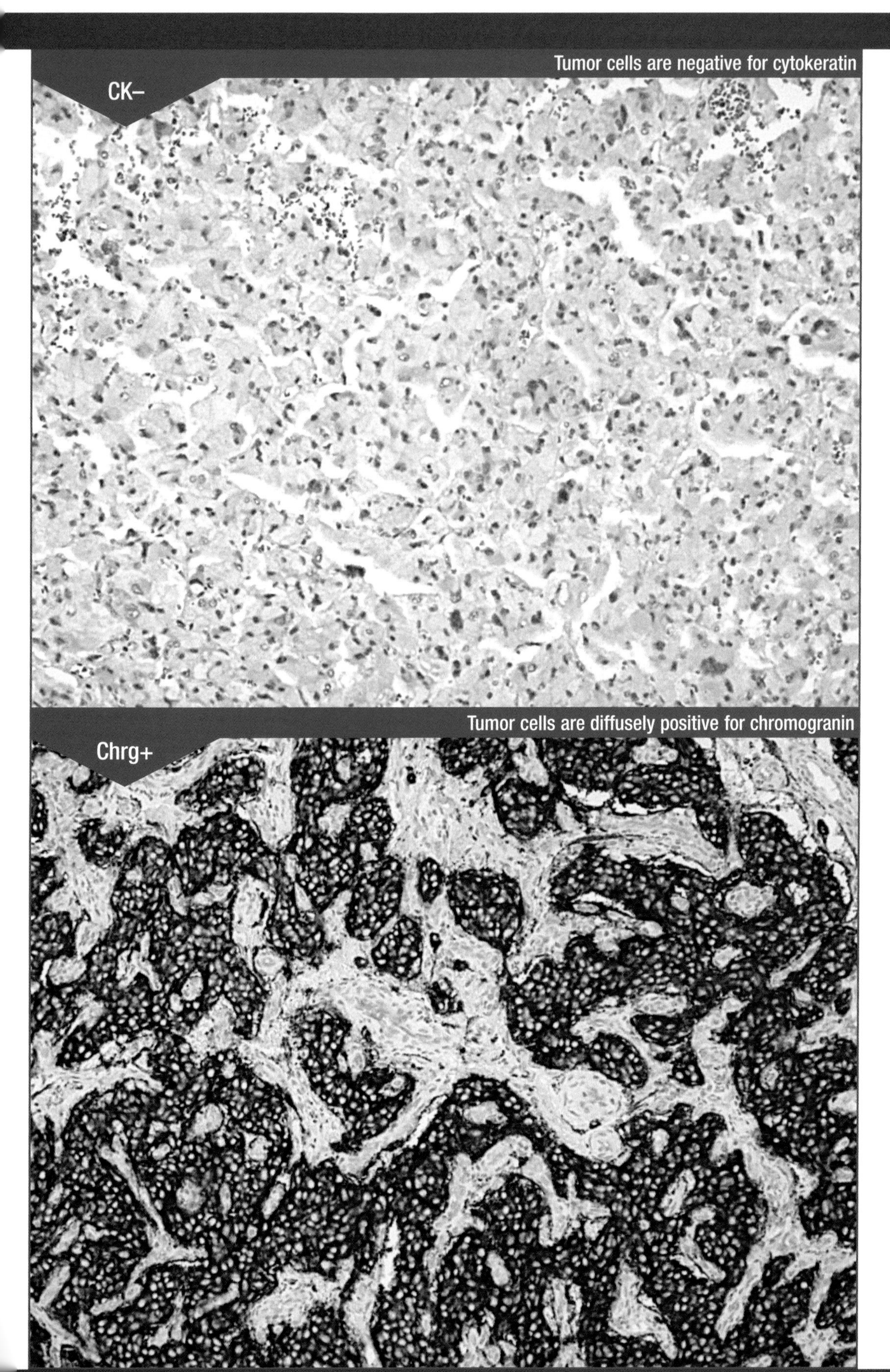

Diagnosis: Pheochromocytoma

Biopsy of tonsillar area

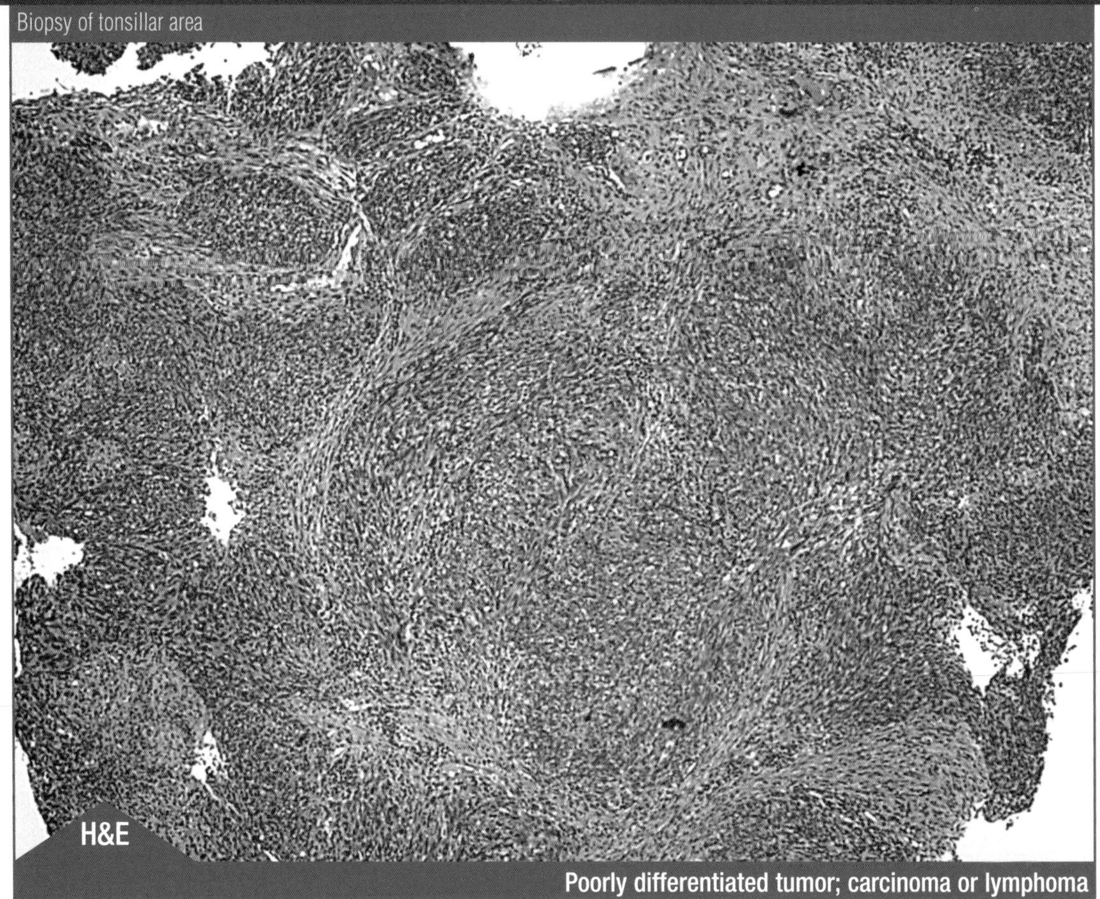

Poorly differentiated tumor; carcinoma or lymphoma

Undifferentiated Nasopharyngeal Carcinoma vs Squamous Cell Carcinoma			
	HLA-DR	BCL-2	Cytokeratin (CK)
Undifferentiated Nasopharyngeal Ca	+	+	+
Squamous Cell Ca	–	–	+

Helpful Hints

Both **HLA-DR** and **BCL-2** are expressed by the majority of undifferentiated nasopharyngeal carcinomas but rarely by squamous cell carcinomas. Interestingly, lymphoepithelial-like carcinomas of the other organs; such as lung, stomach, skin, urinary bladder, etc, share the same immunophenotypic profile.

Thomas 1984, Vera-Sempere 1997.

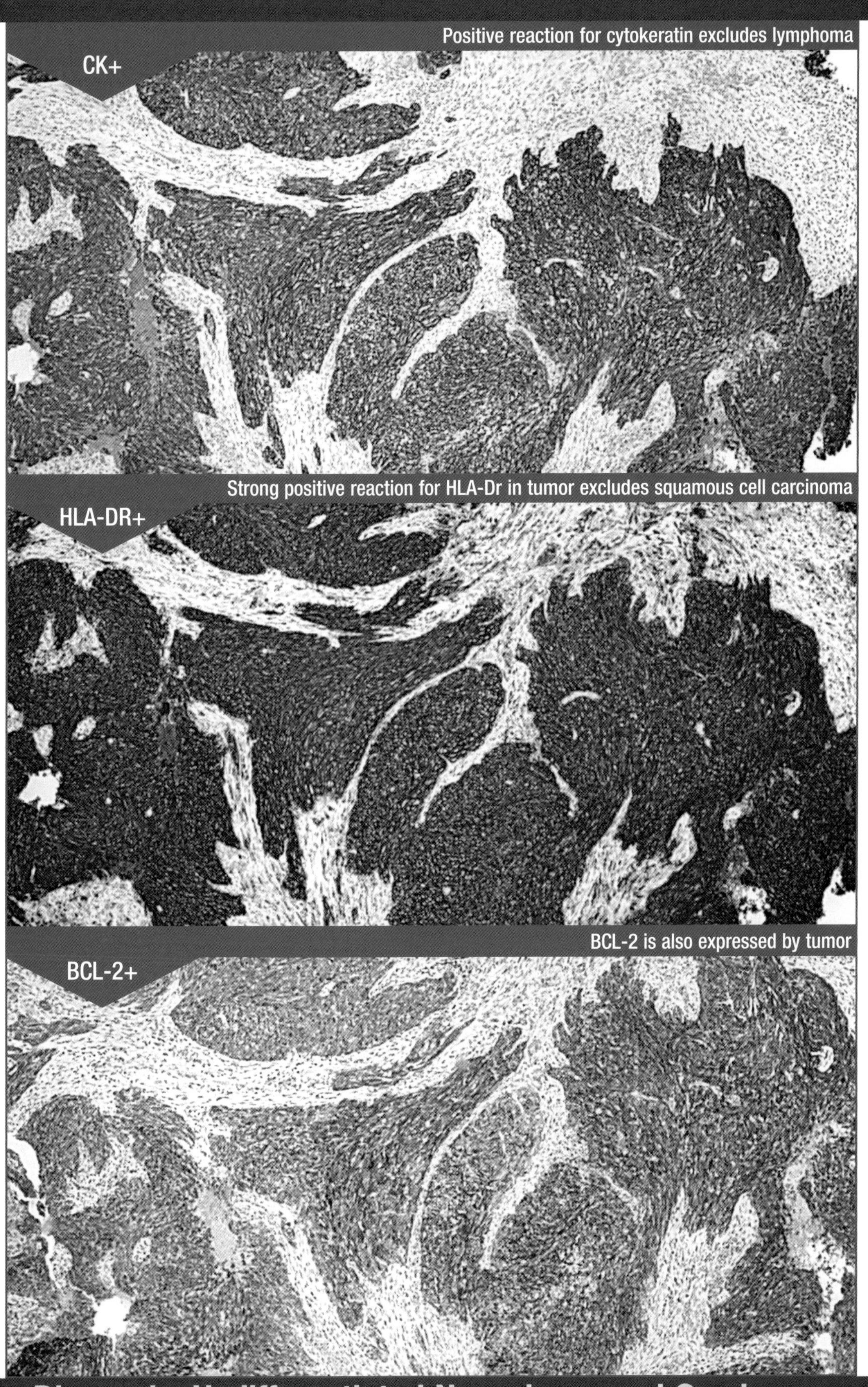

Diagnosis: Undifferentiated Nasopharyngeal Carcinoma

Biopsy of nasopharynx

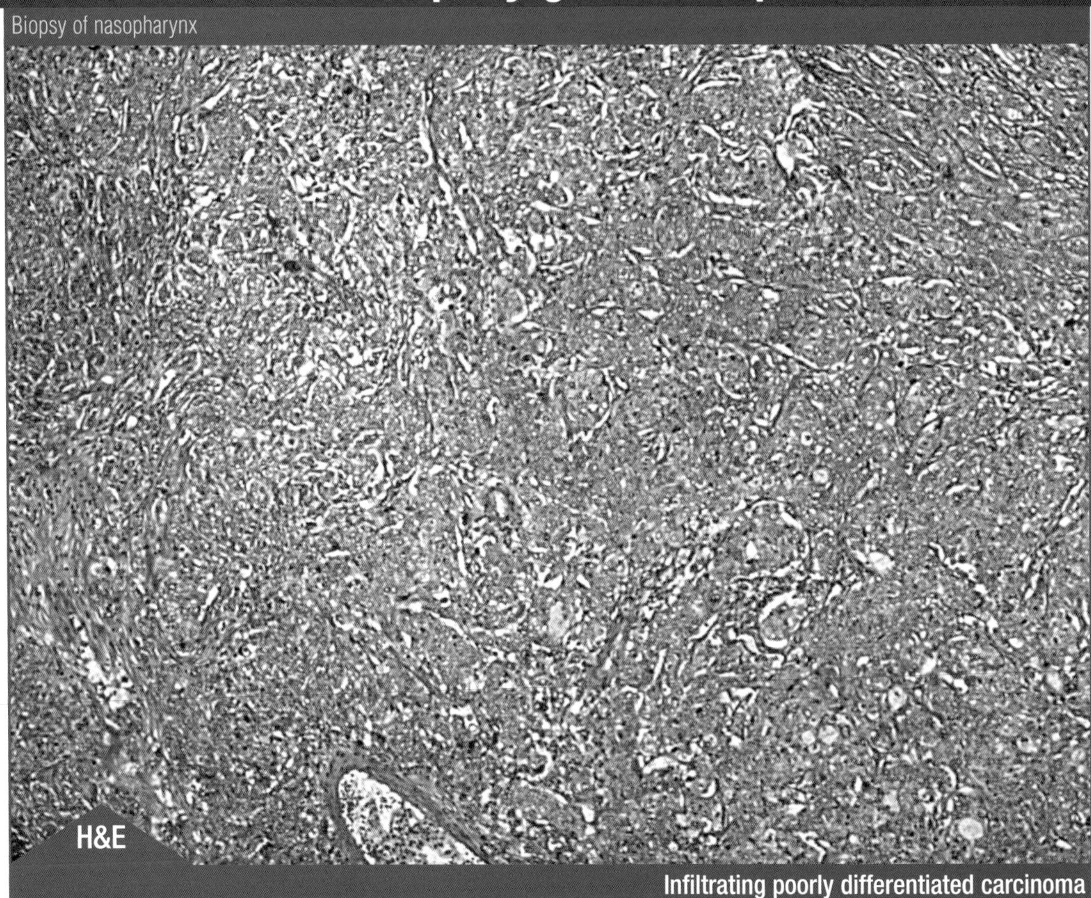

Infiltrating poorly differentiated carcinoma

Undifferentiated Nasopharyngeal Carcinoma vs Squamous Cell Carcinoma			
	HLA-DR	BCL-2	Cytokeratin (CK)
Undifferentiated Nasopharyngeal Ca	+	+	+
Squamous Cell Ca	–	–	+

Helpful Hints

Both **HLA-DR** and **BCL-2** are expressed by the majority of undifferentiated nasopharyngeal carcinomas but rarely by squamous cell carcinomas. Interestingly, lymphoepithelial-like carcinomas of the other organs; such as lung, stomach, skin, urinary bladder, etc, share the same immunophenotypic profile.

Thomas 1984, Vera-Sempere 1997.

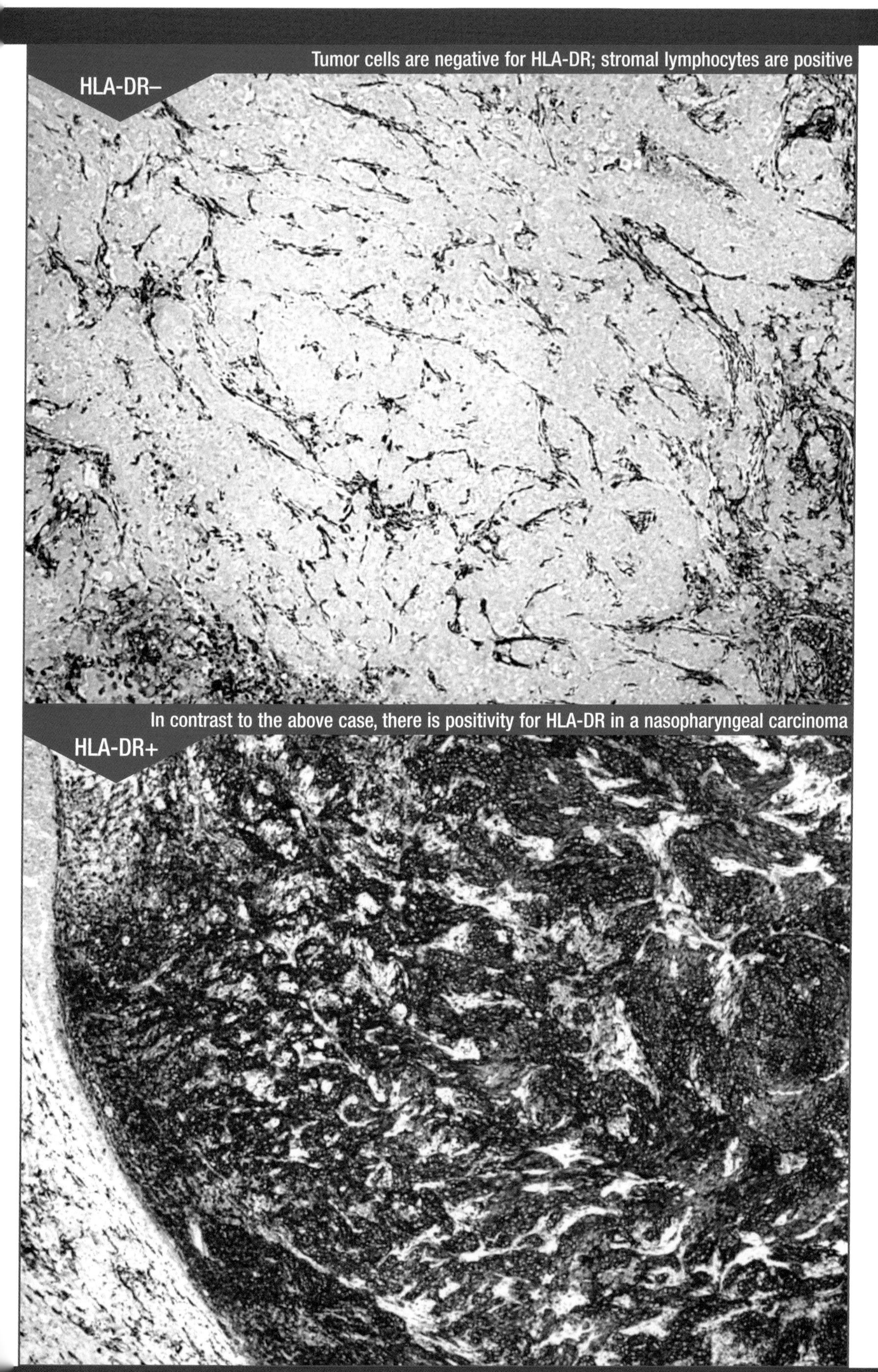

Tumor cells are negative for HLA-DR; stromal lymphocytes are positive

In contrast to the above case, there is positivity for HLA-DR in a nasopharyngeal carcinoma

Diagnosis: Poorly Differentiated Squamous Cell Carcinoma

Lesion of parotid gland

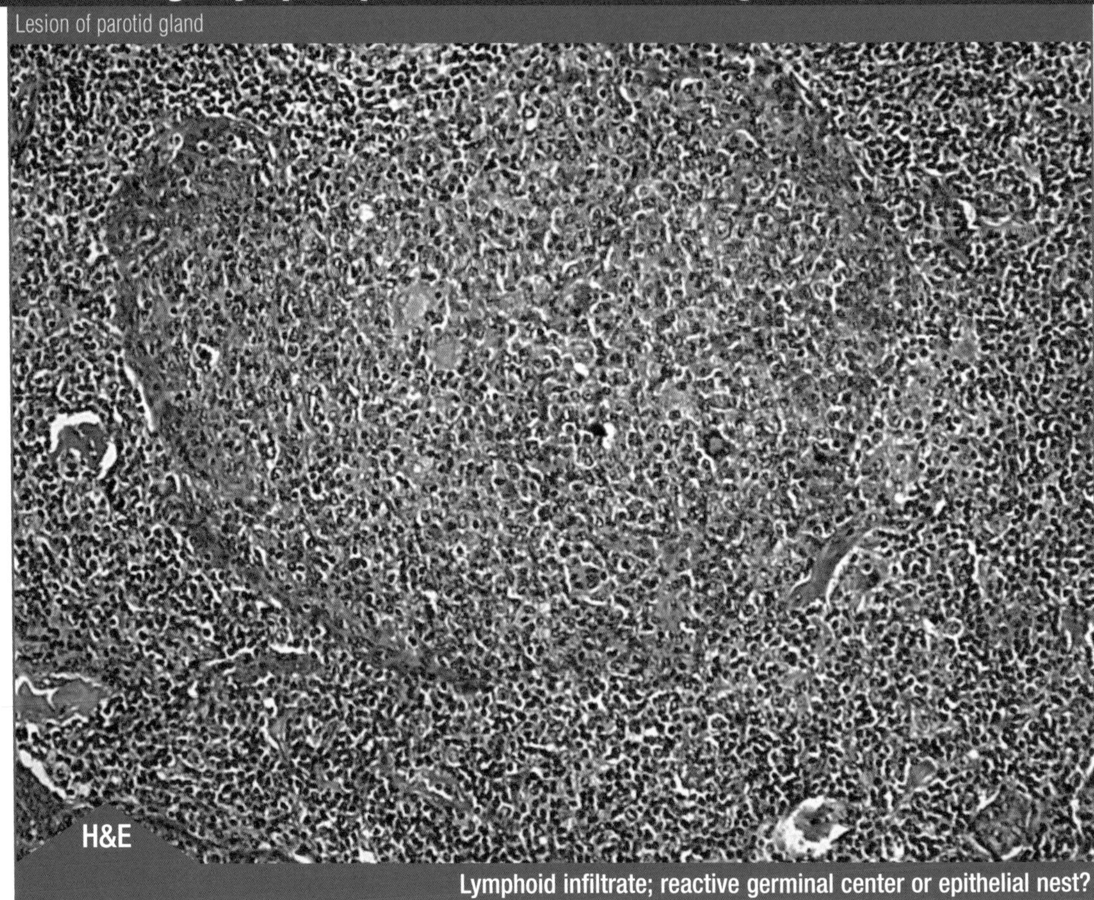

Lymphoid infiltrate; reactive germinal center or epithelial nest?

Benign Lymphoepithelial Lesion vs Malignant Lymphoma		
	Cytokeratin (CK)	p63
Lymphoepithelial Lesion	+	+
Malignant Lymphoma	–	-

Helpful Hints

Because the epithelial elements may not easily be seen by routine stains, benign lymphoepithelial lesions could be mistaken for lymphomas. The epithelial component of this lesion however is easily identified by its positive reaction for **cytokeratin** and **p63**.

Bilal 2003.

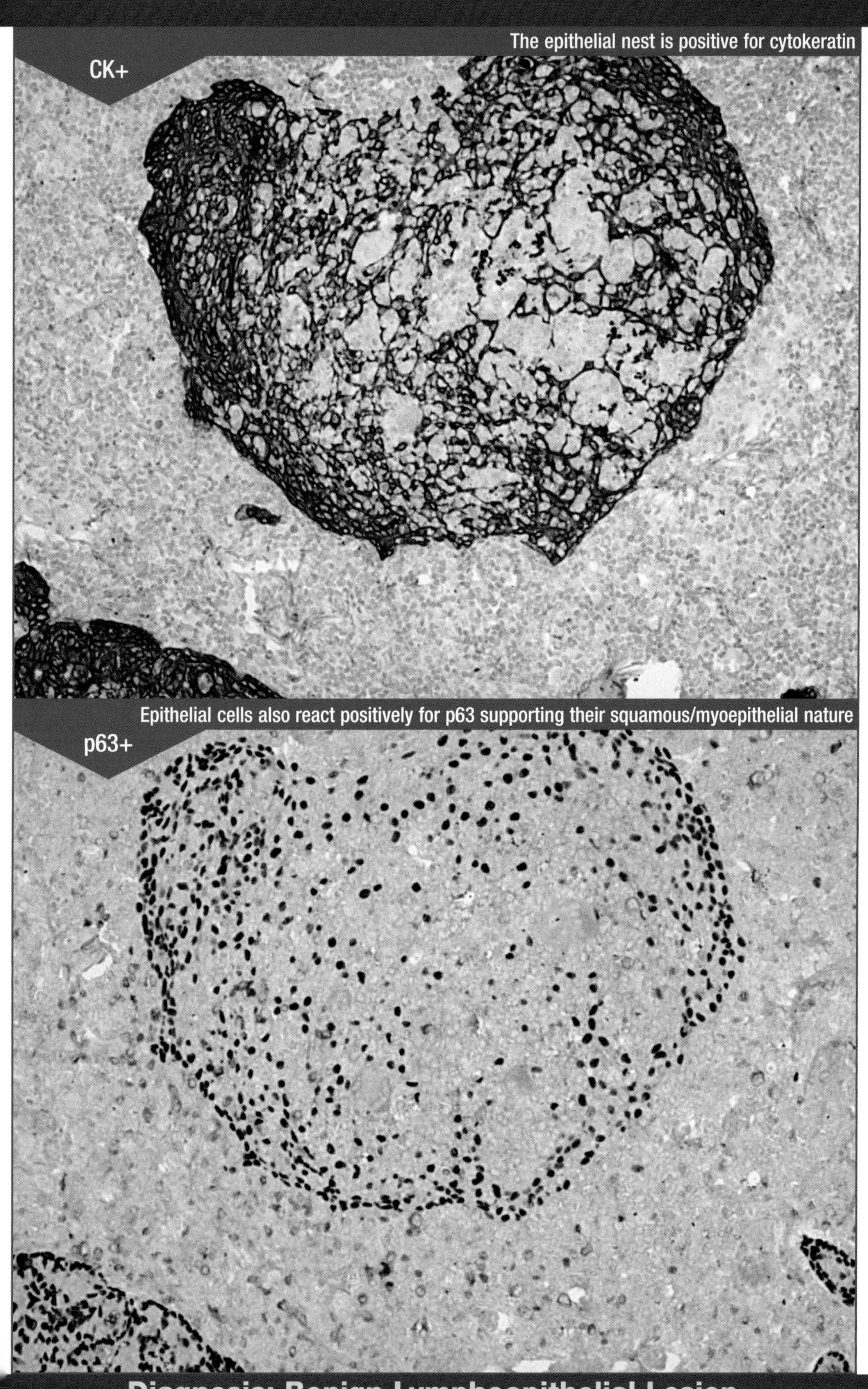

Diagnosis: Benign Lymphoepithelial Lesion

Biopsy of nasal mucosa

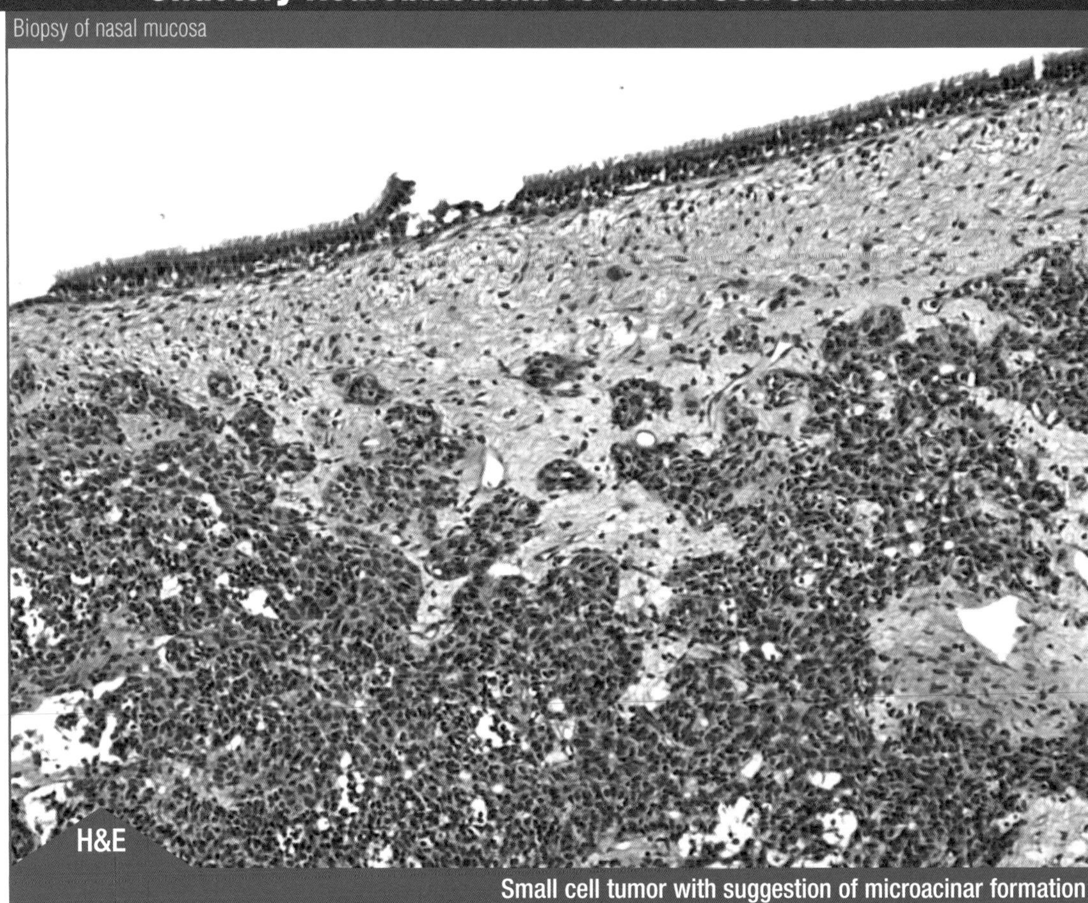

Small cell tumor with suggestion of microacinar formation

Olfactory Neuroblastoma vs Small Cell Carcinoma			
	Cytokeratin (CK)	Chromogranin (Chrg)	Synaptophysin (SP)
Olfactory Neuroblastoma	–	+	+
Small Cell Carcinoma	+	–	–

Helpful Hints

Olfactory neuroblastoma may be difficult to differentiate from other small cell tumors particularly if the biopsy is small and cells are crushed. In the above differential diagnosis, **cytokeratin** stains small cell carcinomas whereas **chromogranin** and **synaptophysin** are expressed by olfactory neuroblastomas.

Devaney 1996.

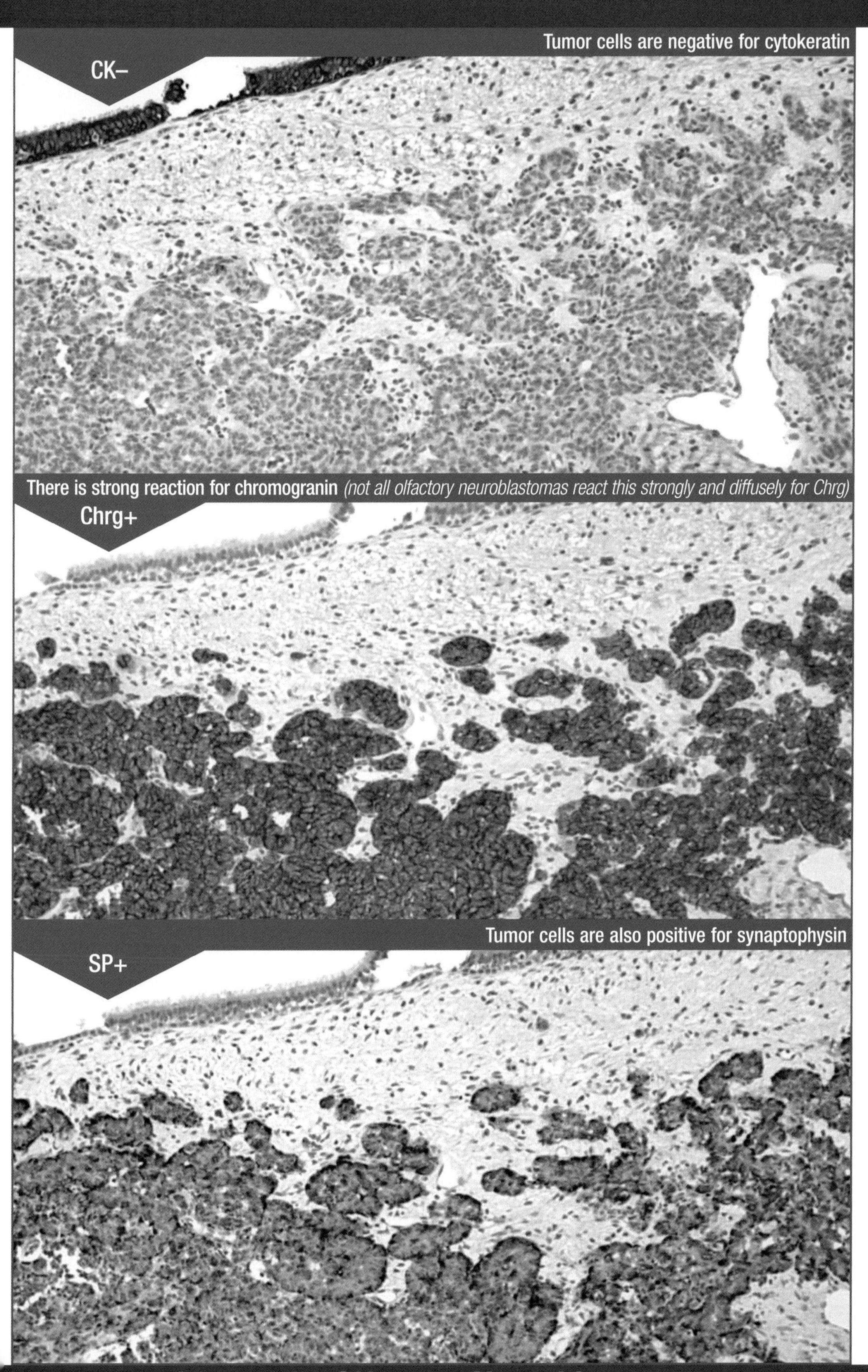
Tumor cells are negative for cytokeratin
CK–
There is strong reaction for chromogranin *(not all olfactory neuroblastomas react this strongly and diffusely for Chrg)*
Chrg+
Tumor cells are also positive for synaptophysin
SP+
Diagnosis: Olfactory Neuroblastoma

Needle core biopsy of thyroid

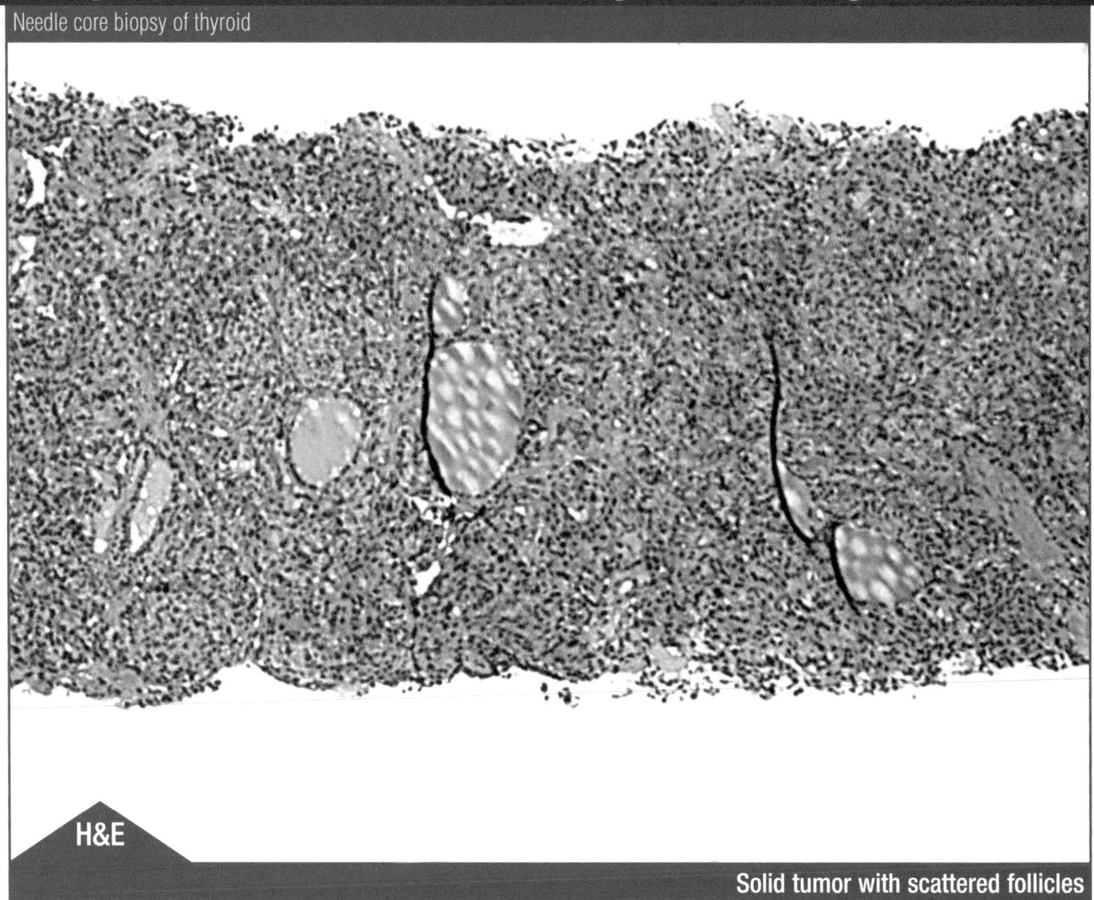

Solid tumor with scattered follicles

Thyroid Follicular Carcinoma vs Thyroid Medullary Carcinoma			
	Thyroglobulin (TGB)	Calcitonin	CEA
Thyroid Follicular Ca	+	–	–
Thyroid Medullary Ca	–	+	+

Helpful Hints

Thyroglobulin is one the most specific markers in tumor immunohistochemistry. It is expressed by all follicular and papillary thyroid carcinomas, but not by any other tumor (struma ovarii, of course, is an exception). Anaplastic thyroid carcinomas however, are usually negative for thyroglobulin, unless they are associated with foci of papillary carcinoma.

For C-cell hyperplasia and medullary thyroid carcinoma, the best markers are **calcitonin** and **carcinoembryonic antigen**; the latter is present in almost 100% of these tumors. Several peptide hormones may be expressed by medullary carcinomas, but they have no diagnostic value. Medullary thyroid carcinomas are frequently positive for chromogranin, whereas follicular tumors are not. **TTF-1** is expressed by both follicular and C-cell tumors of thyroid.

Albores-Saavedra 1983, Sikri 1985.

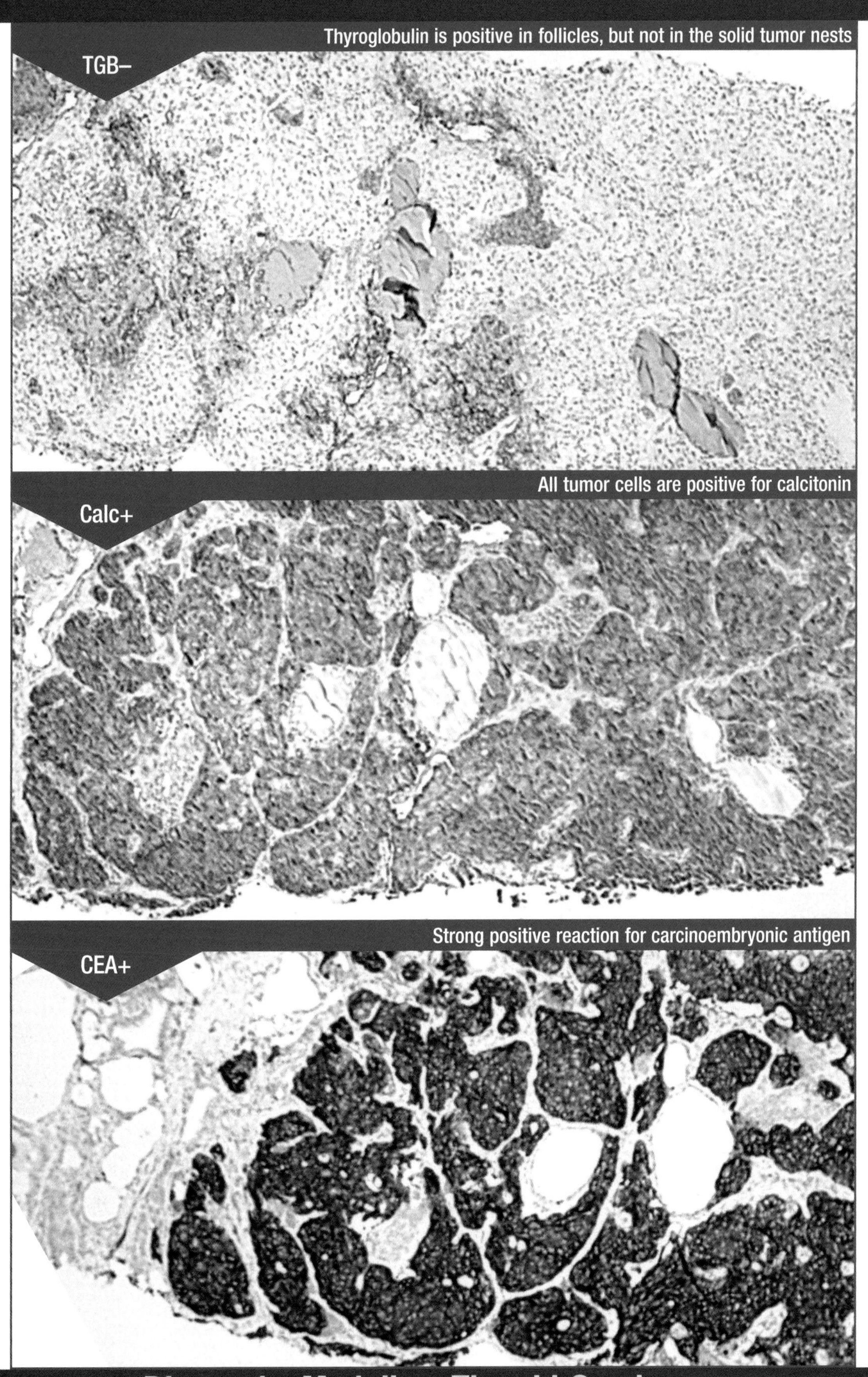

Diagnosis: Medullary Thyroid Carcinoma

Thyroid Follicular Carcinoma vs Thyroid Medullary Carcinoma

Lobectomy for a thyroid nodule

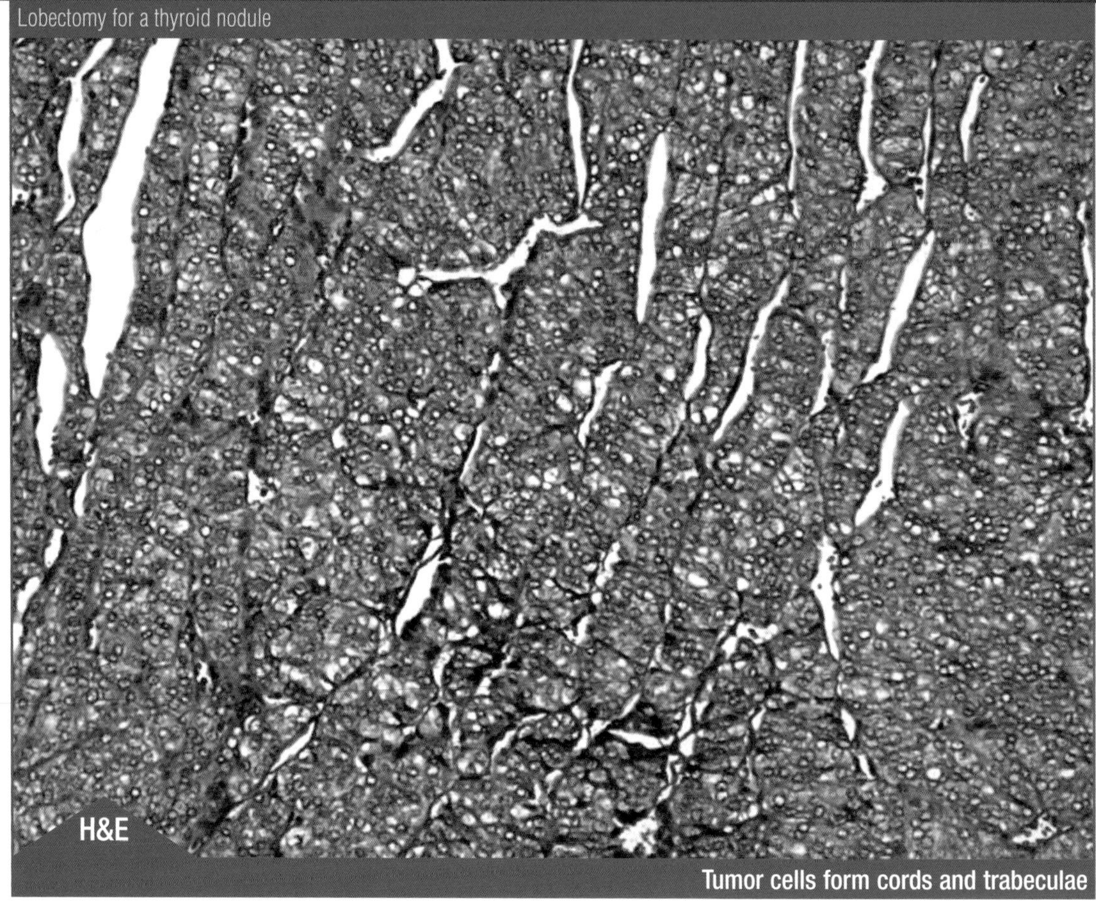

Tumor cells form cords and trabeculae

Thyroid Follicular Carcinoma vs Thyroid Medullary Carcinoma			
	Thyroglobulin (TGB)	Calcitonin	CEA
Thyroid Follicular Ca	+	–	–
Thyroid Medullary Ca	–	+	+

Helpful Hints

Thyroglobulin is one the most specific markers in tumor immunohistochemistry. It is expressed by all follicular and papillary thyroid carcinomas, but not by any other tumor (struma ovarii, of course, is an exception). Anaplastic thyroid carcinomas however, are usually negative for thyroglobulin, unless they are associated with foci of papillary carcinoma.

For C-cell hyperplasia and medullary thyroid carcinoma, the best markers are **calcitonin** and **carcinoembryonic antigen**; the latter is present in almost 100% of these tumors. Several peptide hormones may be expressed by medullary carcinomas, but they have no diagnostic value. Medullary thyroid carcinomas are frequently positive for chromogranin, whereas follicular tumors are not. **TTF-1** is expressed by both follicular and C-cell tumors of thyroid.

Albores-Saavedra 1983, Sikri 1985.

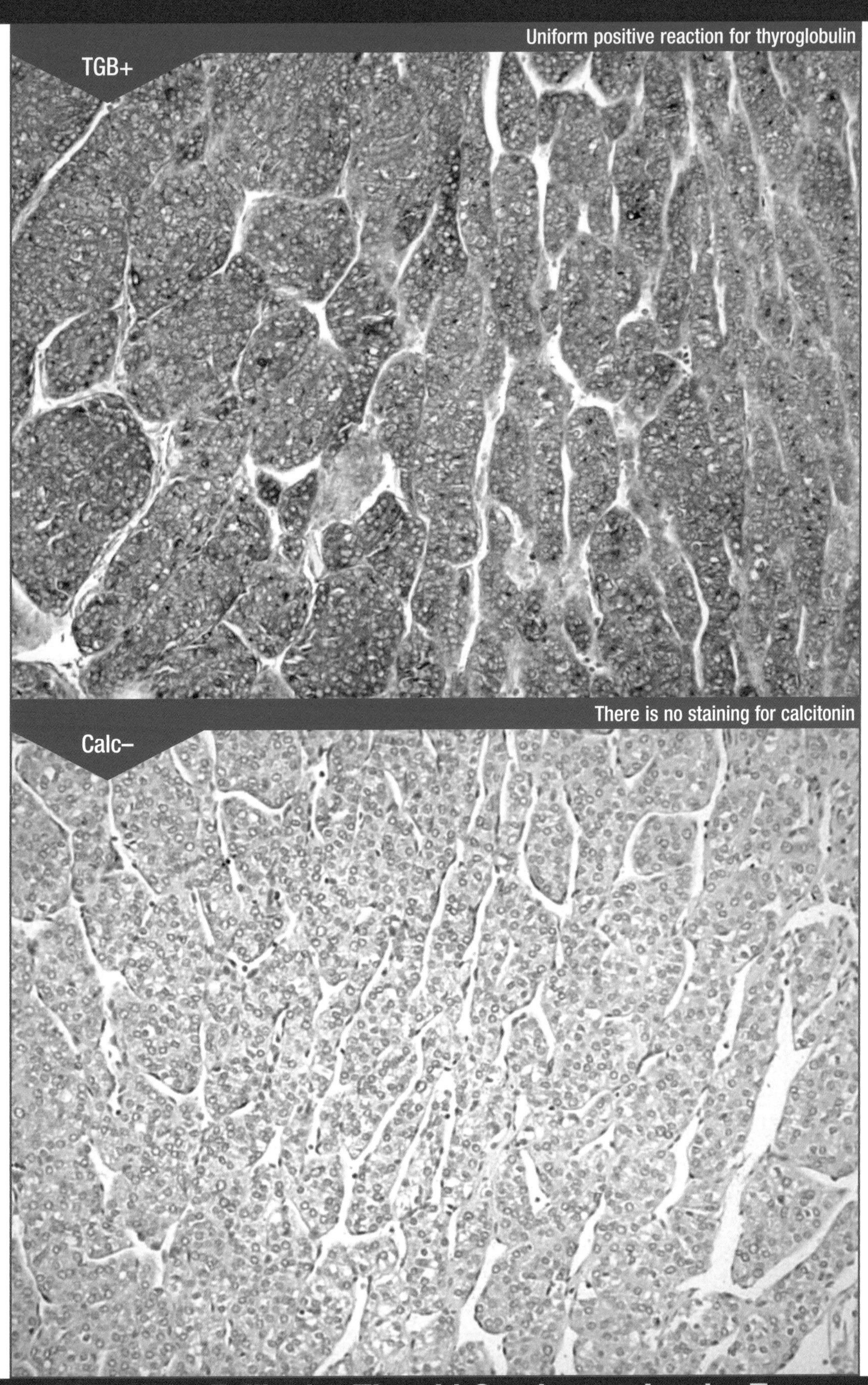

Diagnosis: Follicular Thyroid Carcinoma, Insular Type

Thyroid nodule in a patient explored for hyperparathyroidism

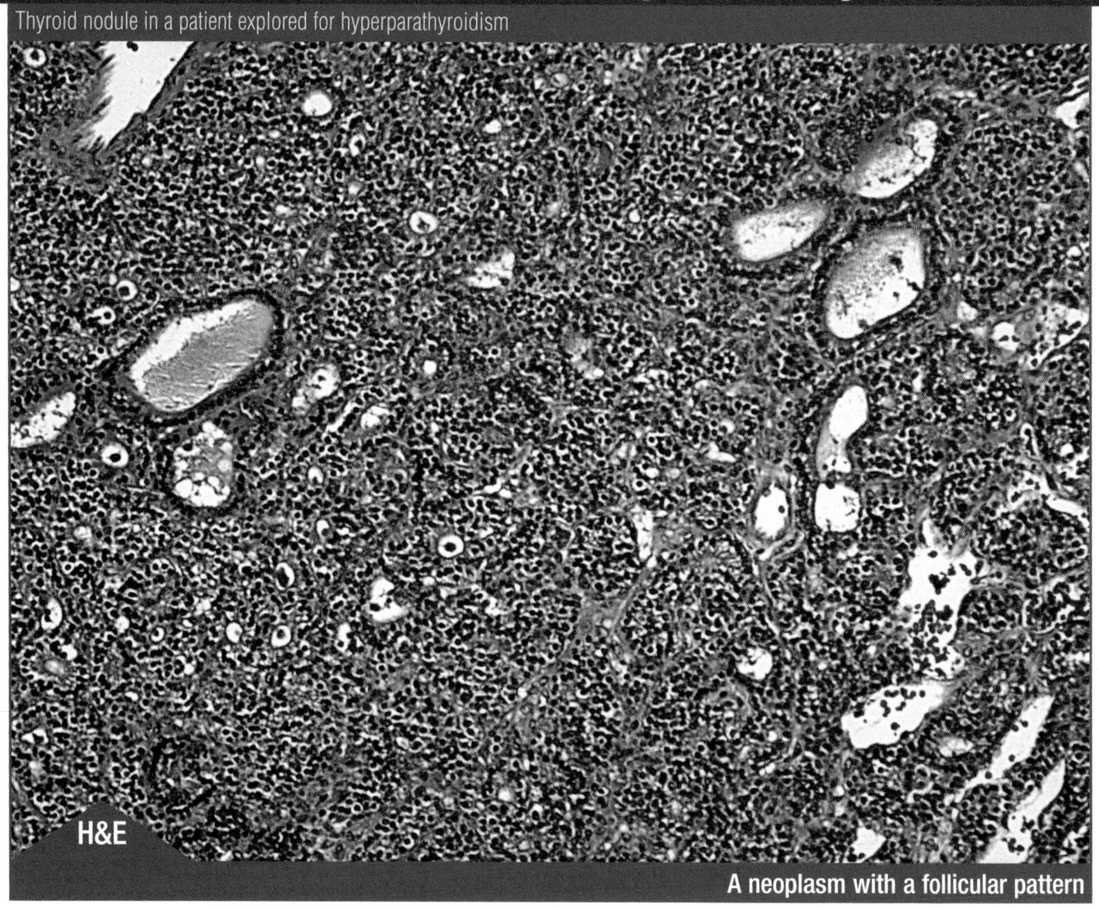

A neoplasm with a follicular pattern

Thyroid Follicular Neoplasm vs Intrathyroid Parathyroid Adenoma		
	Thyroglobulin (TGB)	Parathyroid Hormone (PTH)
Thyroid Follicular Neoplasm	+	–
Intrathyroid Parathyroid Adenoma	–	+

Helpful Hints

Although uncommon, parathyroid adenomas may occasionally occur within thyroid parenchyma and pose a differential diagnosis with thyroid follicular tumors. A combination of parathyroid hormone (**PTH**) for parathyroid and thyroglobulin for follicular neoplasms will establish their histogenesis.

Sawady 1989.

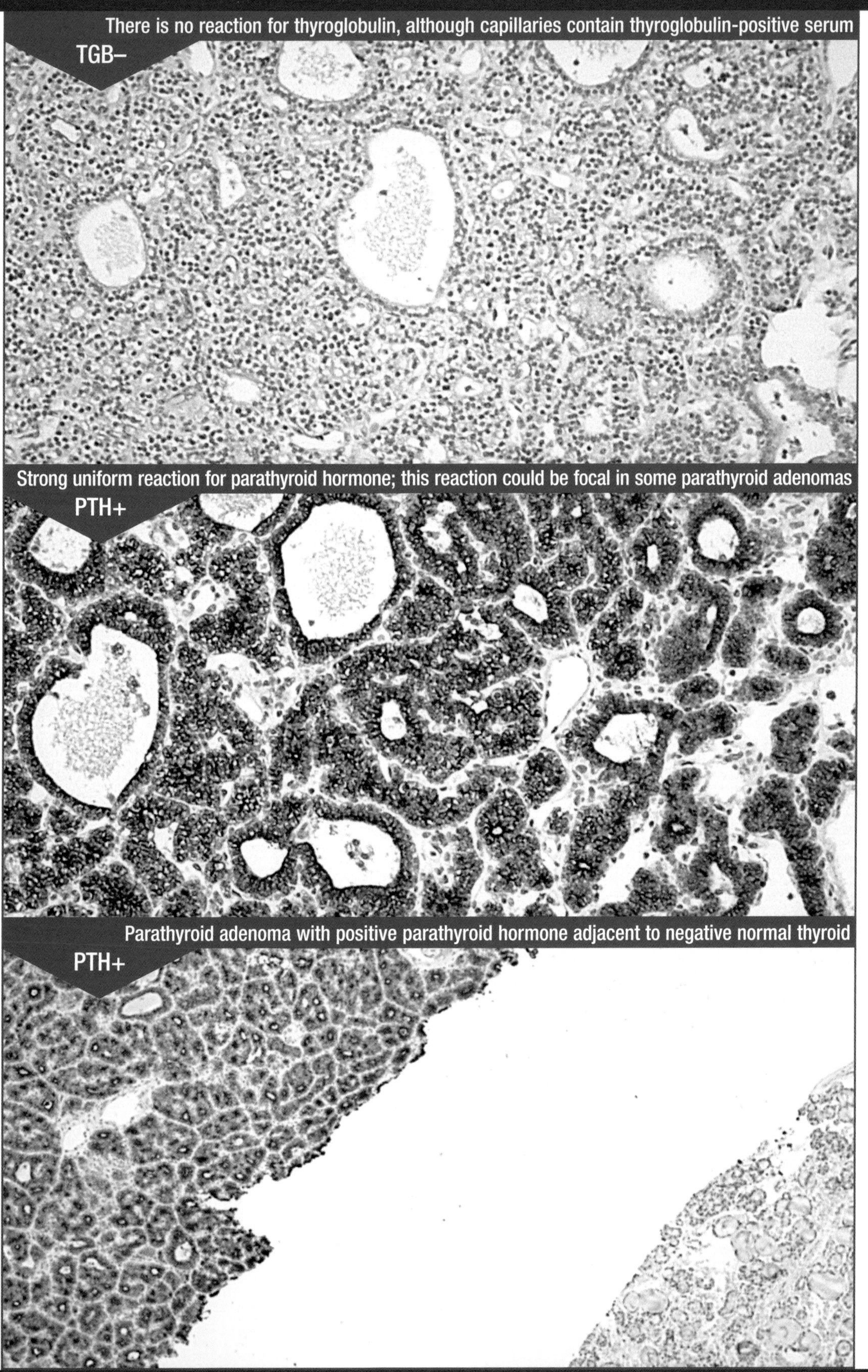

Diagnosis: Intrathyroid Parathyroid Adenoma

Thyroid Clear Cell Carcinoma vs Metastatic Renal Cell Carcinoma

Thyroid lobectomy specimen

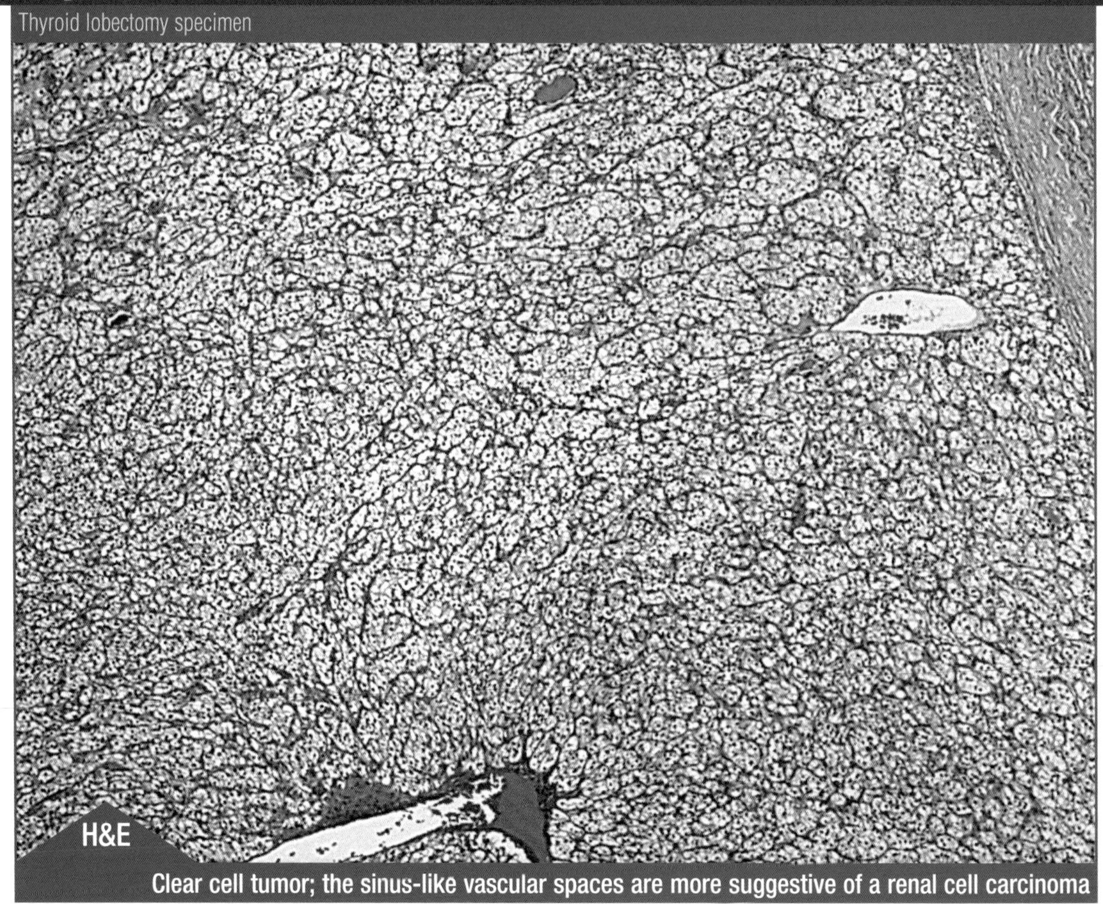

Clear cell tumor; the sinus-like vascular spaces are more suggestive of a renal cell carcinoma

Thyroid Carcinoma vs Metastatic Renal Cell Carcinoma		
	Thyroglobulin (TGB)	RCA
Thyroid Carcinoma	+	–
Metastatic Renal Cell Carcinoma	–	+

Helpful Hints

This is not an uncommon differential diagnostic problem. Metastatic renal cell carcinoma to the thyroid may be the initial presentation of this tumor. Morphologically, they may resemble clear cell or Hurtle cell variants of follicular or papillary thyroid carcinomas.

Renal Cell Antigen is expressed by the great majority of clear cell renal cell carcinomas, whereas **thyroglobulin** is usually present in thyroid follicular cell tumors. **TTF-1** could also be used to confirm a thyroid primary.

Civantos 1984.

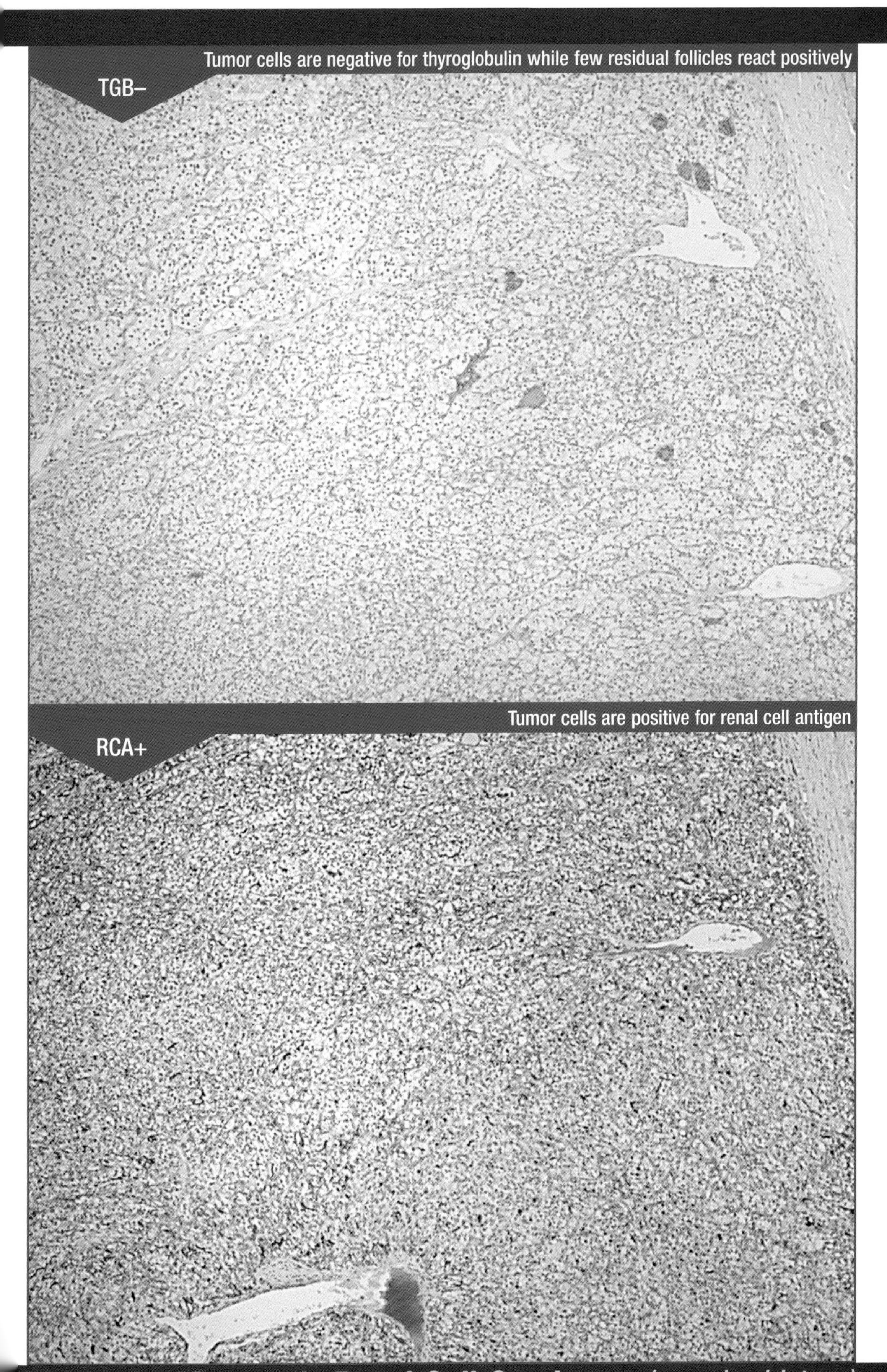

Tumor cells are negative for thyroglobulin while few residual follicles react positively

Tumor cells are positive for renal cell antigen

Diagnosis: Metastatic Renal Cell Carcinoma *(no prior history)*

Cell block of fine needle aspiration of thyroid in a patient with a renal mass

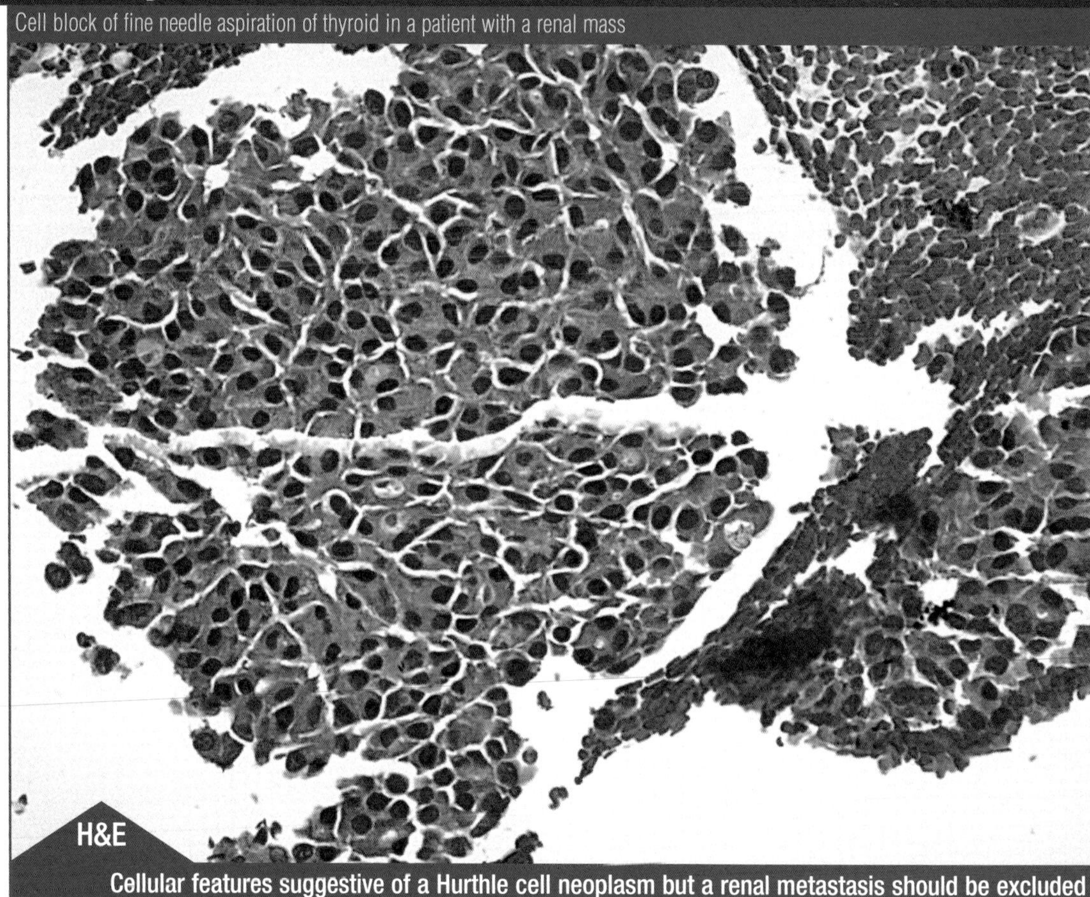

Cellular features suggestive of a Hurthle cell neoplasm but a renal metastasis should be excluded

Thyroid Carcinoma vs Metastatic Renal Cell Carcinoma		
	Thyroglobulin (TGB)	RCA
Thyroid Carcinoma	+	–
Metastatic Renal Cell Carcinoma	–	+

Helpful Hints

This is not an uncommon differential diagnostic problem. Metastatic renal cell carcinoma to the thyroid may be the initial presentation of this tumor. Morphologically, they may resemble clear cell or Hurtle cell variants of follicular or papillary thyroid carcinomas.

Renal Cell Antigen is expressed by the great majority of clear cell renal cell carcinomas, whereas **thyroglobulin** is usually present in thyroid follicular cell tumors. **TTF-1** could also be used to confirm a thyroid primary.

Civantos 1984.

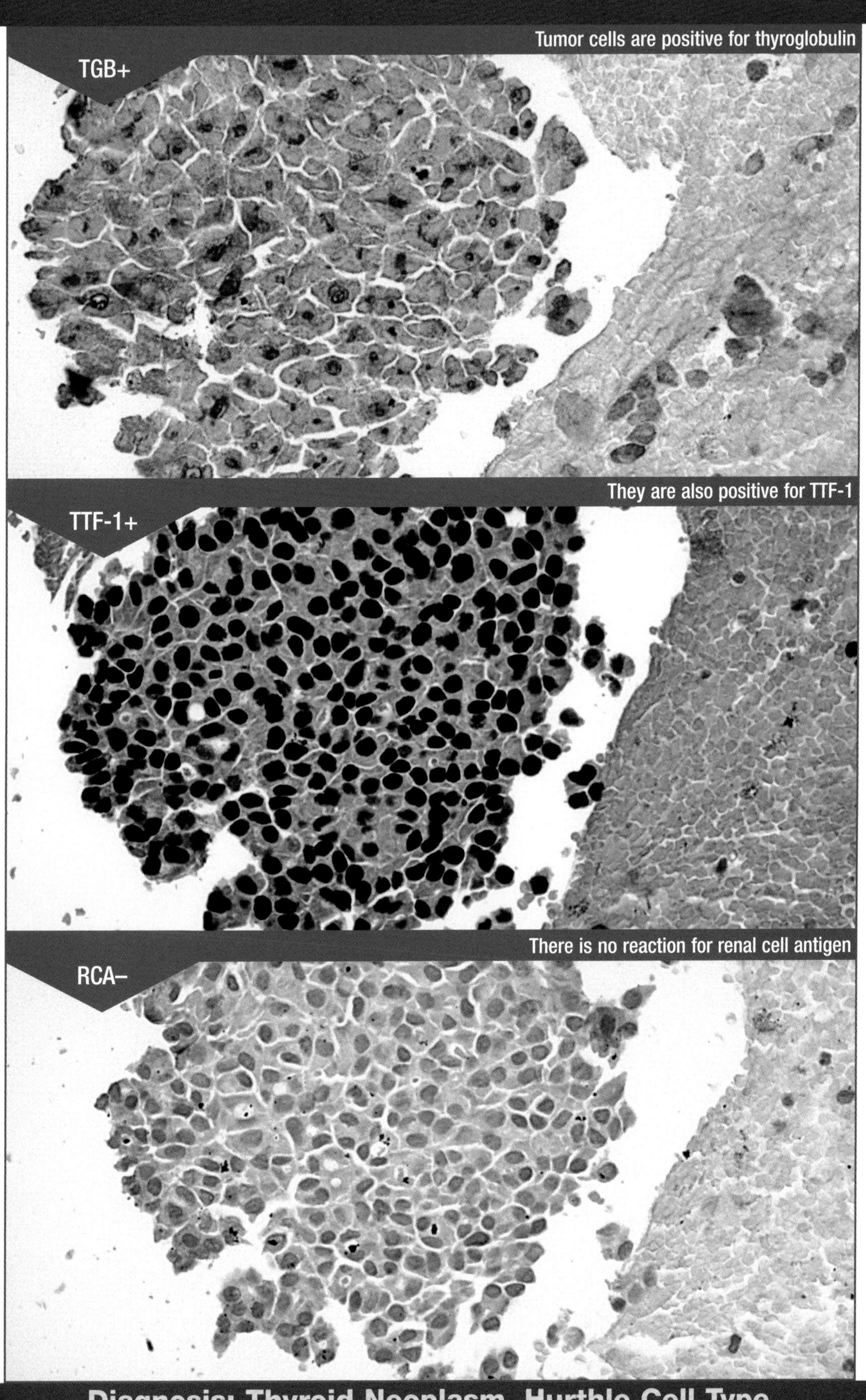

Diagnosis: Thyroid Neoplasm, Hurthle Cell Type

Bronchial biopsy

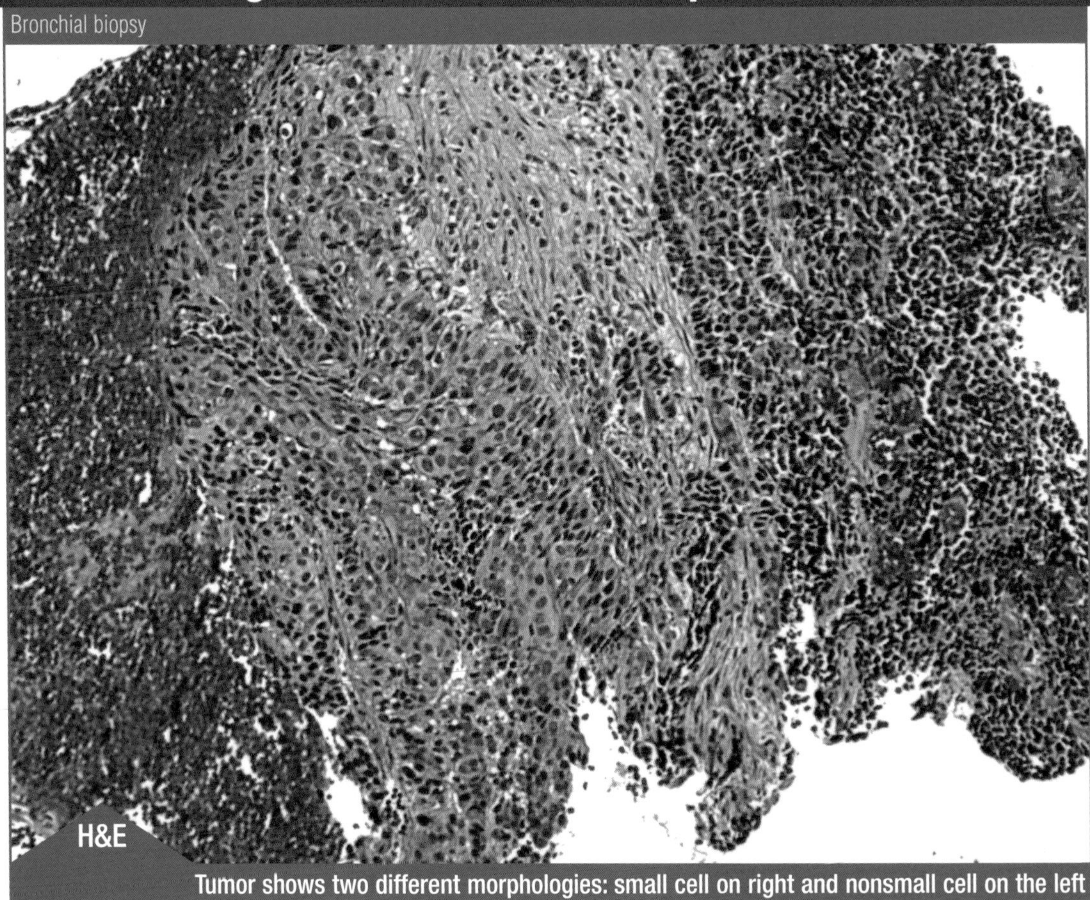

Tumor shows two different morphologies: small cell on right and nonsmall cell on the left

Small Cell Lung Carcinoma vs Basaloid Squamous Cell Carcinoma	TTF-1	p63
Small Cell Lung Carcinoma	+	–
Basaloid Squamous Cell Carcinoma	–	+

Helpful Hints

Basaloid squamous cell carcinomas of the lung may resemble small cell carcinomas particularly in bronchial biopsies. Since basaloid carcinoma is a form of squamous cell carcinoma, it usually does not react for **TTF-1**. On the other hand because squamous cell carcinomas express **p63**, this marker could be used to distinguish them from small cell carcinomas that do not react for p63. Since **chromogranin** is seen in less than 50% of small cell carcinomas, its positivity is helpful, but a negative reaction does not solve the above diagnostic problem.

The pattern of wide spectrum **cytokeratin** staining is also different in small cell and non-small cell lung cancers. While in the latter the reaction is dense and cytoplasmic, the former usually exhibits a perinuclear or punctate staining.

Tan 2003.

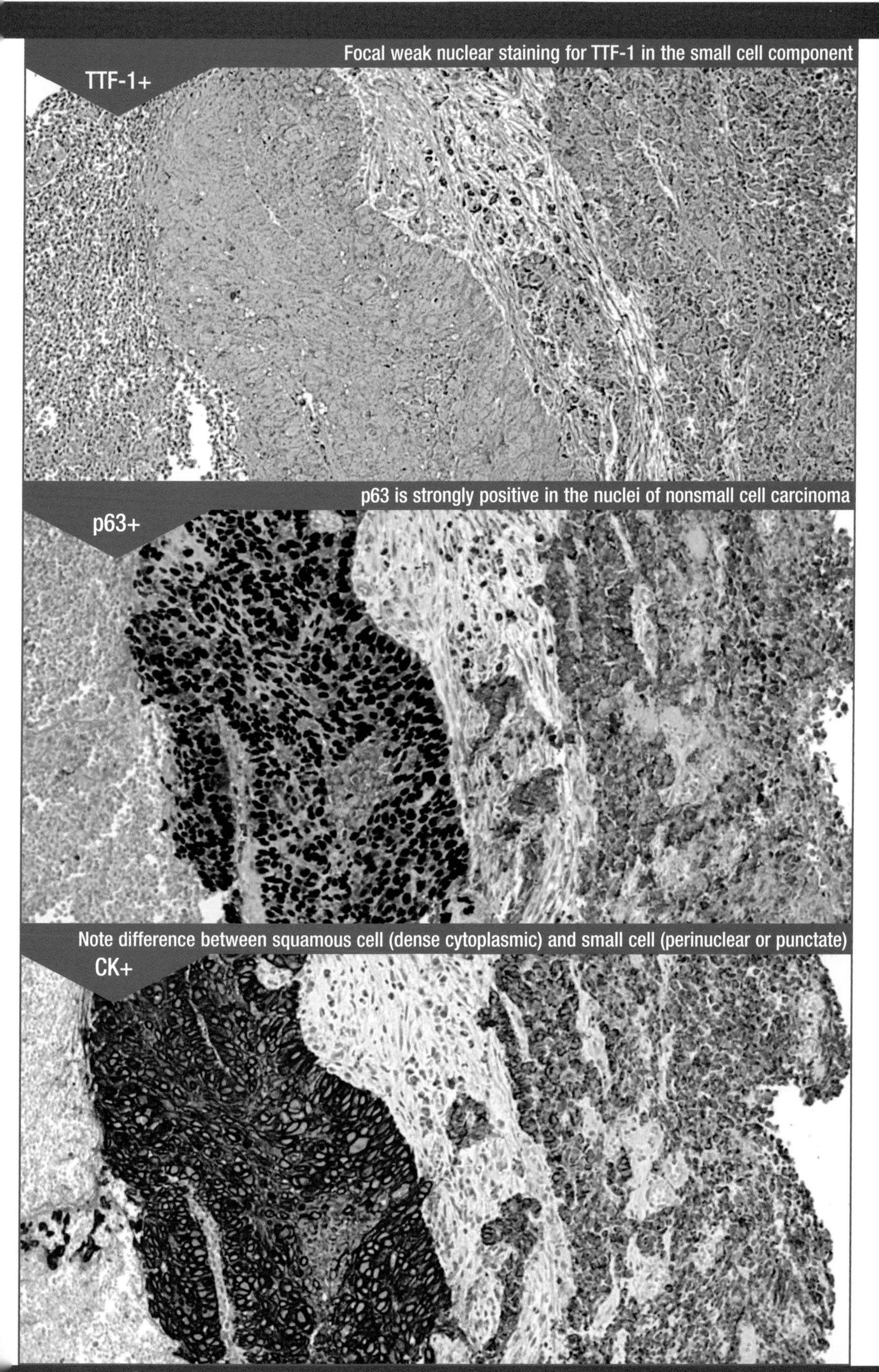

gnosis: Combined Small Cell *(right)* and Squamous Cell Ca *(left)*

Small Cell Lung Carcinoma vs Basaloid Squamous Cell Carcinoma

Bronchial biopsy

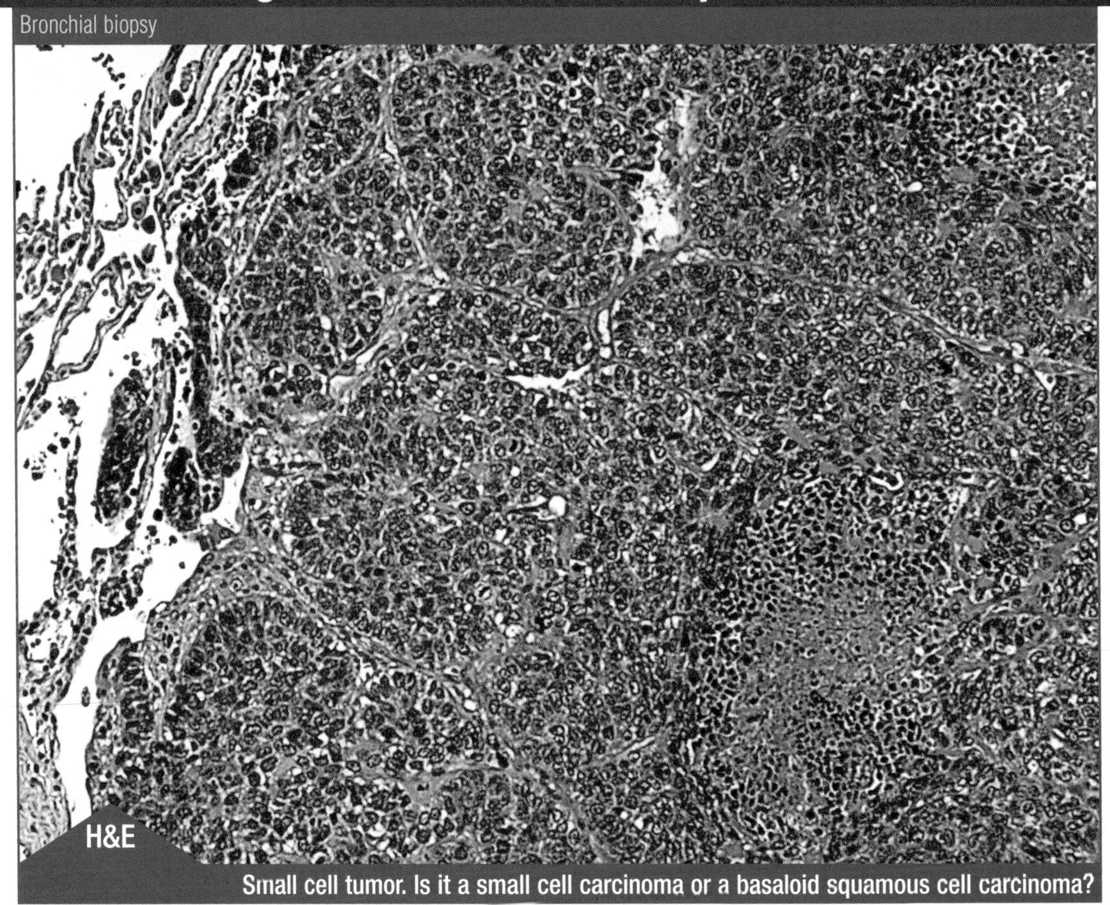

Small cell tumor. Is it a small cell carcinoma or a basaloid squamous cell carcinoma?

Small Cell Lung Carcinoma vs Basaloid Squamous Cell Carcinoma	TTF-1	p63
Small Cell Lung Carcinoma	+	–
Basaloid Squamous Cell Carcinoma	–	+

Helpful Hints

Basaloid squamous cell carcinomas of the lung may resemble small cell carcinomas particularly in bronchial biopsies. Since basaloid carcinoma is a form of squamous cell carcinoma, it usually does not react for **TTF-1**. On the other hand because squamous cell carcinomas express **p63**, this marker could be used to distinguish them from small cell carcinomas that do not react for p63. Since **chromogranin** is seen in less than 50% of small cell carcinomas, its positivity is helpful, but a negative reaction does not solve the above diagnostic problem.

The pattern of wide spectrum **cytokeratin** staining is also different in small cell and non-small cell lung cancers. While in the latter the reaction is dense and cytoplasmic, the former usually exhibits a perinuclear or punctate staining.

Tan 2003.

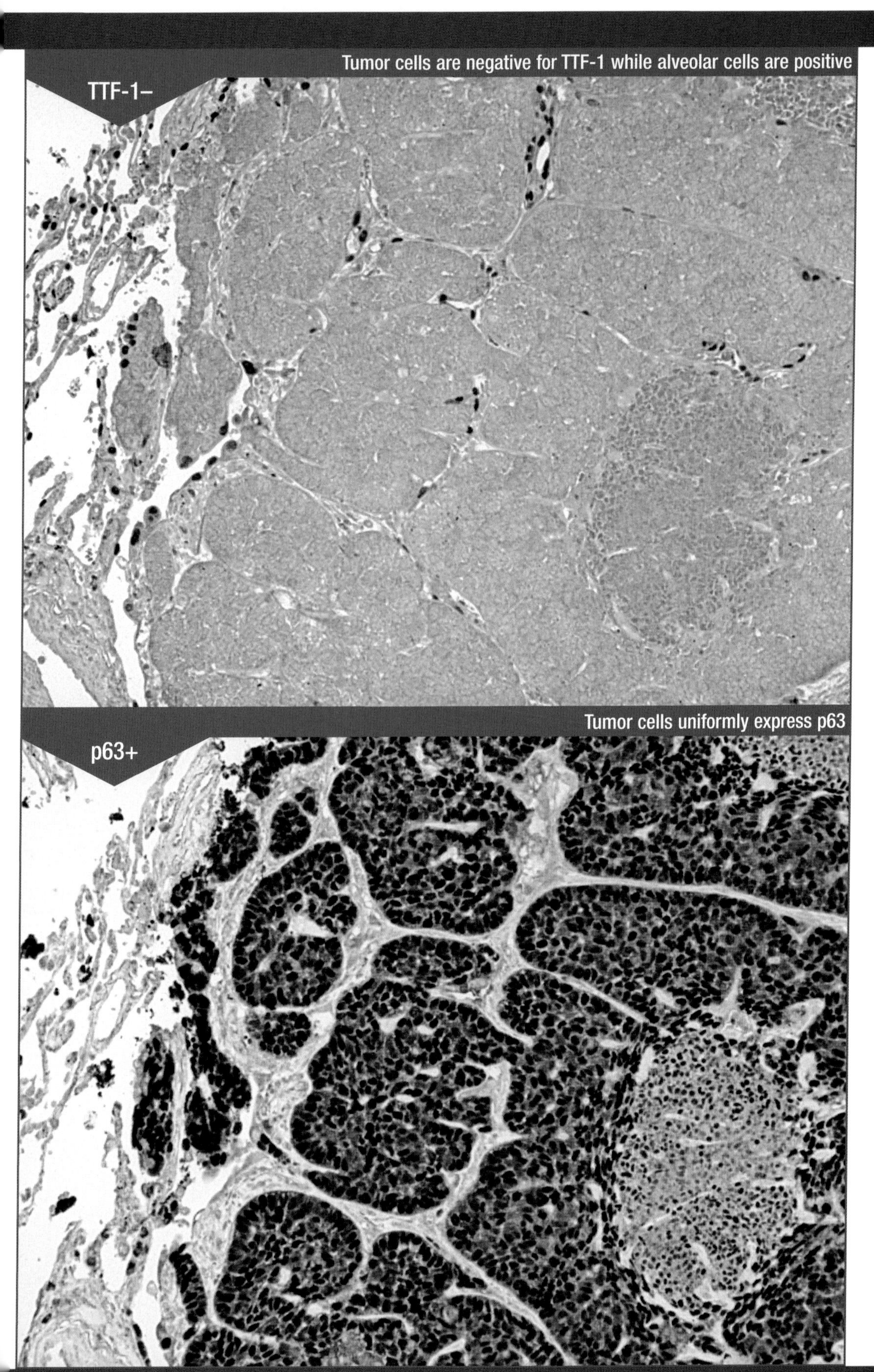

Diagnosis: Basaloid Squamous Cell Carcinoma

Bronchial biopsy in a patient with history of colonic carcinoma

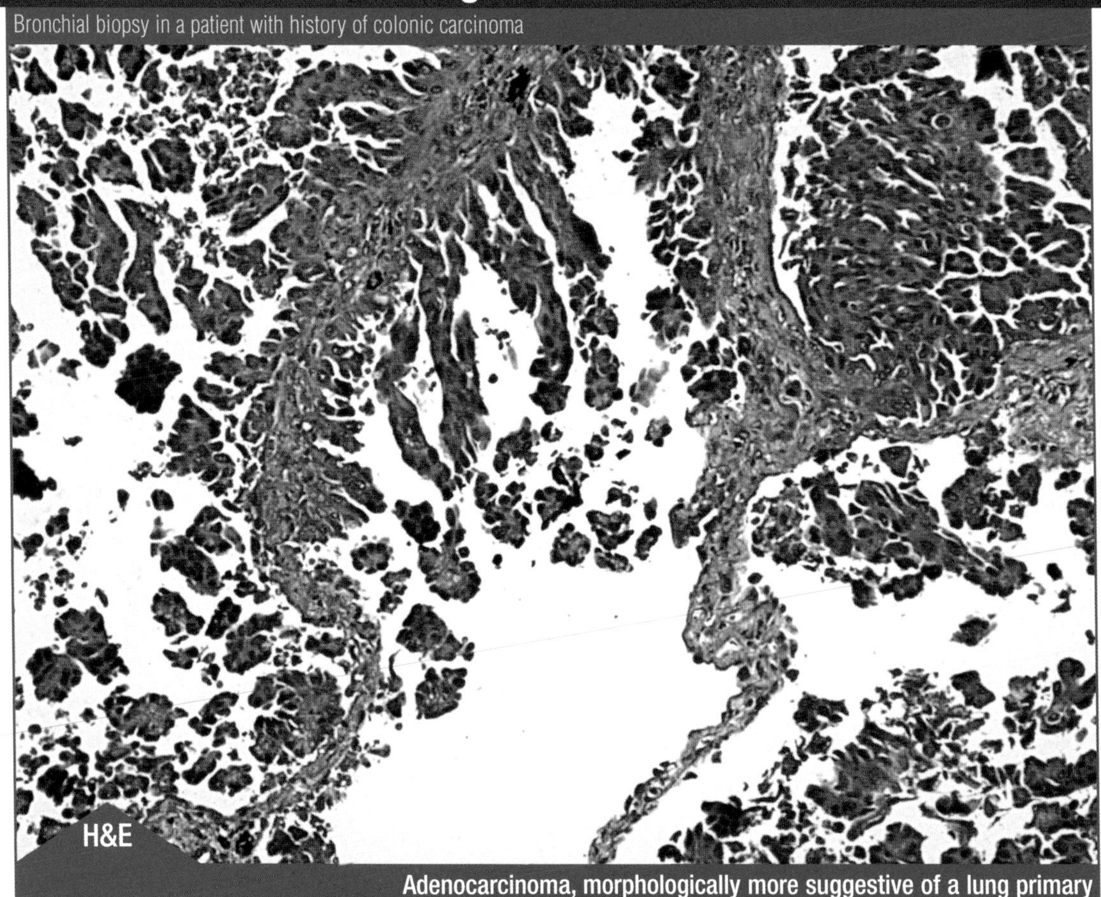

Adenocarcinoma, morphologically more suggestive of a lung primary

Adenocarcinoma of Lung vs Metastatic Colonic Carcinoma		
	TTF-1	CK20
Adenocarcinoma of Lung	+	–
Met Colonic Carcinoma	–	+

Helpful Hints

The majority of adenocarcinomas of the lung are positive for **TTF-1** and **CK20**. The exception is the mucinous type of bronchioloalveolar carcinoma, which in addition to TTF-1-negativity, may be positive for CK20. These tumors, however, are usually positive for **CK7** whereas metastatic colonic carcinomas to the lung are usually negative for CK7.

Lau 2002a.

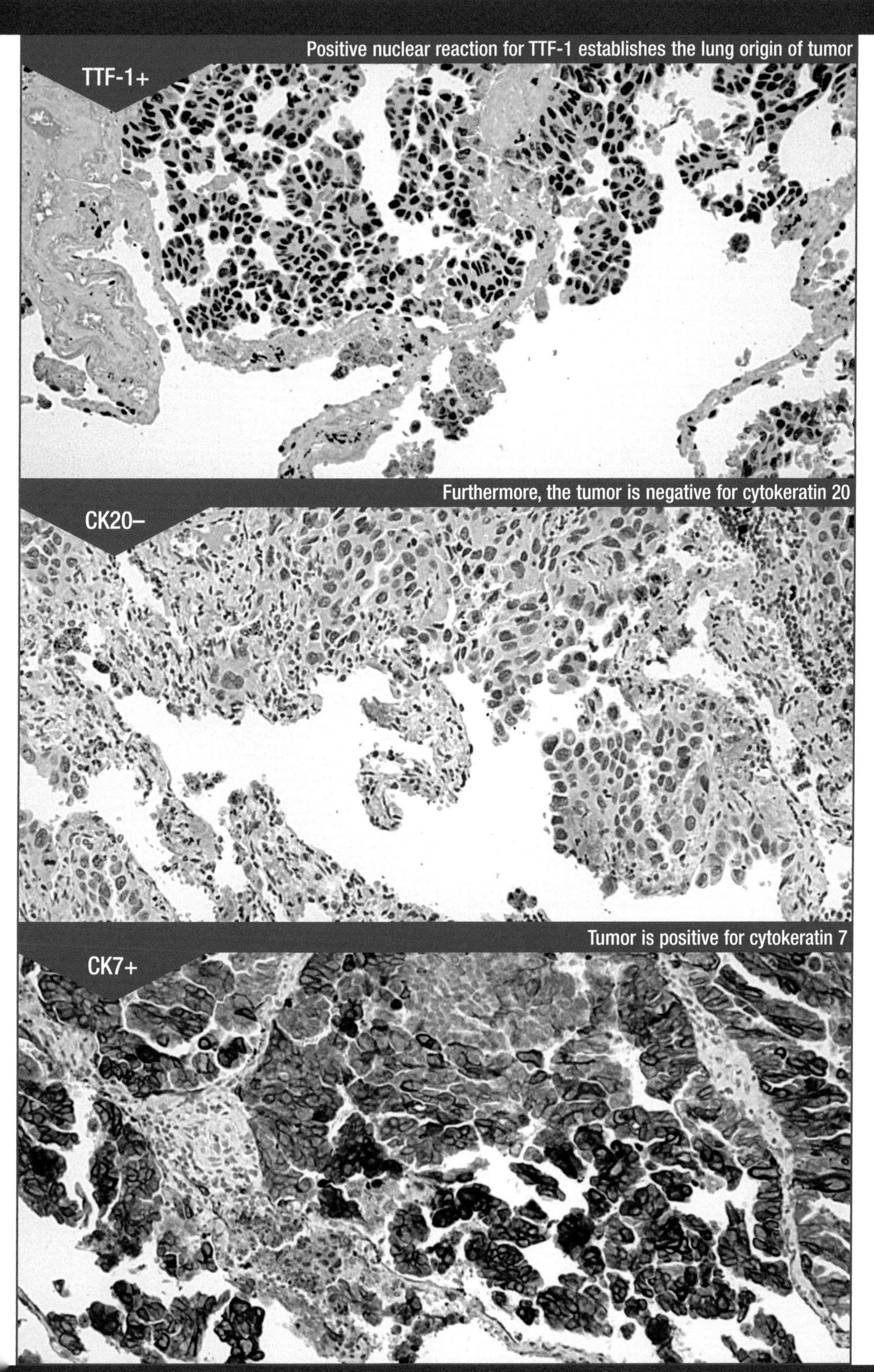

Diagnosis: Adenocarcinoma of Lung

Wedge resection of lung in a patient with history of colon cancer

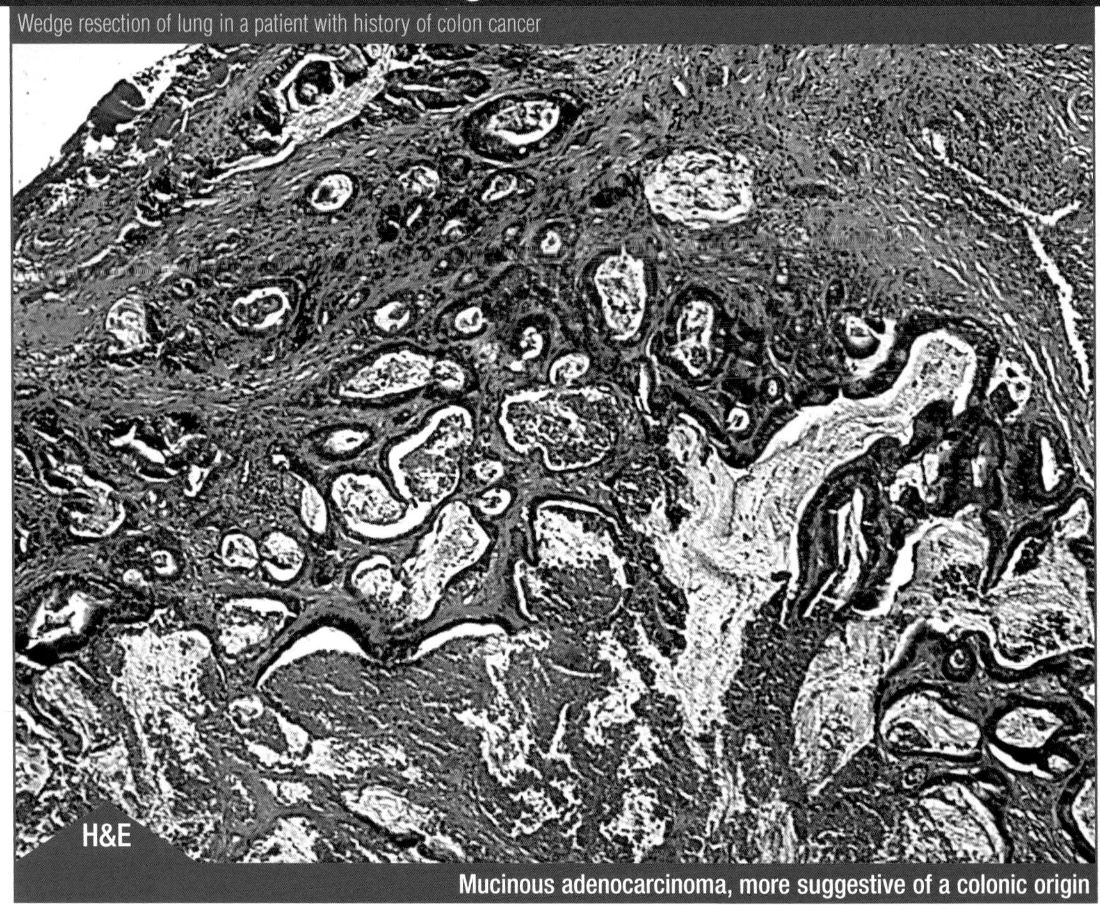

Mucinous adenocarcinoma, more suggestive of a colonic origin

Adenocarcinoma of Lung vs Metastatic Colonic Carcinoma			
	TTF-1	CK20	CK7
Adenocarcinoma of Lung	+	–	+
Met Colonic Carcinoma	–	+	–

Helpful Hints

The majority of adenocarcinomas of the lung are positive for **TTF-1**. The exception is the mucinous type of bronchioloalveolar carcinoma, which in addition to TTF-1-negativity, may be positive for **CK20**. These tumors, however, are usually positive for **CK7** whereas metastatic colonic carcinomas to the lung are usually negative for CK7.

Lau 2002a.

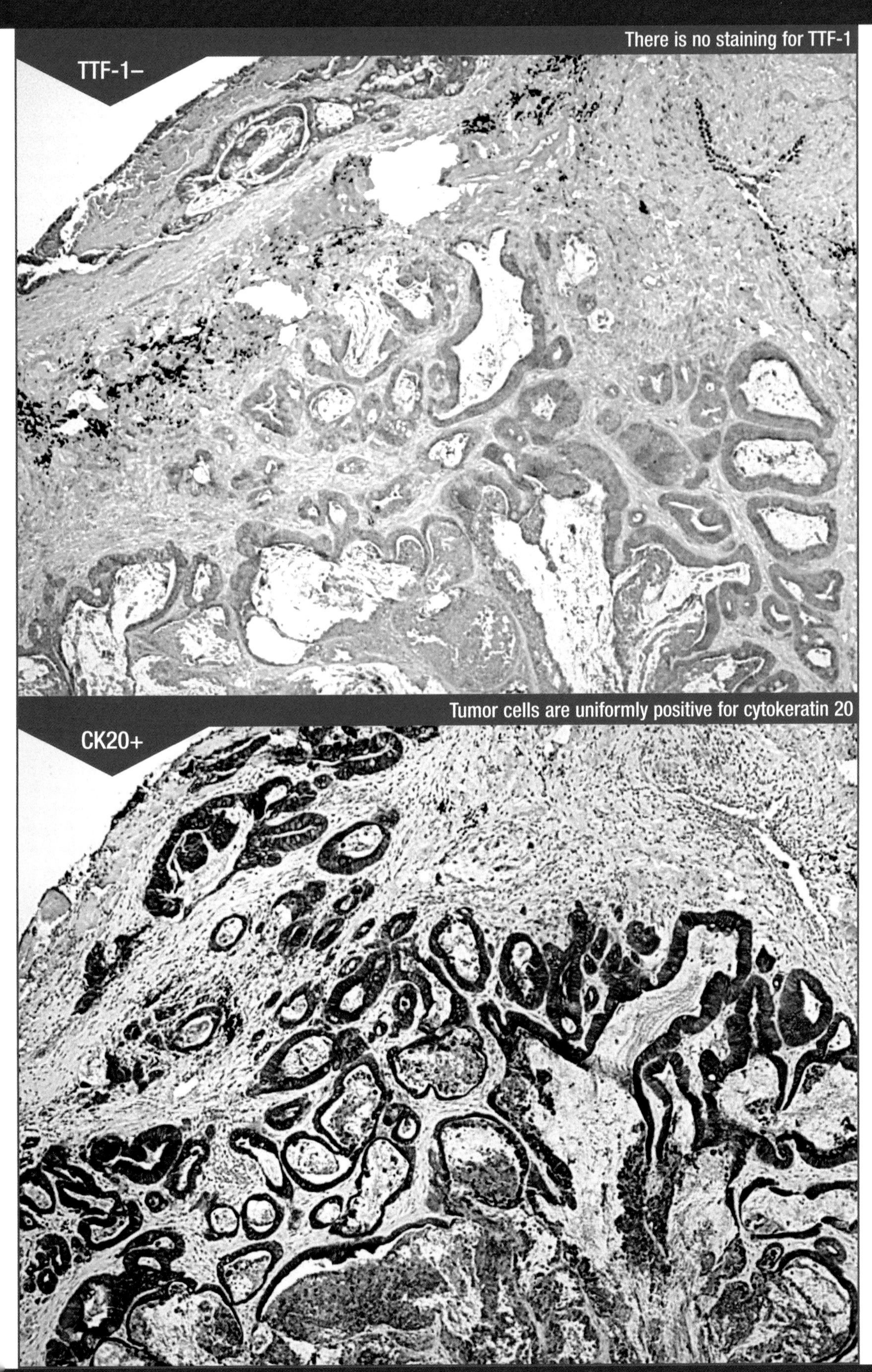

Diagnosis: Metastatic Colonic Carcinoma

Adenocarcinoma of Lung vs Metastatic Renal Cell Carcinoma

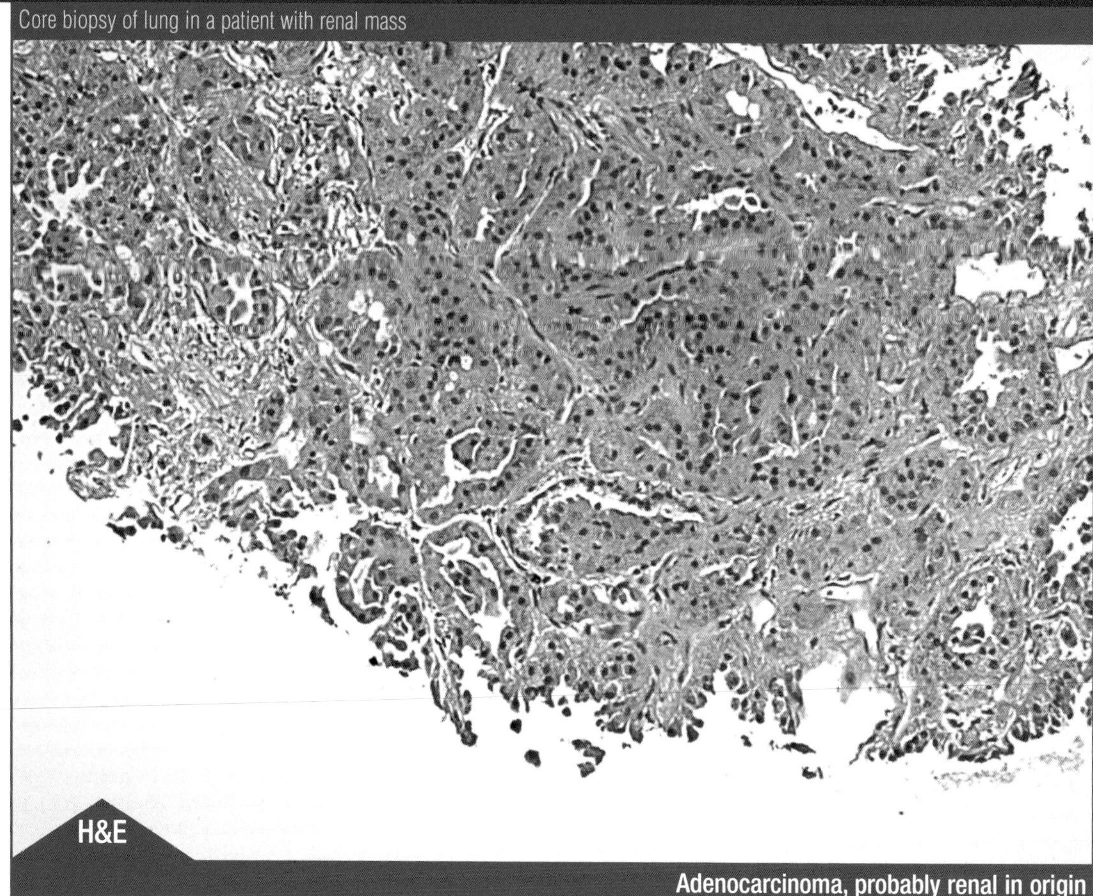

Adenocarcinoma, probably renal in origin

Adenocarcinoma of Lung vs Metastatic Renal Cell Carcinoma			
	TTF-1	CEA	RCA
Adenocarcinoma of Lung	+	+	–
Mets Renal Cell Carcinoma	–	–	+

Helpful Hints

While most adenocarcinomas of the lung react positively for **TTF-1** and **carcinoembryonic antigen** (**CEA**), renal cell carcinomas are always negative for these antigens. Cytokeratin subtypes and epithelial membrane antigen are not helpful in this differential diagnosis. **Renal cell antigen** (**RCA**) is more frequently expressed by the clear cell type of renal cell carcinomas but other variants may also be positive. Adenocarcinomas of the lung are always negative for renal cell antigen.

Moldvay 2004.

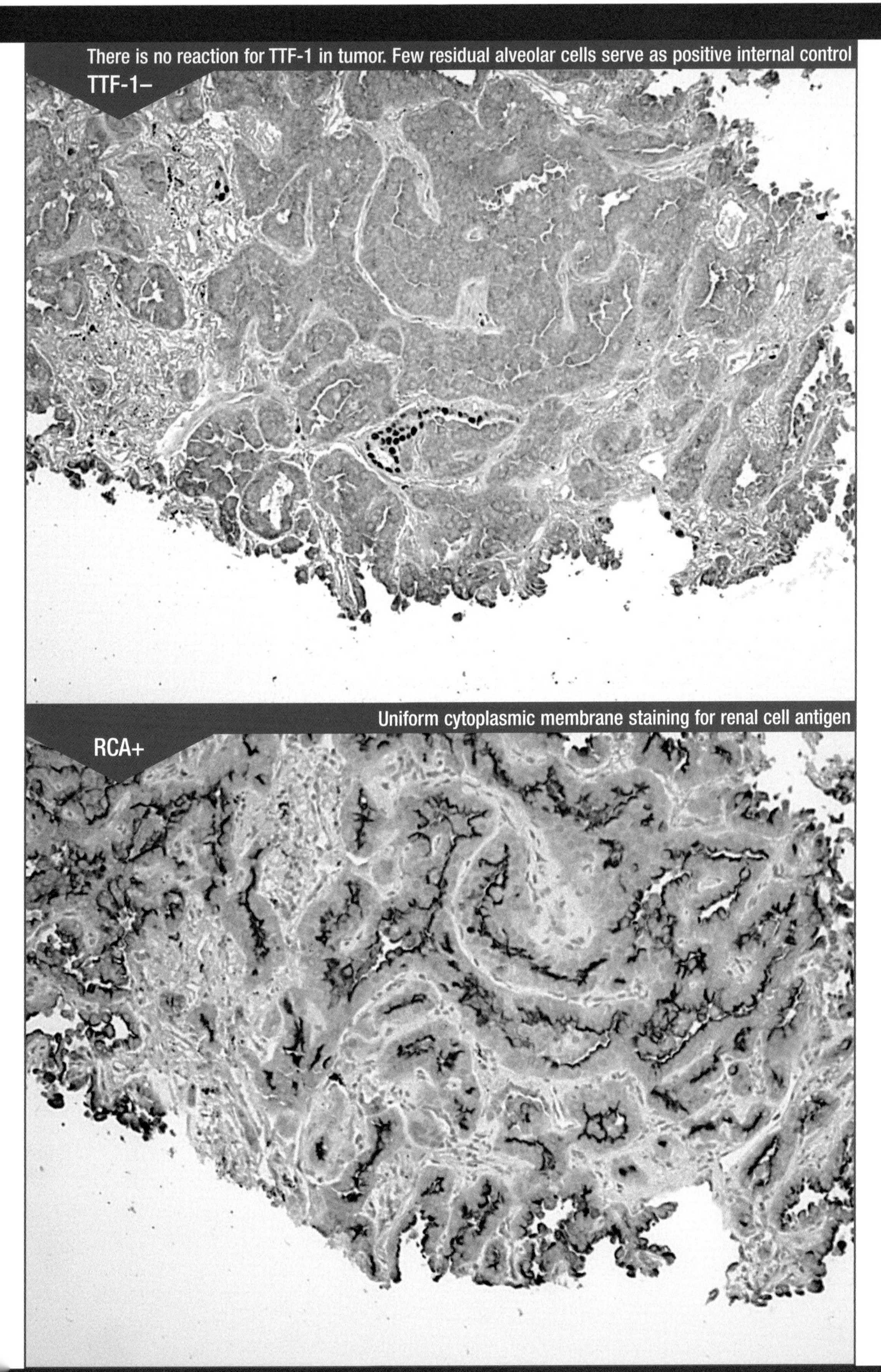

Diagnosis: Metastatic Renal Cell Carcinoma

Lobectomy specimen; no history of renal tumor

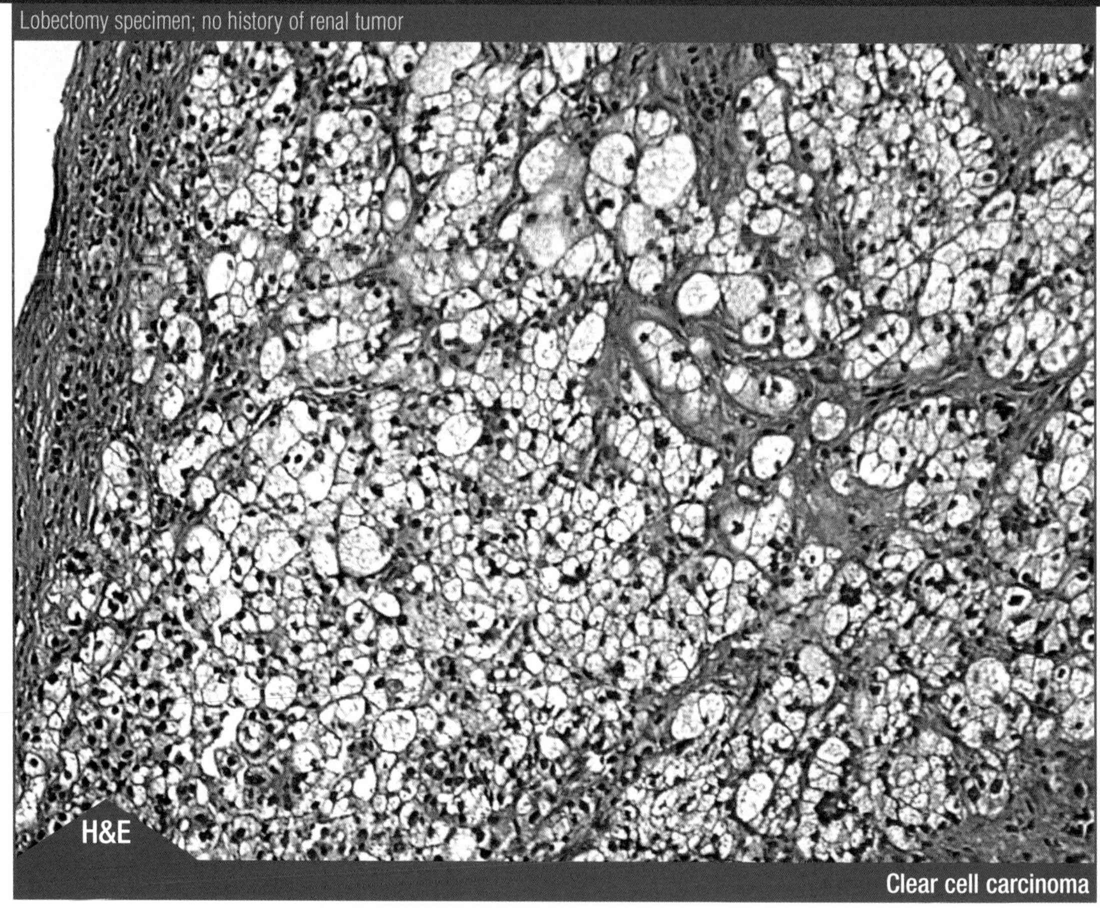

Clear cell carcinoma

Adenocarcinoma of Lung vs Metastatic Renal Cell Carcinoma			
	TTF-1	CEA	RCA
Adenocarcinoma of Lung	+	+	–
Mets Renal Cell Carcinoma	–	–	+

Helpful Hints

While most adenocarcinomas of the lung react positively for **TTF-1** and **carcinoembryonic antigen (CEA)**, renal cell carcinomas are always negative for these antigens. Cytokeratin subtypes and epithelial membrane antigen are not helpful in this differential diagnosis. **Renal cell antigen (RCA)** is more frequently expressed by the clear cell type of renal cell carcinomas but other variants may also be positive. Adenocarcinomas of the lung are always negative for renal cell antigen.

Moldvay 2004.

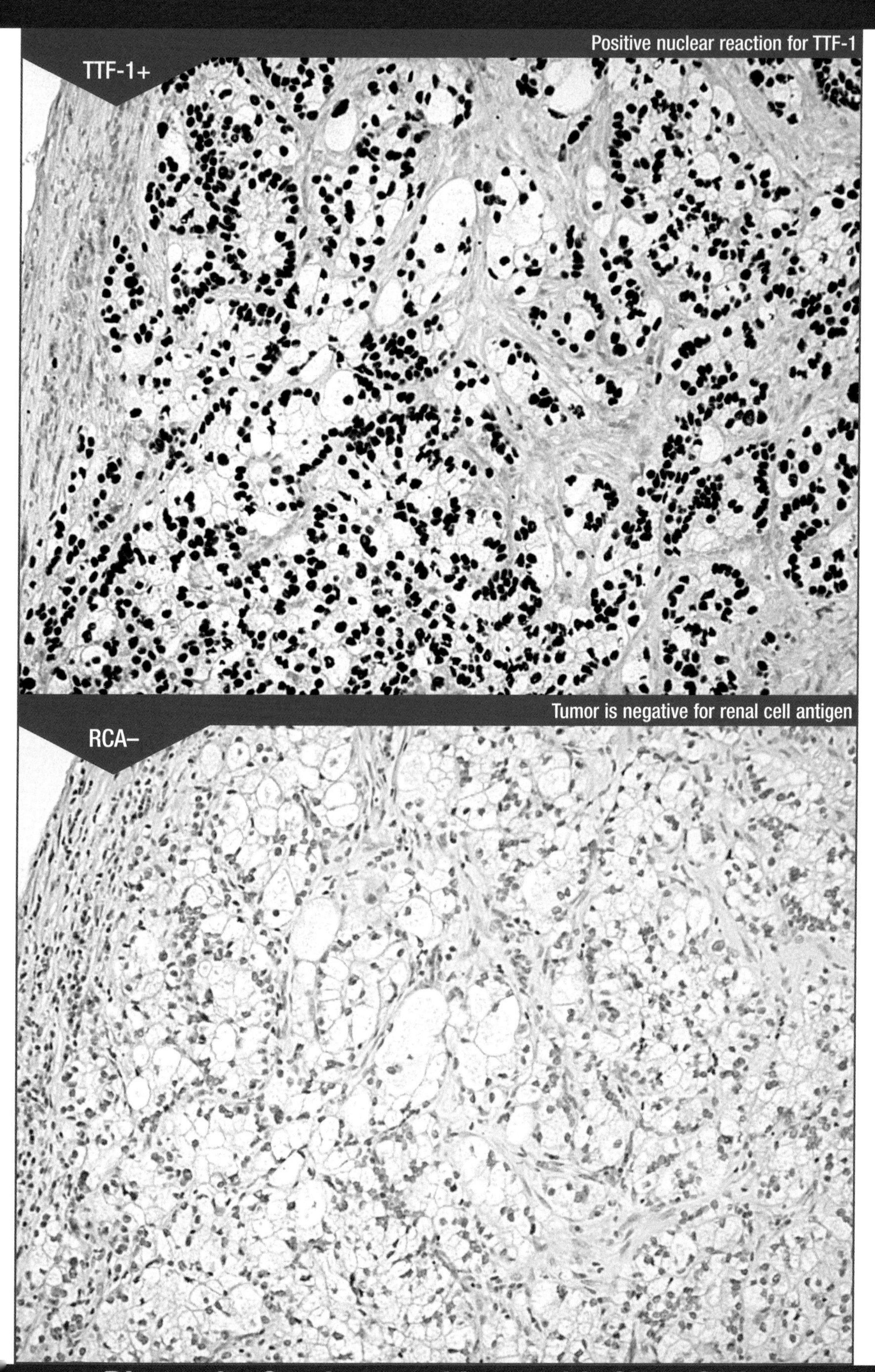

Diagnosis: Carcinoma of Lung with Clear Cells

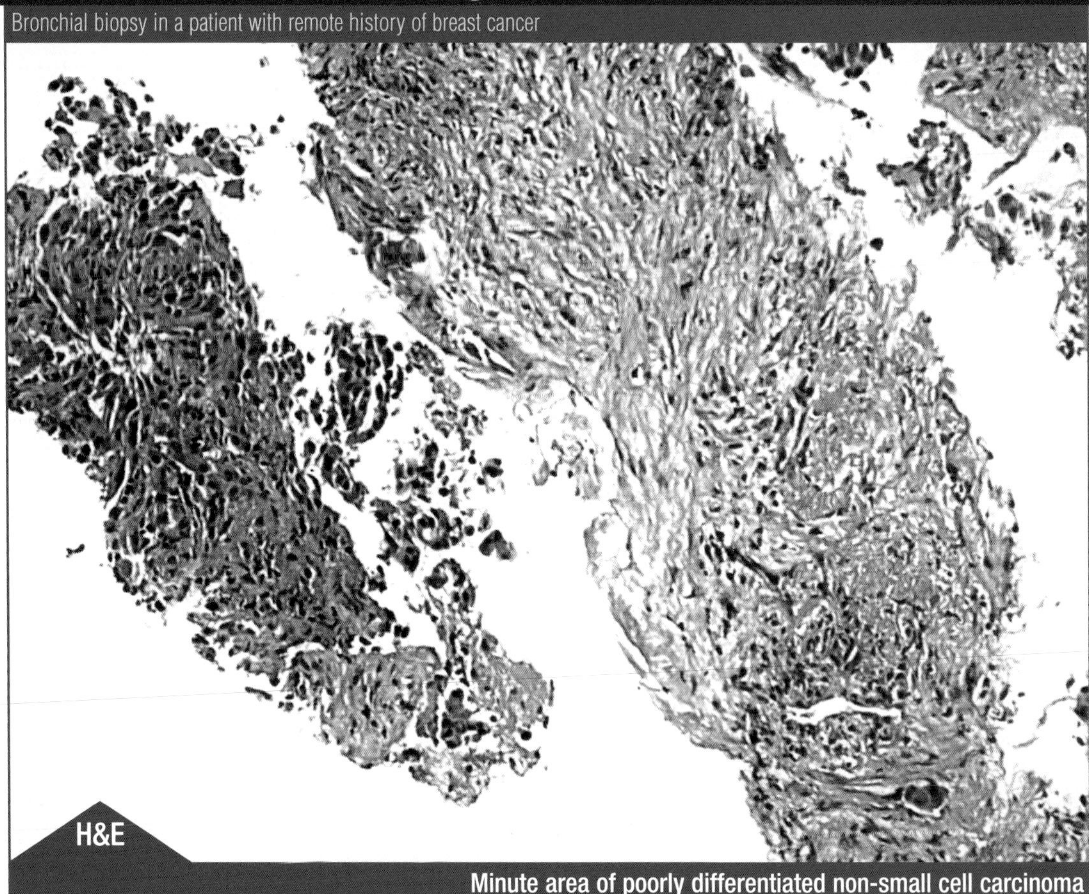

Bronchial biopsy in a patient with remote history of breast cancer

Minute area of poorly differentiated non-small cell carcinoma

Adenocarcinoma of Lung vs Metastatic Breast Carcinoma		
	TTF-1	Estrogen Receptor (ER)
Adenocarcinoma of Lung	+	–
Metastatic Breast Carcinoma	–	S

Helpful Hints

This is not an uncommon differential diagnostic problem; a bronchial biopsy from a patient with distant history of breast cancer. Unlike the aggressive ER-negative types of breast cancer that metastasize early, late metastasis from a breast primary is usually ER-positive. TTF-1 is not expressed by mammary carcinomas and hence, the combination of estrogen receptor and TTF-1 is usually sufficient to resolve this diagnostic problem. With antibody ER-1D5, lung carcinomas are ordinarily negative for estrogen receptor.

Nadji 2005.

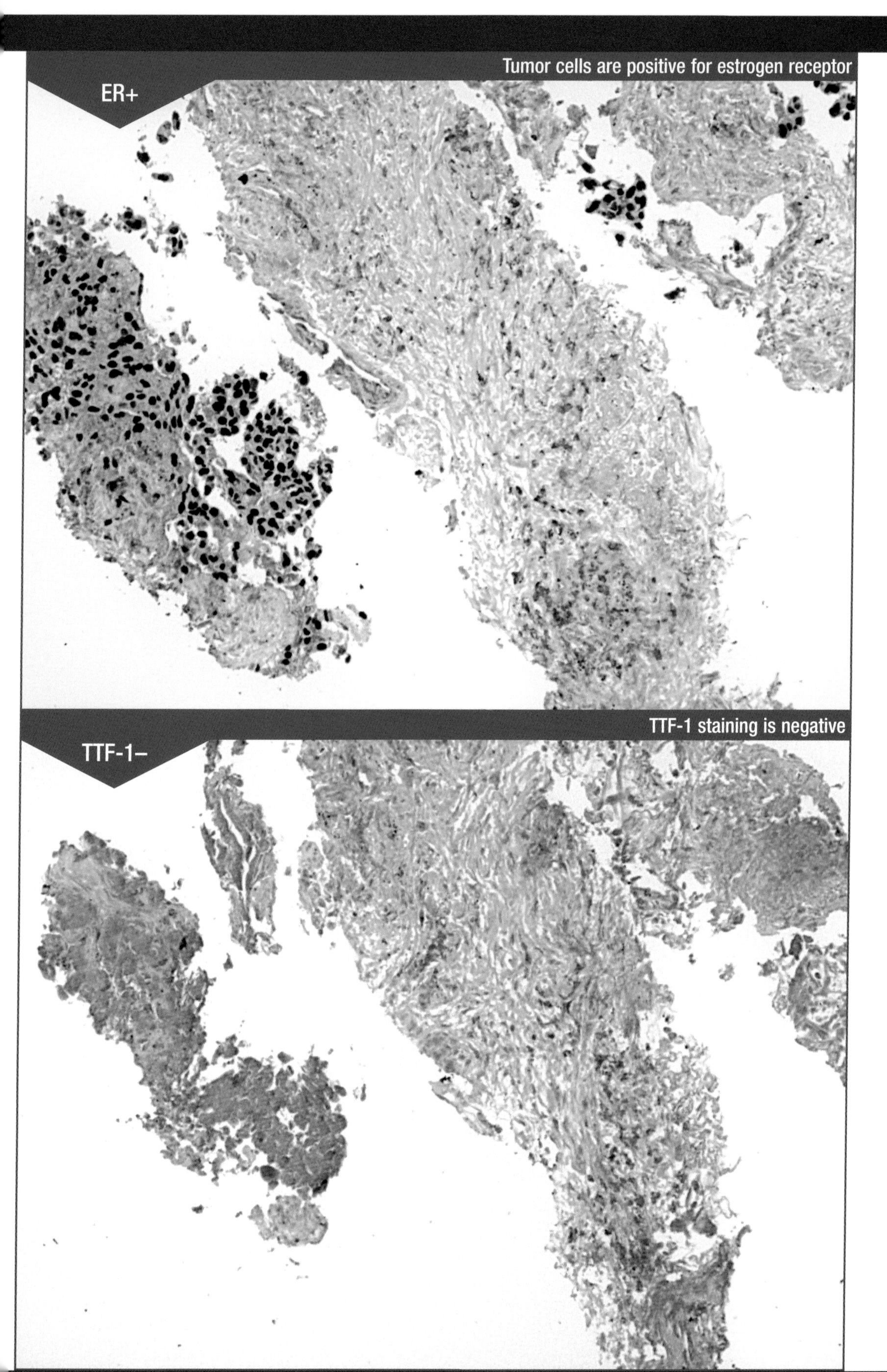

Diagnosis: Metastatic Breast Carcinoma

Bronchial biopsy

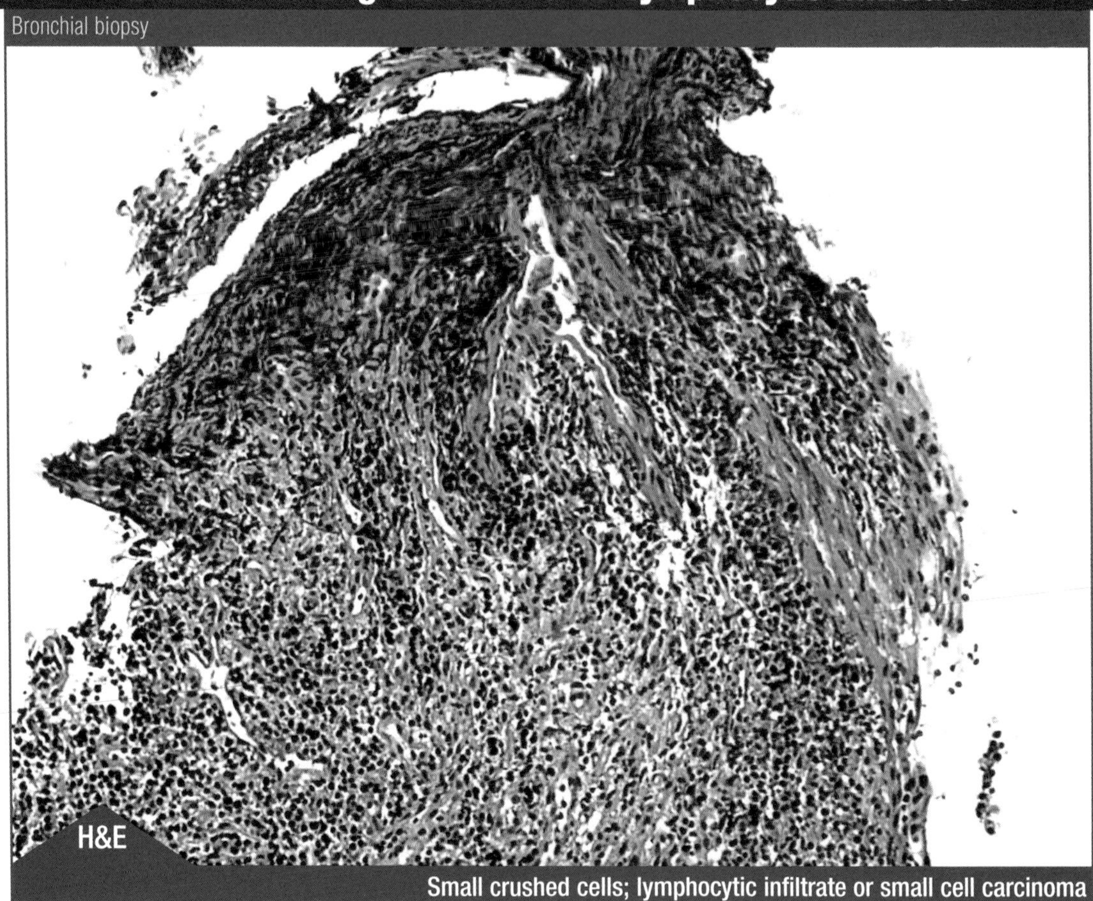

Small crushed cells; lymphocytic infiltrate or small cell carcinoma

Small Cell Lung Carcinoma vs Lymphocytic Infiltrate		
	Cytokeratin (CK)	CD45
Small Cell Lung Carcinoma	+	–
Lymphocytic Infiltrate	–	+

Helpful Hints

This is a very common diagnostic problem in small, crushed biopsies of the lung. **CD45** stains lymphocytic infiltrate while cytokeratin shows a punctate or perinuclear reaction in small cell carcinomas. Rarely, when cytokeratin reaction is equivocal, one may use epithelial membrane antigen for identifying small cell carcinomas. **TTF-1** is also helpful because more than 80% of small cell lung cancers are positive for this marker.

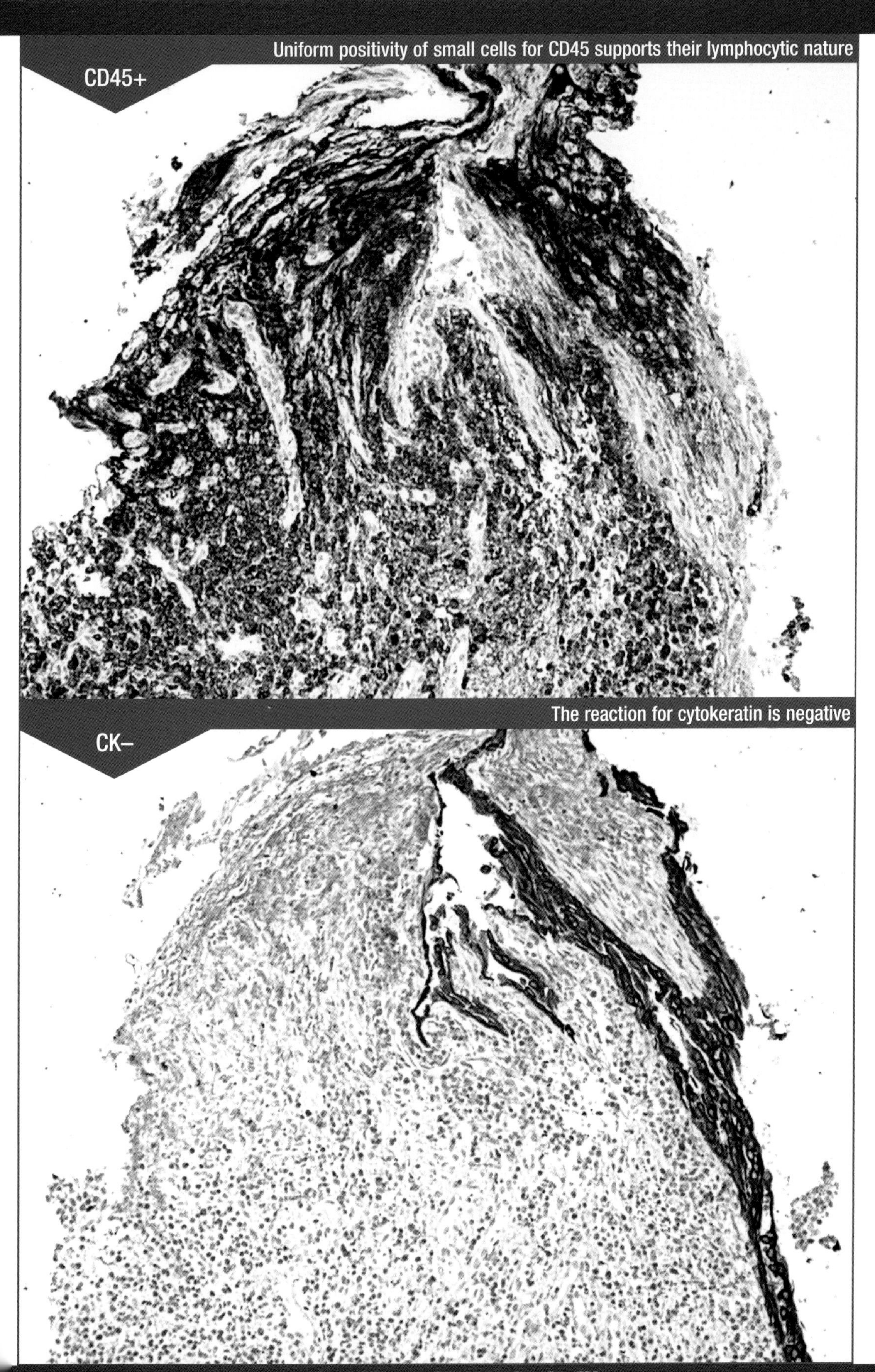

Diagnosis: Lymphocytic Infiltrate

Bronchial biopsy

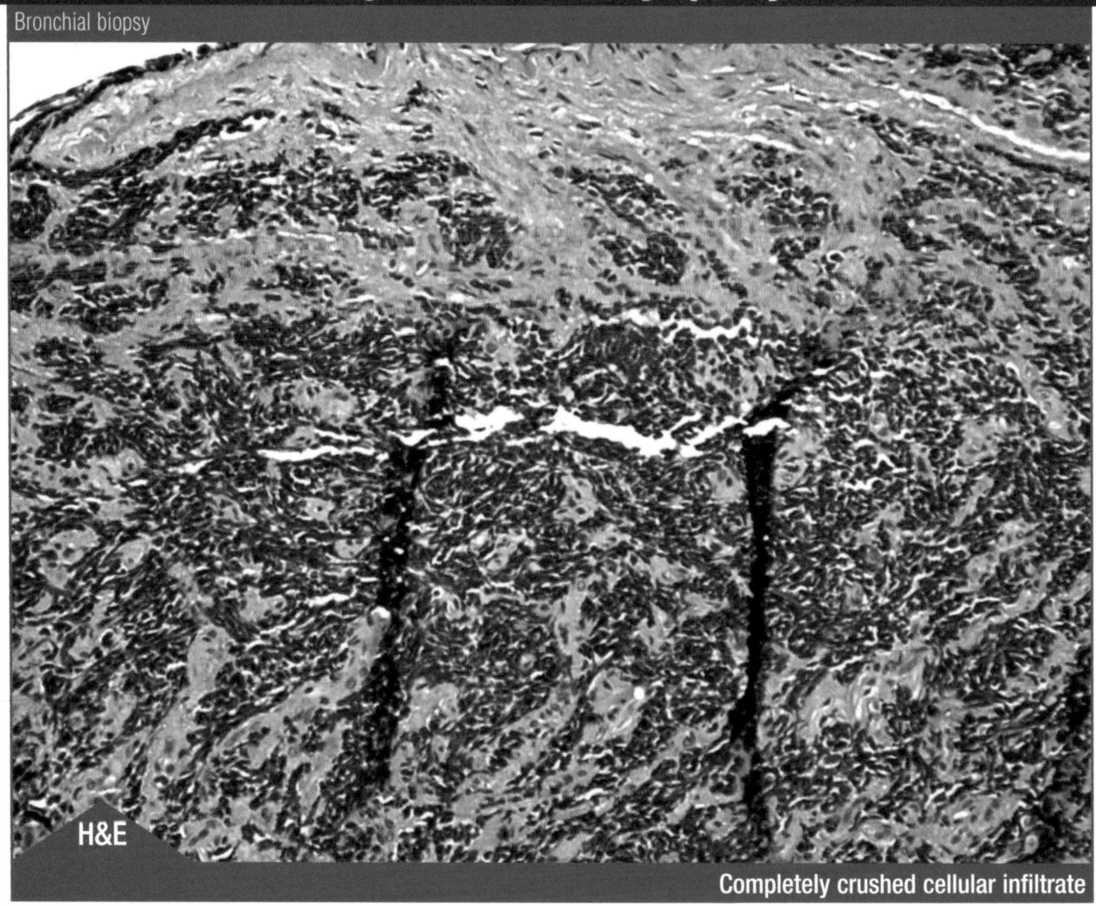

Completely crushed cellular infiltrate

Small Cell Lung Carcinoma vs Lymphocytic Infiltrate		
	Cytokeratin (CK)	CD45
Small Cell Lung Carcinoma	+	–
Lymphocytic Infiltrate	–	+

Helpful Hints

This is a very common diagnostic problem in small, crushed biopsies of the lung. **CD45** stains lymphocytic infiltrate while cytokeratin shows a punctate or perinuclear reaction in small cell carcinomas. Rarely, when cytokeratin reaction is equivocal, one may use epithelial membrane antigen for identifying small cell carcinomas. **TTF-1** is also helpful because more than 80% of small cell lung cancers are positive for this marker.

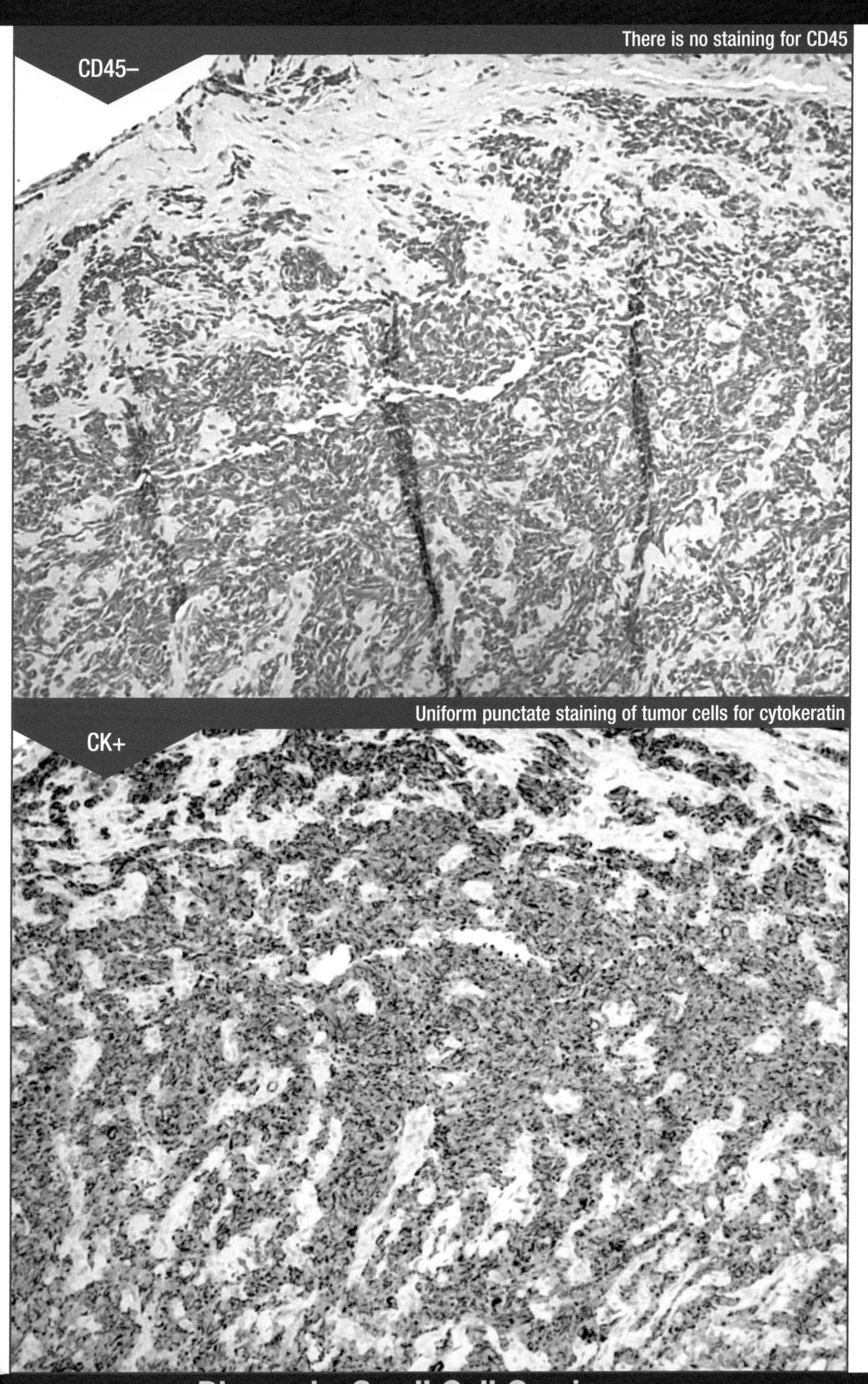

Diagnosis: Small Cell Carcinoma

Segmental resection of lung in a young adult with history of Ewing sarcoma

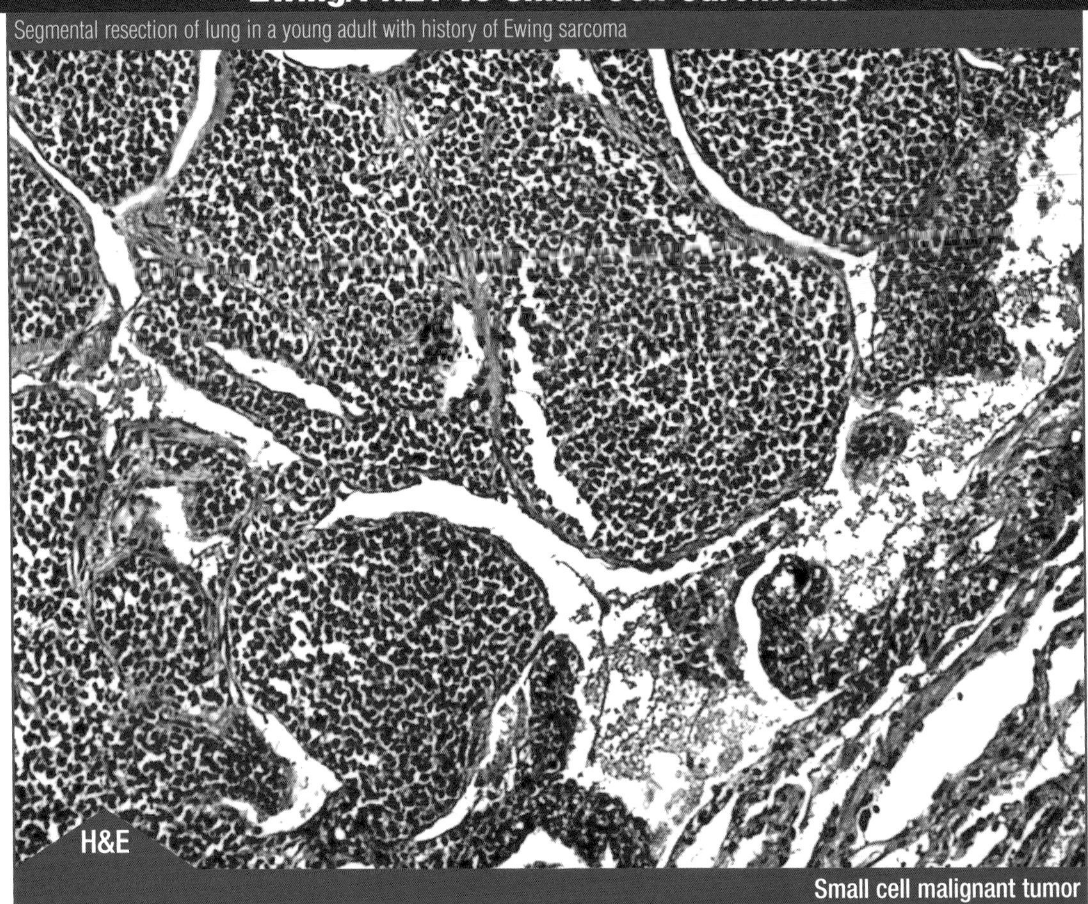

Small cell malignant tumor

Ewing/PNET in Lung vs Small Cell Carcinoma		
	CD99	Cytokeratin (CK)
Ewing/PNET	+	–
Small Cell Carcinoma	–	+

Helpful Hints

Although small cell carcinomas are extremely rare in children, Ewing sarcoma/PNET may occur in adults and hence create a differential diagnosis problem. The above choice of markers will help in separating these morphologic entities.

Wick 2000.

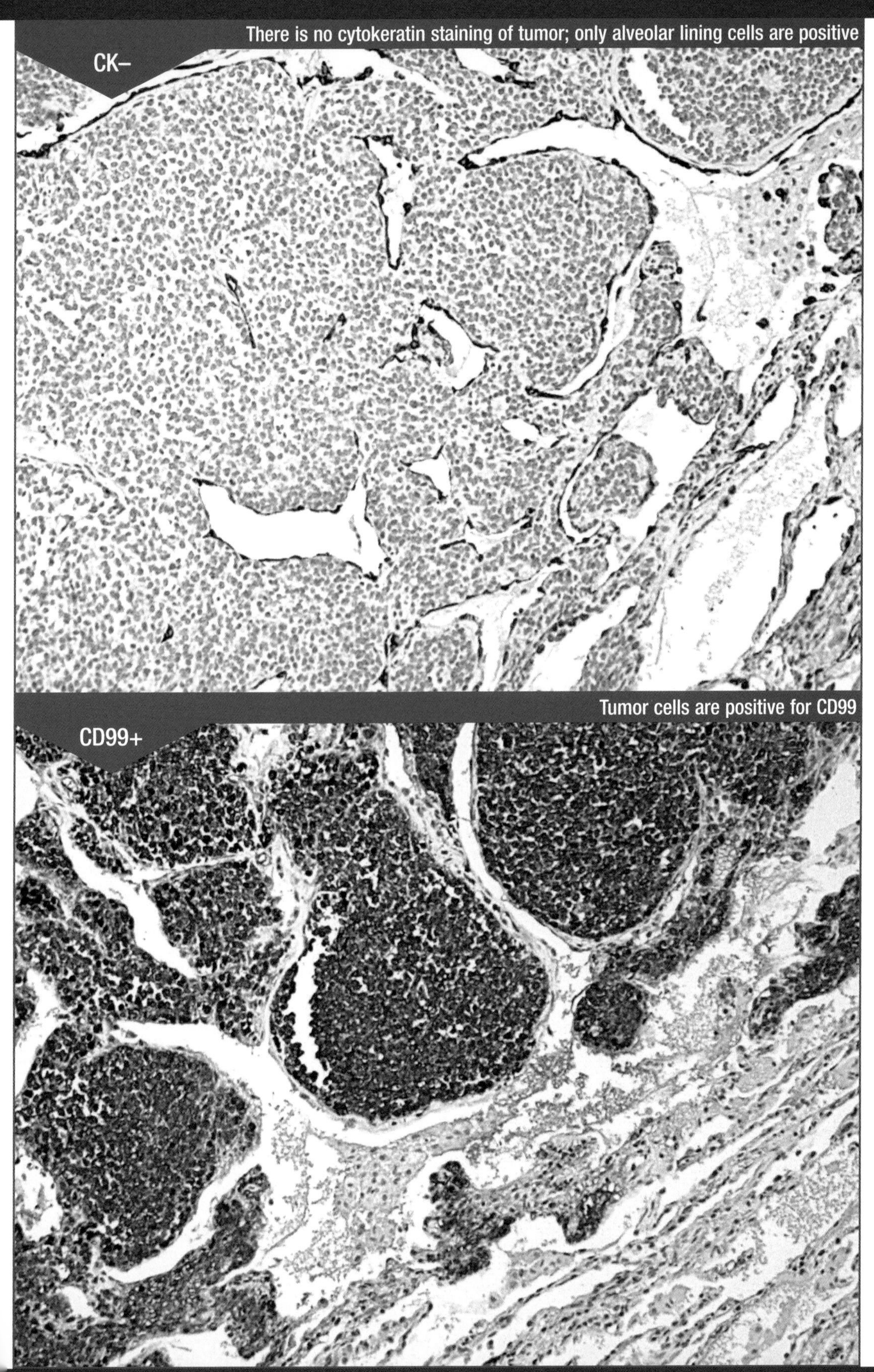

Diagnosis: Metastatic Ewing Sarcoma in Lung

Segmental resection of the lung

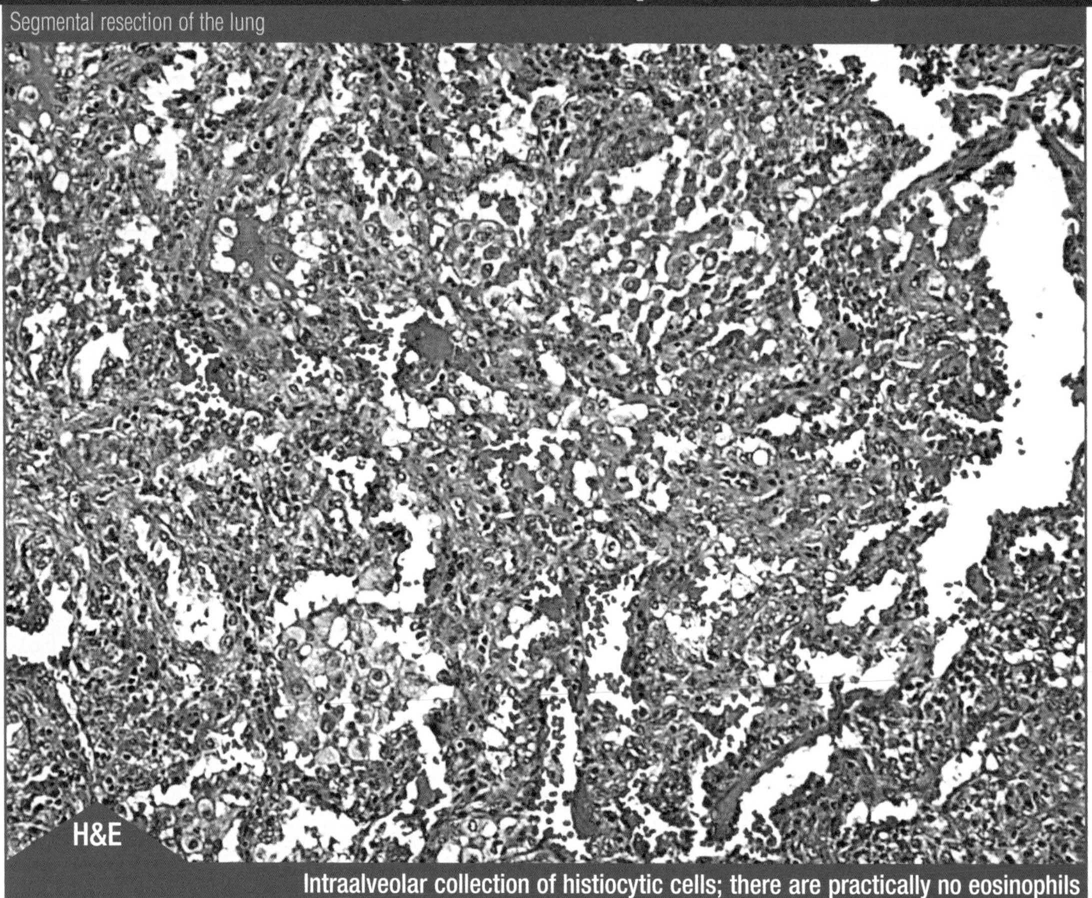

Intraalveolar collection of histiocytic cells; there are practically no eosinophils

Langerhans Cell Histiocytosis vs Nonspecific Histiocytic Infiltrate		
	CD1a	S100
Langerhans Cell Histiocytosis	+	+
Nonspecific Histiocytic Infiltrate	–	–

Helpful Hints

Langerhans Cell Histiocytosis of the lung (eosinophilic granuloma) may be difficult to diagnose on the basis of histology alone. These lesions often lack a population of eosinophils and may be mistaken for a collection of alveolar macrophages. Clinical suspicion is very important in using the **CD1a** and **S100 protein** in such lesions.

Pileri 2002.

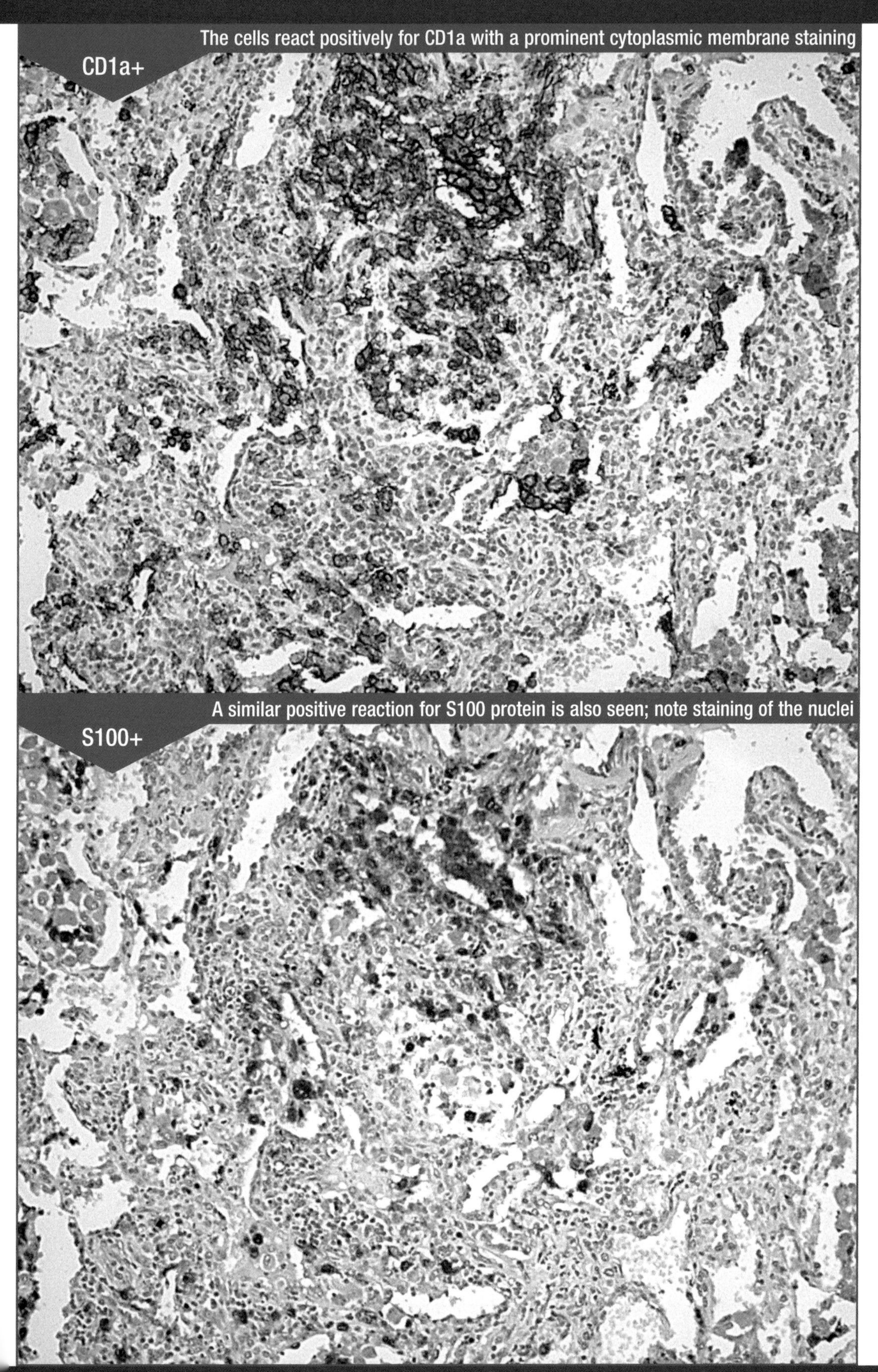

Diagnosis: Langerhans Cell Histiocytosis

Biopsy of a tumor mass involving pleura and pericardium

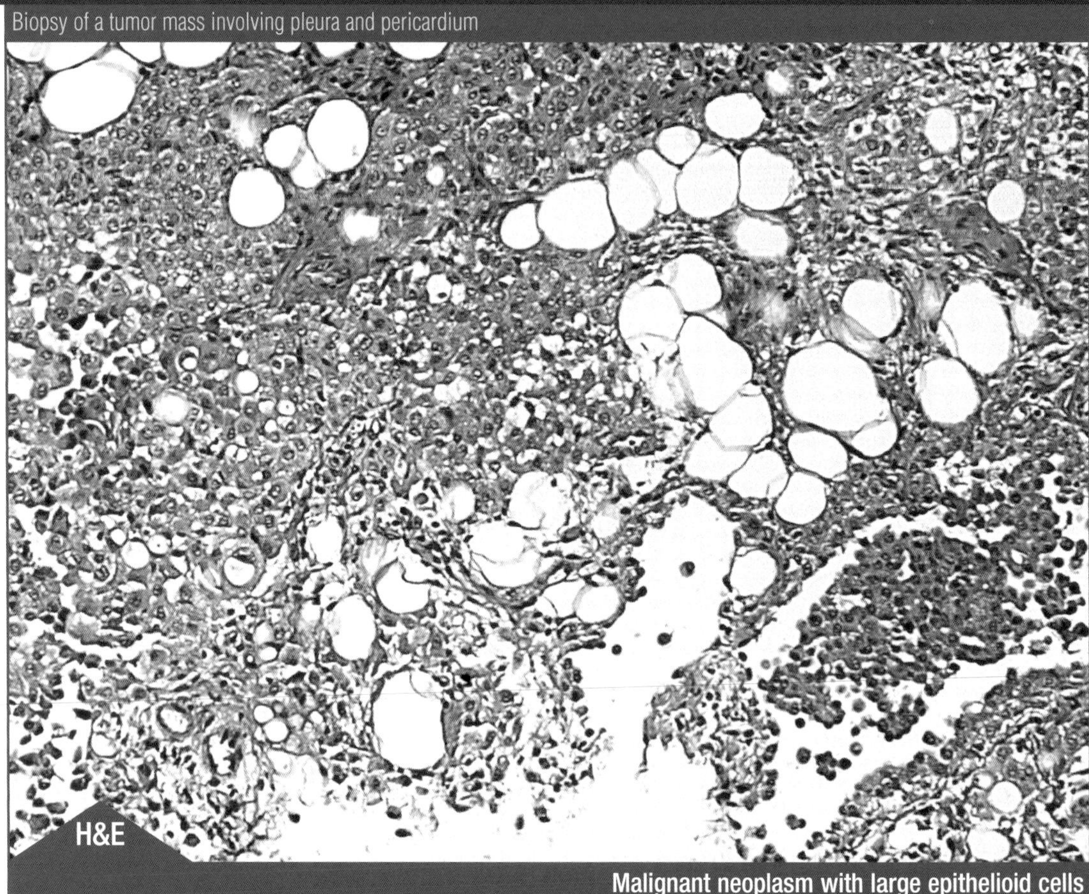

Malignant neoplasm with large epithelioid cells

Malignant Mesothelioma vs Adenocarcinoma of Lung	Calretinin	TTF-1	CEA
Malignant Mesothelioma	+	–	–
Adenocarcinoma of Lung	–	+	+

Helpful Hints

The differential diagnosis of malignant mesotheliomas from the look-alike lesions depends on the location of the tumor and morphologic subtype of mesothelioma. For example, malignant epithelial mesotheliomas of the pleura should be separated from adenocarcinomas, particularly from those of lung origin. While most adenocarcinomas of the lung express **carcinoembryonic antigen** (**CEA**) and **TTF-1**, mesotheliomas are always negative. Conversely, **calretinin** is seen in epithelial mesotheliomas but not in adenocarcinomas. It should be noted that the characteristic calretinin staining of malignant mesotheliomas is both nuclear and cytoplasmic. Cytoplasmic reaction alone is not diagnostic because it may be seen in some adenocarcinomas. Although there are a large group of markers purported to be helpful in the above differential diagnosis, the three markers suggested here resolve the majority of such differentials.

Comin 2001.

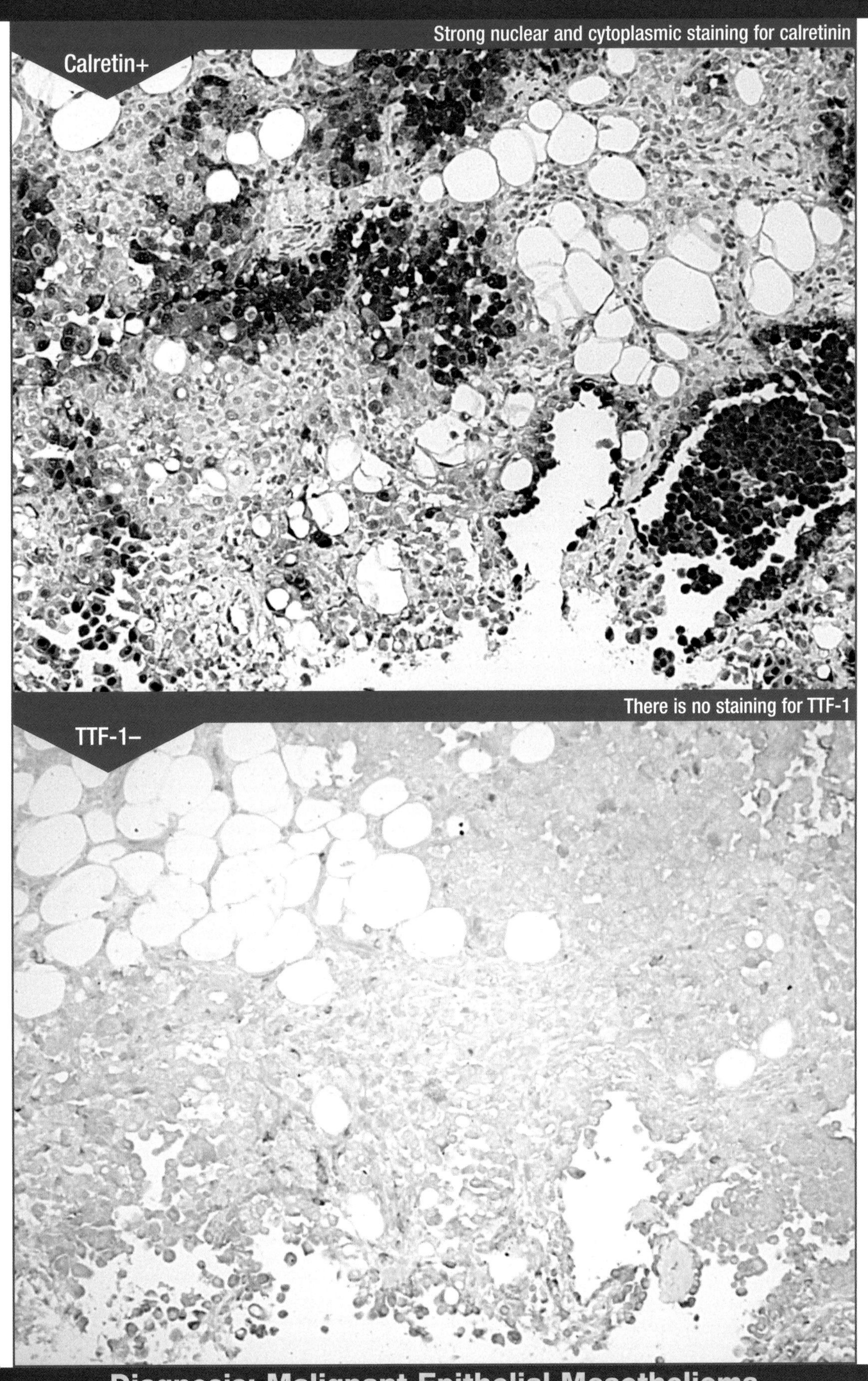

Diagnosis: Malignant Epithelial Mesothelioma

Pleural biopsy

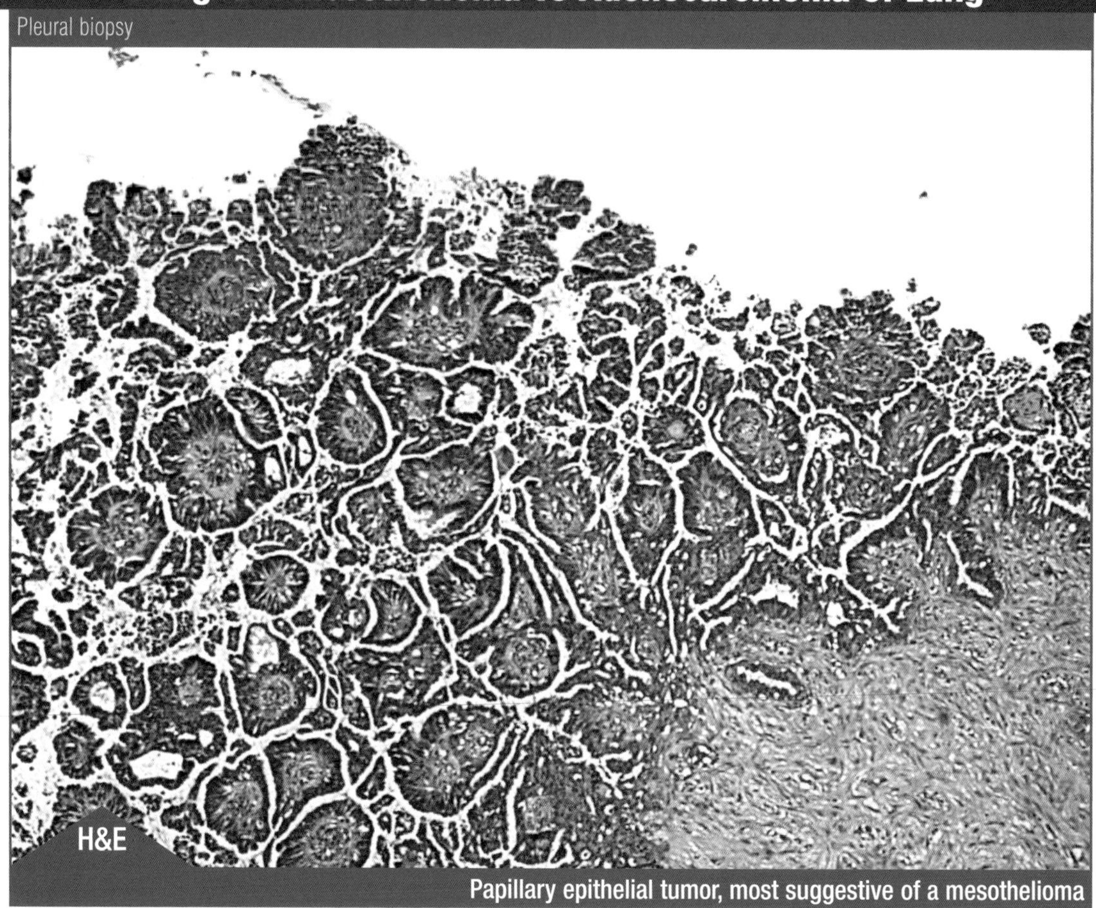

Papillary epithelial tumor, most suggestive of a mesothelioma

Malignant Mesothelioma vs Adenocarcinoma of Lung			
	Calretinin	TTF-1	CEA
Malignant Mesothelioma	+	–	–
Adenocarcinoma of Lung	–	+	+

Helpful Hints

The differential diagnosis of malignant mesotheliomas from the look-alike lesions depends on the location of the tumor and morphologic subtype of mesothelioma. For example, malignant epithelial mesotheliomas of the pleura should be separated from adenocarcinomas, particularly from those of lung origin. While most adenocarcinomas of the lung express **carcinoembryonic antigen** (**CEA**) and **TTF-1**, mesotheliomas are always negative. Conversely, **calretinin** is seen in epithelial mesotheliomas but not in adenocarcinomas. It should be noted that the characteristic calretinin staining of malignant mesotheliomas is both nuclear and cytoplasmic. Cytoplasmic reaction alone is not diagnostic because it may be seen in some adenocarcinomas. Although there are a large group of markers purported to be helpful in the above differential diagnosis, the three markers suggested here resolve the majority of such differentials.

Comin 2001.

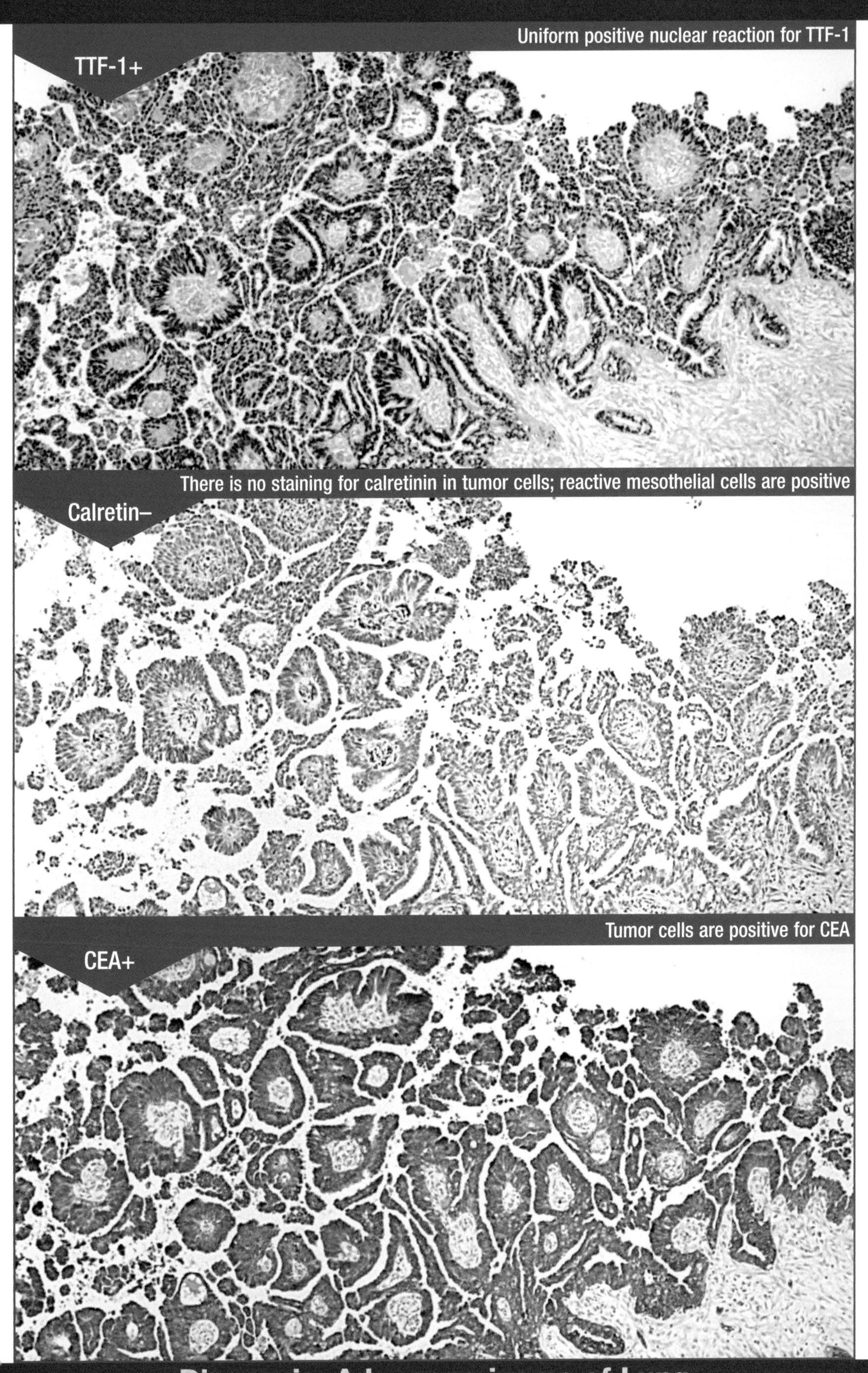

Diagnosis: Adenocarcinoma of Lung

Pleural mass

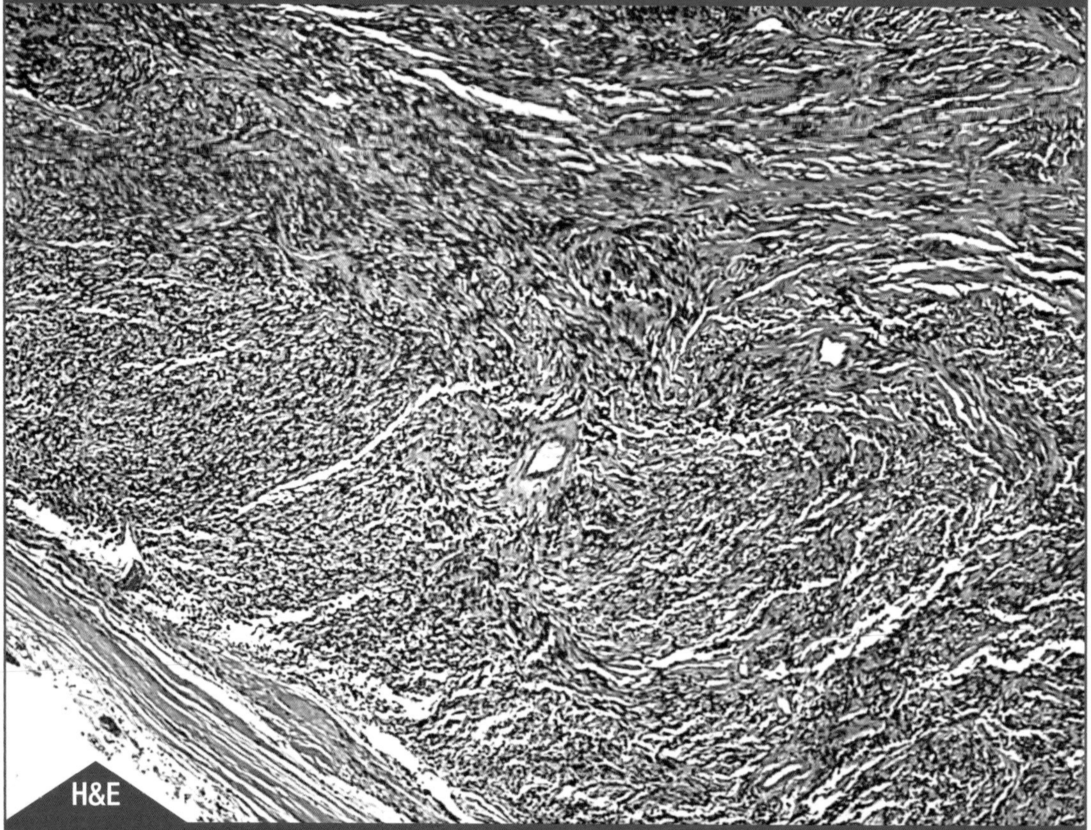

H&E

Spindle cell neoplasm more suggestive of a solitary fibrous tumor

Desmoplastic Mesothelioma vs Solitary Fibrous Tumor		
	Cytokeratin (CK)	CD34
Desmoplastic Mesothelioma	+	−
Solitary Fibrous Tumor	−	+

Helpful Hints

The desmoplastic variant of malignant mesotheliomas should be separated from solitary fibrous tumors of the pleura. The latter is always positive for **CD34** but negative for **cytokeratin**. Desmoplastic mesotheliomas on the other hand express cytokeratin but are negative for CD34.

The differential diagnosis between desmoplastic mesothelioma and post inflammatory pleural reaction with entrapped mesothelial cells may be difficult and cannot be resolved by immunohistochemistry alone.

van de Rijn 1994.

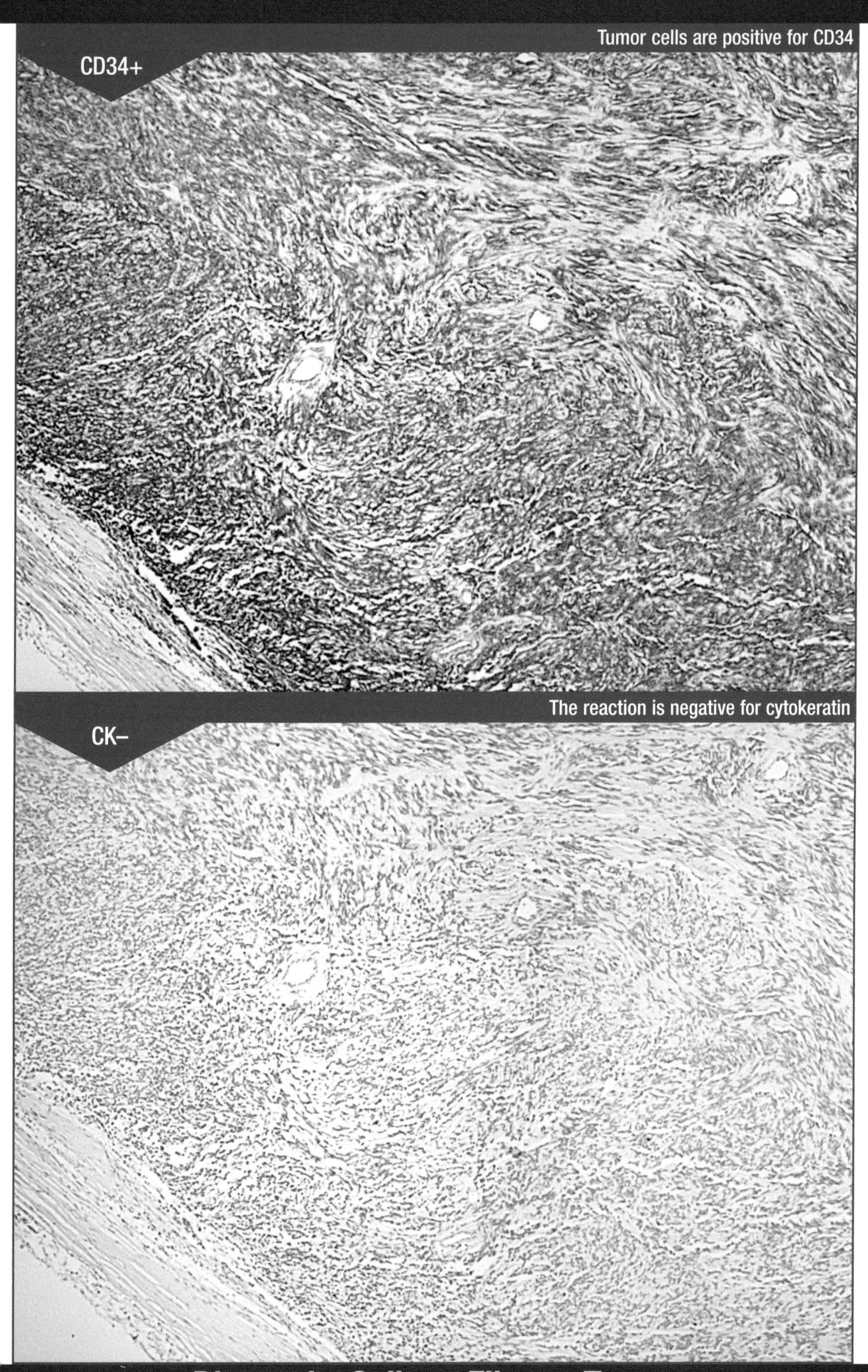

Diagnosis: Solitary Fibrous Tumor

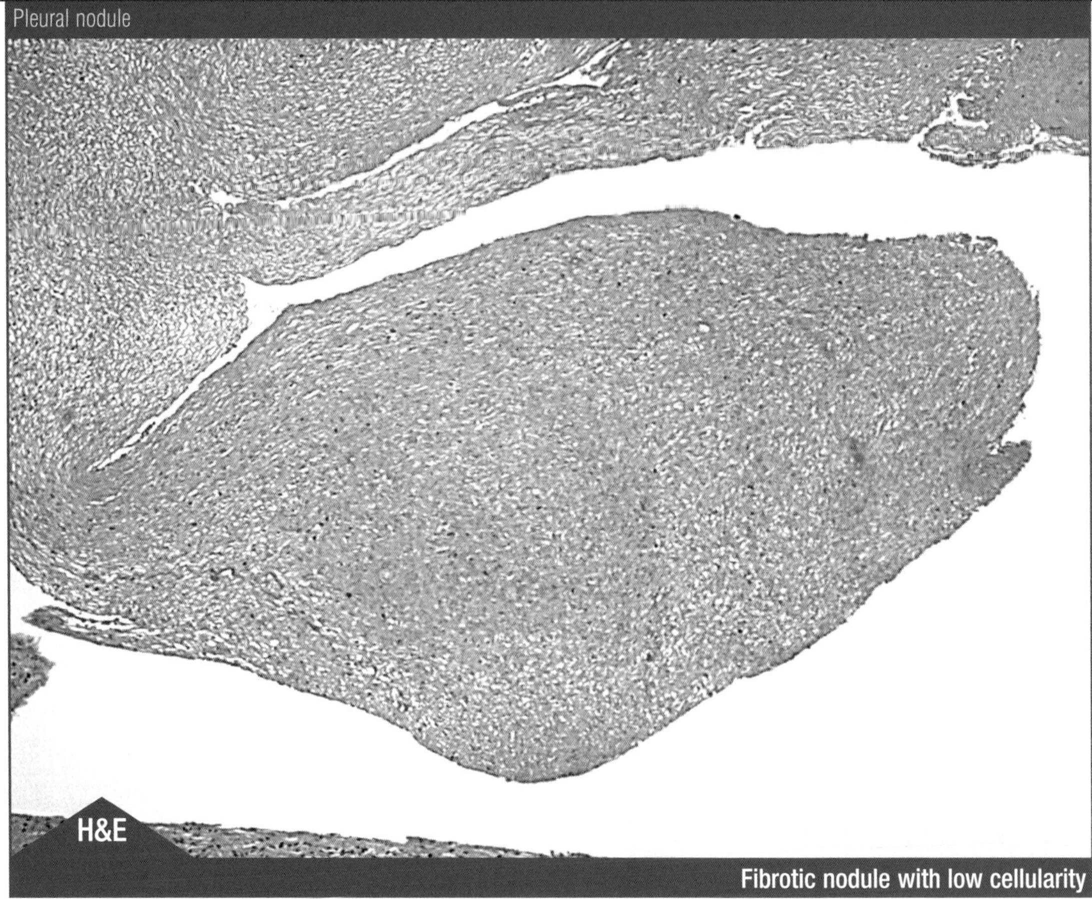

Fibrotic nodule with low cellularity

Desmoplastic Mesothelioma vs Solitary Fibrous Tumor		
	Cytokeratin (CK)	CD34
Desmoplastic Mesothelioma	+	–
Solitary Fibrous Tumor	–	+

Helpful Hints

The desmoplastic variant of malignant mesotheliomas should be separated from solitary fibrous tumors of the pleura. The latter is always positive for **CD34** but negative for **cytokeratin**. Desmoplastic mesotheliomas on the other hand express cytokeratin but are negative for CD34.

The differential diagnosis between desmoplastic mesothelioma and post inflammatory pleural reaction with entrapped mesothelial cells may be difficult and cannot be resolved by immunohistochemistry alone.

van de Rijn 1994.

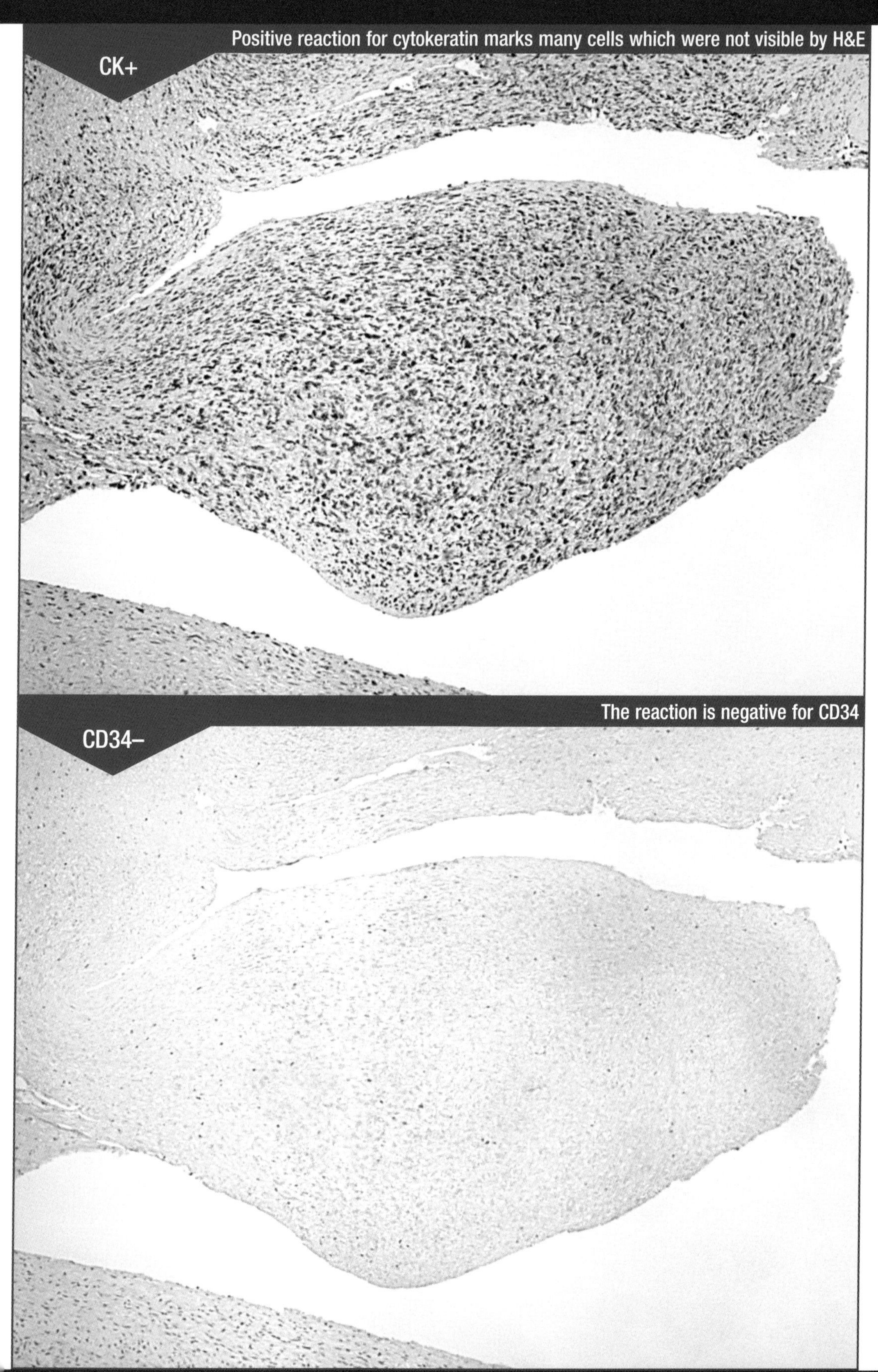

Diagnosis: Desmoplastic Malignant Mesothelioma

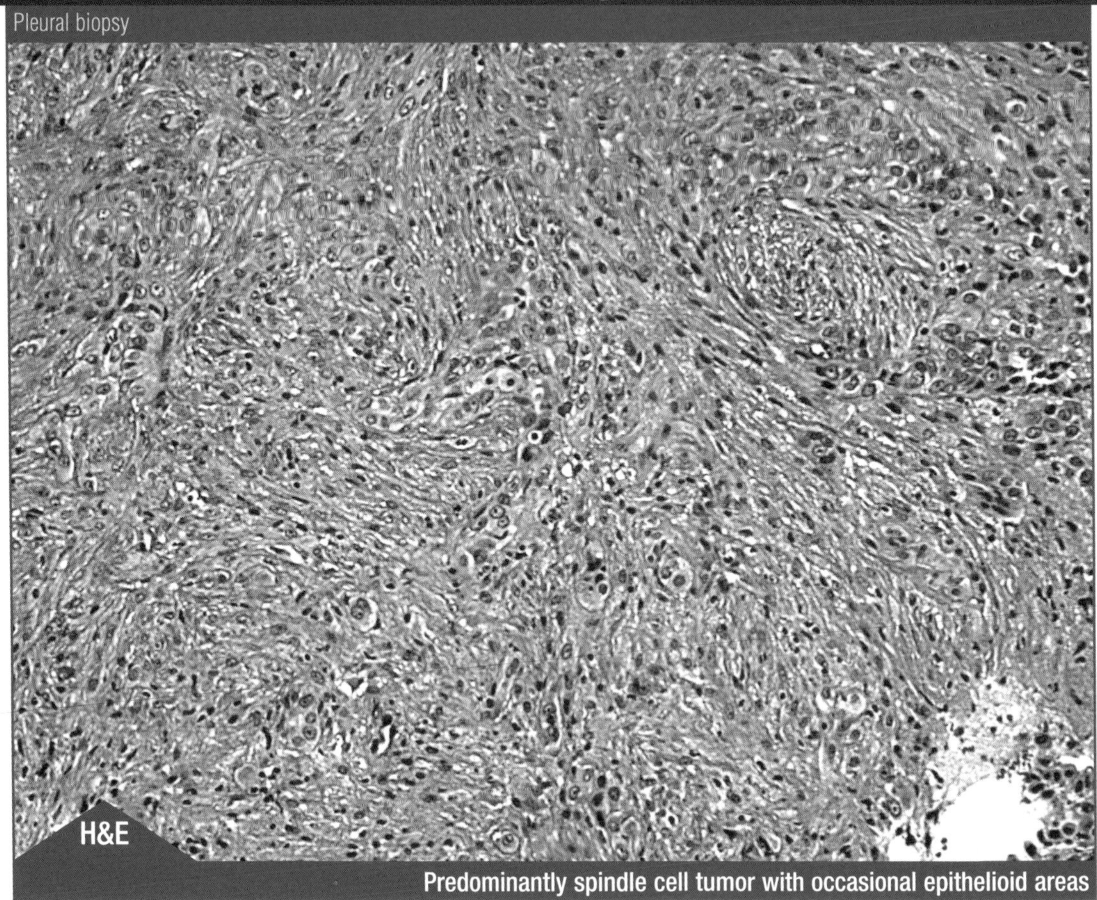

Predominantly spindle cell tumor with occasional epithelioid areas

Sarcomatoid Mesothelioma vs Synovial Sarcoma of Pleura			
	Cytokeratin (CK)	CD99	Calretinin
Sarcomatoid Mesothelioma	+	–	–
Synovial Sarcoma of Pleura	+	+	–

Helpful Hints

Unlike desmoplastic mesotheliomas, sarcomatoid malignant mesotheliomas are usually very cellular with little if any fibrous stoma. Their main differential diagnosis is with sarcomas of the pleura. Most sarcomas of the pleura are negative for **cytokeratin** whereas sarcomatoid mesotheliomas are always positive. The exception is synovial sarcoma of pleura that also expresses cytokeratin. This distinction is difficult, but staining for **CD99** and **BCL-2** could be helpful; they are expected to be expressed by synovial sarcomas but not by sarcomatoid mesotheliomas. Those sarcomas with specific markers, such as leiomyosarcomas (**H-Caldesmon**) and neurogenic sarcomas (**S100 protein**) can be distinguished by the expression of their respective markers.

Calretinin is usually present focally in biphasic mesotheliomas but absent in sarcomatoid mesotheliomas. The latter is therefore, difficult to differentiate from spindle cell carcinomas of the lung. This is because they both express cytokeratin but are negative for calretinin and TTF-1. Spindle cell carcinomas of lung may express **p63**.

Nicholson 1998.

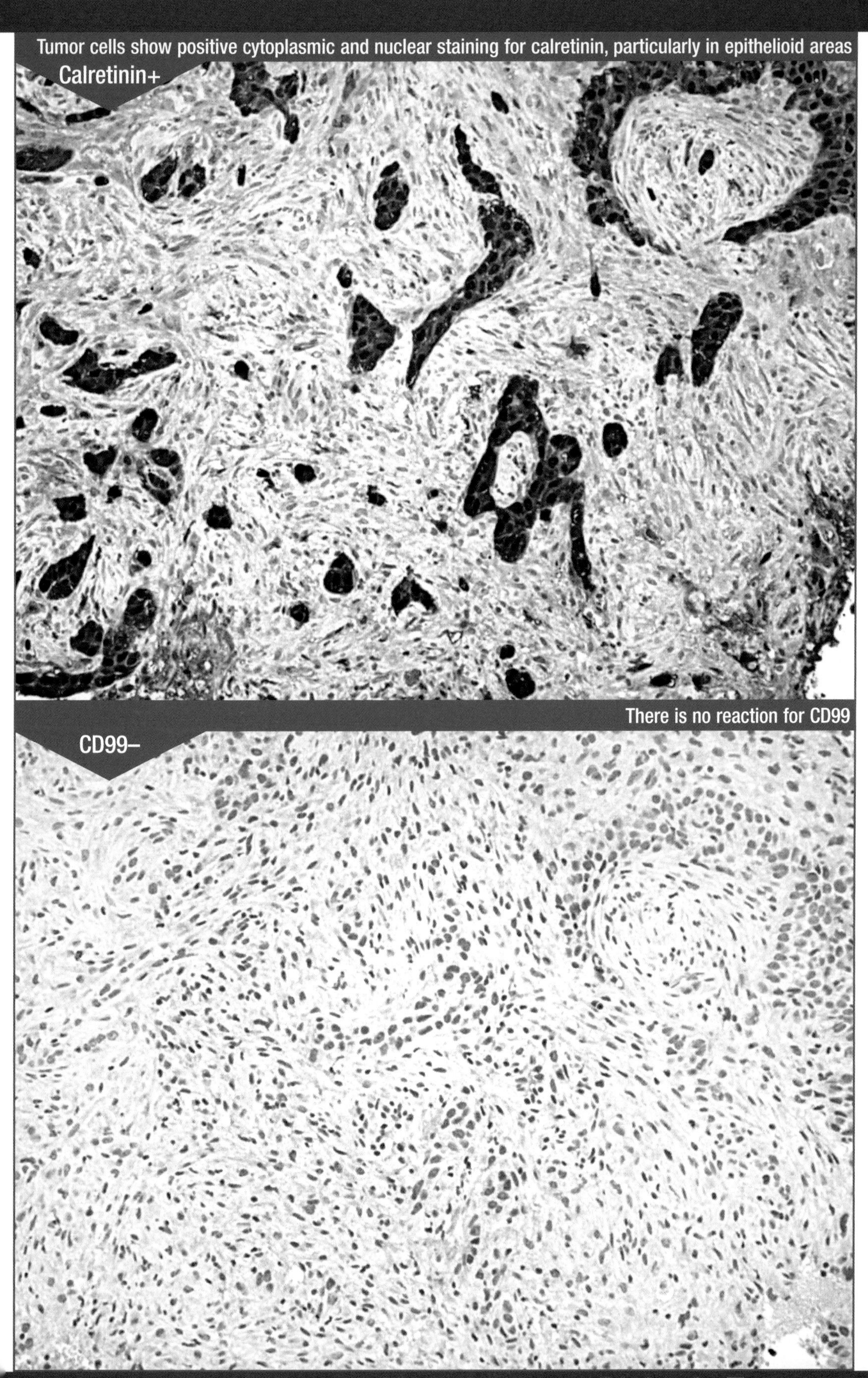

Diagnosis: Malignant Mesothelioma, Biphasic Type

Pleural tumor

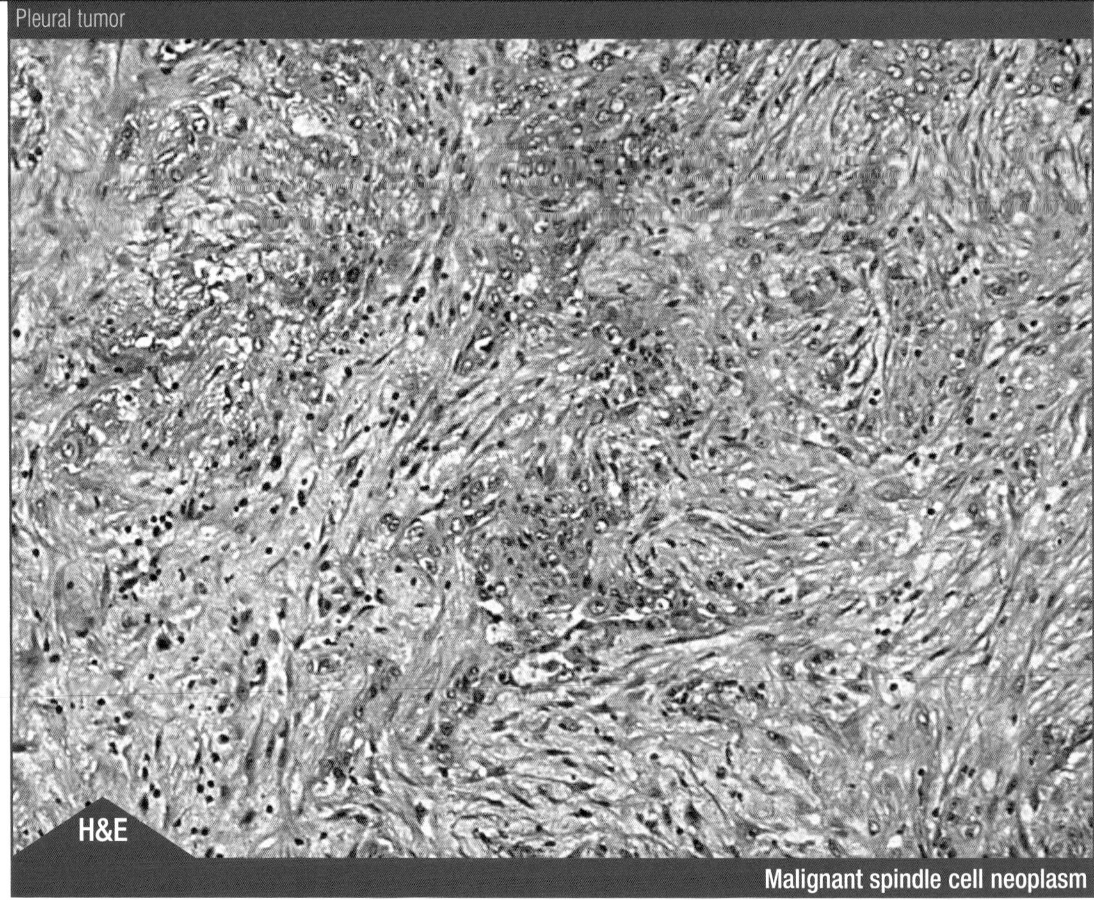

Malignant spindle cell neoplasm

Biphasic Mesothelioma vs Synovial Sarcoma of Pleura			
	Cytokeratin (CK)	CD99	Calretinin
Biphasic Mesothelioma	+	–	S
Synovial Sarcoma of Pleura	–	+	–

Helpful Hints

Unlike desmoplastic mesotheliomas, sarcomatoid malignant mesotheliomas are usually very cellular with little if any fibrous stoma. Their main differential diagnosis is with sarcomas of the pleura. Most sarcomas of the pleura are negative for **cytokeratin** whereas sarcomatoid mesotheliomas are always positive. The exception is synovial sarcoma of pleura that also expresses cytokeratin. This distinction is difficult, but staining for **CD99** and **BCL-2** could be helpful; they are expected to be expressed by synovial sarcomas but not by sarcomatoid mesotheliomas. Those sarcomas with specific markers, such as leiomyosarcomas (**H-Caldesmon**) and neurogenic sarcomas (**S100 protein**) can be distinguished by the expression of their respective markers.

Calretinin is usually present focally in biphasic mesotheliomas but absent in sarcomatoid mesotheliomas. The latter is therefore, difficult to differentiate from spindle cell carcinomas of the lung. This is because they both express cytokeratin but are negative for calretinin and TTF-1. Spindle cell carcinomas of lung may express **p63**.

Nicholson 1998.

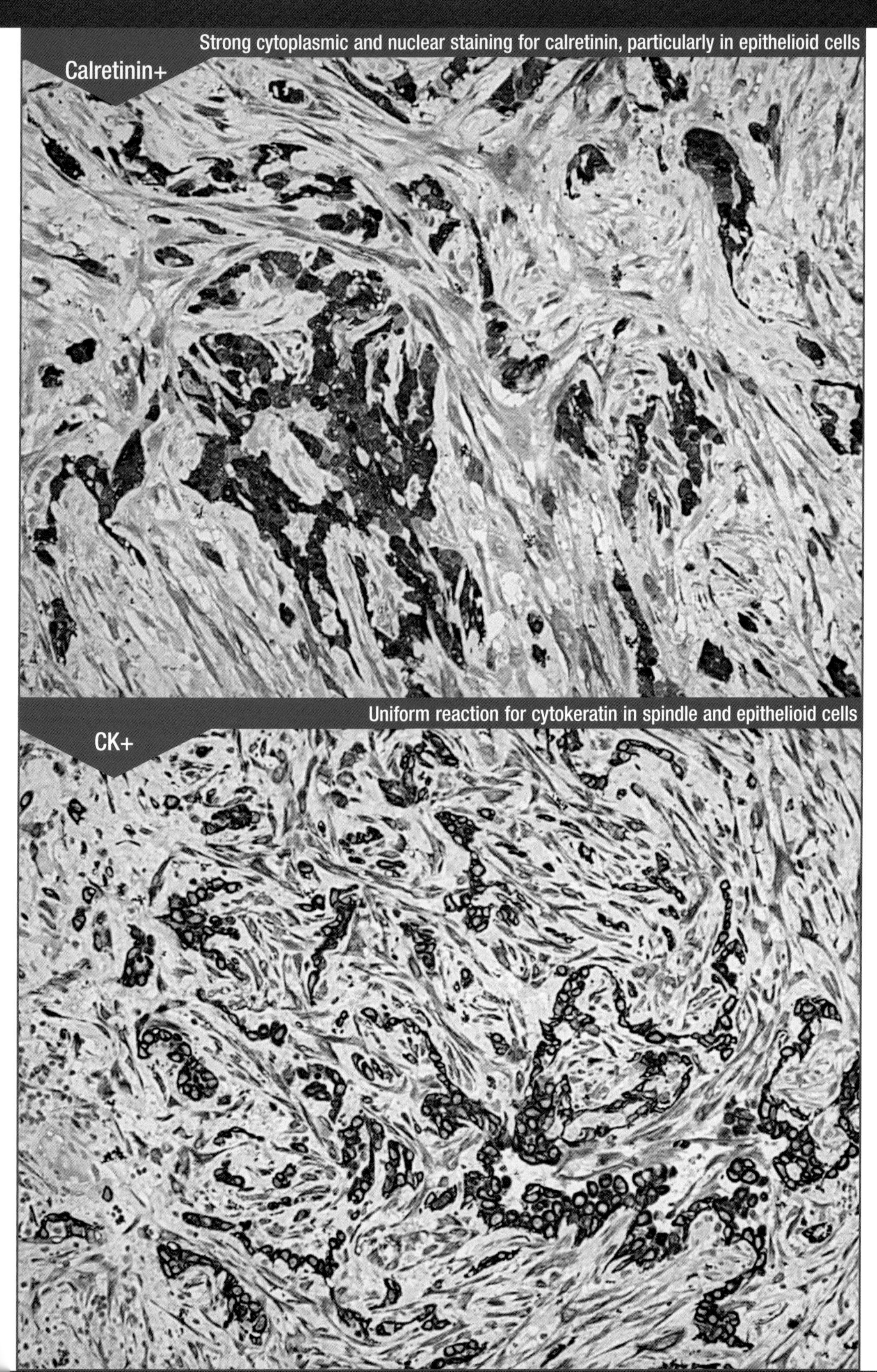

Diagnosis: Malignant Mesothelioma, Biphasic Type

Cell block preparation from pleural fluid

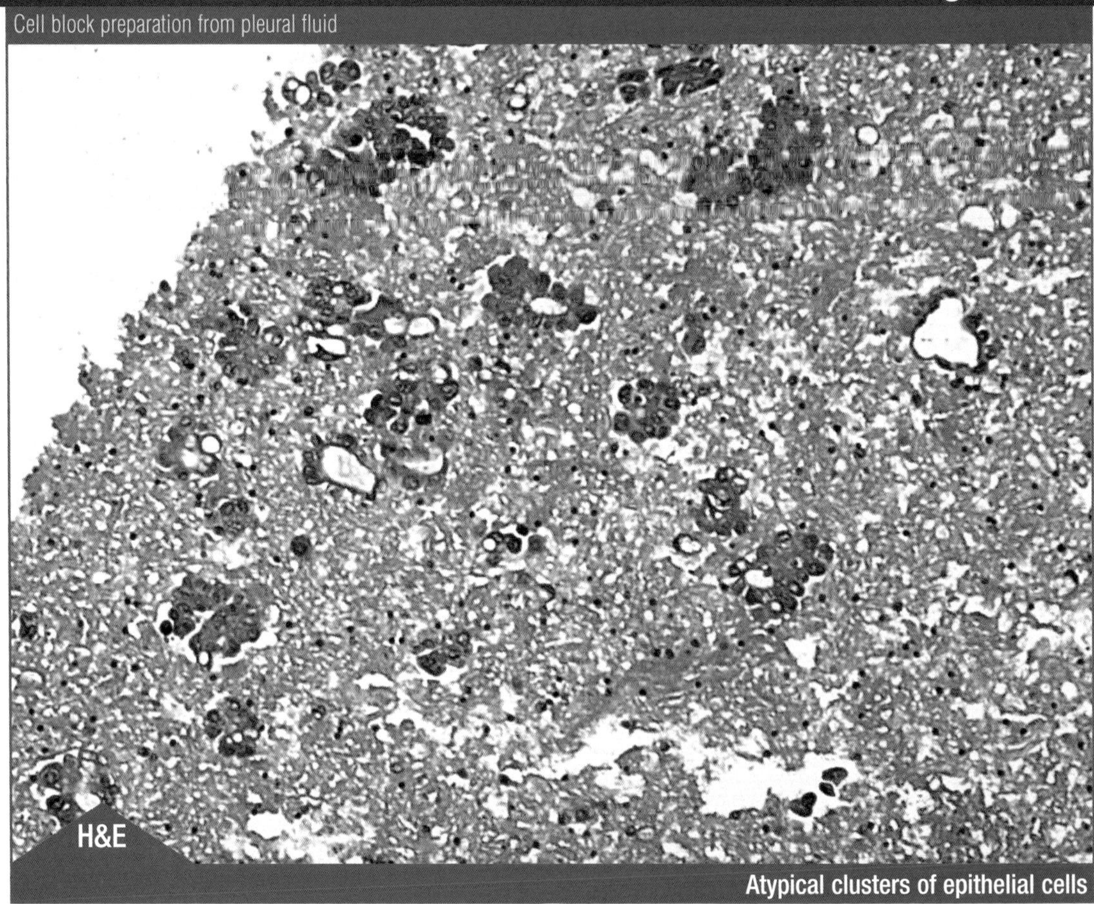

Atypical clusters of epithelial cells

Reactive Mesothelium vs Adenocarcinoma of Lung			
	Calretinin	TTF-1	CEA
Reactive Mesothelium	+	–	–
Adenocarcinoma of Lung	–	+	+

Helpful Hints

This is a common differential diagnosis problem in body cavity fluid cytology. The choices of markers are the same used for separating malignant mesotheliomas from adenocarcinomas of the lung. The staining for those markers can be performed either on cell blocks or on properly fixed cell smears or centrifuged specimens. Air-dried cell preparations are unsuitable for immunocytochemistry of the above markers. Currently, there are no markers that distinguish cells of malignant mesothelioma from reactive mesothelium in fluid cytology.

Nadji 1990.

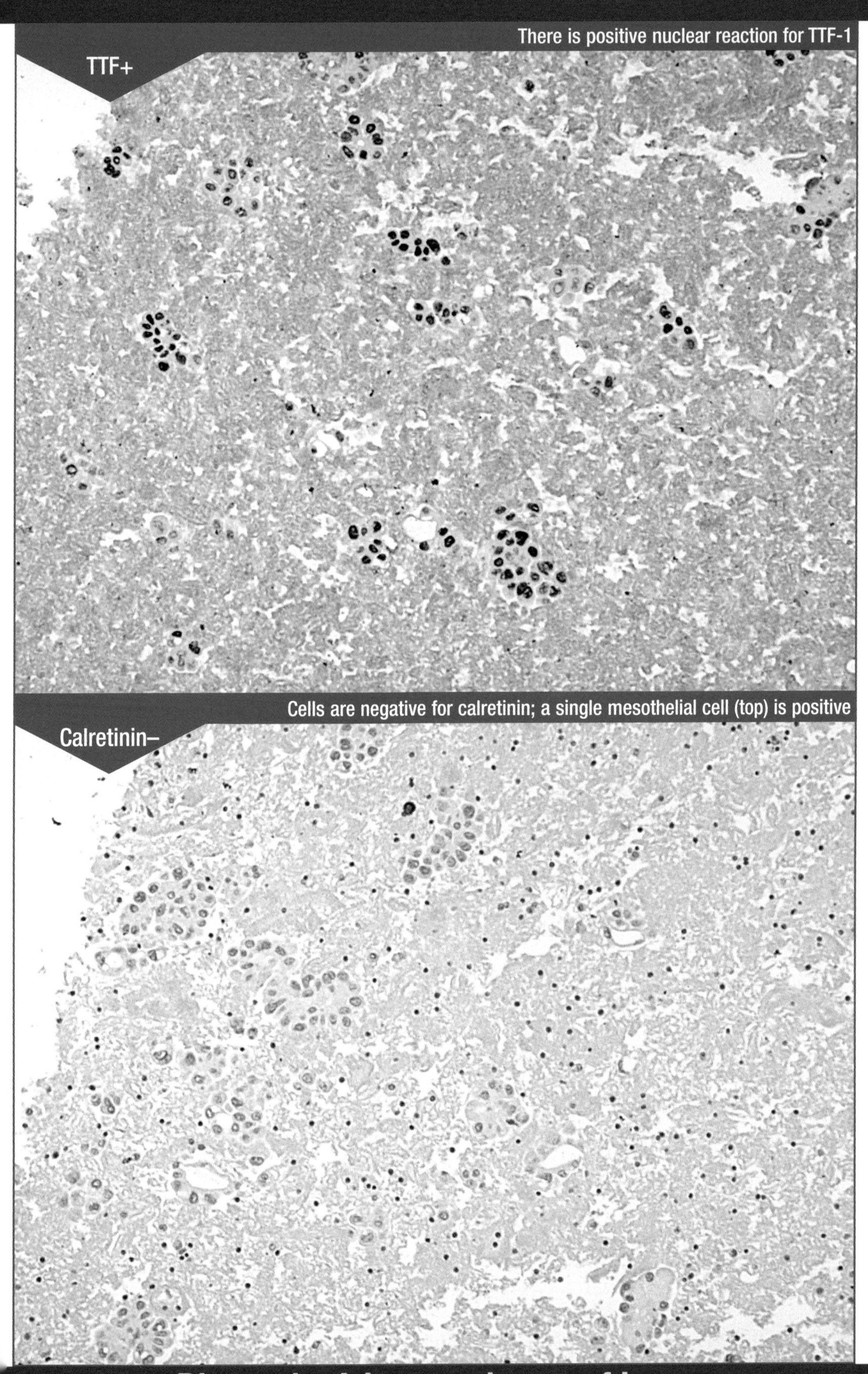

There is positive nuclear reaction for TTF-1

Cells are negative for calretinin; a single mesothelial cell (top) is positive

Diagnosis: Adenocarcinoma of Lung

Cell block preparation of pleural fluid

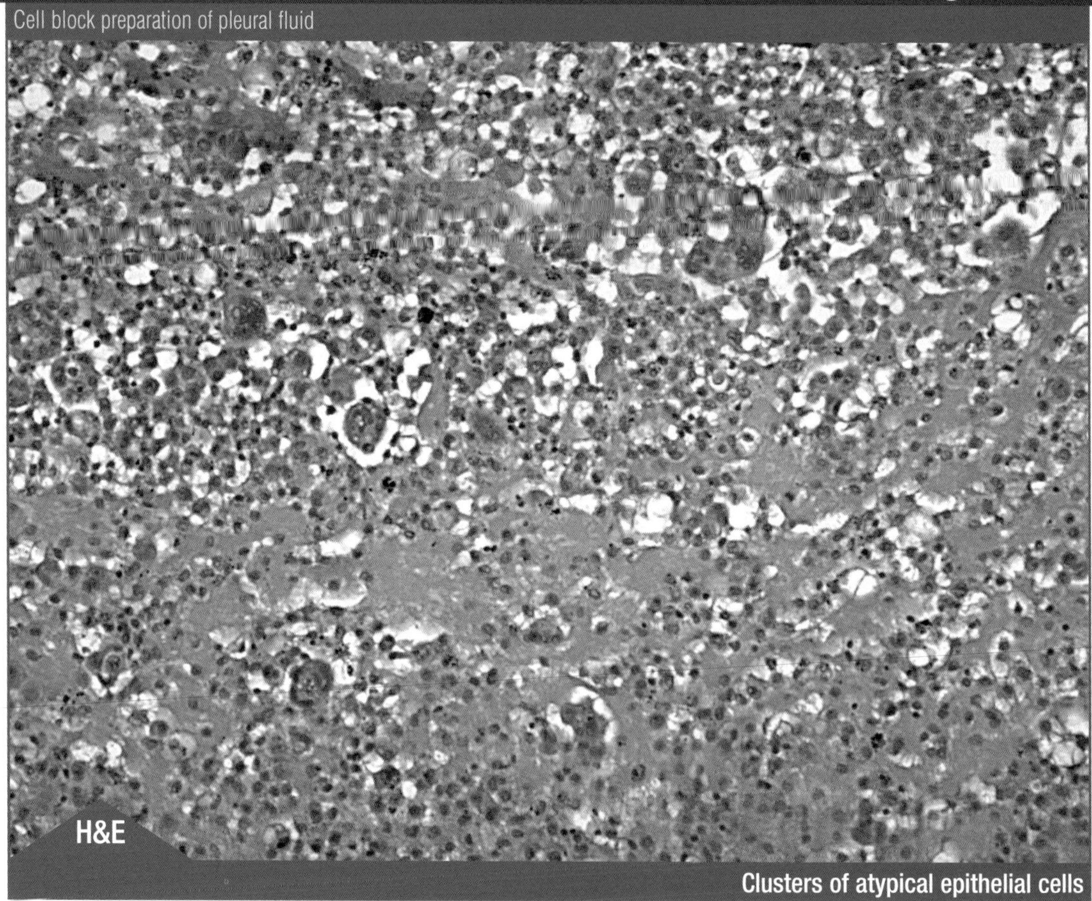

Clusters of atypical epithelial cells

Reactive Mesothelium vs Adenocarcinoma of Lung			
	Calretinin	TTF-1	CEA
Reactive Mesothelium	+	–	–
Adenocarcinoma of Lung	–	+	+

Helpful Hints

This is a common differential diagnosis problem in body cavity fluid cytology. The choices of markers are the same used for separating malignant mesotheliomas from adenocarcinomas of the lung. The staining for those markers can be performed either on cell blocks or on properly fixed cell smears or centrifuged specimens. Air-dried cell preparations are unsuitable for immunocytochemistry of the above markers. Currently, there are no markers that distinguish cells of malignant mesothelioma from reactive mesothelium in fluid cytology. **Calretinin** establishes mesothelial origin but does not differentiate between benign and malignant mesothelial cells.

Nadji 1990.

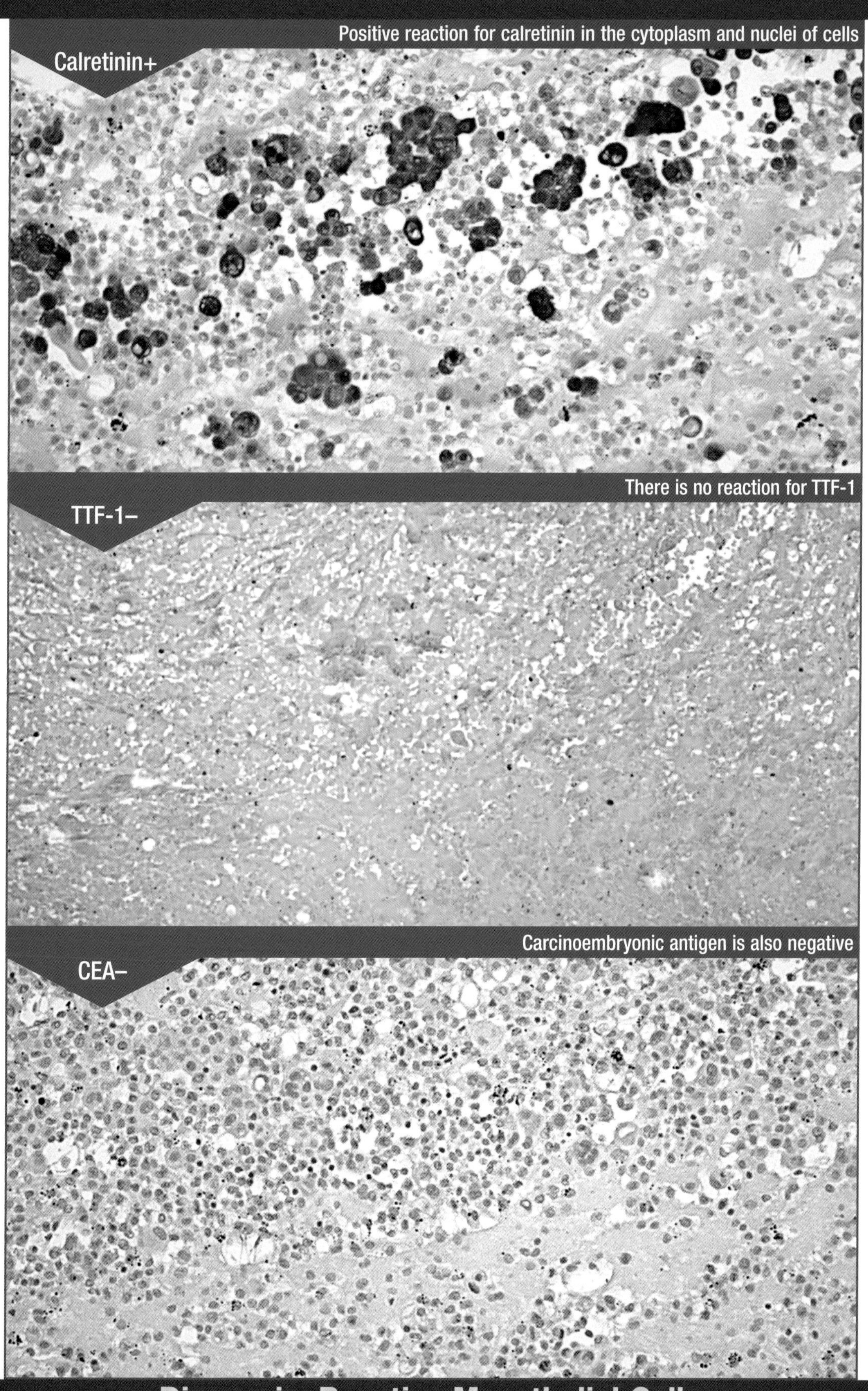

Diagnosis: Reactive Mesothelial Cells

Core biopsies of a mediastinal mass

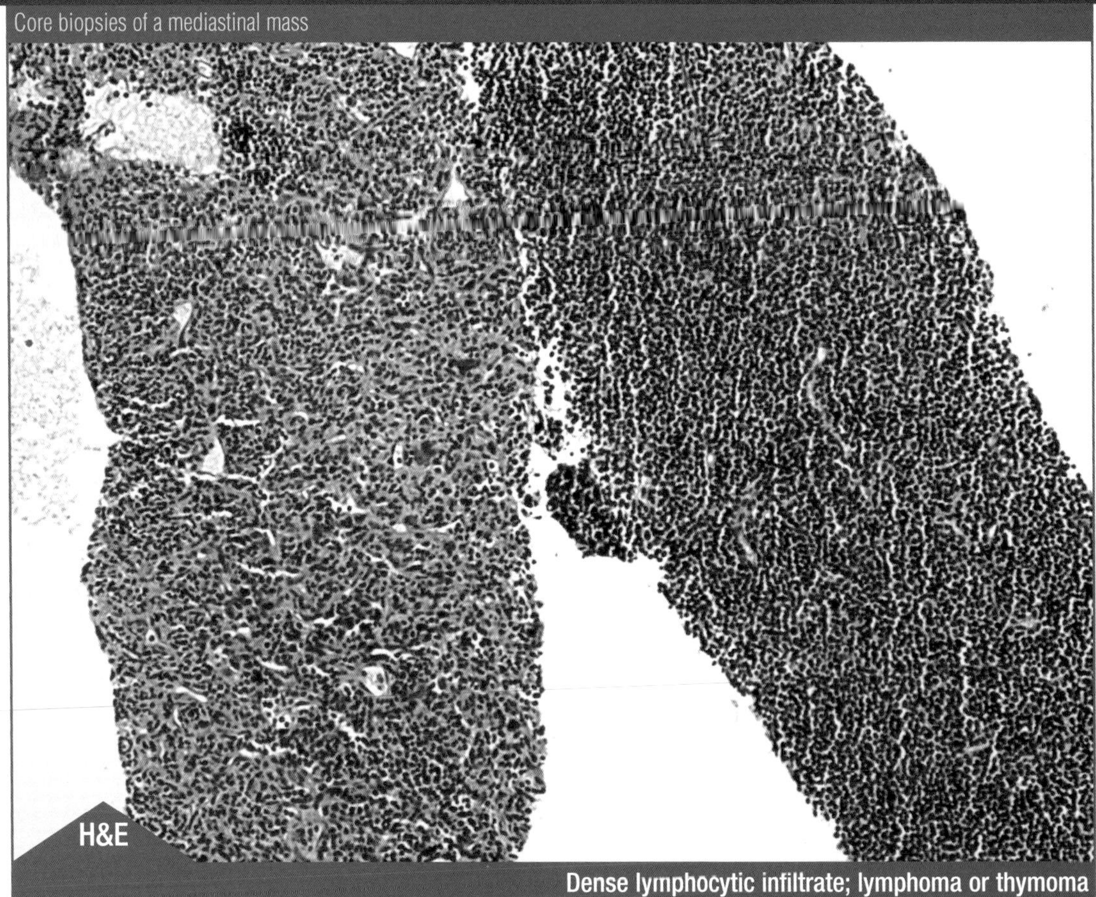

Dense lymphocytic infiltrate; lymphoma or thymoma

Thymoma vs Lymphoma	
	Cytokeratin (CK)
Thymoma	+
Lymphoma	–

Helpful Hints

This differential diagnosis may be difficult in small mediastinal biopsies. The epithelial component of thymomas is highlighted in a characteristic trabecular or reticular pattern by **cytokeratin** stain. This pattern is not seen in normal thymus.

The use of **CD45** is not helpful for the above differential diagnosis. Similarly, because thymomas are composed mainly of T lymphocytes, **CD3** cannot be used to differentiate T cell lymphomas from thymomas. **CD20** however, may help to identify mediastinal B cell lymphomas. If Hodgkin lymphoma is suspected, **CD30** and **CD15** could be used.

Ring 1986.

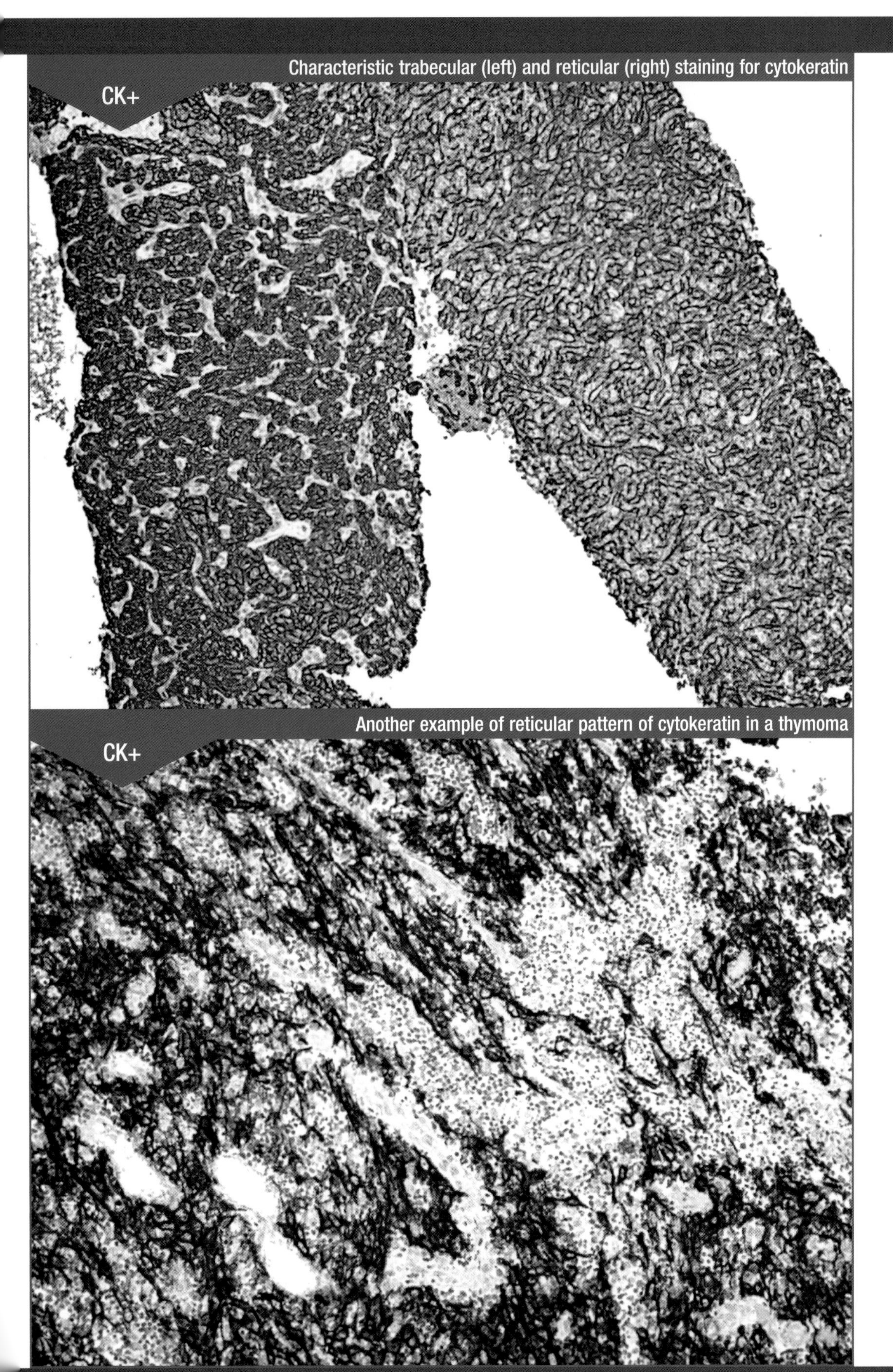

Characteristic trabecular (left) and reticular (right) staining for cytokeratin

Another example of reticular pattern of cytokeratin in a thymoma

Diagnosis: Thymoma

Mediastinal mass

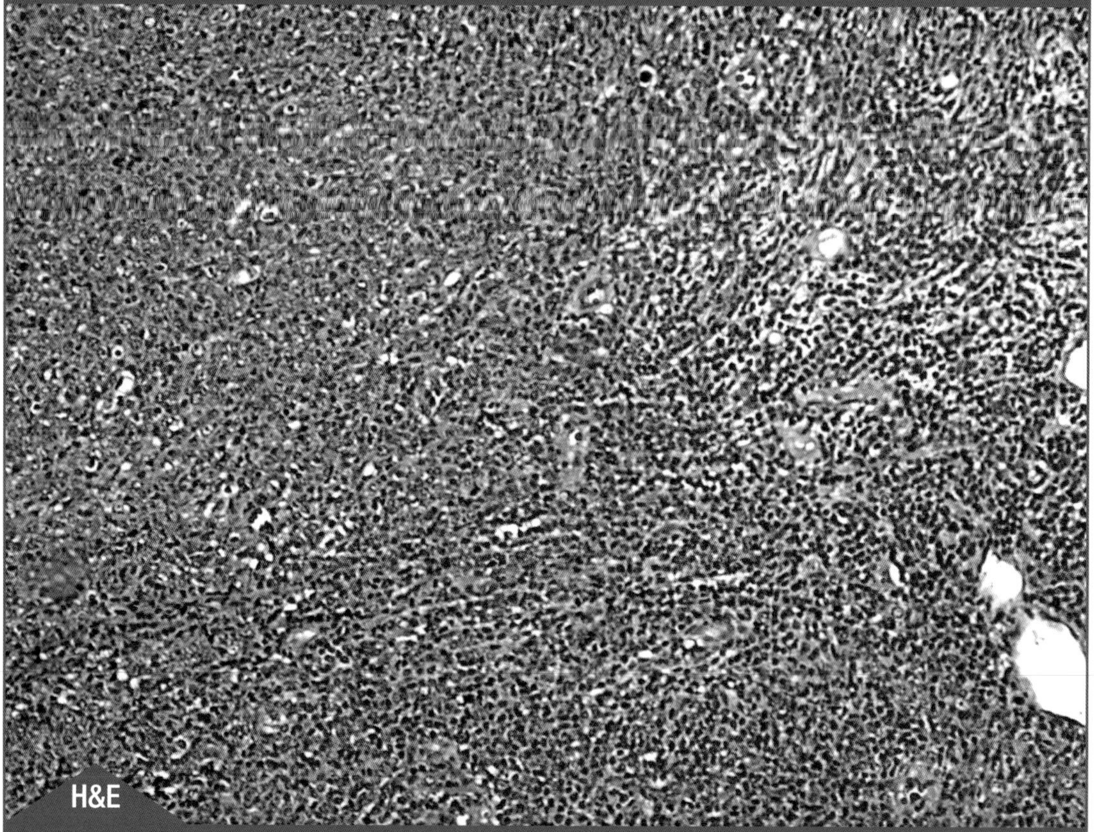

H&E

Lymphocytic infiltrate more suggestive of a lymphoma

Thymoma vs Lymphoma	Cytokeratin (CK)	CD20	CD30/CD15
Thymoma	+	–	–
Lymphoma	–	+	S

Helpful Hints

This differential diagnosis may be difficult in small mediastinal biopsies. The epithelial component of thymomas is highlighted in a characteristic trabecular or reticular pattern by **cytokeratin** stain. This pattern is not seen in normal thymus.

The use of **CD45** is not helpful for the above differential diagnosis. Similarly, because thymomas are composed mainly of T lymphocytes, **CD3** cannot be used to differentiate T cell lymphomas from thymomas. **CD20** however, may help to identify mediastinal B cell lymphomas. If Hodgkin lymphoma is suspected, **CD30** and **CD15** could be used.

Ring 1986.

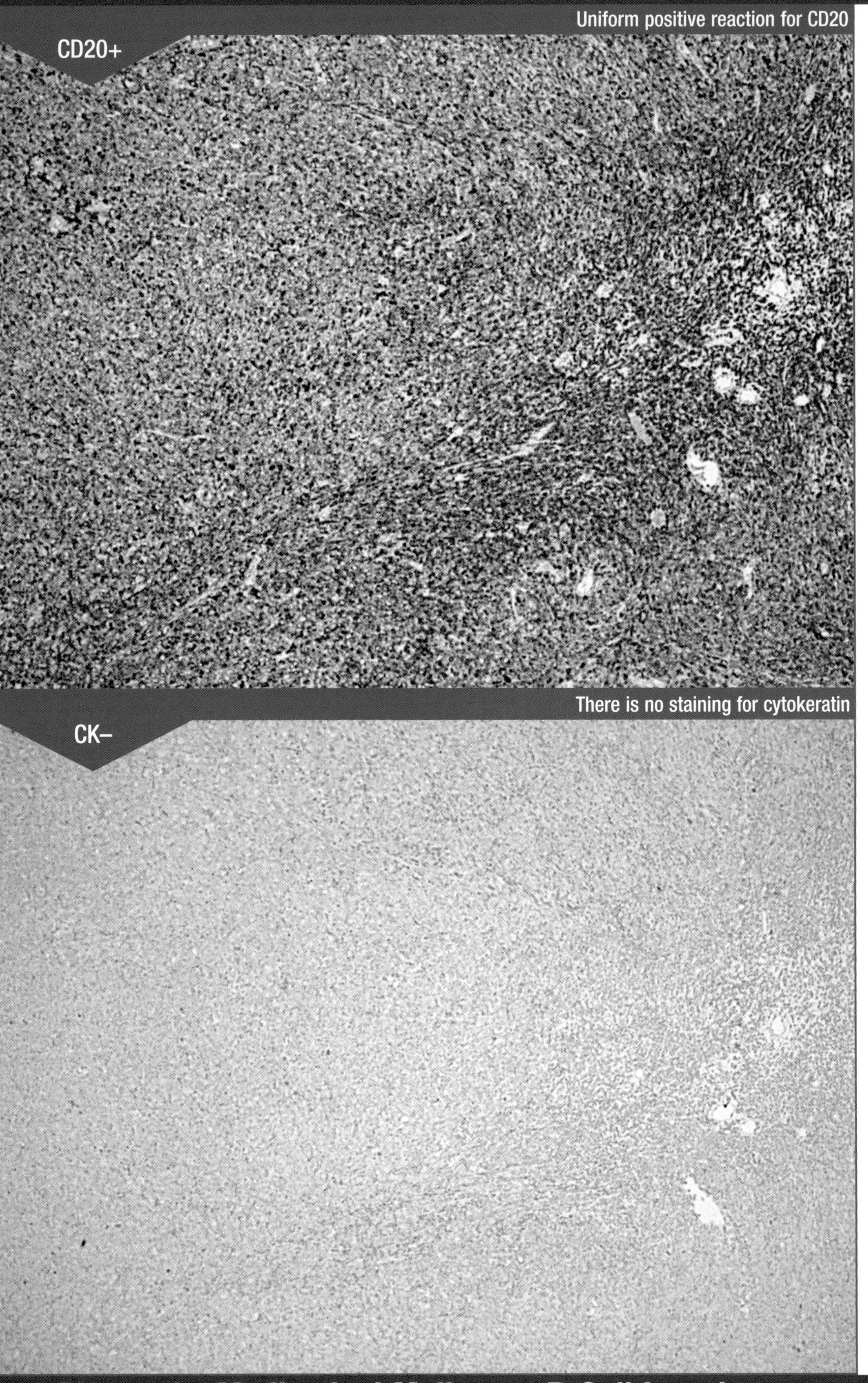
Uniform positive reaction for CD20
CD20+
There is no staining for cytokeratin
CK–
Diagnosis: Mediastinal Malignant B Cell Lymphoma

Mediastinal biopsy

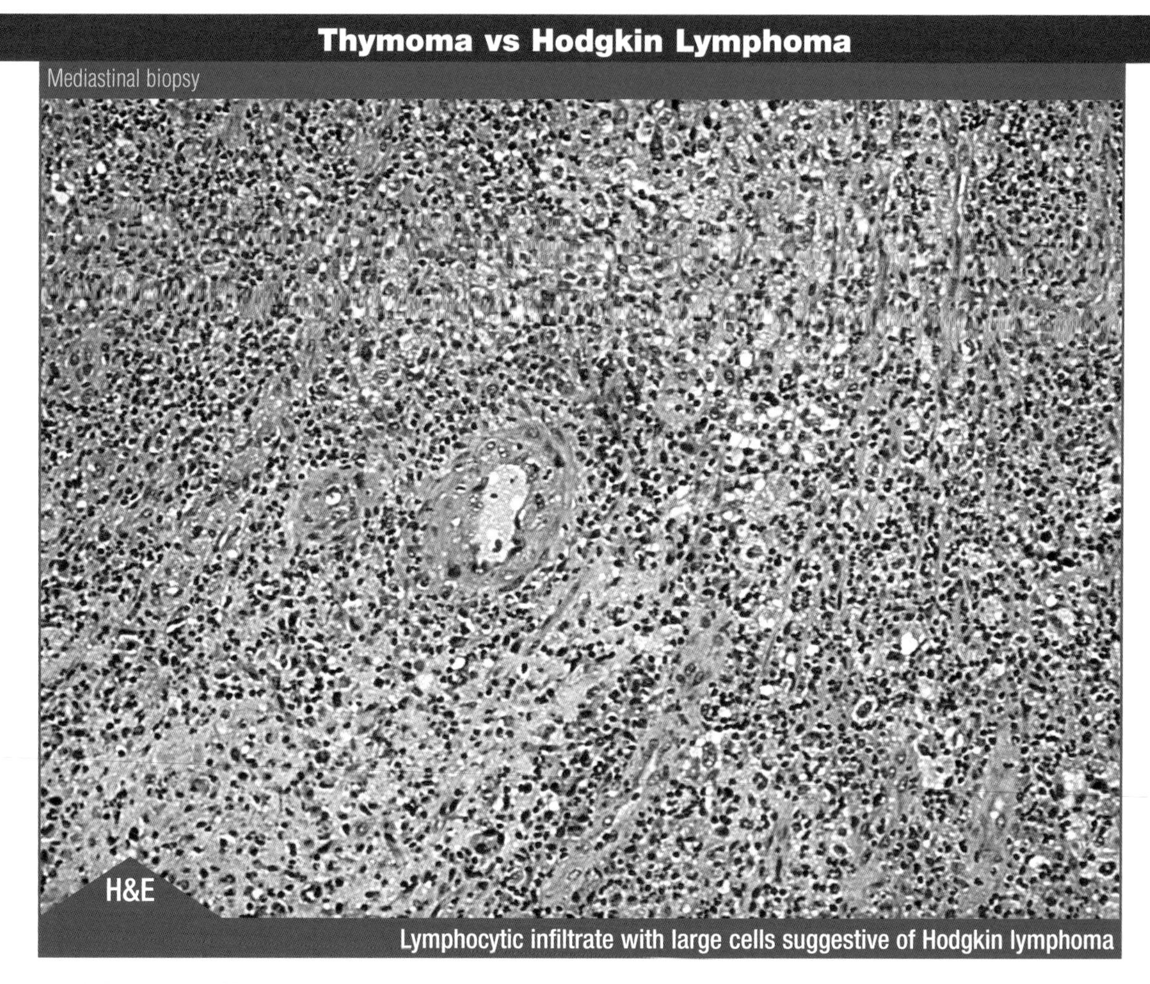

Lymphocytic infiltrate with large cells suggestive of Hodgkin lymphoma

Thymoma vs Hodgkin Lymphoma		
	Cytokeratin (CK)	CD30/CD15
Thymoma	+	–
Hodgkin Lymphoma	–	+

Helpful Hints

This differential diagnosis may be difficult in small mediastinal biopsies. The epithelial component of thymomas is highlighted in a characteristic trabecular or reticular pattern by **cytokeratin** stain. This pattern is not seen in normal thymus.

The use of **CD45** is not helpful for the above differential diagnosis. Similarly, because thymomas are composed mainly of T lymphocytes, **CD3** cannot be used to differentiate T cell lymphomas from thymomas. **CD20** however, may help to identify mediastinal B cell lymphomas. If Hodgkin lymphoma is suspected, **CD30** and **CD15** could be used.

Ring 1986.

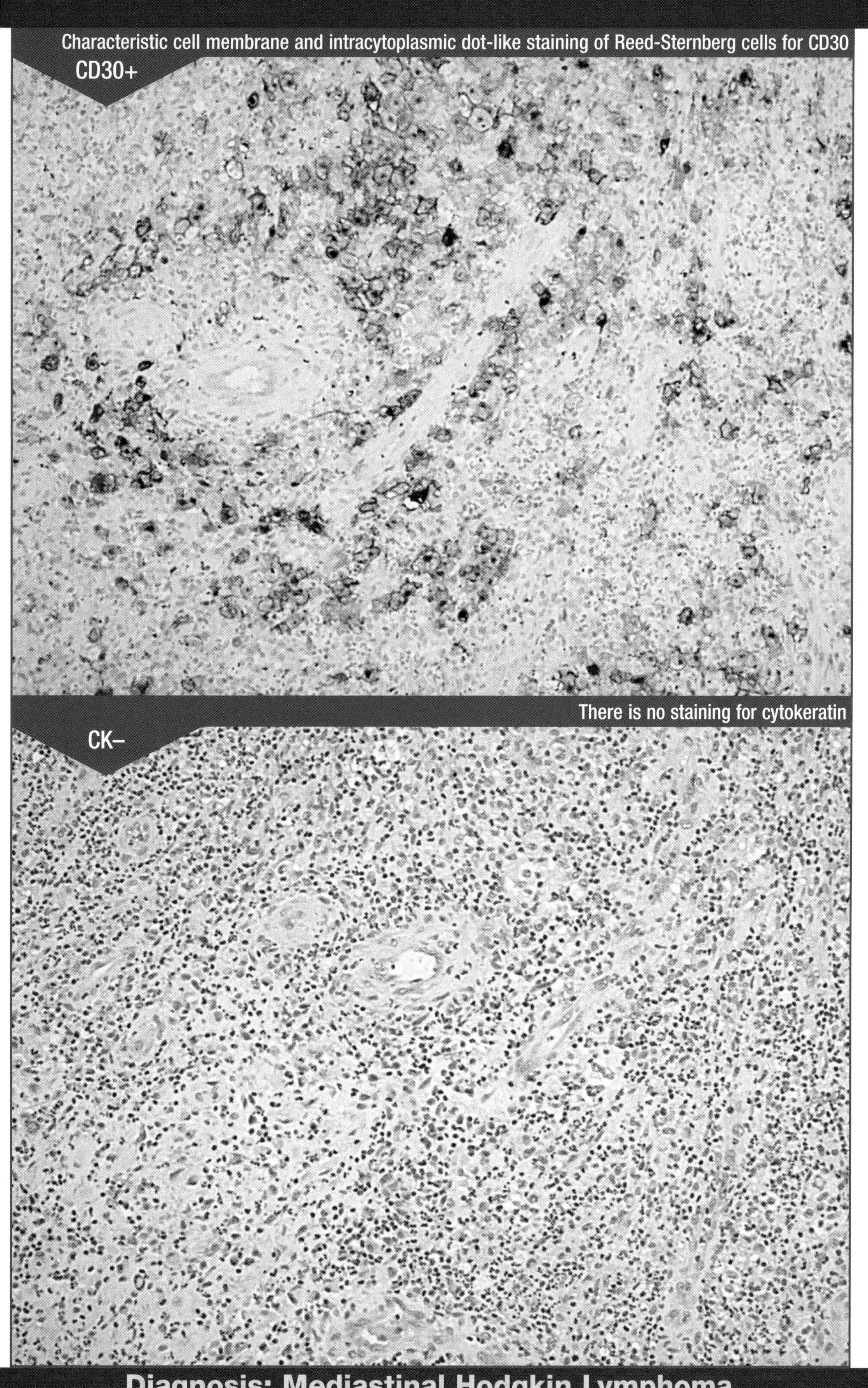

Diagnosis: Mediastinal Hodgkin Lymphoma

Pelvic mass in a young female

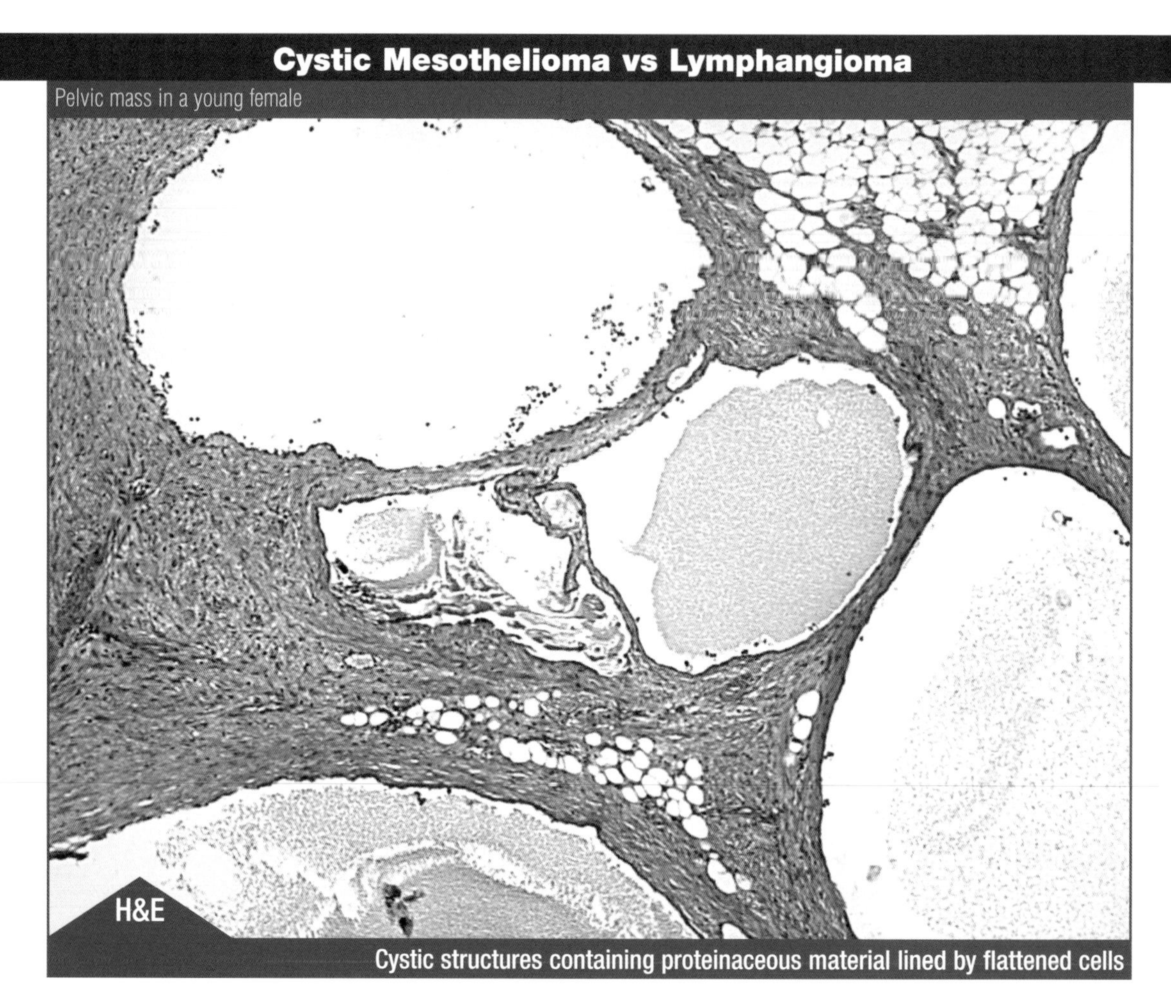

Cystic structures containing proteinaceous material lined by flattened cells

Cystic Mesothelioma vs Lymphangioma			
	Calretinin	Cytokeratin (CK)	CD31
Cystic Mesothelioma	+	+	–
Lymphangioma	–	–	+

Helpful Hints

Benign cystic mesotheliomas may morphologically mimic cystic lymphangiomas. The lining of the cysts, however, stains positive for cytokeratin and calretinin in cystic mesotheliomas. The endothelial lining of lymphangiomas can be identified by either CD31 or D2-40.

Sawh 2003.

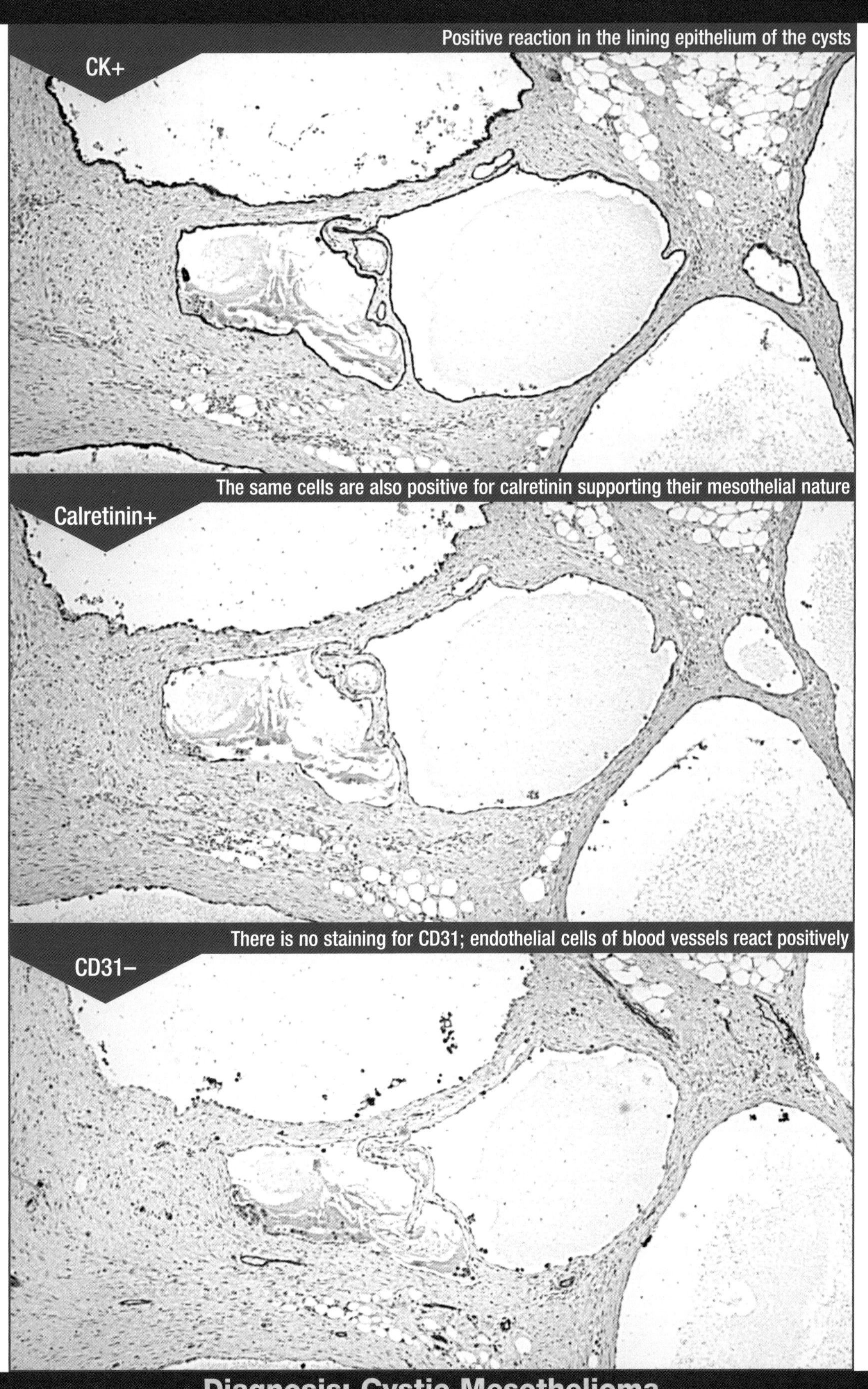

Diagnosis: Cystic Mesothelioma

Cell block preparation from the ascitic fluid of patient with abdominal carcinomatosis

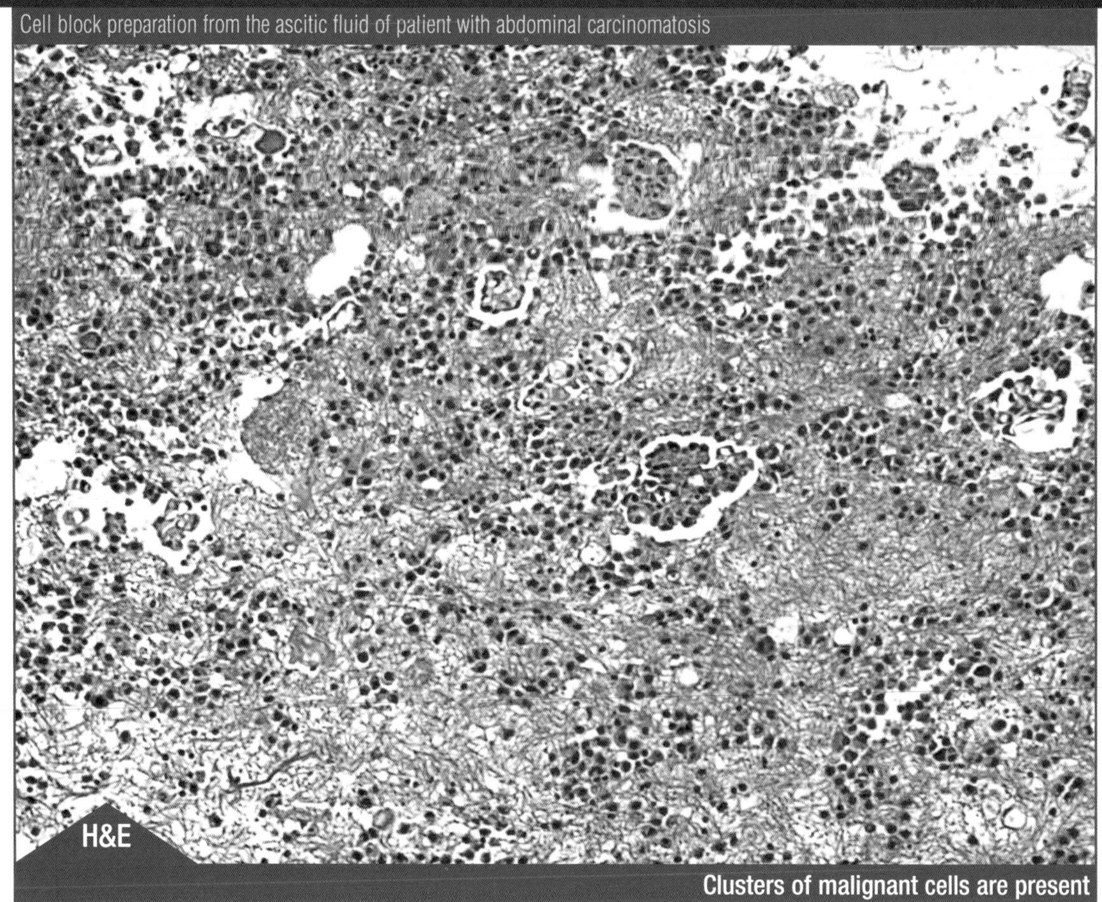

Clusters of malignant cells are present

Peritoneal Mesothelioma vs Ovarian Carcinoma		
	Calretinin	Estrogen Receptor (ER)
Peritoneal Mesothelioma	+	–
Ovarian Carcinoma	–	S

Helpful Hints

The differential diagnosis of the malignant mesotheliomas in the abdominal cavity is with a different group of neoplasms than those that occur in the pleura. In the female the most common diagnostic possibilities include gynecologic/ovarian carcinomas.

Unlike breast carcinomas that are either diffusely positive or completely negative for estrogen receptor (when ER antibody ID5 is used), carcinomas of the ovary may show only **focal ER-positivity**. But the estrogen receptor expression by ovarian tumors is limited to endometrioid and serous variants; mucinous ovarian carcinomas are usually negative for estrogen receptor. Mucinous tumors however are frequently positive for carcinoembryonic antigen, while mesotheliomas are negative. All subtypes of ovarian epithelial tumors are negative for **calretinin**. One should not use **CA-125** as a marker for gynecologic/ovarian tumor as the majority of malignant mesotheliomas are also positive for this antigen.

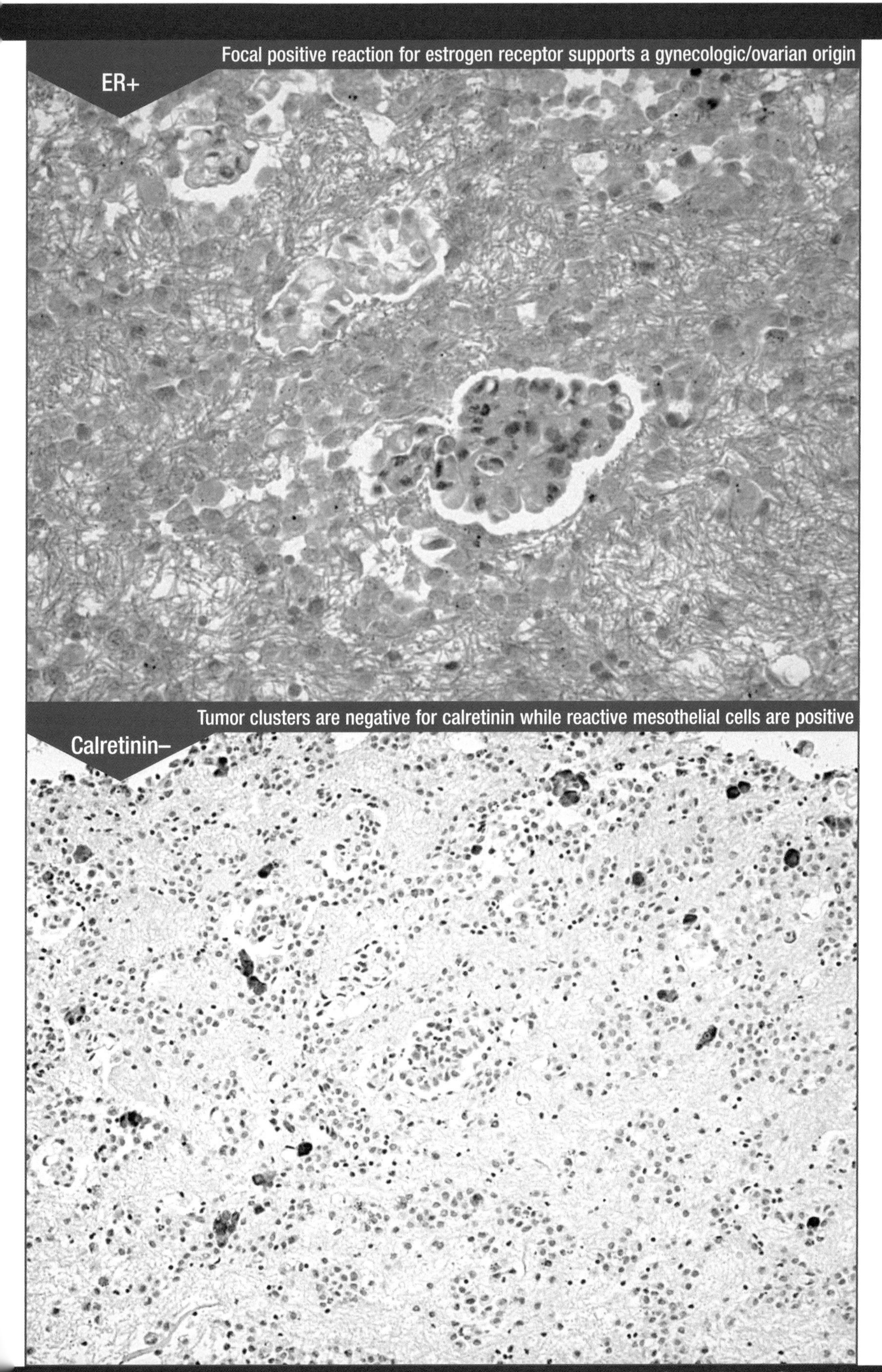

Diagnosis: Adenocarcinoma Consistent with Ovarian Origin

Cell block preparation from ascitic fluid

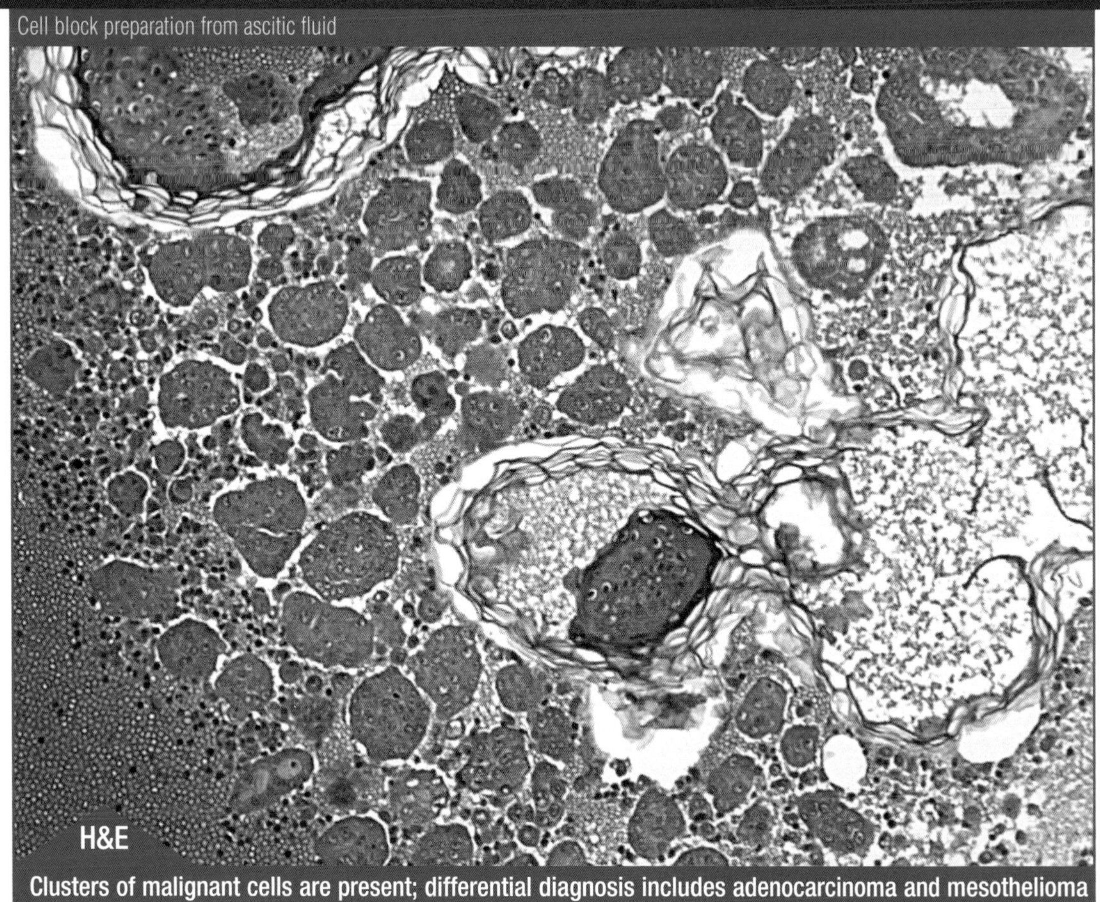

Clusters of malignant cells are present; differential diagnosis includes adenocarcinoma and mesothelioma

Peritoneal Mesothelioma vs Ovarian Carcinoma		
	Calretinin	Estrogen Receptor (ER)
Peritoneal Mesothelioma	+	–
Ovarian Carcinoma	–	S

Helpful Hints

The differential diagnosis of the malignant mesotheliomas in the abdominal cavity is with a different group of neoplasms than those that occur in the pleura. In the female the most common diagnostic possibilities include gynecologic/ovarian carcinomas.

Unlike breast carcinomas that are either diffusely positive or completely negative for estrogen receptor (when ER antibody ID5 is used), carcinomas of the ovary may show only **focal ER-positivity**. But the estrogen receptor expression by ovarian tumors is limited to endometrioid and serous variants; mucinous ovarian carcinomas are usually negative for estrogen receptor. Mucinous tumors however are frequently positive for carcinoembryonic antigen, while mesotheliomas are negative. All subtypes of ovarian epithelial tumors are negative for **calretinin**. One should not use **CA-125** as a marker for gynecologic/ovarian tumor as the majority of malignant mesotheliomas are also positive for this antigen.

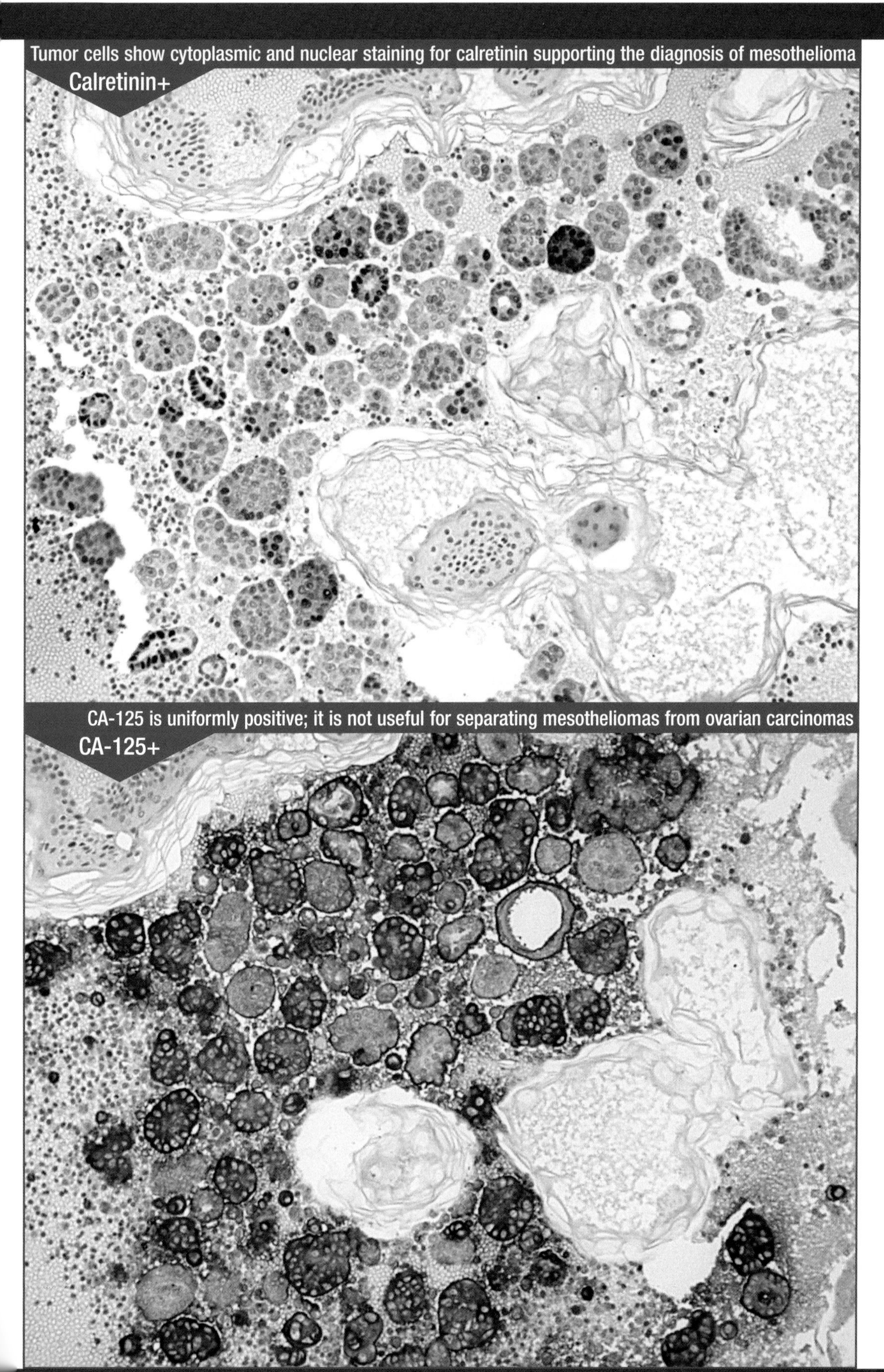

Diagnosis: Malignant Mesothelioma

Omental mass in an 11 year-old

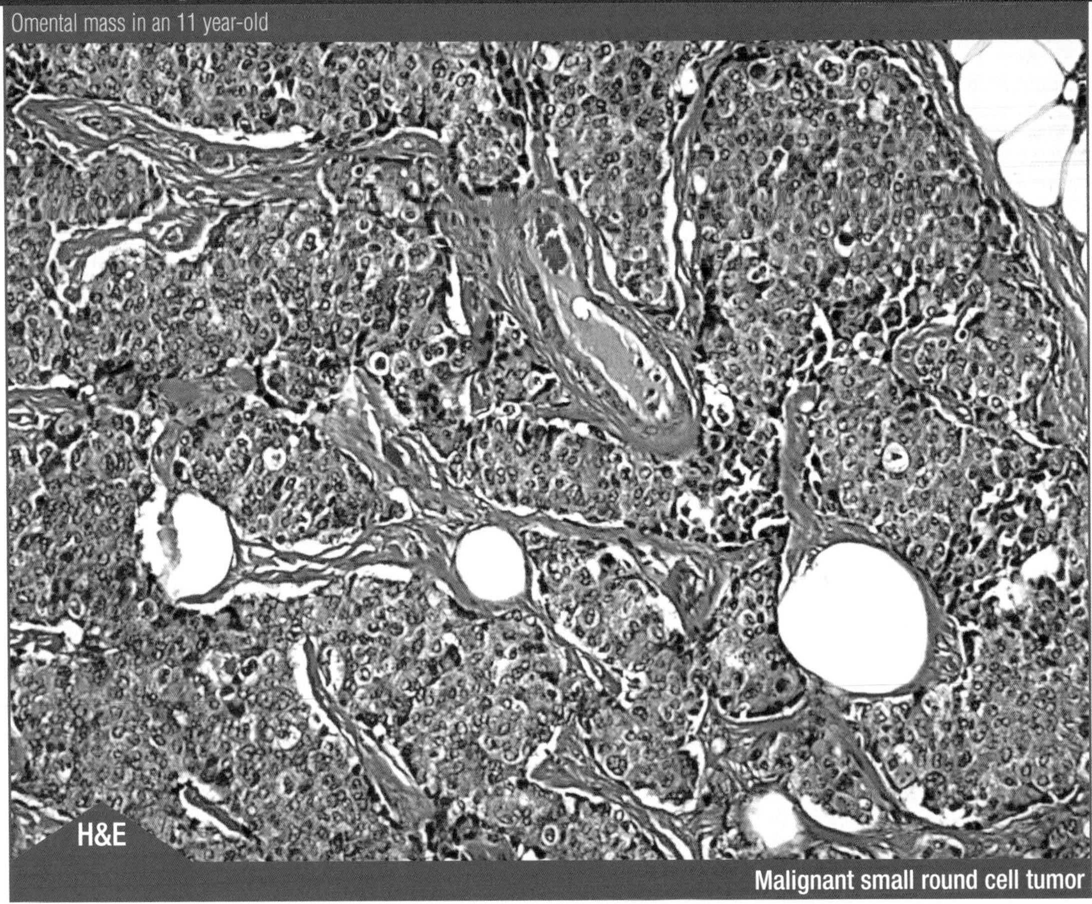

Malignant small round cell tumor

Desmoplastic Small Cell Tumor			
	Cytokeratin (CK)	Desmin	Chromogranin (Chrg)
Desmoplastic Small Cell Tumor	+	+	S

Helpful Hints

Desmoplastic small cell tumors are morphologically in the differential diagnosis of other small round cell neoplasm. The combination of **cytokeratin** and **desmin** positivity along with focal reactivity for **chromogranin** and occasionally other markers such as **epithelial membrane antigen**, distinguishes desmoplastic small round cell tumors from morphologically similar neoplasm. The positive reaction for the above markers could be focal and therefore on a small biopsy it may not be possible to appreciate the combined reactivity.

Lae 2002.

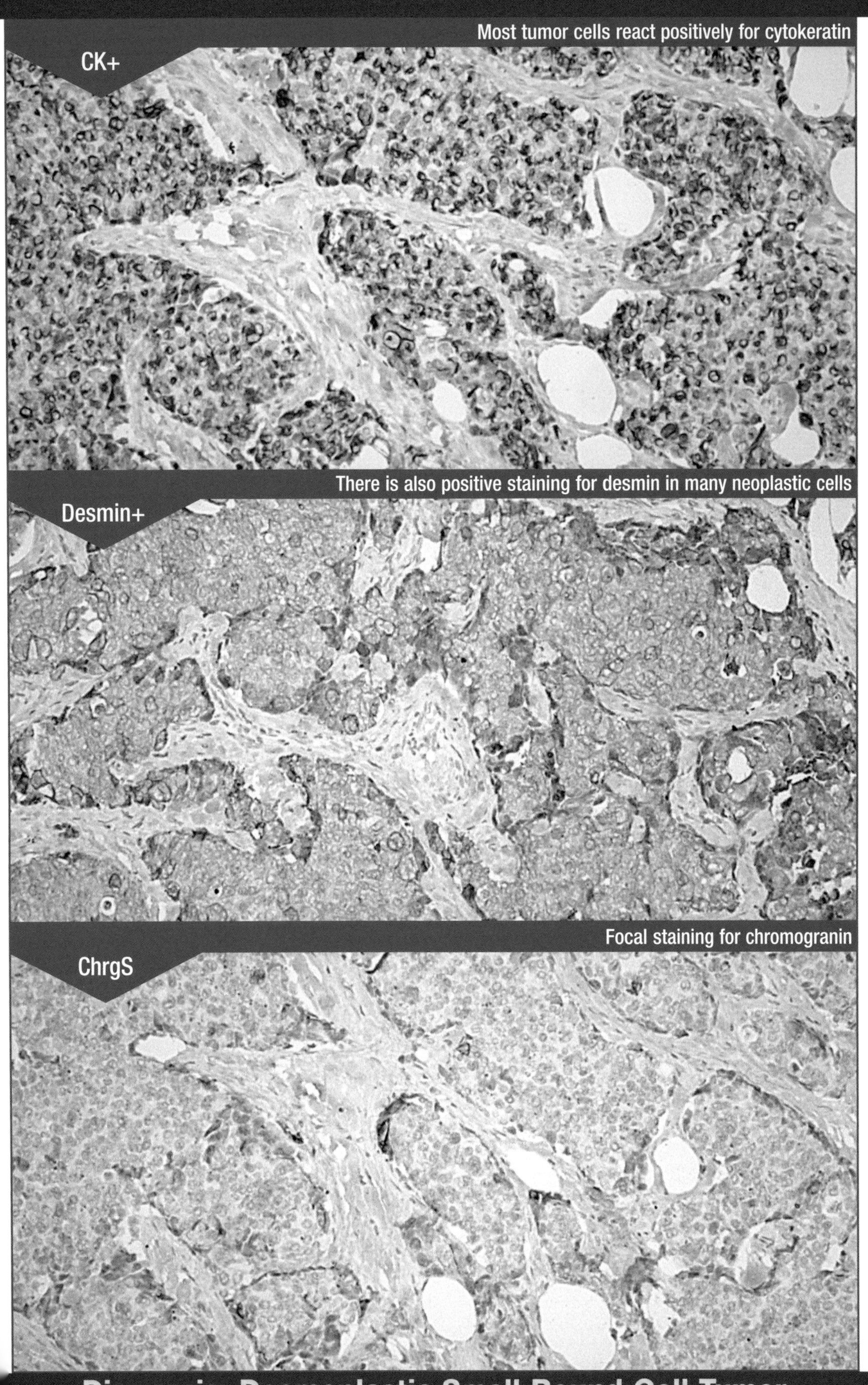

Diagnosis: Desmoplastic Small Round Cell Tumor

Pelvic tumor involving mesosalpinx

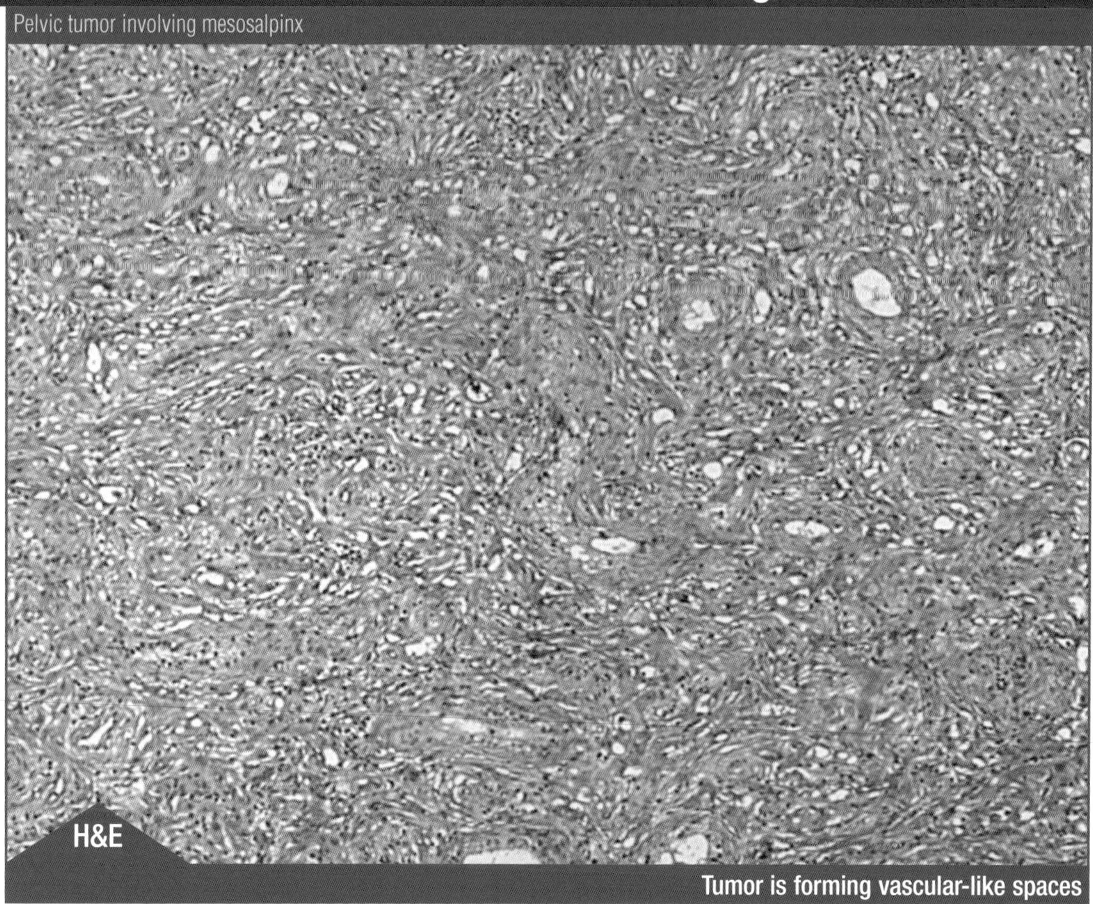

Tumor is forming vascular-like spaces

Adenomatoid Tumor vs Hemangioma			
	Cytokeratin (CK)	Calretinin	CD31
Adenomatoid Tumor	+	+	–
Hemangioma	–	–	+

Helpful Hints

In majority of cases, the above lesions could be distinguished from each other by routine stains. If immunohistochemistry is needed, the use of **cytokeratin**, **calretinin**, and **CD31** distinguishes adenomatoid tumors from hemangiomas.

Nogales 2002.

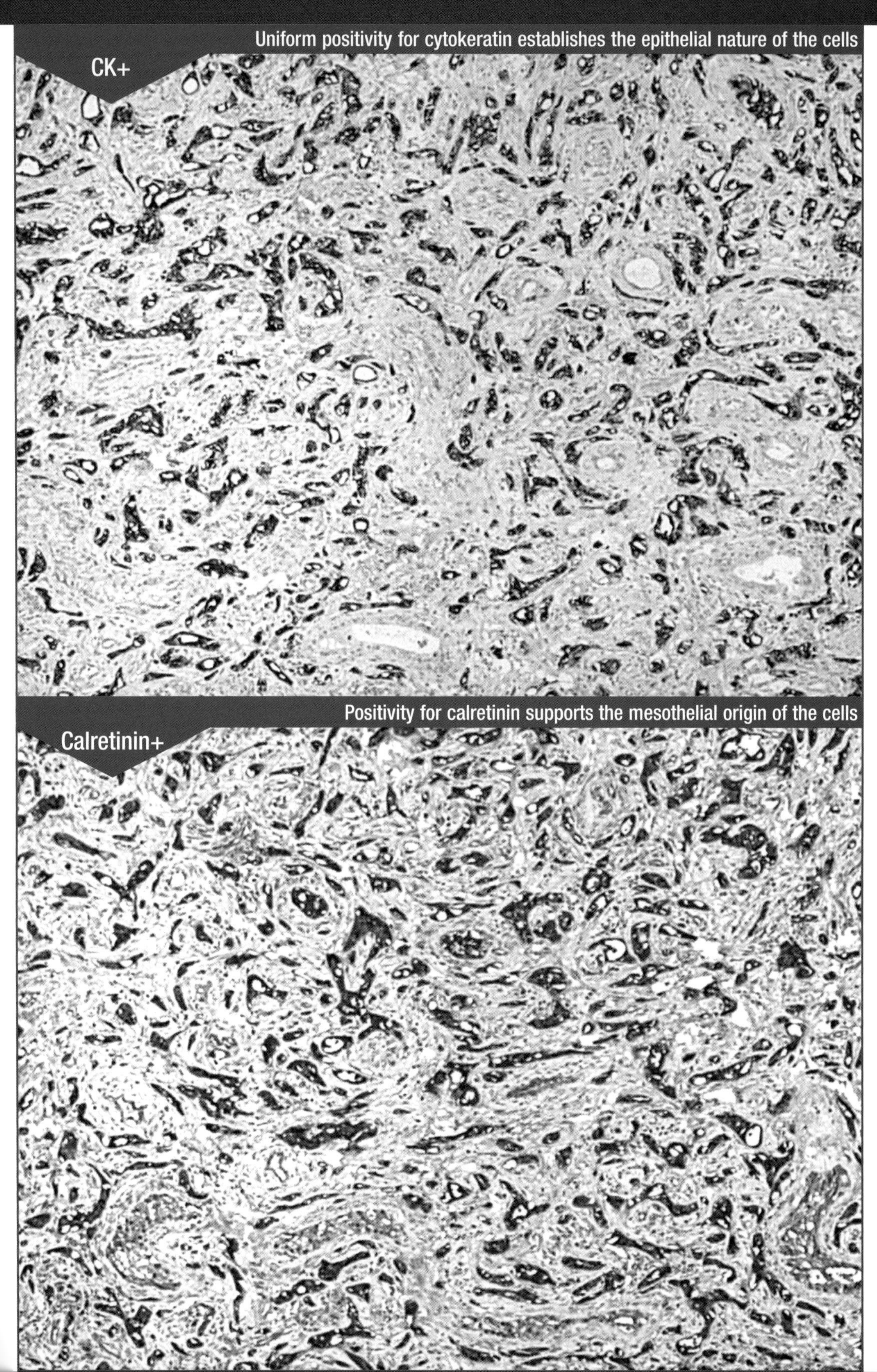

Diagnosis: Adenomatoid Tumor

Abdominal tumor in a child, clinically, neuroblastoma was suspected

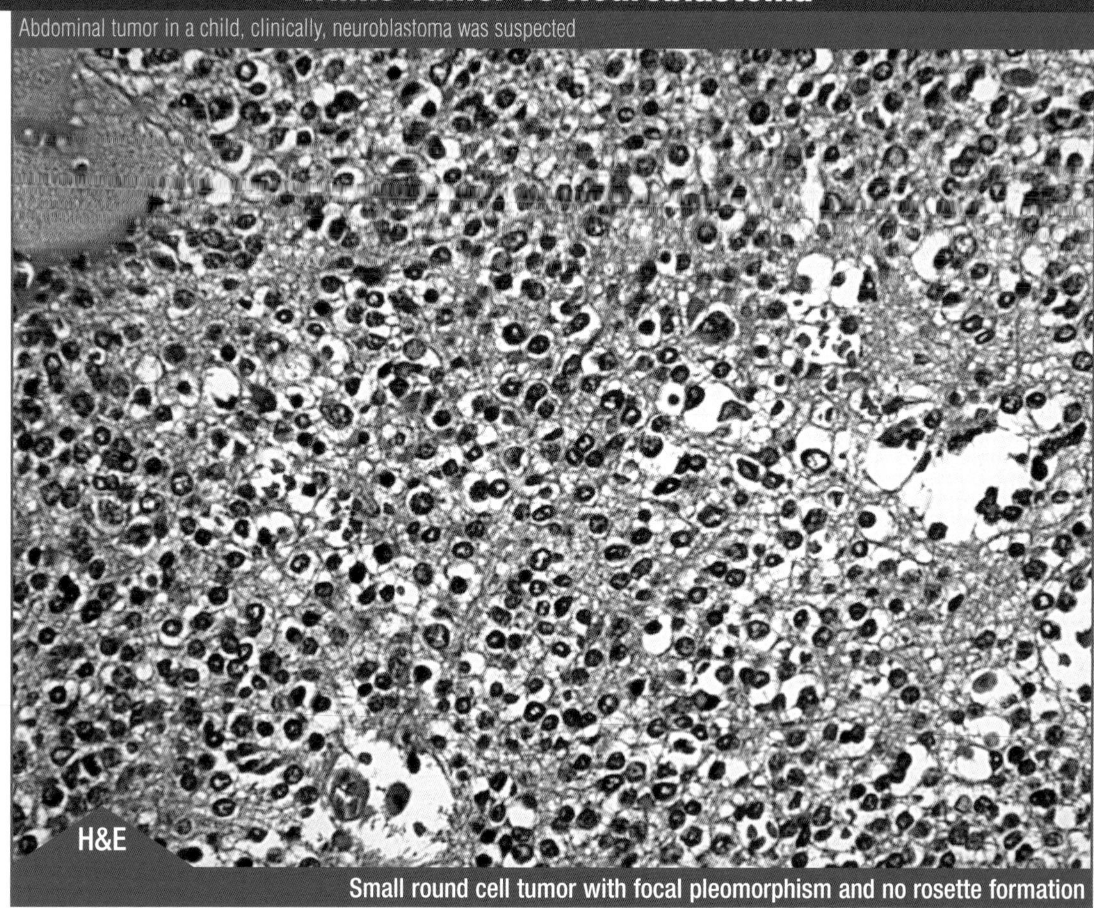

Small round cell tumor with focal pleomorphism and no rosette formation

Wilms Tumor vs Neuroblastoma			
	WT-1	Desmin	NB84
Wilms Tomor	+	S	–
Neuroblastoma	–	–	+

Helpful Hints

Neuroblastoma antigen (**NB84**) is expressed by primitive and differentiating neuroblasts. Therefore, most neuroblastomas and ganglioneuroblastomas are positive for this marker. Wilms tumors are negative for this antigen, but are focally positive for keratin and desmin, reflecting their epithelial and muscle differentiation. All Wilms tumors are positive for **WT-1**.

Thomas 1991, Ghanem 2000.

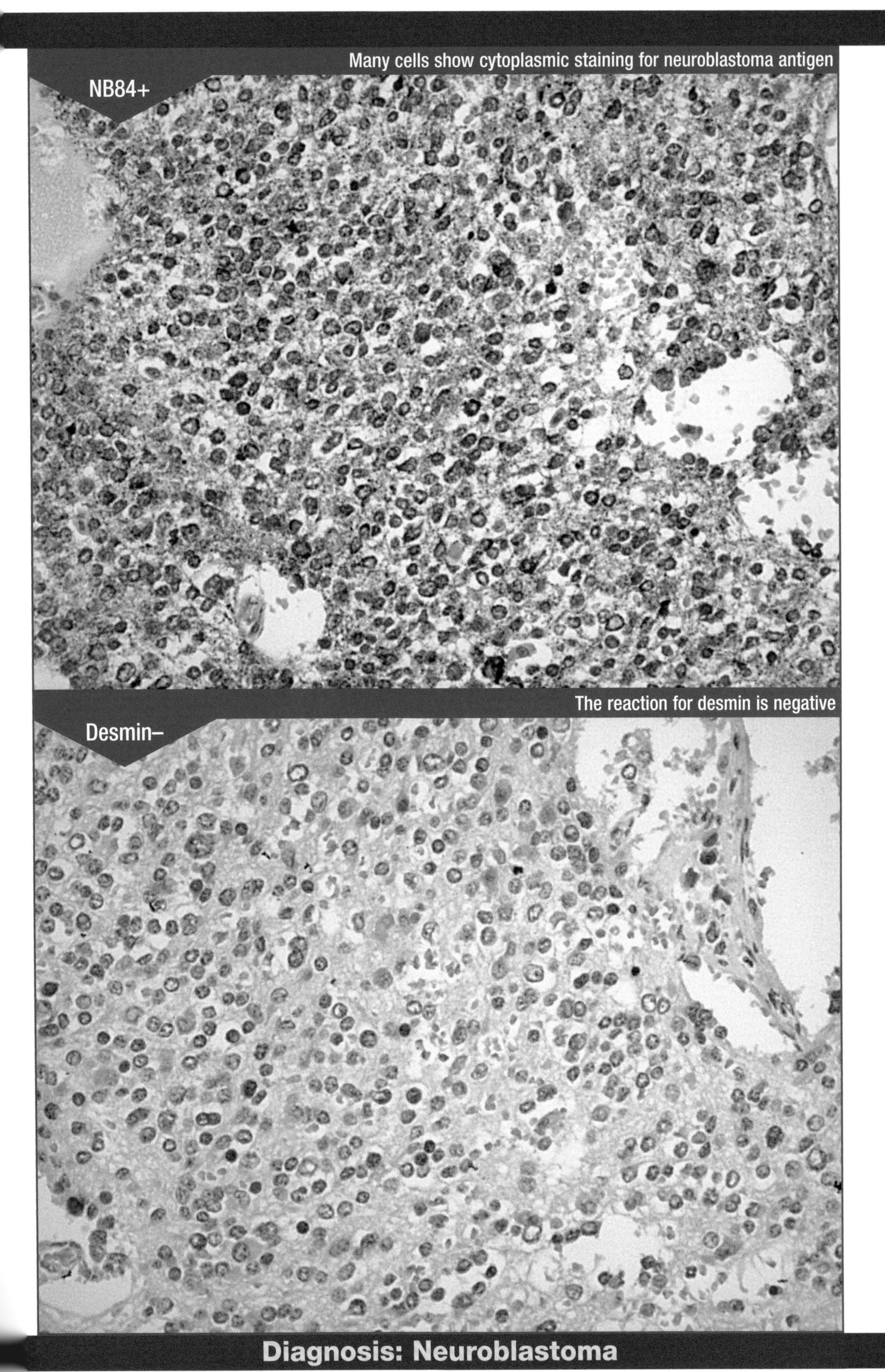

Diagnosis: Neuroblastoma

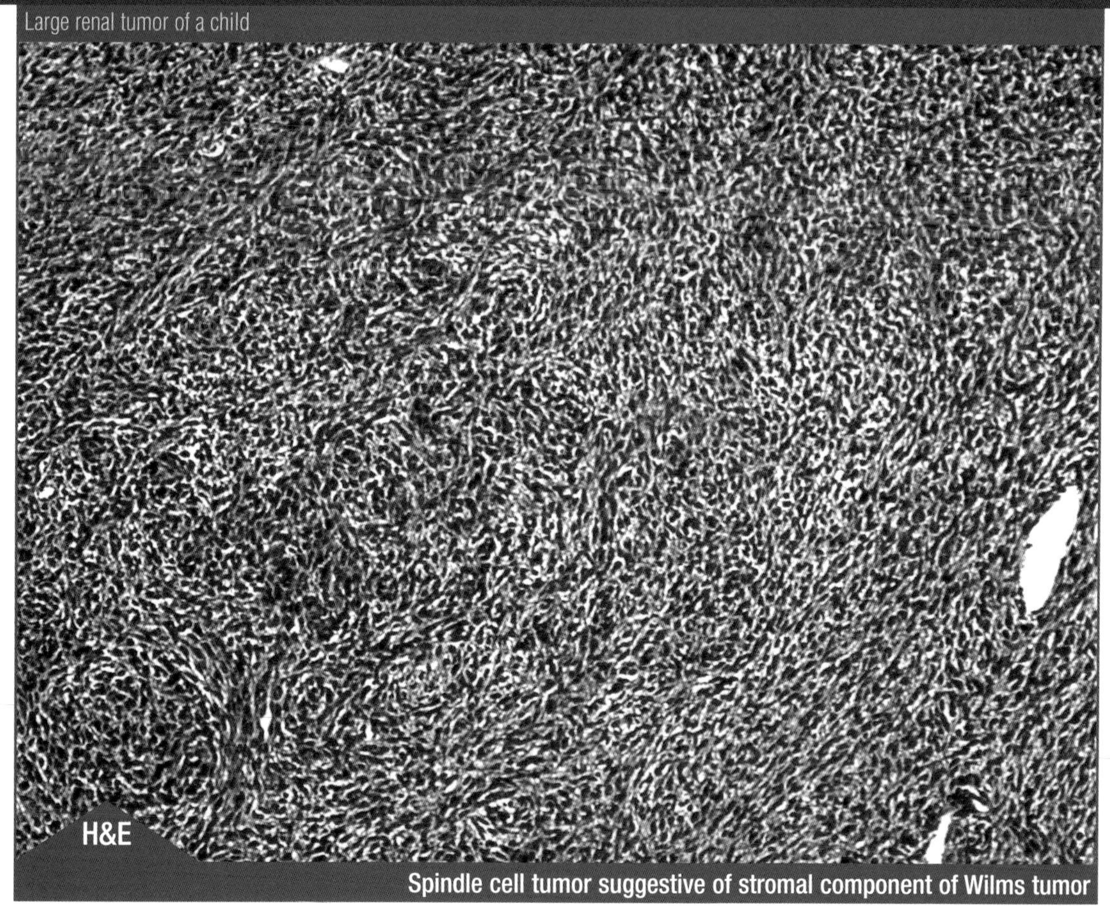

Spindle cell tumor suggestive of stromal component of Wilms tumor

Wilms Tumor vs Neuroblastoma			
	WT-1	Desmin	NB84
Wilms Tomor	+	S	–
Neuroblastoma	–	–	+

Helpful Hints

Neuroblastoma antigen (**NB84**) is expressed by primitive and differentiating neuroblasts. Therefore, most neuroblastomas and ganglioneuroblastomas are positive for this marker. Wilms tumors are negative for this antigen, but are focally positive for keratin and desmin, reflecting their epithelial and muscle differentiation. All Wilms tumors are positive for **WT-1**.

Thomas 1991, Ghanem 2000.

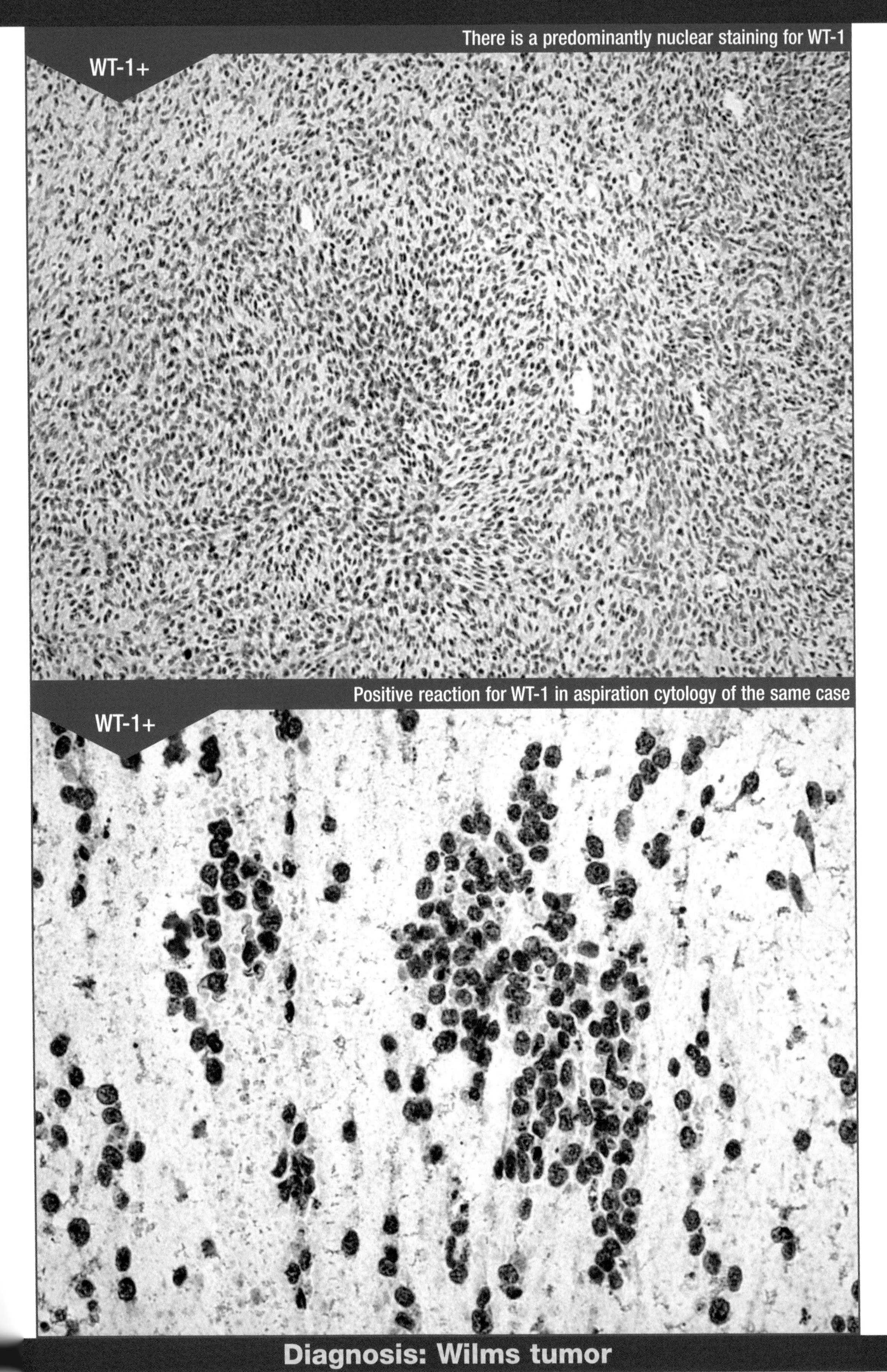

Diagnosis: Wilms tumor

Uterine tumor

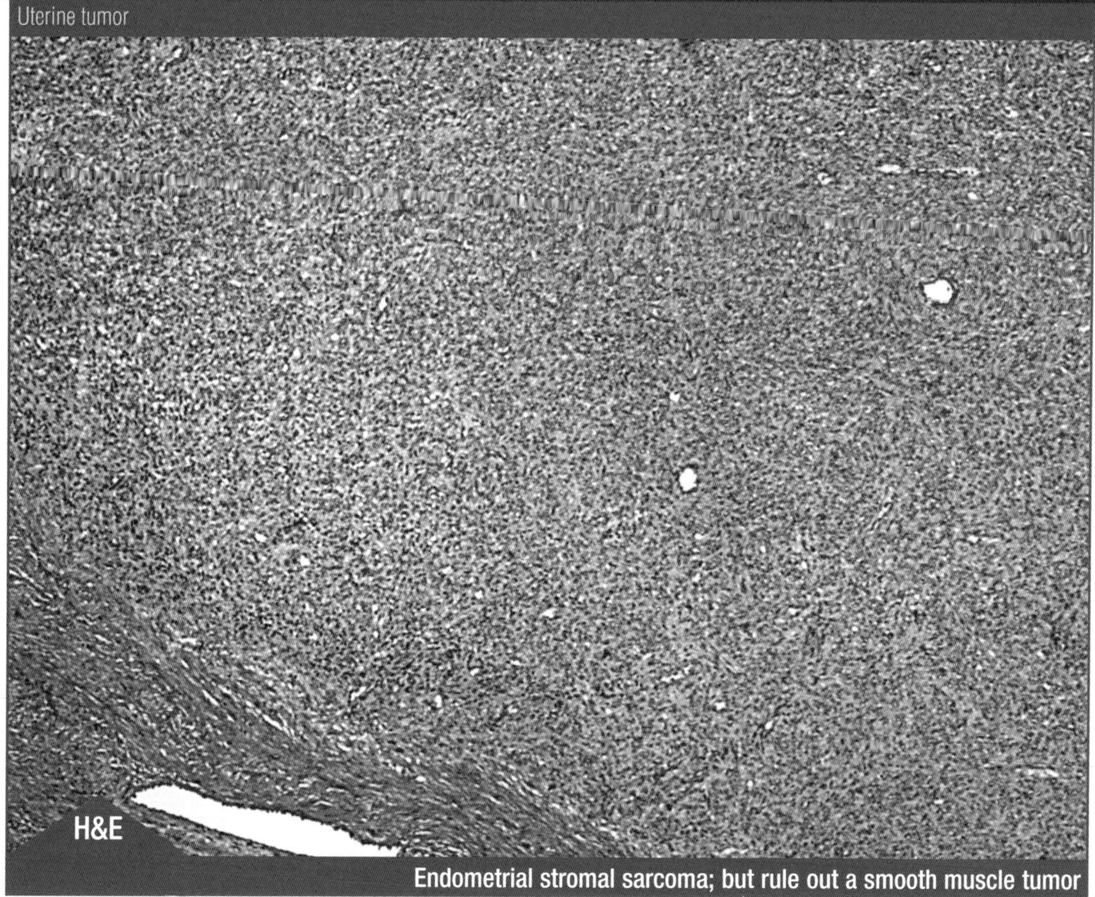

Endometrial stromal sarcoma; but rule out a smooth muscle tumor

Uterine Leiomyosarcoma vs Endometrial Stromal Sarcoma			
	CD10	H-Caldesmon (HCD)	Estrogen Receptor (ER)
Uterine Leiomyosarcoma	–	+	S
Endometrial Stromal Sarcoma	+	–	+

Helpful Hints

Endometrial stromal sarcomas are positive for **CD10** while leiomyosarcomas are not. On the other hand, **H-Caldesmon** (**HCD**) is expressed by leiomyosarcomas but not by stromal sarcomas. It should be noted that focal desmin positivity can be seen in some stromal sarcomas of the uterus.

Both stromal sarcomas and leiomyosarcomas may be positive for **estrogen receptor** (**ER**). The reaction is more uniform and diffuse in stromal sarcomas.

Toki 2002, Zhu 2004.

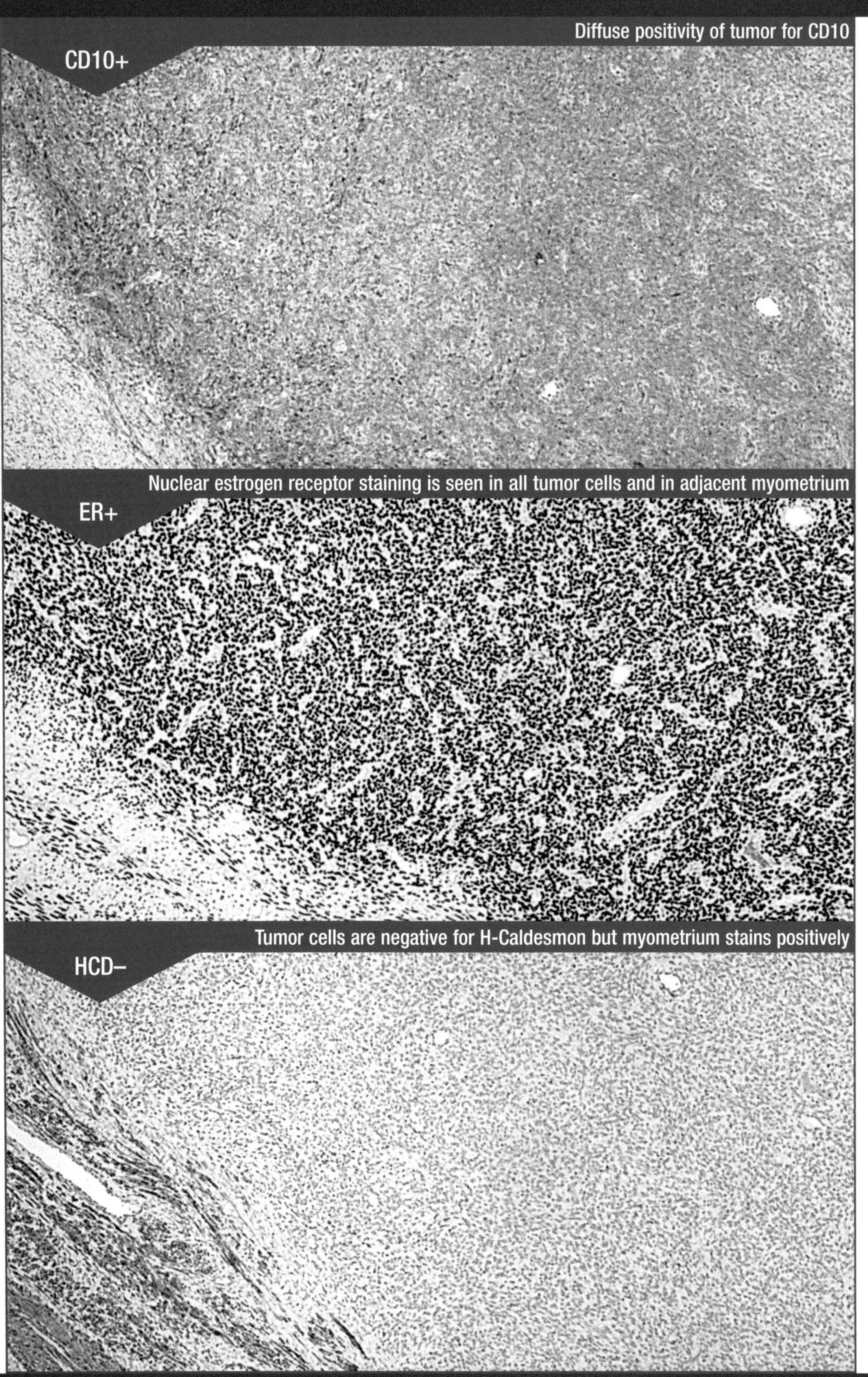

Diagnosis: Stromal Sarcoma of Uterus

Polypoid lesion in the uterine cavity

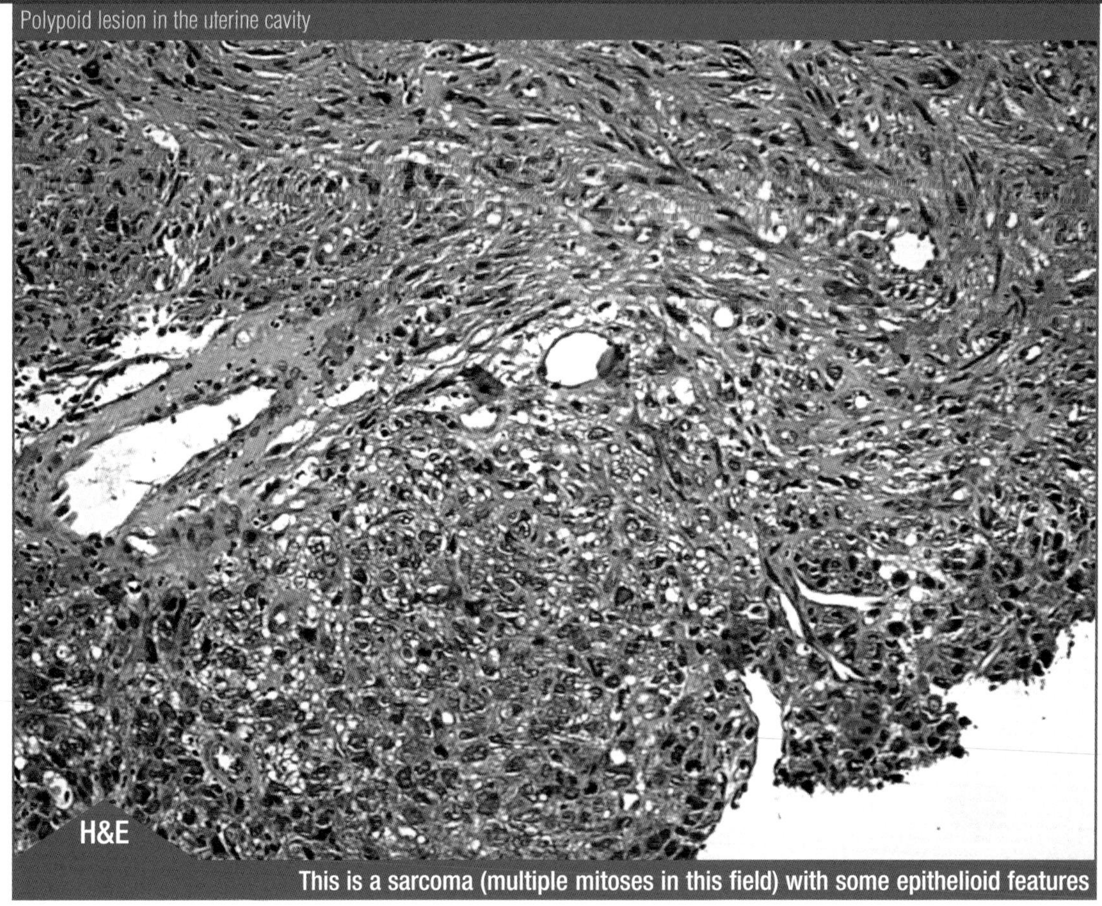

This is a sarcoma (multiple mitoses in this field) with some epithelioid features

Uterine Leiomyosarcoma vs Endometrial Stromal Sarcoma			
	CD10	H-Caldesmon (HCD)	Estrogen Receptor (ER)
Uterine Leiomyosarcoma	–	+	S
Endometrial Stromal Sarcoma	+	–	+

Helpful Hints

Endometrial stromal sarcomas are positive for **CD10** while leiomyosarcomas are not. On the other hand, **H-Caldesmon** (**HCD**) is expressed by leiomyosarcomas but not by stromal sarcomas. It should be noted that focal desmin positivity can be seen in some stromal sarcomas of the uterus.

Both stromal sarcomas and leiomyosarcomas may be positive for **estrogen receptor** (**ER**). The reaction is more uniform and diffuse in stromal sarcomas.

Toki 2002, Zhu 2004.

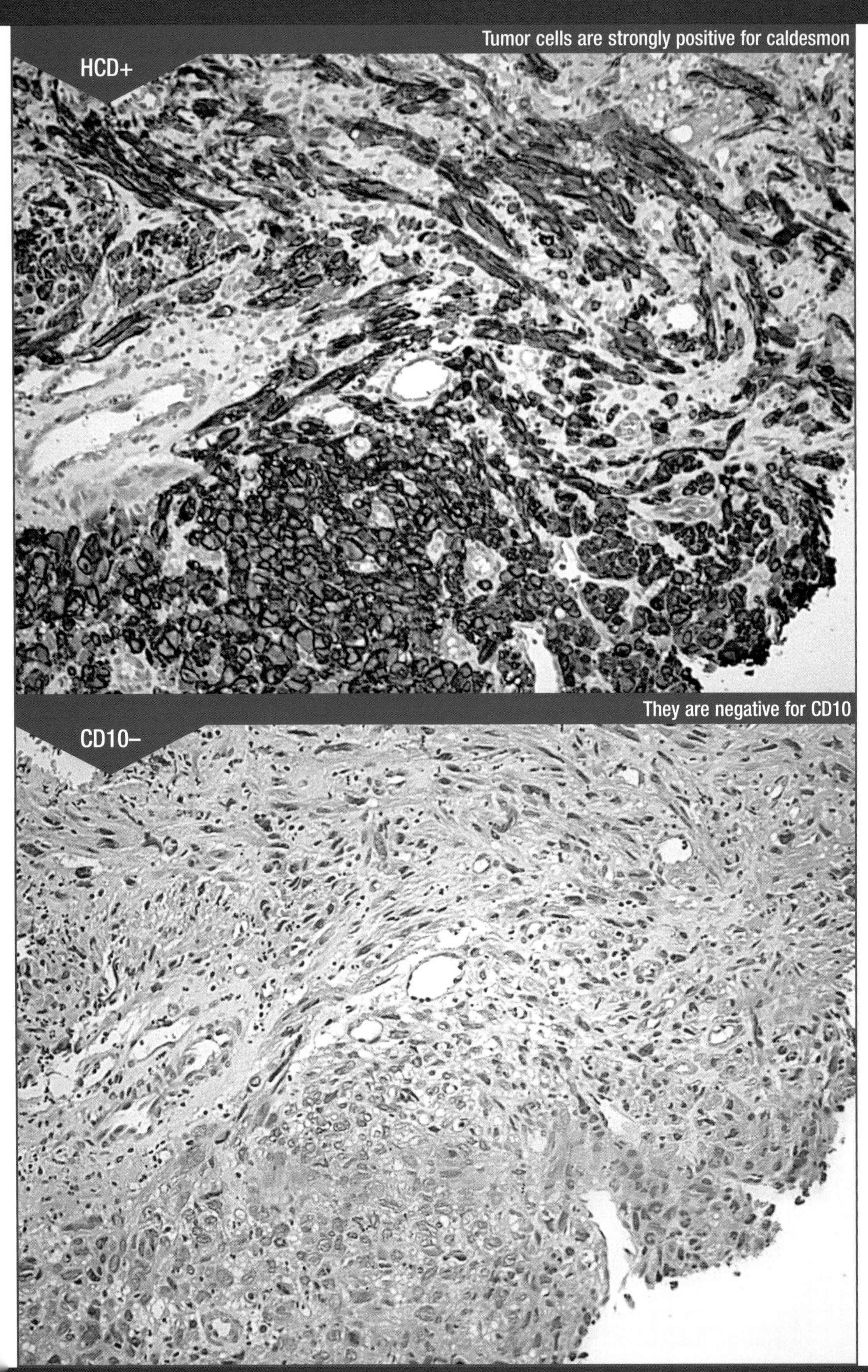

Diagnosis: Leiomyosarcoma, Epithelioid Type

Cone biopsy of cervix

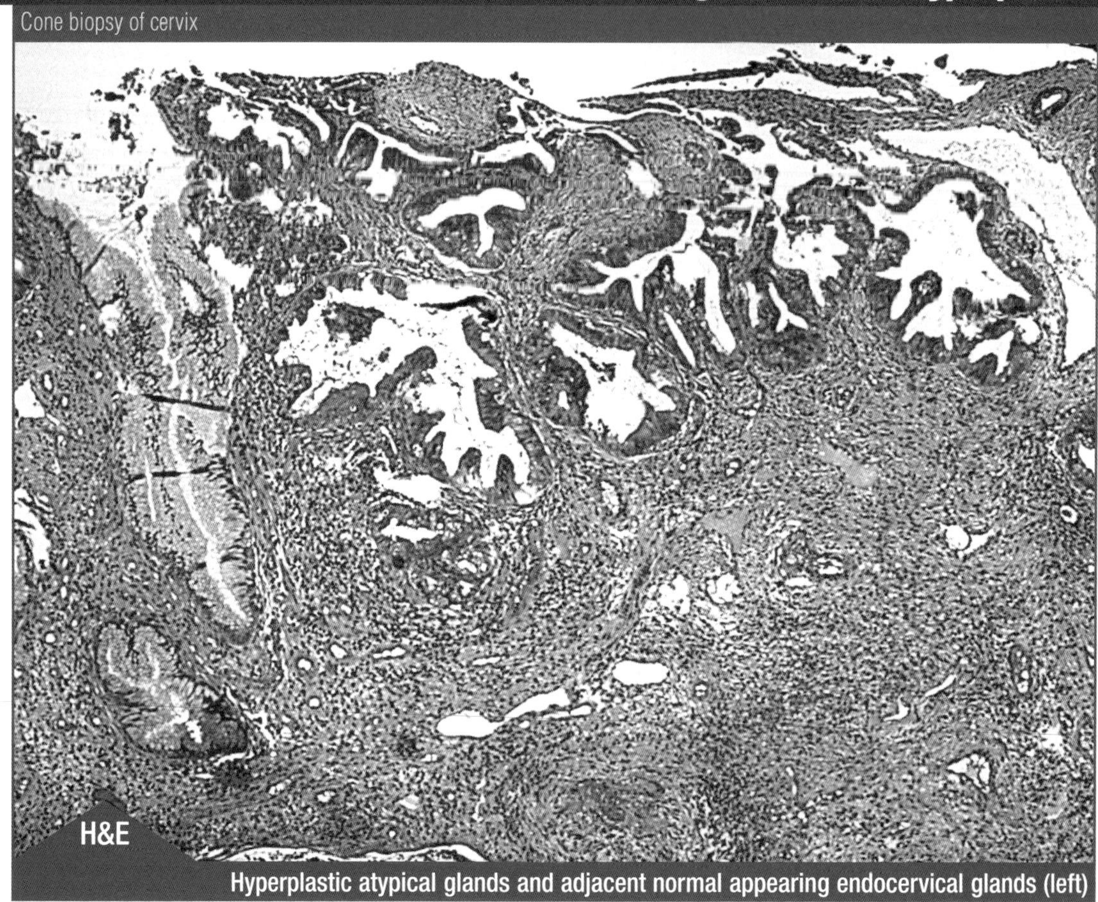

Hyperplastic atypical glands and adjacent normal appearing endocervical glands (left)

Adenocarcinoma of Uterine Cervix vs Benign Glandular Hyperplasia		
	p16	p63
Adenocarcinoma of Cervix	+	–
Benign Glandular Hyperplasia	–	+

Helpful Hints

p16 is an oncogene expressed, at least focally, by a number of different tumors. It is uniformly expressed by all HPV-related precancerous or cancerous lesions of the uterine cervix. Most adenocarcinomas of cervix are HPV-related and therefore express p16. In cervical cancer, whether squamous or glandular, staining for p16 is strong and diffuse and is present in the both the cytoplasms and nuclei of tumor cells. P16 reaction in non-HPV related cancers, such as those of endometrium, is usually focal in distribution. Benign glandular hyperplasias of the cervix are negative for p16. **p63** is present in the basal cells of the metaplastic squamous epithelium and hence is positive in benign glandular hyperplasias with or without squamous metaplasia. It is absent in adenocarcinomas.

Negri 2003, Schorge 2004.

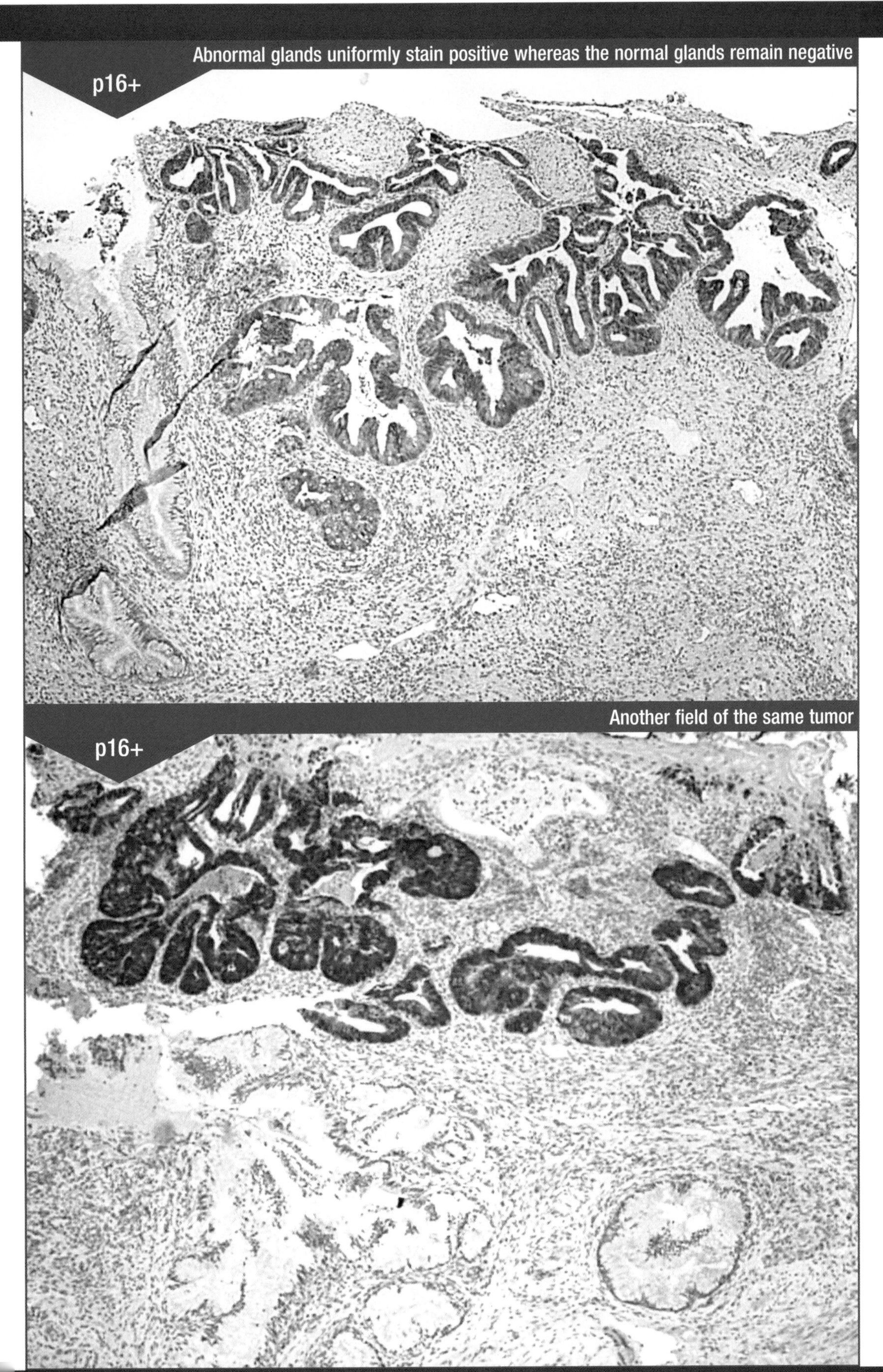

Diagnosis: Adenocarcinoma of Cervix

Endocervical polyp

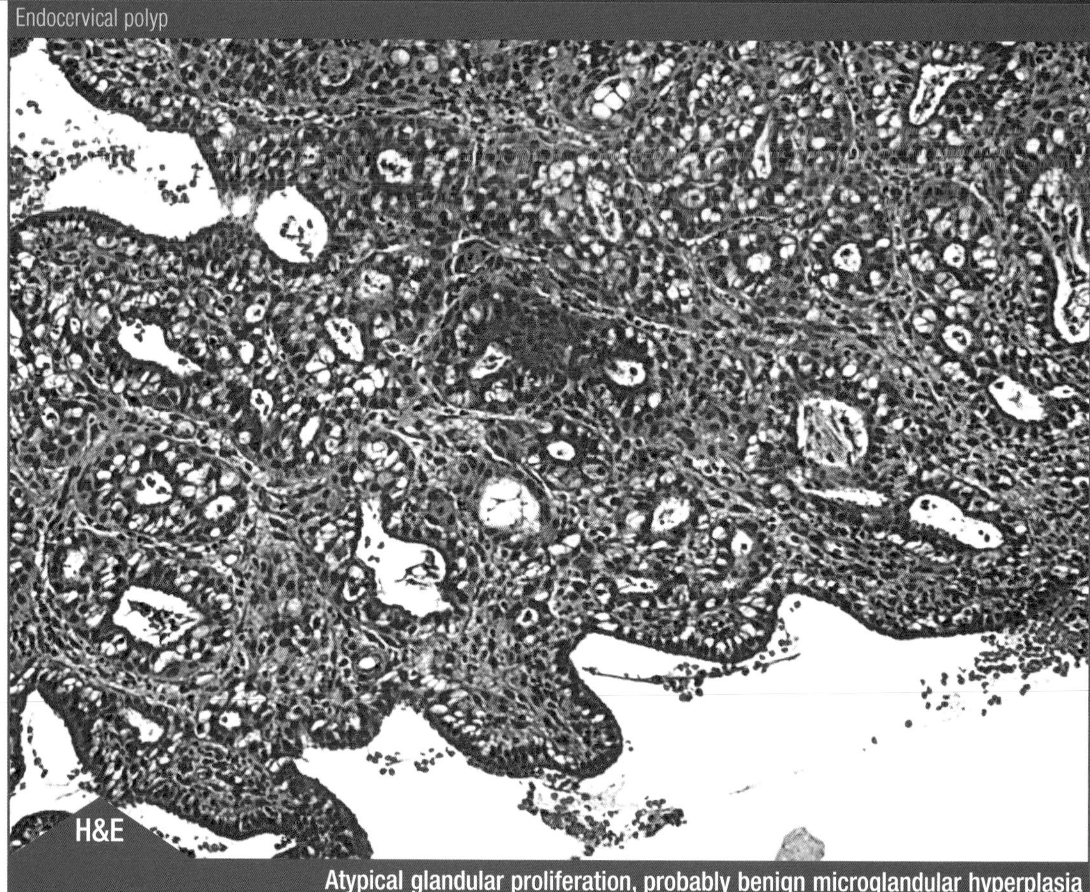

Atypical glandular proliferation, probably benign microglandular hyperplasia

Adenocarcinoma of Uterine Cervix vs Benign Glandular Hyperplasia		
	p16	p63
Adenocarcinoma of Cervix	+	–
Benign Glandular Hyperplasia	–	+

Helpful Hints

p16 is an oncogene expressed, at least focally, by a number of different tumors. It is uniformly expressed by all HPV-related precancerous or cancerous lesions of the uterine cervix. Most adenocarcinomas of cervix are HPV-related and therefore express p16. In cervical cancer, whether squamous or glandular, staining for p16 is strong and diffuse and is present in the both the cytoplasms and nuclei of tumor cells. P16 reaction in non-HPV related cancers, such as those of endometrium, is usually focal in distribution. Benign glandular hyperplasias of the cervix are negative for p16. **p63** is present in the basal cells of the metaplastic squamous epithelium and hence is positive in benign glandular hyperplasias with or without squamous metaplasia. It is absent in adenocarcinomas.

Negri 2003, Schorge 2004.

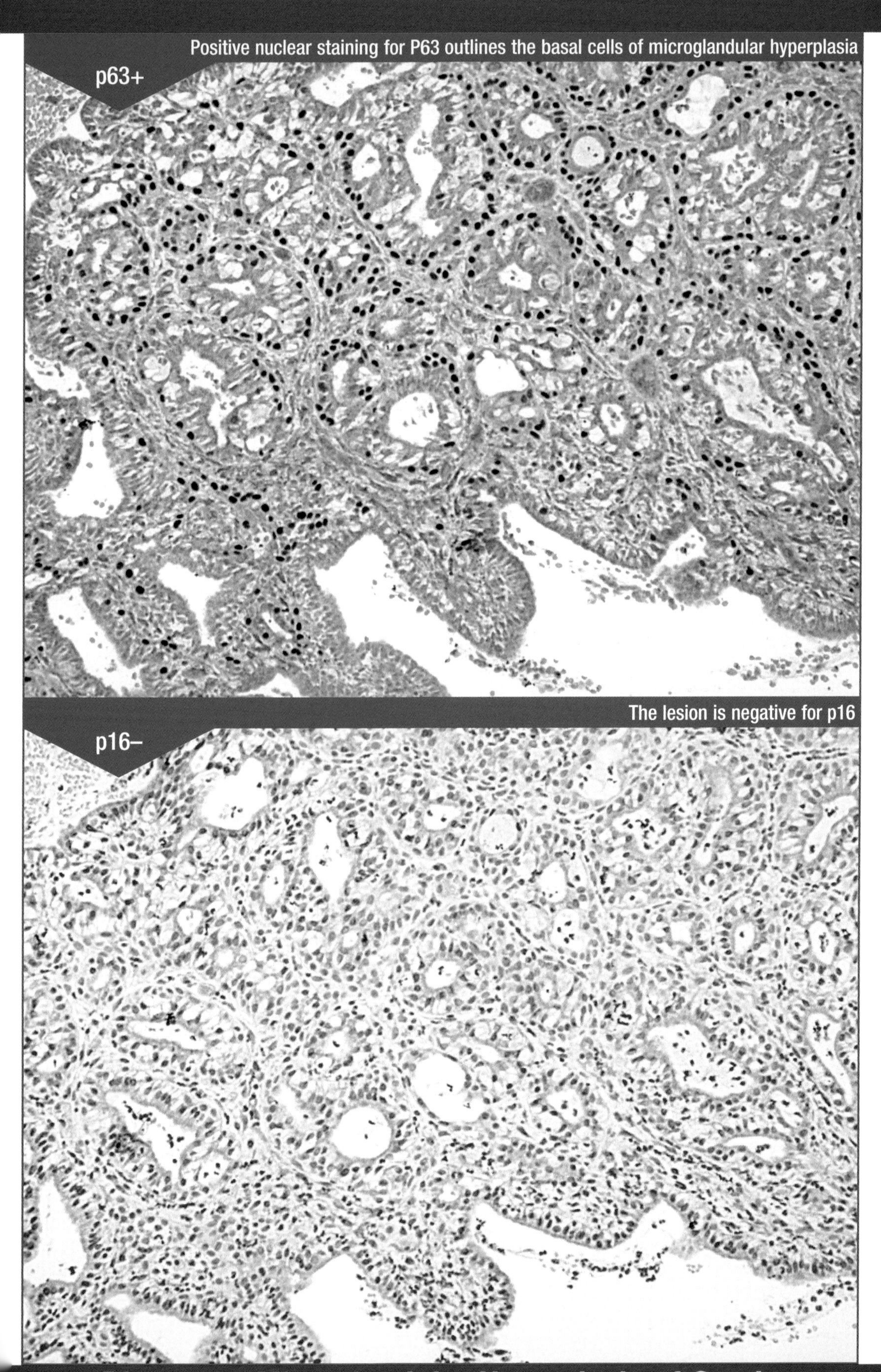

Diagnosis: Microglandular Hyperplasia of Cervix

Hysterectomy specimen

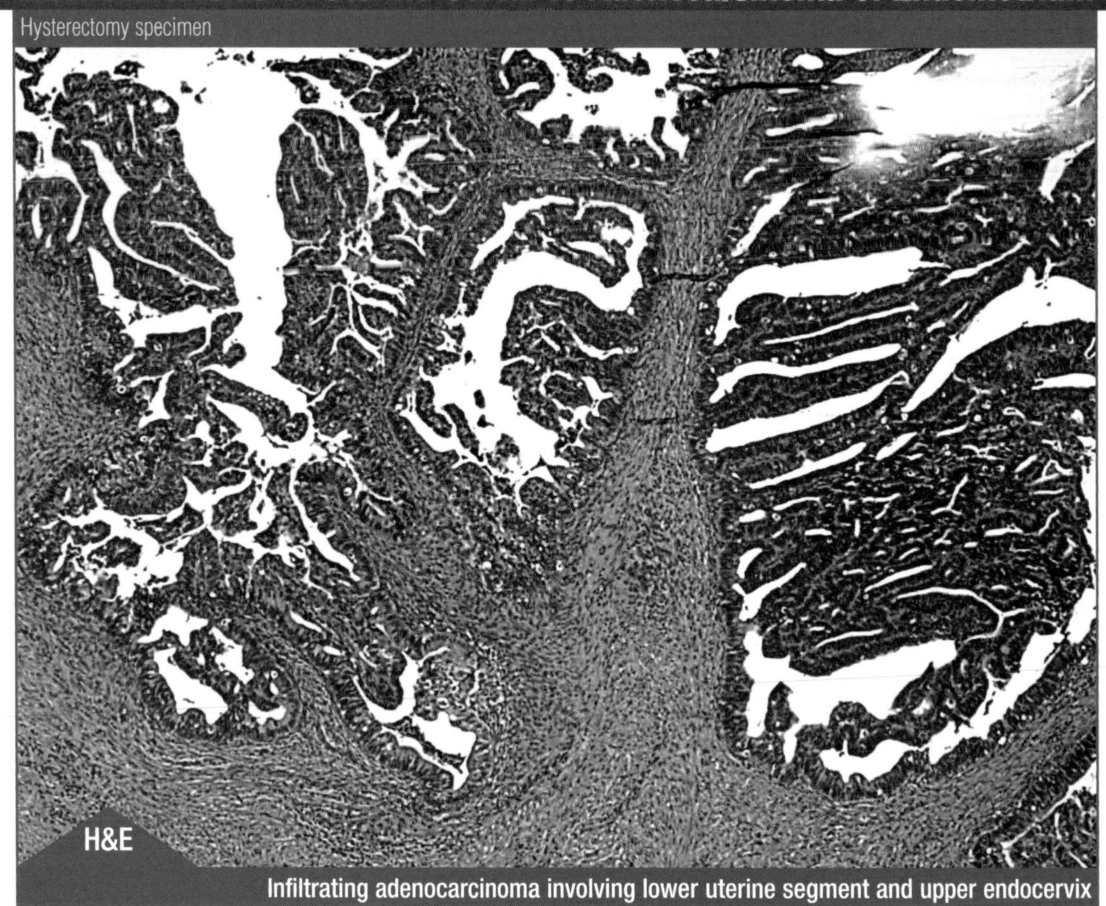

Infiltrating adenocarcinoma involving lower uterine segment and upper endocervix

Adenocarcinoma of Uterine Cervix vs Adenocarcinoma of Endometrium		
	p16	Estrogen Receptor (ER)
Adenocarcinoma of Cervix	+	S
Endometrial Adenocarcinoma	S	+

Helpful Hints

The immunohistochemical differential diagnosis between endometrial and endocervical adenocarcinoma is difficult. This is because the expression of markers in Müllerian epithelial-derived tumors is "cell type"-dependant and not "site"-dependant.

A combination of **p16** and **estrogen receptor** (**ER**) as suggested above may be helpful in some cases but not at all times. The expression of p16 in HPV-related cervical cancers is uniform and strong throughout the tumor. However, p16 may be expressed by a number of other tumors including endometrial carcinomas. In most such cases, the reaction for p16 is only focal. Conversely, most endometrial carcinomas express estrogen receptor whereas in endocervical adenocarcinomas the reaction may be focal or negative.

McCluggage 2003.

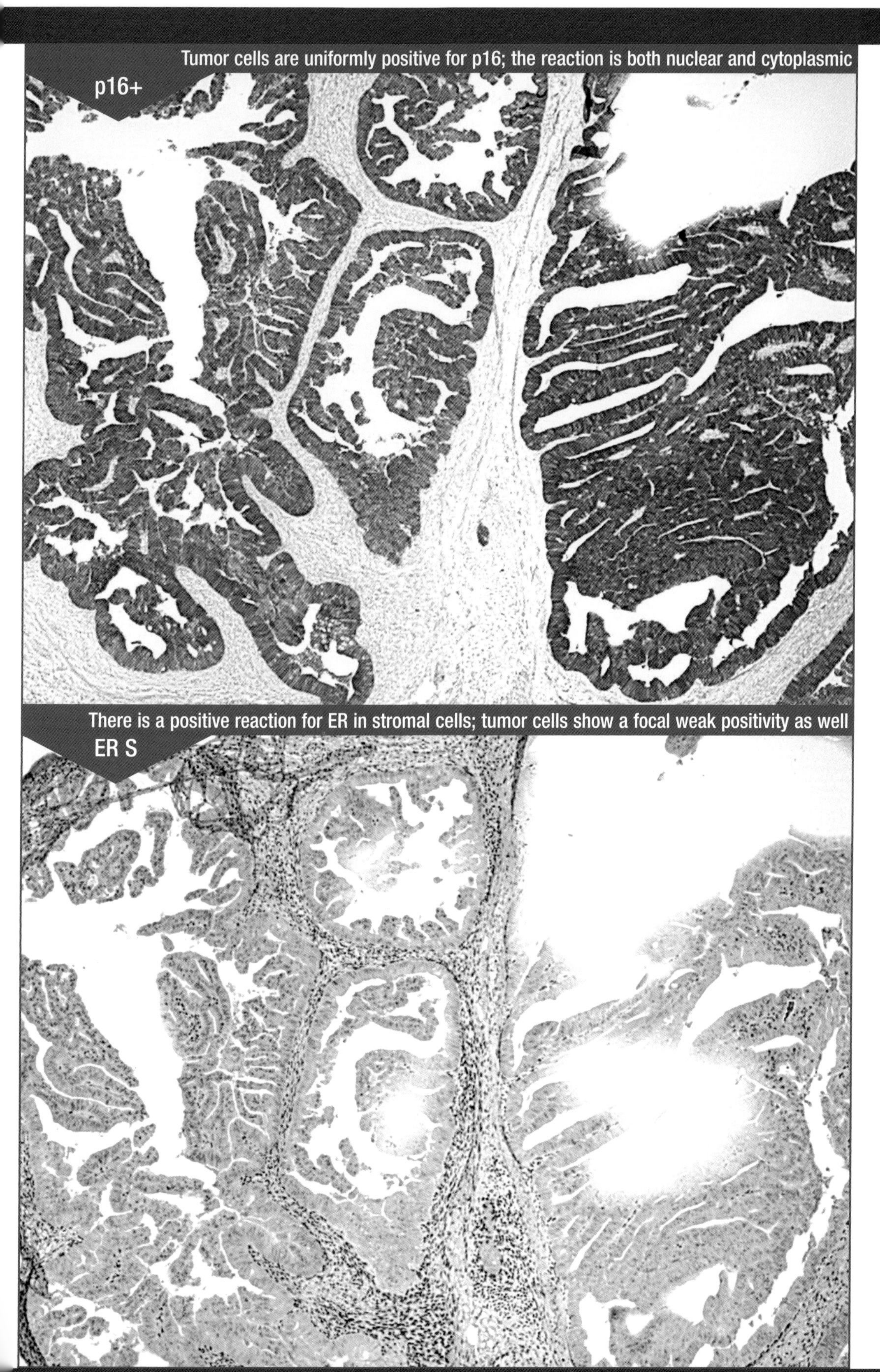

Tumor cells are uniformly positive for p16; the reaction is both nuclear and cytoplasmic

There is a positive reaction for ER in stromal cells; tumor cells show a focal weak positivity as well

Diagnosis: Endocervical Adenocarcinoma

Hysterectomy for endometrial adenocarcinoma

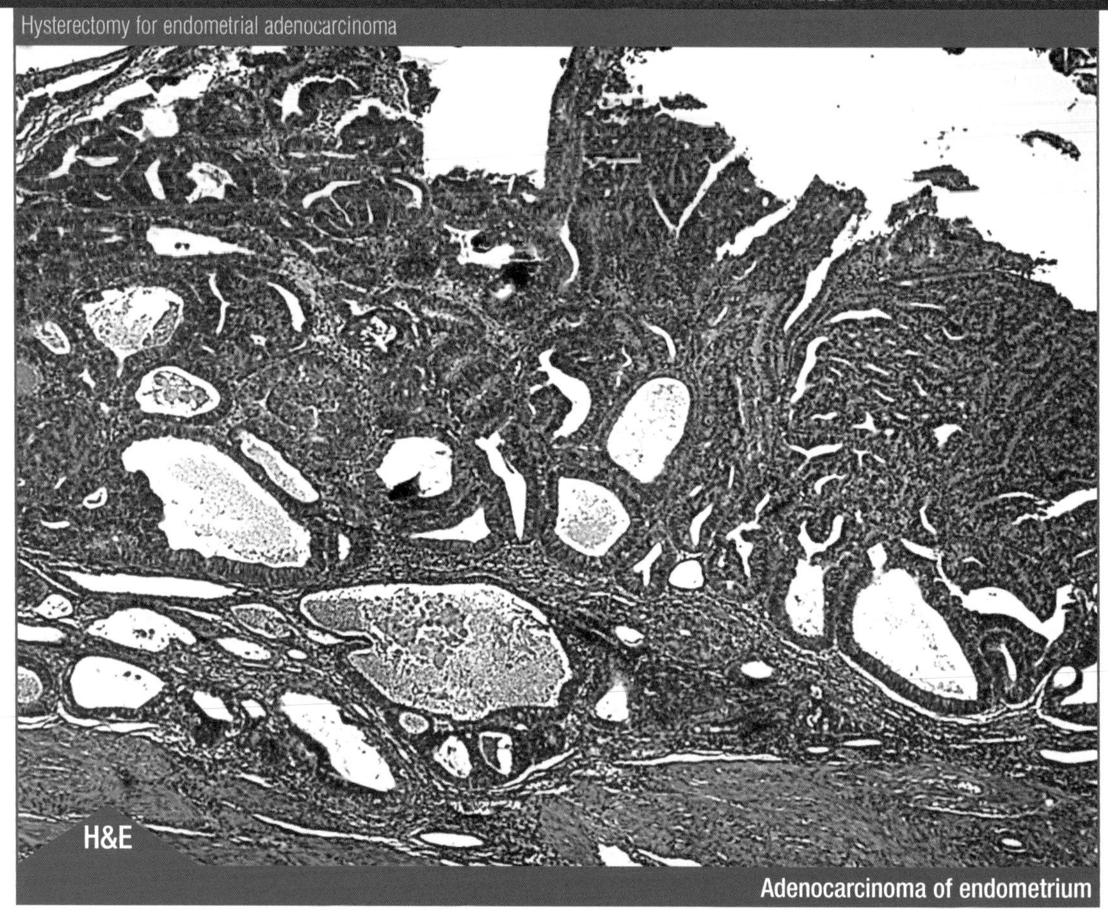

Adenocarcinoma of endometrium

Adenocarcinoma of Uterine Cervix vs Adenocarcinoma of Endometrium		
	p16	Estrogen Receptor (ER)
Adenocarcinoma of Cervix	+	S
Endometrial Adenocarcinoma	S	+

Helpful Hints

The immunohistochemical differential diagnosis between endometrial and endocervical adenocarcinoma is difficult. This is because the expression of markers in Müllerian epithelial-derived tumors is "cell type"-dependant and not "site"-dependant.

A combination of **p16** and **estrogen receptor** (**ER**) as suggested above may be helpful in some cases but not at all times. The expression of p16 in HPV-related cervical cancers is uniform and strong throughout the tumor. However, p16 may be expressed by a number of other tumors including endometrial carcinomas. In most such cases, the reaction for p16 is only focal. Conversely, most endometrial carcinomas express estrogen receptor whereas in endocervical adenocarcinomas the reaction may be focal or negative.

McCluggage 2003.

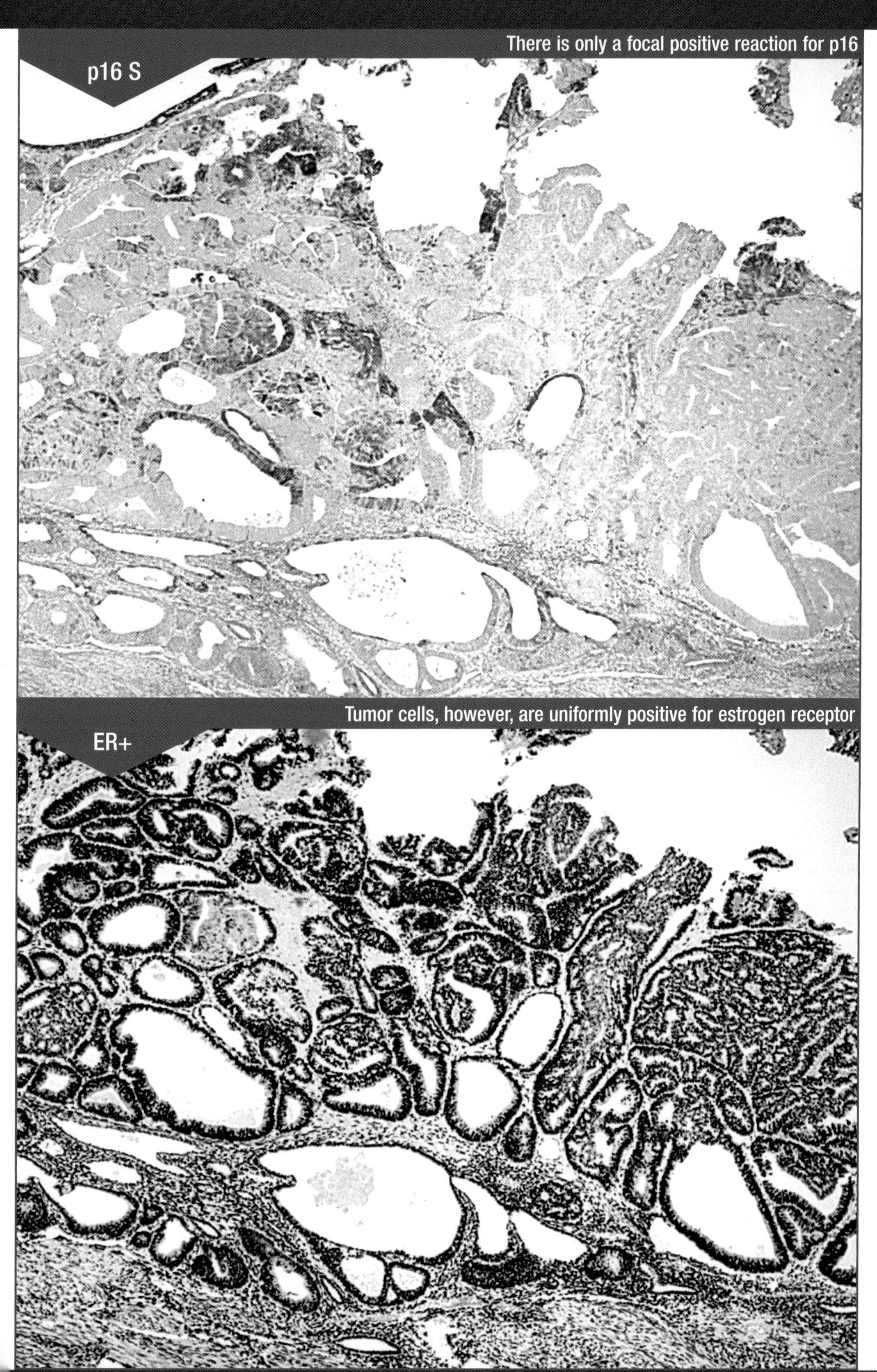

Diagnosis: Endometrial Adenocarcinoma

Specimen labeled as products of conception

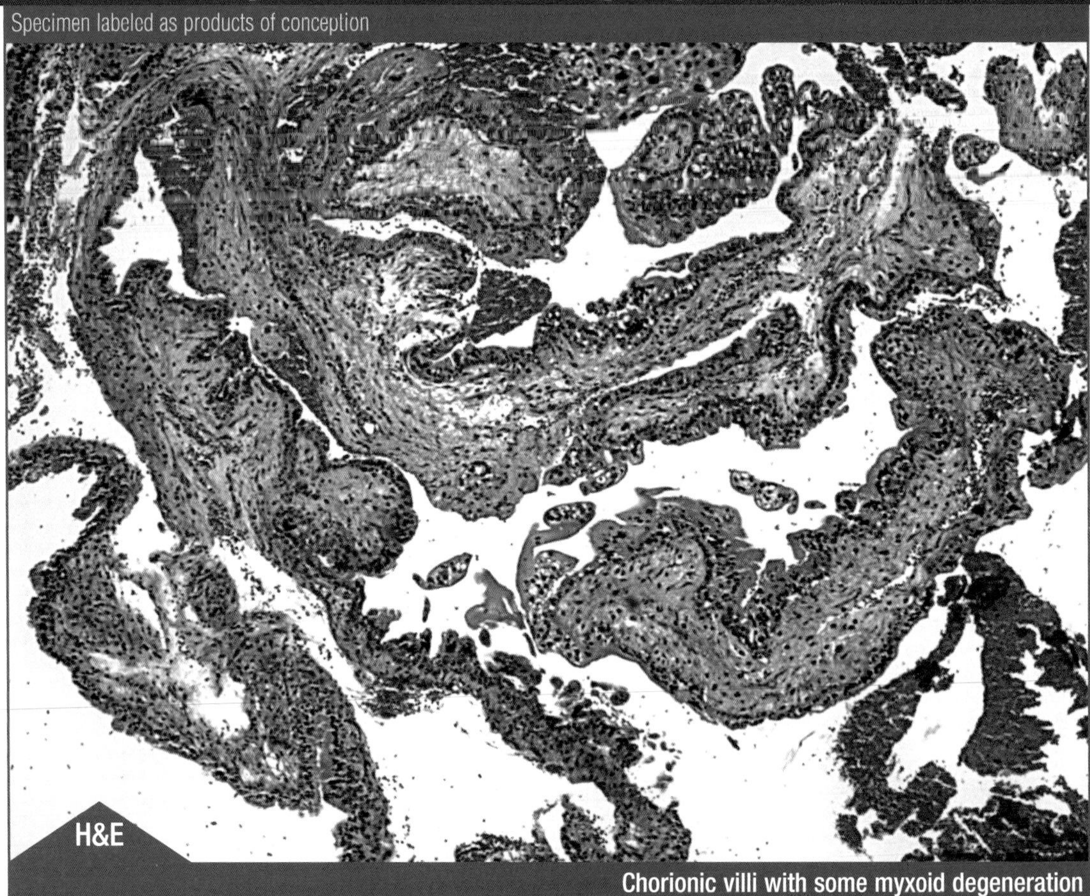

Chorionic villi with some myxoid degeneration

Hydatidiform Mole vs Hydropic Abortion	
	p57 in villi
Hydatidiform Mole	–
Hydropic Abortion	+

Helpful Hints

This is not an uncommon differential diagnosis; it can be resolved by the use of **p57** staining. This nuclear marker is a cyclin-dependent kinase inhibitor expressed by maternal and not by paternal derived cells. It therefore, stains deciduas, stroma of villi, and trophoblasts of hydropic abortions. It is not expressed by the stroma or cytotrophoblasts of the molar villi (paternally derived). Syncytiotrophoblasts in molar pregnancies and hydropic abortions are always positive for p57.

When correctly classified as molar pregnancy by p57, further separation into complete and partial moles becomes irrelevant because the clinical management, follow up and biologic behavior is practically the same.

Romaguera 2005.

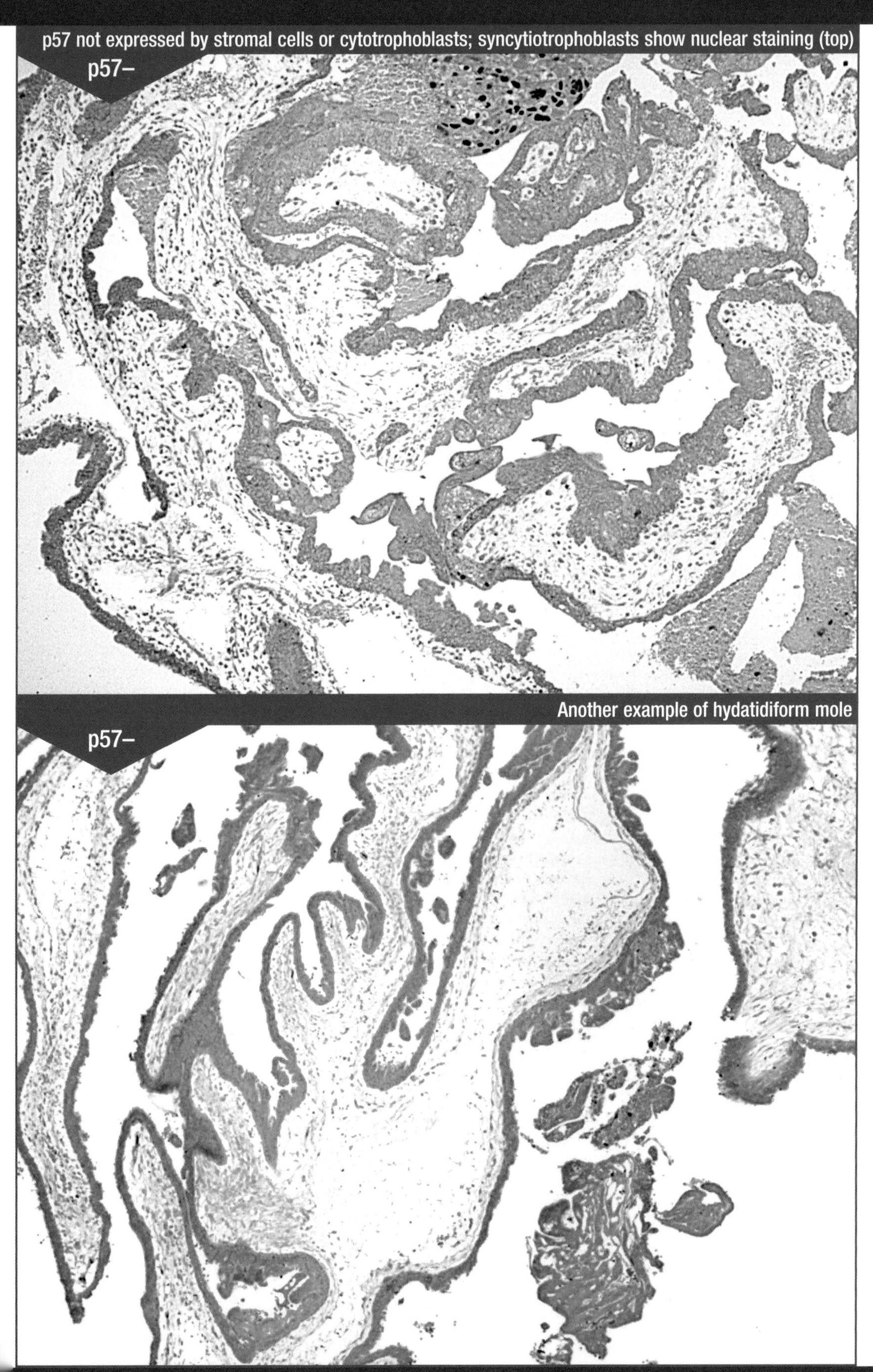

Diagnosis: Molar Pregnancy

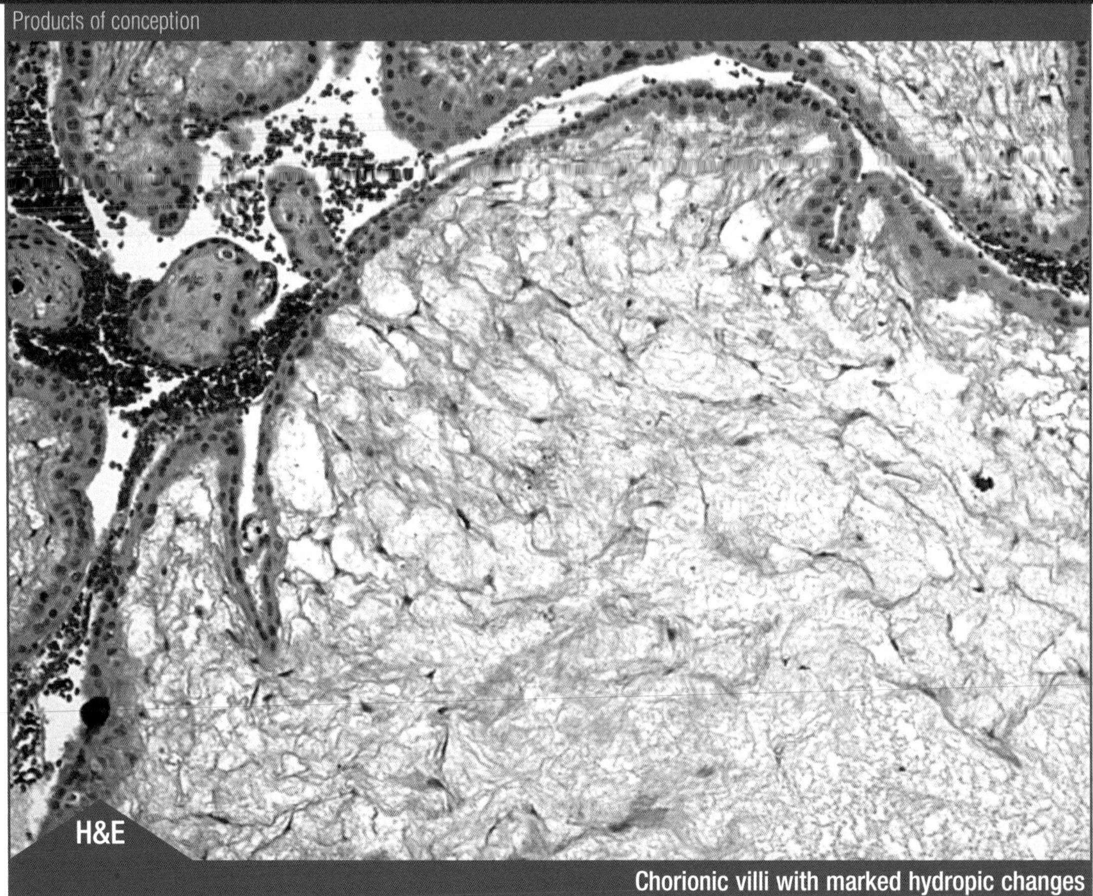

Chorionic villi with marked hydropic changes

Hydatidiform Mole vs Hydropic Abortion	
	p57 in villi
Hydatidiform Mole	–
Hydropic Abortion	+

Helpful Hints

This is not an uncommon differential diagnosis; it can be resolved by the use of **p57** staining. This nuclear marker is a cyclin-dependent kinase inhibitor expressed by maternal and not by paternal derived cells. It therefore, stains deciduas, stroma of villi, and trophoblasts of hydropic abortions. It is not expressed by the stroma or cytotropholasts of the molar villi (paternally derived). Syncytiotrophoblasts in molar pregnancies and hydropic abortions are always positive for p57.

When correctly classified as molar pregnancy by p57, further separation into complete and partial moles becomes irrelevant because the clinical management, follow up and biologic behavior is practically the same.

Romaguera 2005.

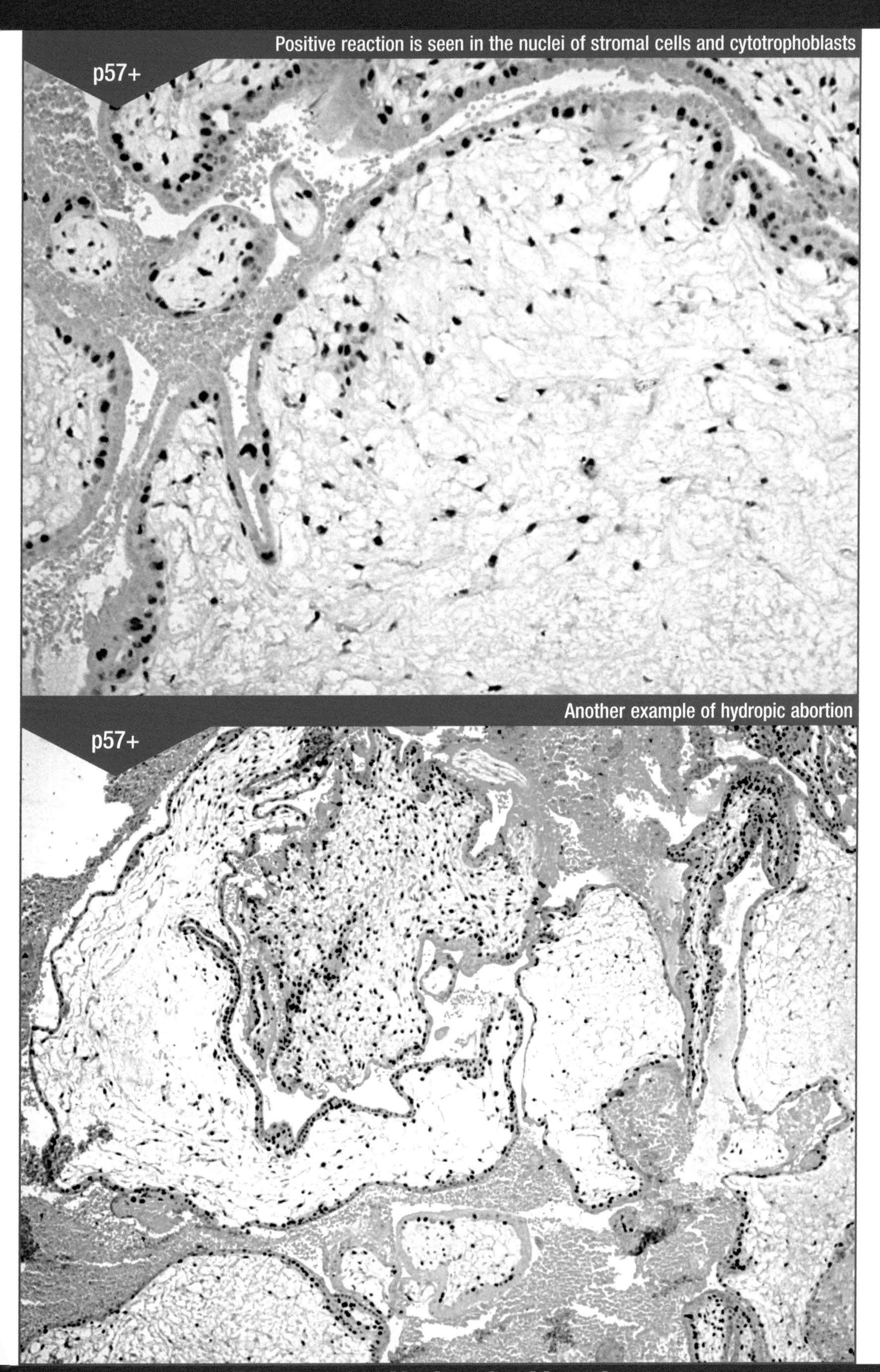

Diagnosis: Hydropic Abortion

Solid ovarian tumor

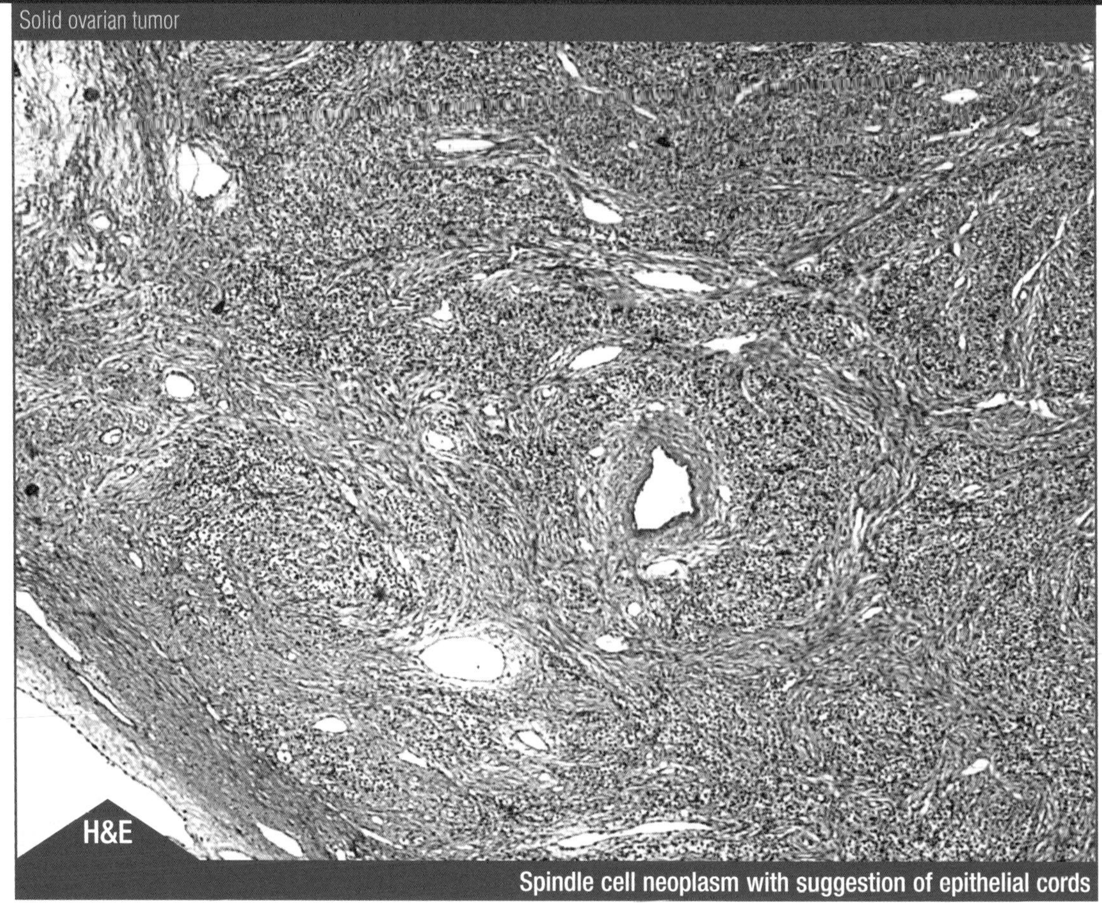

Spindle cell neoplasm with suggestion of epithelial cords

Ovarian Epithelial Tumor vs Sex Cord Stromal Tumor		
	Inhibin	Cytokeratin (CK)
Ovarian Epithelial Tumor	–	+
Sex Cord Stromal Tumor	+	–

Helpful Hints

Granulosa cell and Sertoli-Leydig cell tumors of the ovary can occasionally present with morphologic features similar to those of ovarian epithelial tumors. Most ovarian sex cord stromal tumors are positive for **inhibin** while epithelial tumors of the ovary are not. On the other hand, with rare exception of tubular areas of Sertoli-Leydig cell tumors, sex cord stromal neoplasms of the ovary do not express **cytokeratins**.

Endometrioid and serous carcinomas of the ovary ordinarily show at least a focal staining for ER while sex cord stromal tumors are usually negative.

Calretinin is also present in most sex cord stromal tumors, usually more prominent in the leuteinized stroma or in Leydig cells.

Deavers 2003.

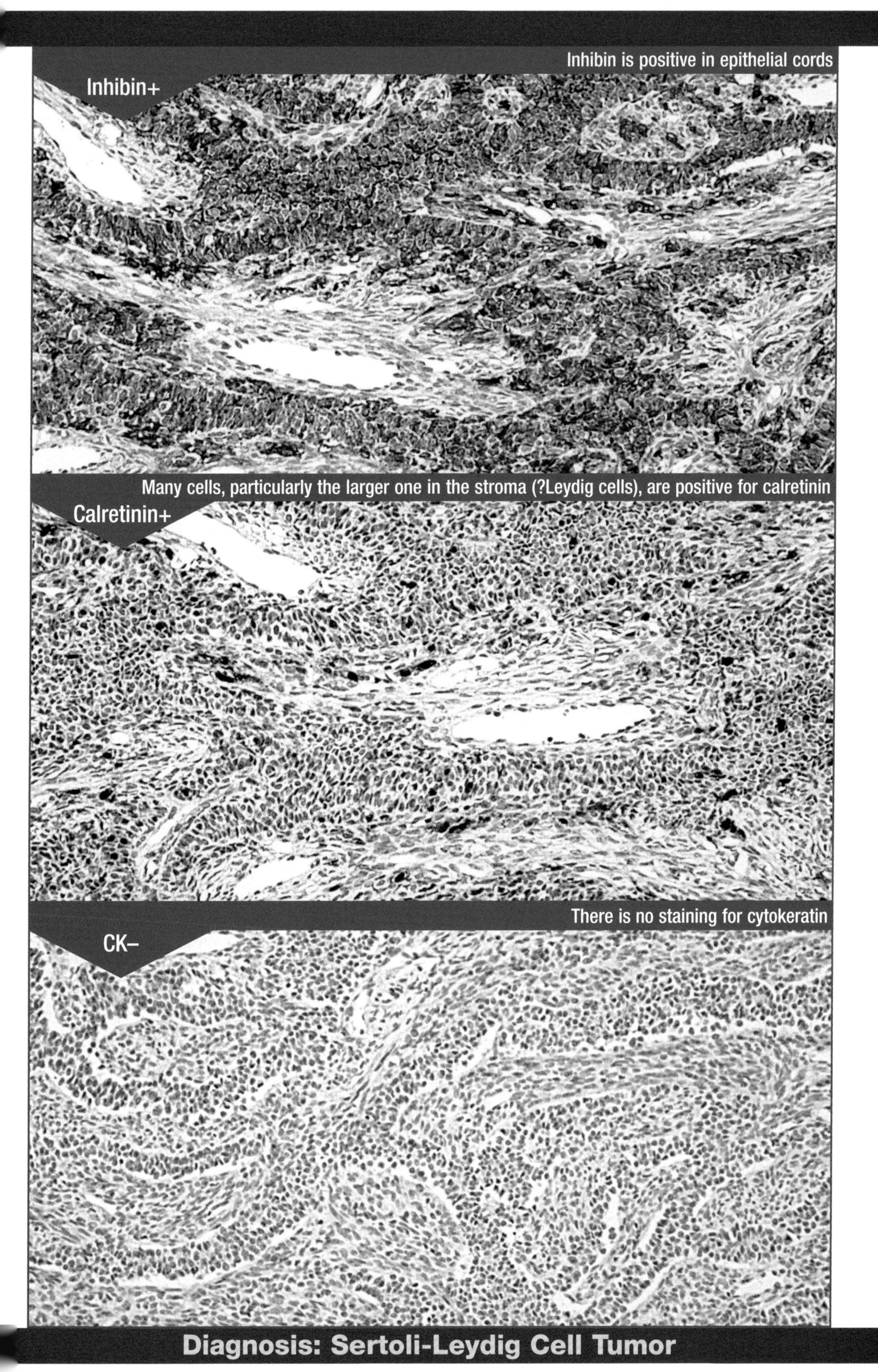

Diagnosis: Sertoli-Leydig Cell Tumor

Ovarian tumor

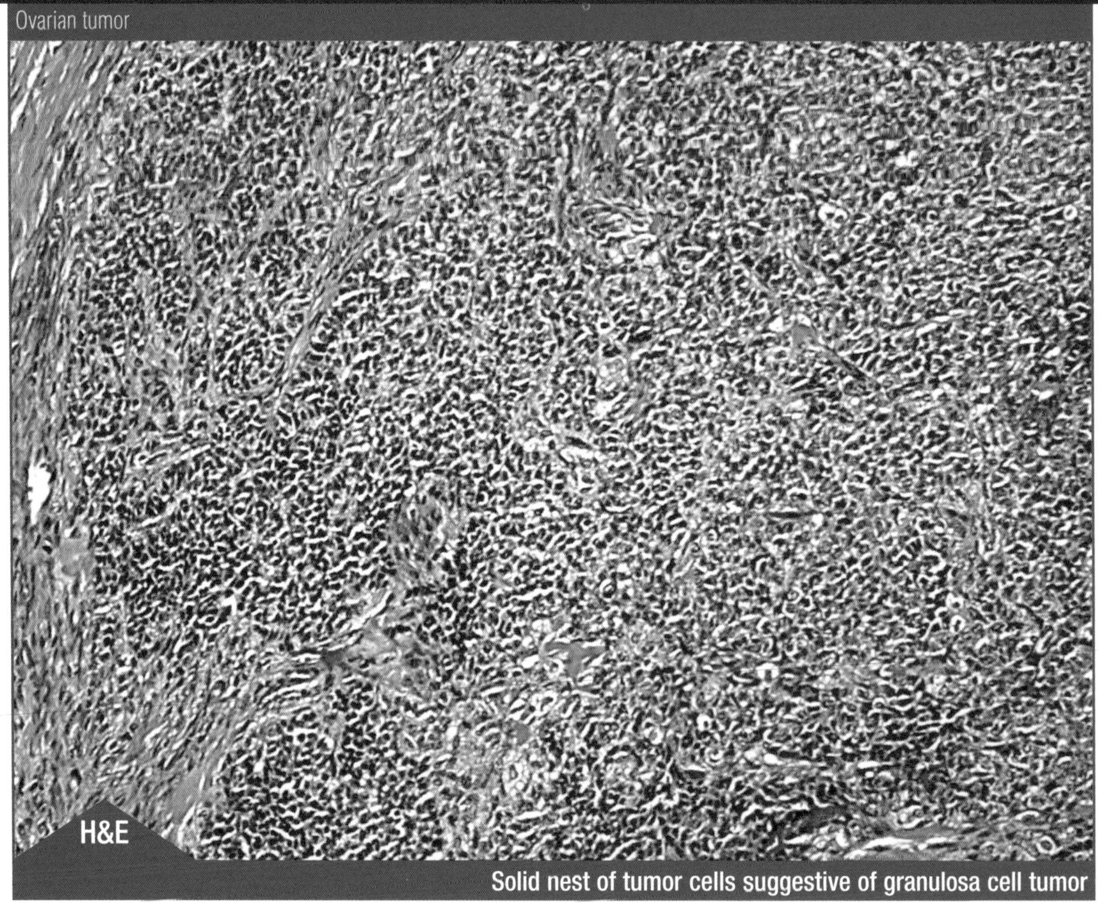

Solid nest of tumor cells suggestive of granulosa cell tumor

Ovarian Epithelial Tumor vs Sex Cord Stromal Tumor		
	Inhibin	Cytokeratin (CK)
Ovarian Epithelial Tumor	–	+
Sex Cord Stromal Tumor	+	–

Helpful Hints

Granulosa cell and Sertoli-Leydig cell tumors of the ovary can occasionally present with morphologic features similar to those of ovarian epithelial tumors. Most ovarian sex cord stromal tumors are positive for **inhibin** while epithelial tumors of the ovary are not. On the other hand, with rare exception of tubular areas of Sertoli-Leydig cell tumors, sex cord stromal neoplasms of the ovary do not express **cytokeratins**.

Endometrioid and serous carcinomas of the ovary ordinarily show at least a focal staining for ER while sex cord stromal tumors are usually negative.

Calretinin is also present in most sex cord stromal tumors, usually more prominent in the leuteinized stroma or in Leydig cells.

Deavers 2003.

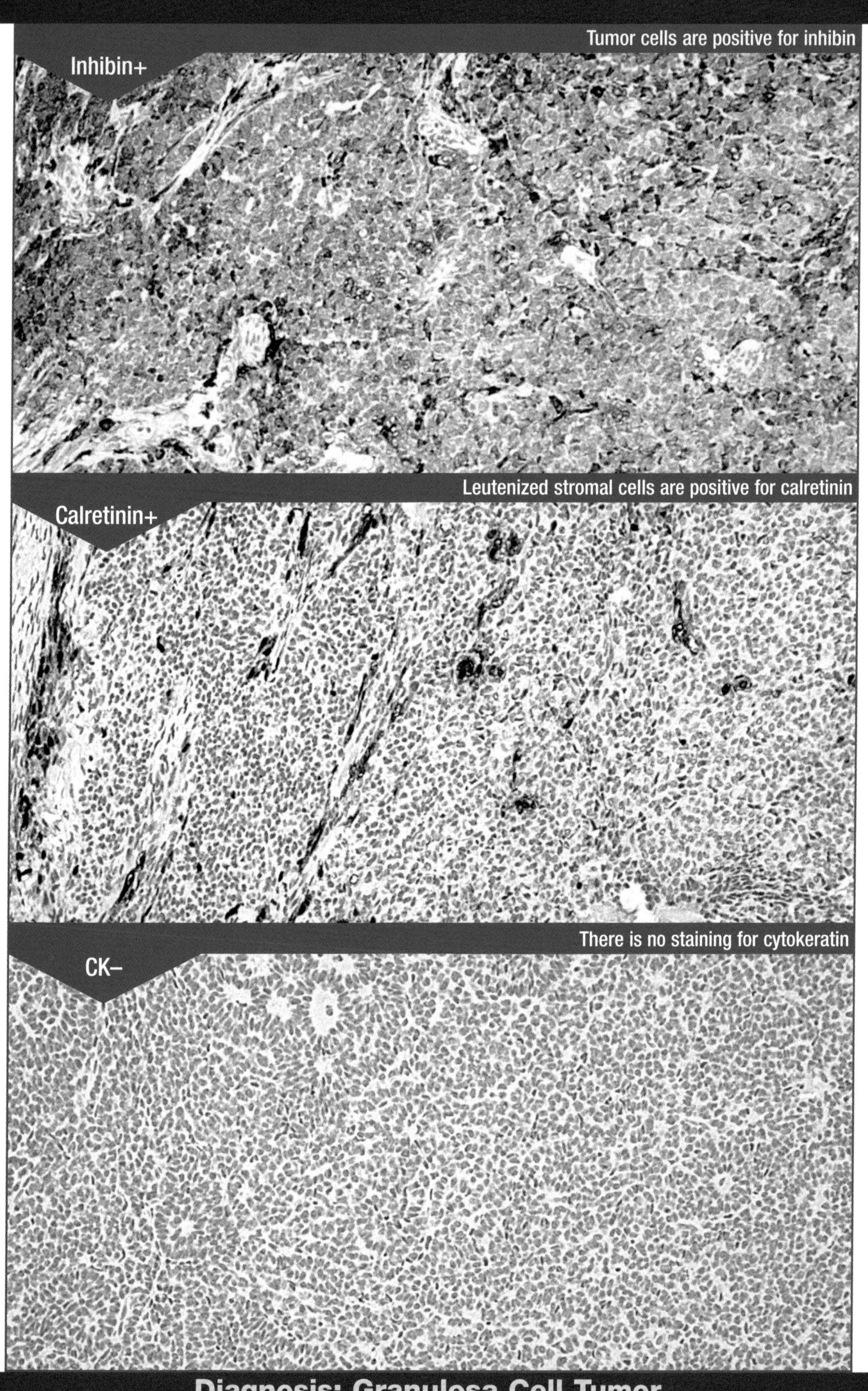

Diagnosis: Granulosa Cell Tumor

Ovarian Carcinoma vs Metastatic Colonic Carcinoma

Partially cystic unilateral ovarian tumor

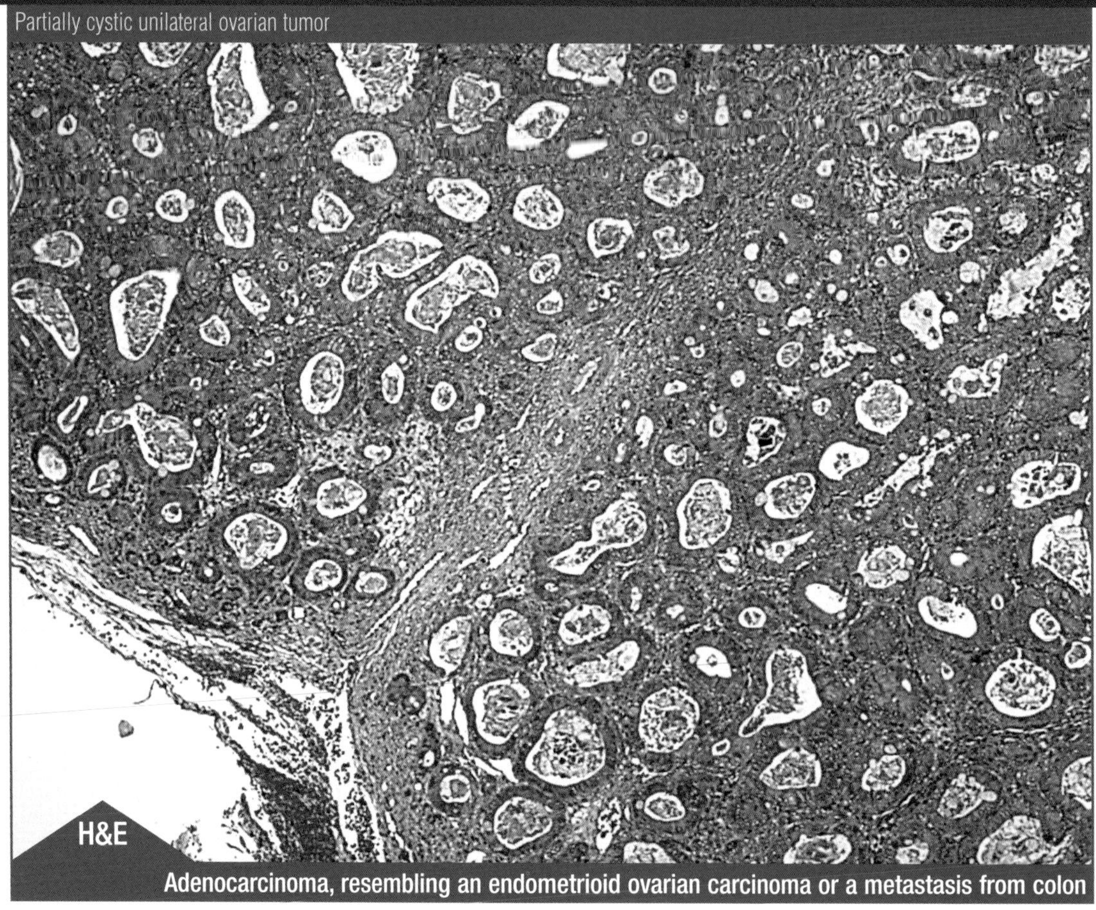

Adenocarcinoma, resembling an endometrioid ovarian carcinoma or a metastasis from colon

Ovarian Carcinoma vs Metastatic Colonic Carcinoma			
	CK7	CK20	Estrogen Receptor (ER)
Ovarian Carcinoma	+	–	S
Colonic Carcinoma	–	+	–

Helpful Hints

Unilateral or bilateral metastatic colonic carcinomas in the ovary are usually cystic and may grossly and microscopically resemble ovarian carcinomas, particularly the endometrioid type. Most cases can be resolved by a combination of **cytokeratin 20** (positive in colon cancer) and **cytokeratin 7** (positive in ovarian cancer). One may add **estrogen receptor** (**ER**) to the panel to identify ovarian carcinomas, but it should be remembered that mucinous ovarian carcinomas are always negative for estrogen receptor.

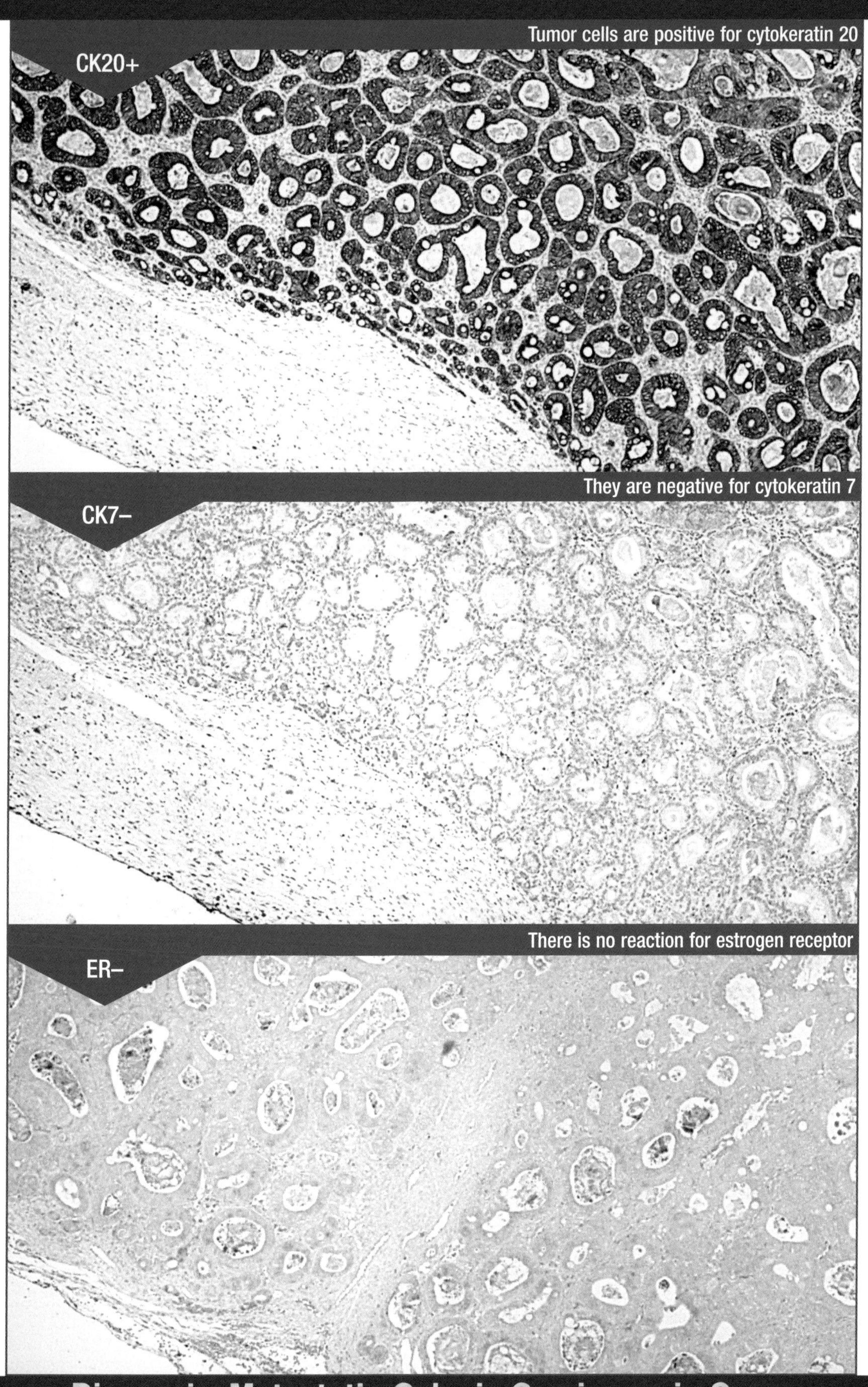

Diagnosis: Metastatic Colonic Carcinoma in Ovary

Partially cystic ovarian tumor

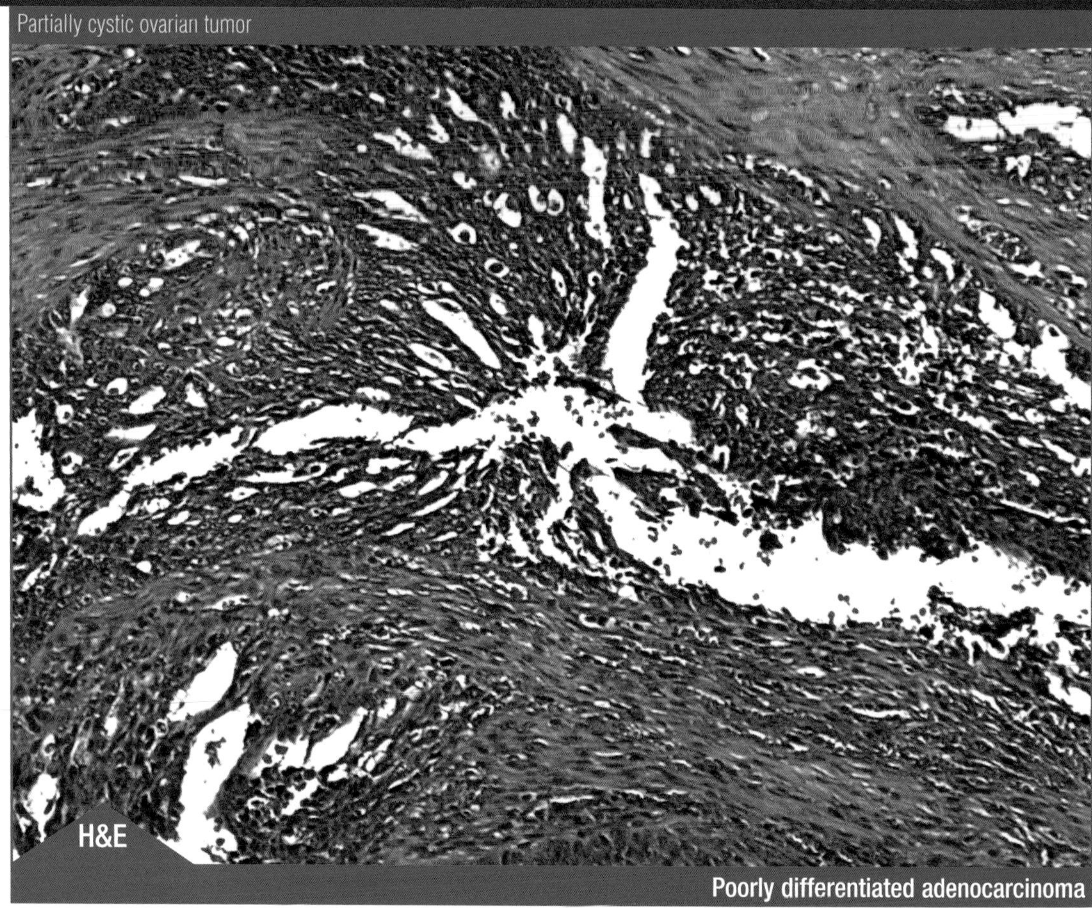

Poorly differentiated adenocarcinoma

Ovarian Carcinoma vs Metastatic Colonic Carcinoma			
	CK7	CK20	Estrogen Receptor (ER)
Ovarian Carcinoma	+	–	S
Colonic Carcinoma	–	+	–

Helpful Hints

Unilateral or bilateral metastatic colonic carcinomas in the ovary are usually cystic and may grossly and microscopically resemble ovarian carcinomas, particularly the endometrioid type. Most cases can be resolved by a combination of **cytokeratin 20** (positive in colon cancer) and **cytokeratin 7** (positive in ovarian cancer). One may add **estrogen receptor** (**ER**) to the panel to identify ovarian carcinomas, but it should be remembered that mucinous ovarian carcinomas are always negative for estrogen receptor.

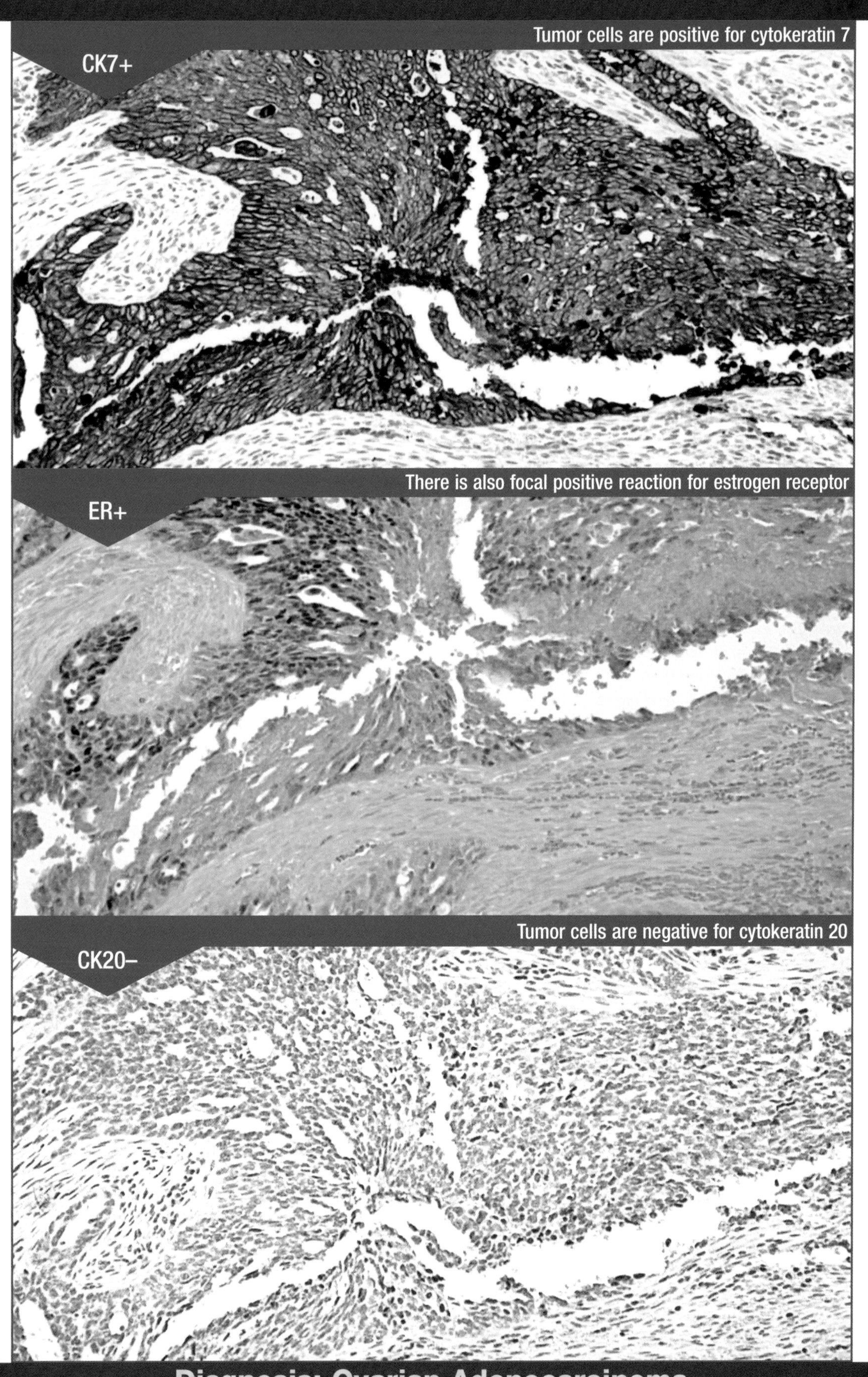

Diagnosis: Ovarian Adenocarcinoma

Core needle biopsy of breast

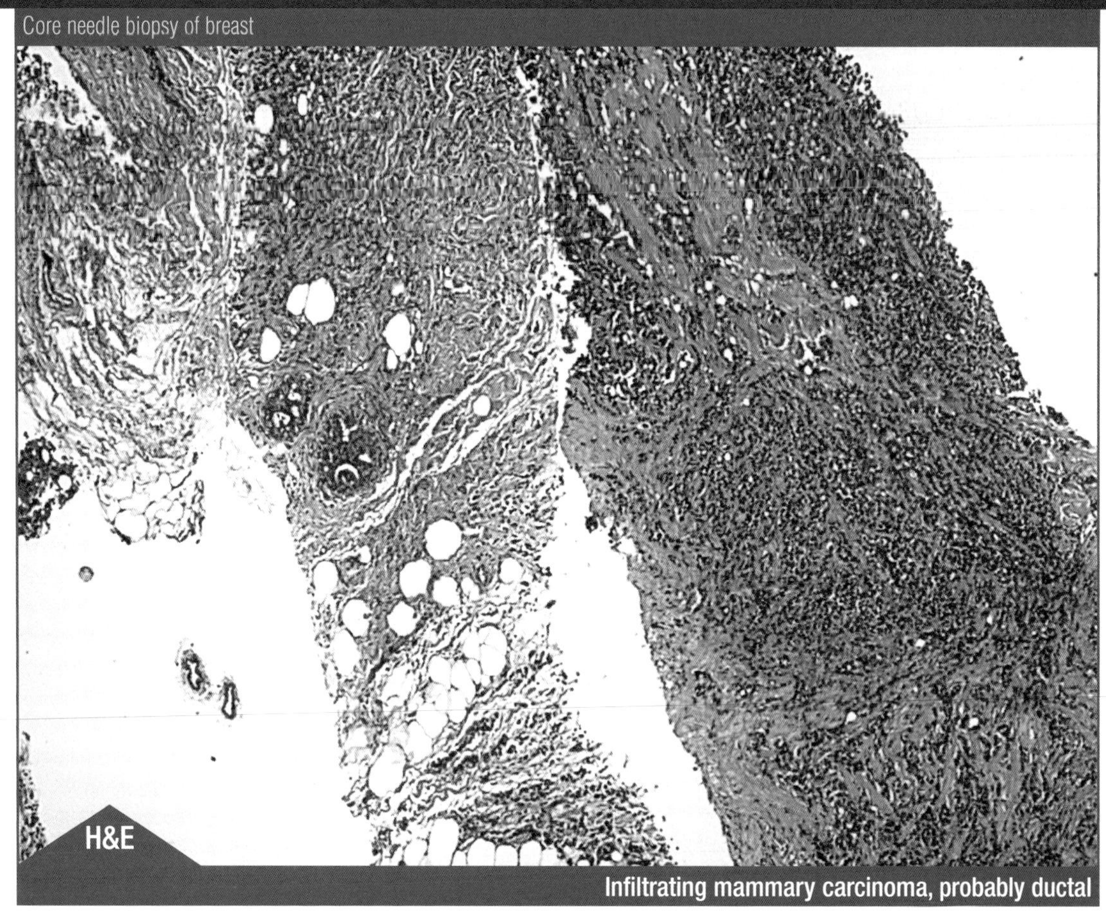

Infiltrating mammary carcinoma, probably ductal

Lobular Carcinoma of Breast vs Ductal Carcinoma of Breast	
	E-Cadherin
Lobular Carcinoma of Breast	–
Ductal Carcinoma of Breast	+

Helpful Hints

Both in situ and invasive ductal carcinomas are usually strongly positive for **E-Cadherin** whereas lobular carcinomas are mostly negative. It should be noted that focal staining for this antigen could be seen in lobular carcinomas.

Acs 2001.

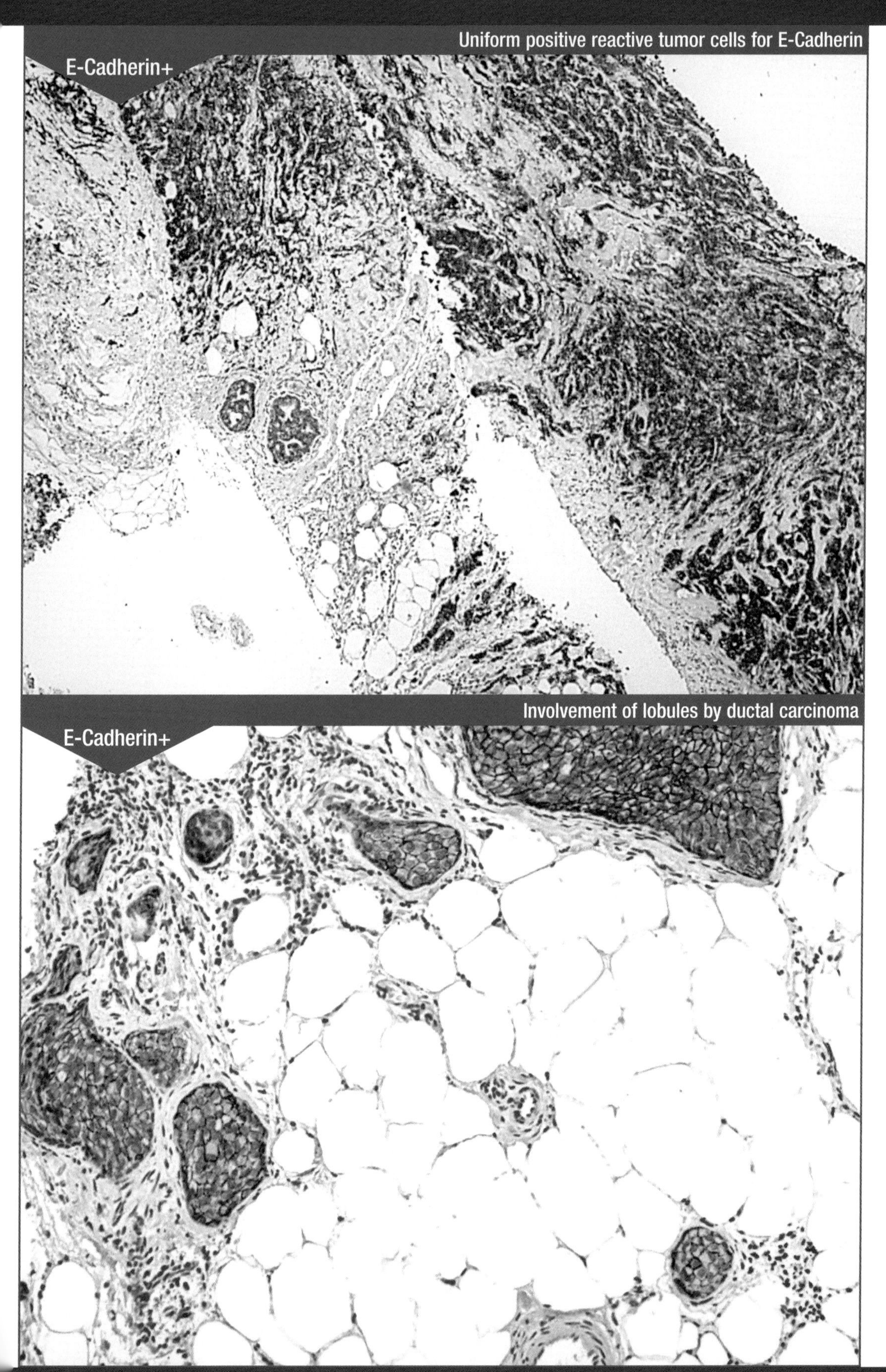

Diagnosis: Infiltrating Ductal Carcinoma

Core biopsy of breast

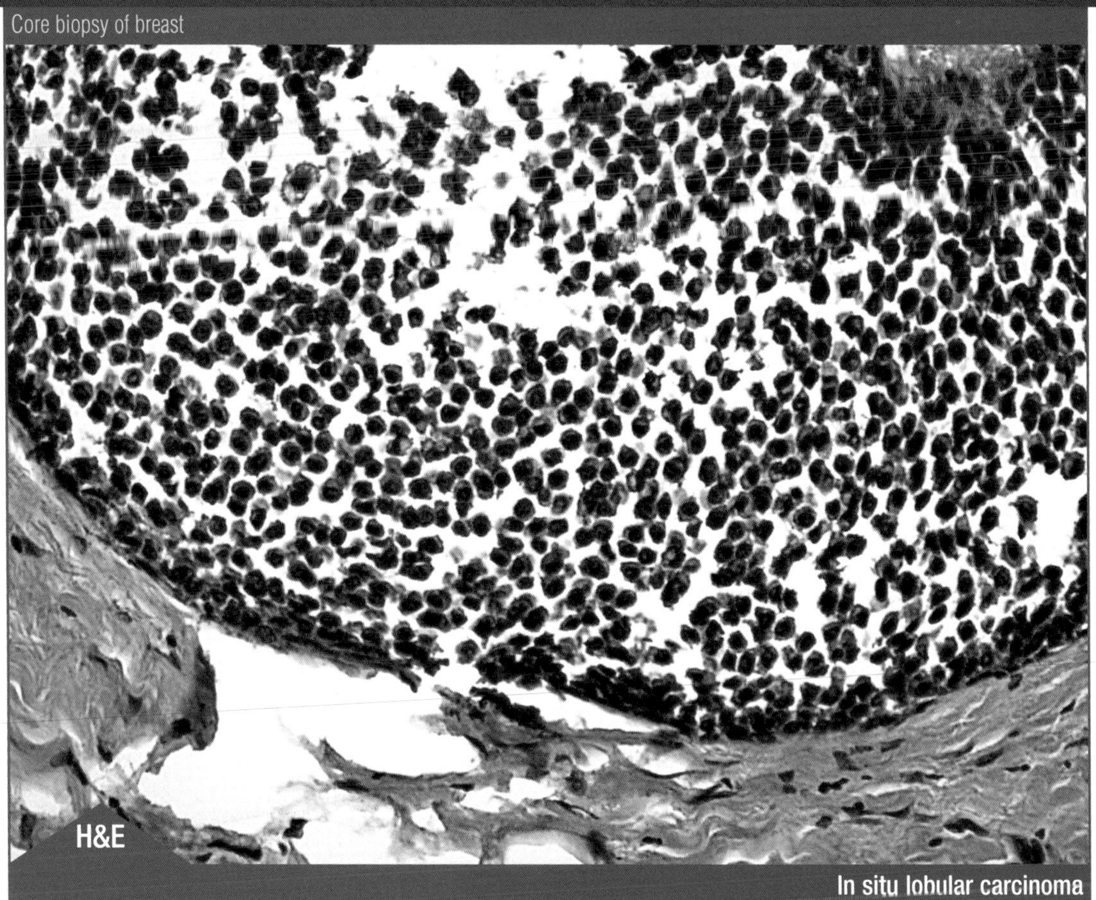

In situ lobular carcinoma

Lobular Carcinoma of Breast vs Ductal Carcinoma of Breast	
	E-Cadherin
Lobular Carcinoma of Breast	–
Ductal Carcinoma of Breast	+

Helpful Hints

Both in situ and invasive ductal carcinomas are usually strongly positive for **E-Cadherin** whereas lobular carcinomas are mostly negative. It should be noted that focal staining for this antigen could be seen in lobular carcinomas.

Acs 2001.

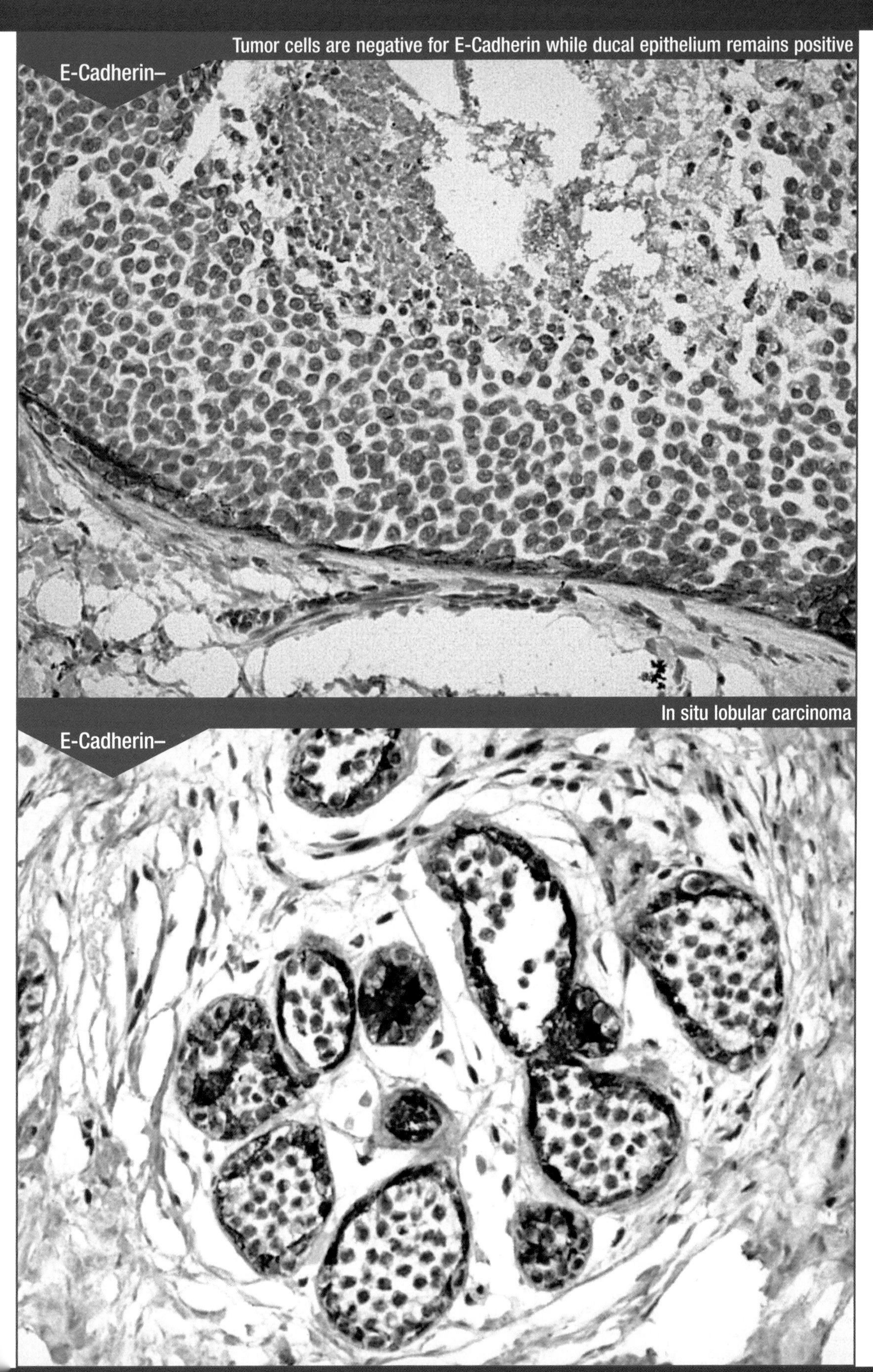

Diagnosis: In Situ Lobular Carcinoma

Excisional biopsy of a breast mass

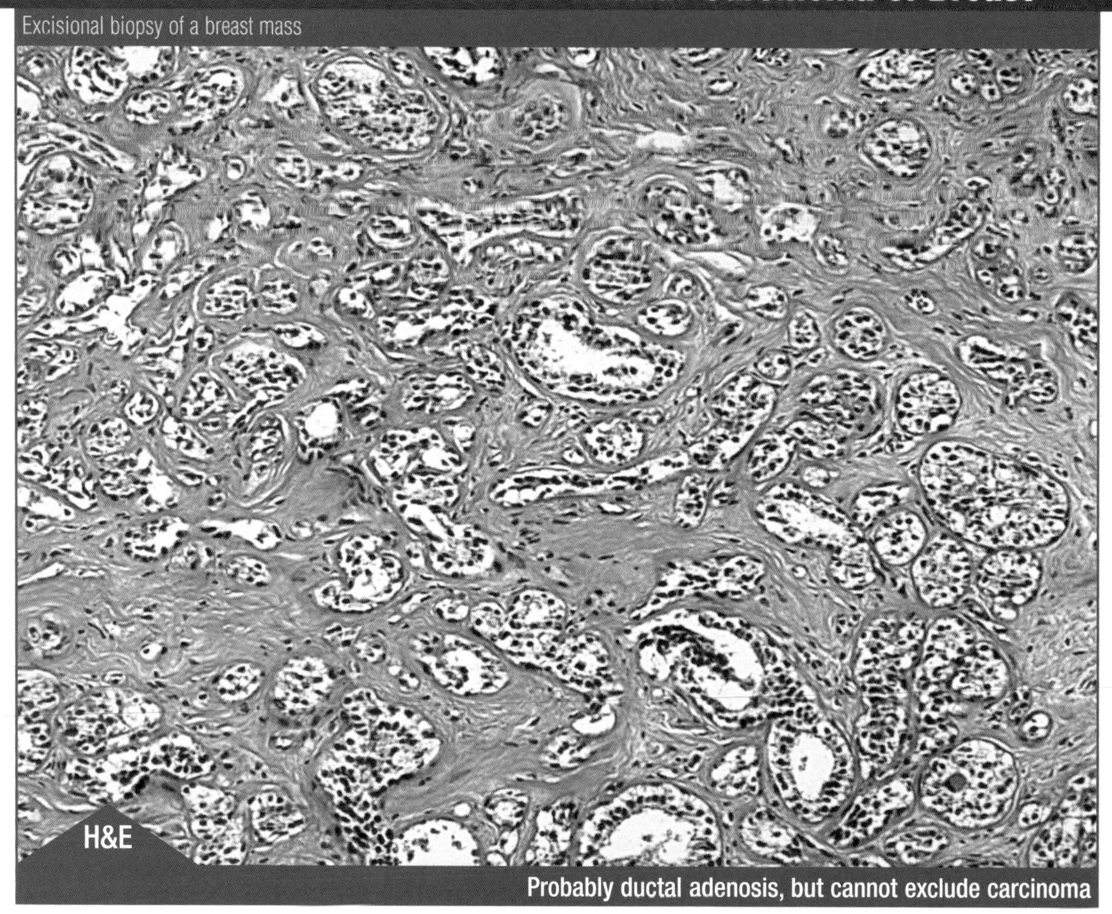

Probably ductal adenosis, but cannot exclude carcinoma

Ductal Adenosis of Breast vs Tubular Carcinoma of Breast		
	p63	HMWK
Ductal Adenosis of Breast	+	+
Tubular Carcinoma of Breast	–	–

Helpful Hints

As markers of basal and myoepithelial cells, both **p63** and **high molecular weight keratin** (**HMWK**) are positive in adenosis but negative in tubular carcinoma. These markers however, are not particularly useful in differentiating atypical ductal hyperplasia from intraductal carcinoma as both lesions contain basal/myoepithelial cells.

Use of other markers such as **actins** and **calponin** has been advocated in this differential diagnosis but they are not as useful as p63 and high molecular weight keratin.

Wang 2002.

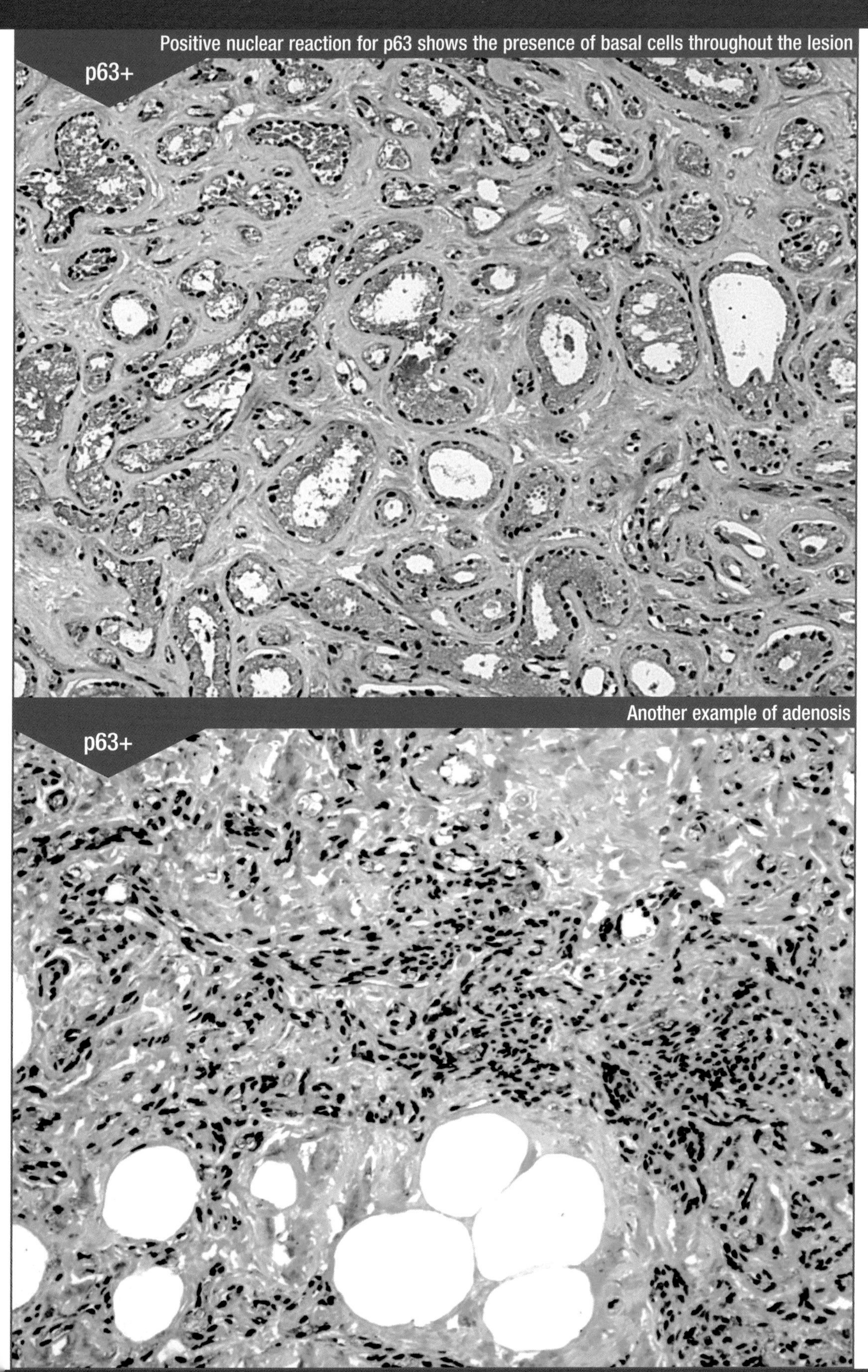

Diagnosis: Ductal Adenosis of Breast

Core biopsy of breast

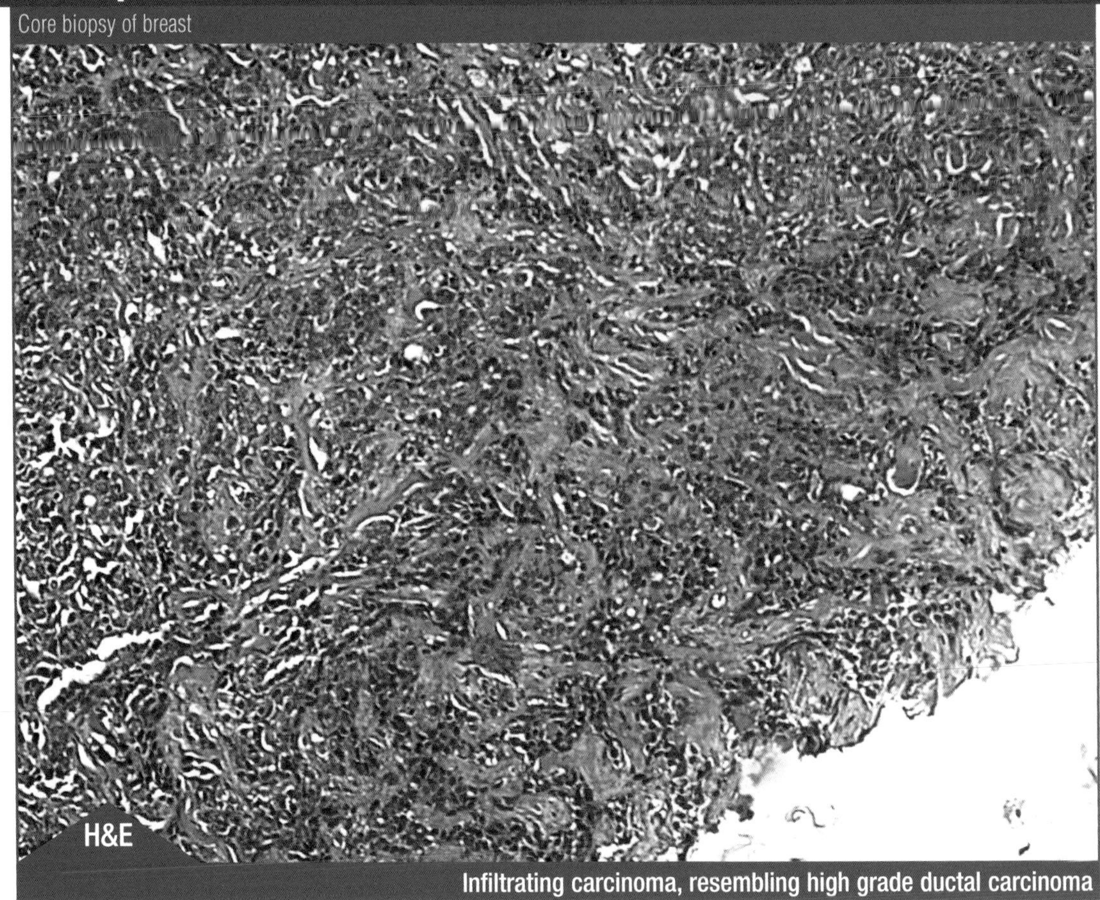

Infiltrating carcinoma, resembling high grade ductal carcinoma

Metaplastic Carcinoma of Breast vs Ductal Carcinoma of Breast	
	p63
Metaplastic Carcinoma of Breast	+
Ductal Carcinoma of Breast	–

Helpful Hints

Metaplastic breast cancers are a group of basal/myoepithelial cell-derived tumors and as such express markers of these cells. Their morphologic spectrum ranges from squamous carcinomas to spindle cell and sarcomatoid carcinomas. These tumors are always negative for estrogen receptor and HER2 but at least focally express **p63**.

Wang 2002.

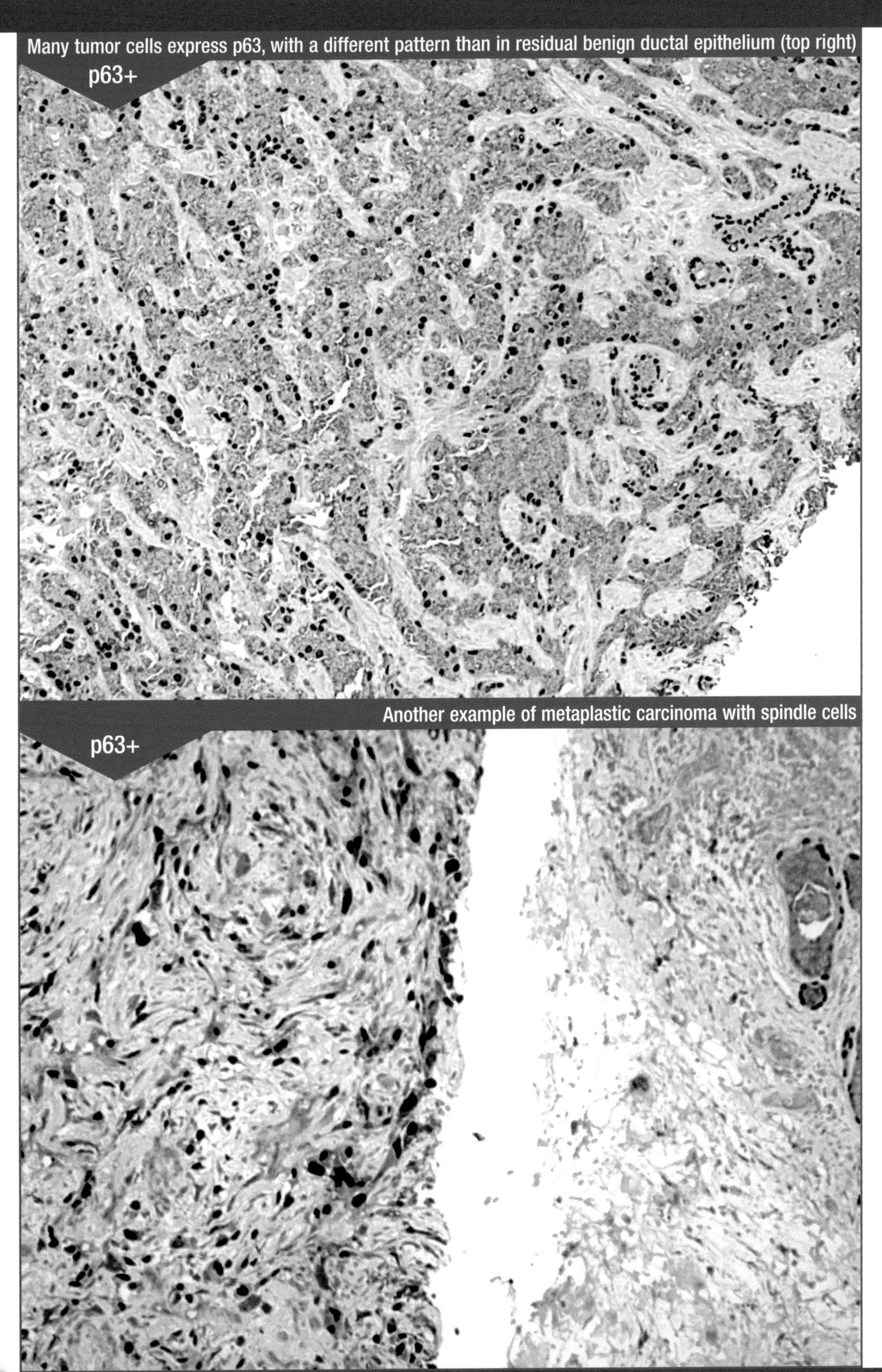

Diagnosis: Metaplastic Carcinoma of Breast

Excisional biopsy of breast

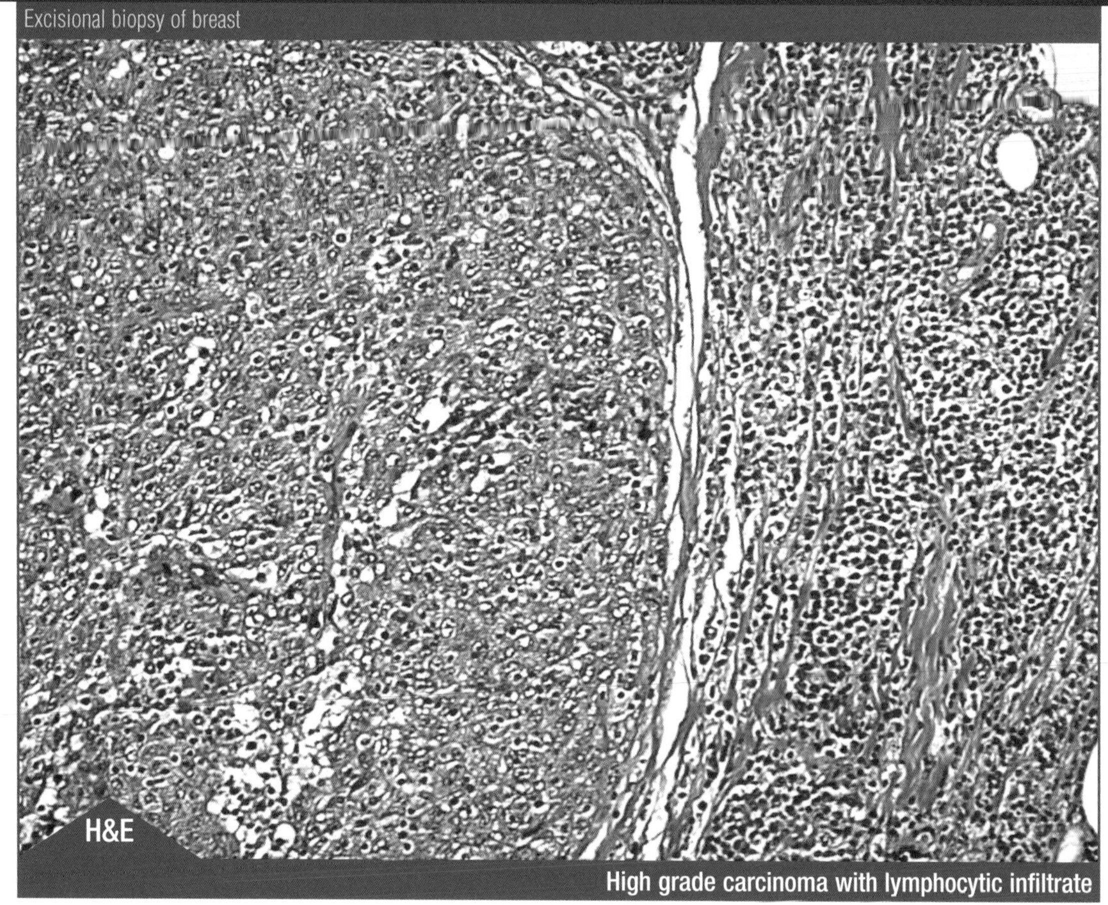

High grade carcinoma with lymphocytic infiltrate

Medullary Carcinoma of Breast vs Ductal Carcinoma of Breast		
	HLA-DR	Estrogen Receptor (ER)
Medullary Carcinoma	+	–
Ductal Carcinoma	–	S

Helpful Hints

True medullary carcinomas of breast are sometimes difficult to differentiate from poorly differentiated ductal carcinomas with lymphoid infiltrate. Medullary carcinomas are always positive for **HLA-DR** but ductal carcinomas are rarely positive. Furthermore, true medullary carcinomas are never positive for **estrogen receptor** (**ER**) or HER2, whereas ductal carcinomas could be positive for either or both.

Because host lymphoreticular cells are always strongly positive for HLA-DR, the interpretation of this reaction in tumor cells should be limited to the areas distant from host's cellular infiltrate.

Feinmesser 2000.

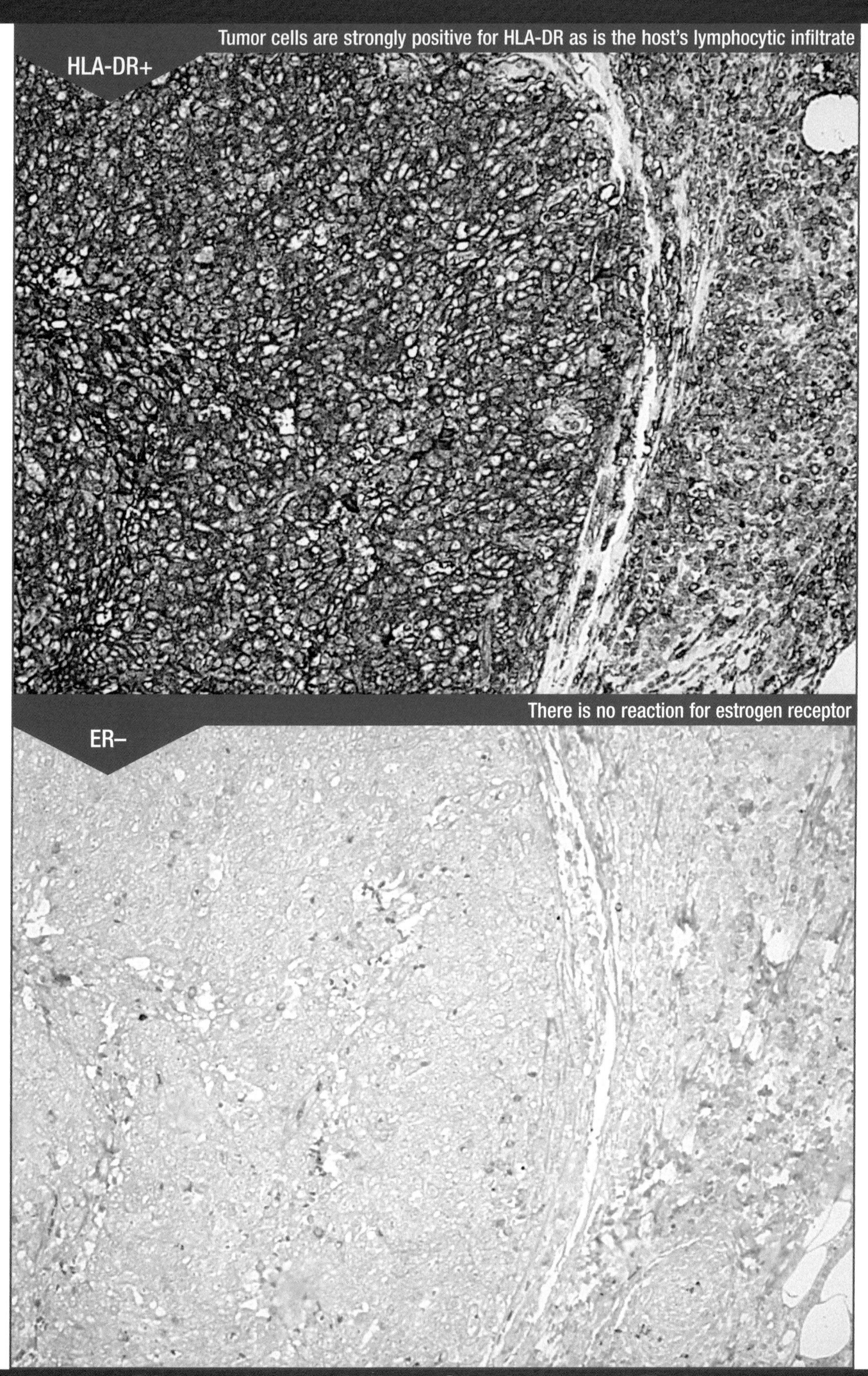

Diagnosis: Medullary Carcinoma of Breast

Transurethral resection of bladder in a patient with suspected recurrent cancer

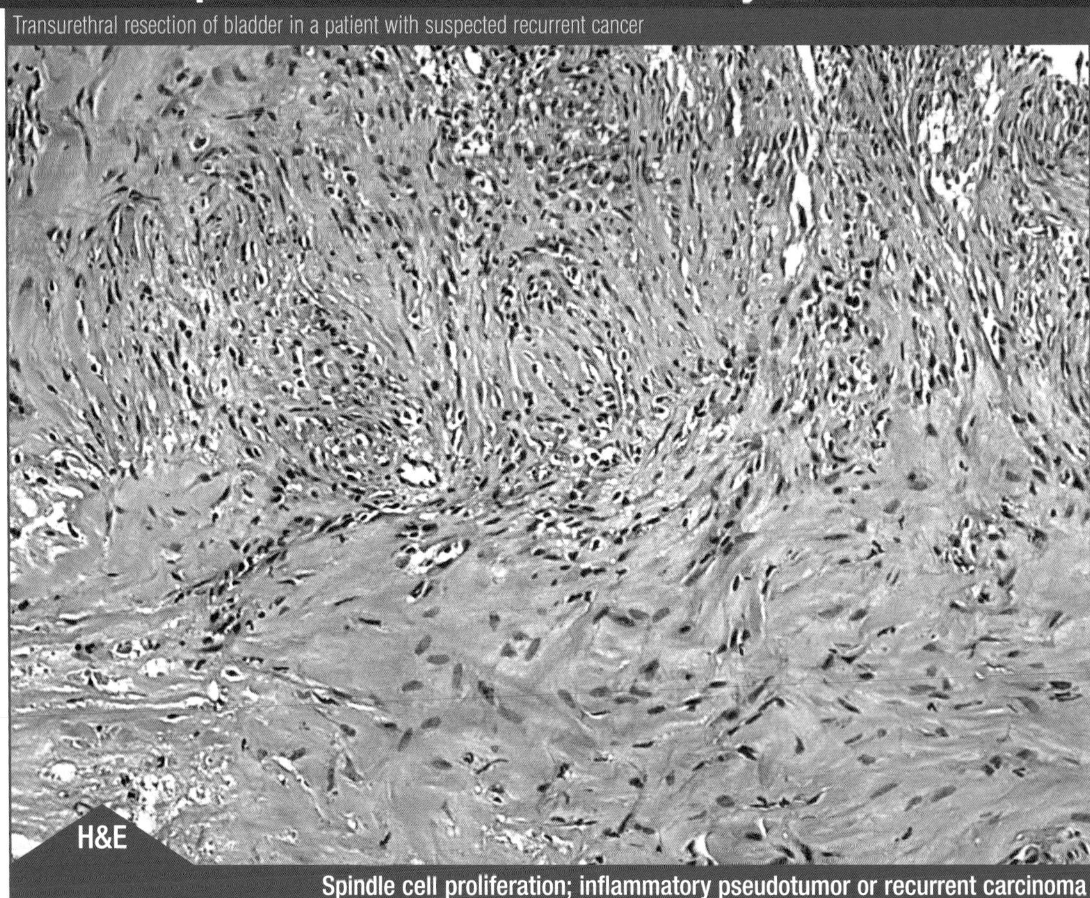

Spindle cell proliferation; inflammatory pseudotumor or recurrent carcinoma

Metaplastic Carcinoma vs Inflammatory Pseudotumor		
	Cytokeratin (CK)	p63
Metaplastic Carcinoma	+	S
Inflammatory Pseudotumor	–	–

Helpful Hints

Metaplastic carcinomas of the urinary bladder (carcinomas with sarcoma-like areas) may be difficult to distinguish from sarcomas or inflammatory pseudotumors, particularly in small biopsies. Metaplastic carcinomas are usually at least focally positive for **cytokeratin** while inflammatory pseudosarcomas remain negative. **Anaplastic Lymphoma Kinase** (**ALK**) is suggested as a potential marker for pseudosarcomas but the frequency of its expression is unpredictable. One may also use **p63** in this differential diagnosis; any positivity favors a metaplastic carcinoma.

Chan 2001, Coffin 1995.

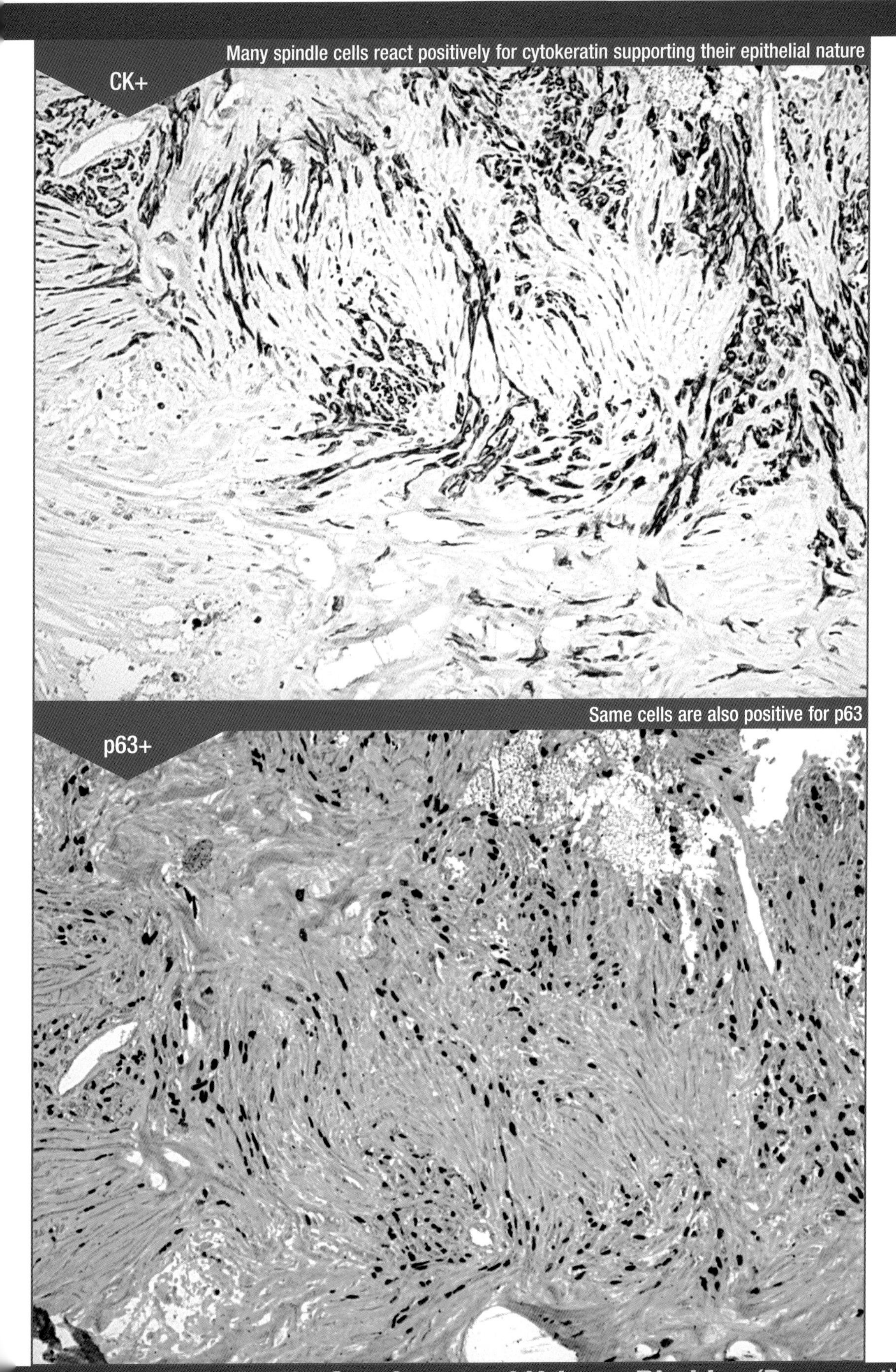

iagnosis: Metaplastic Carcinoma of Urinary Bladder *(Recurrent)*

Transurethral resection of prostatic urethra

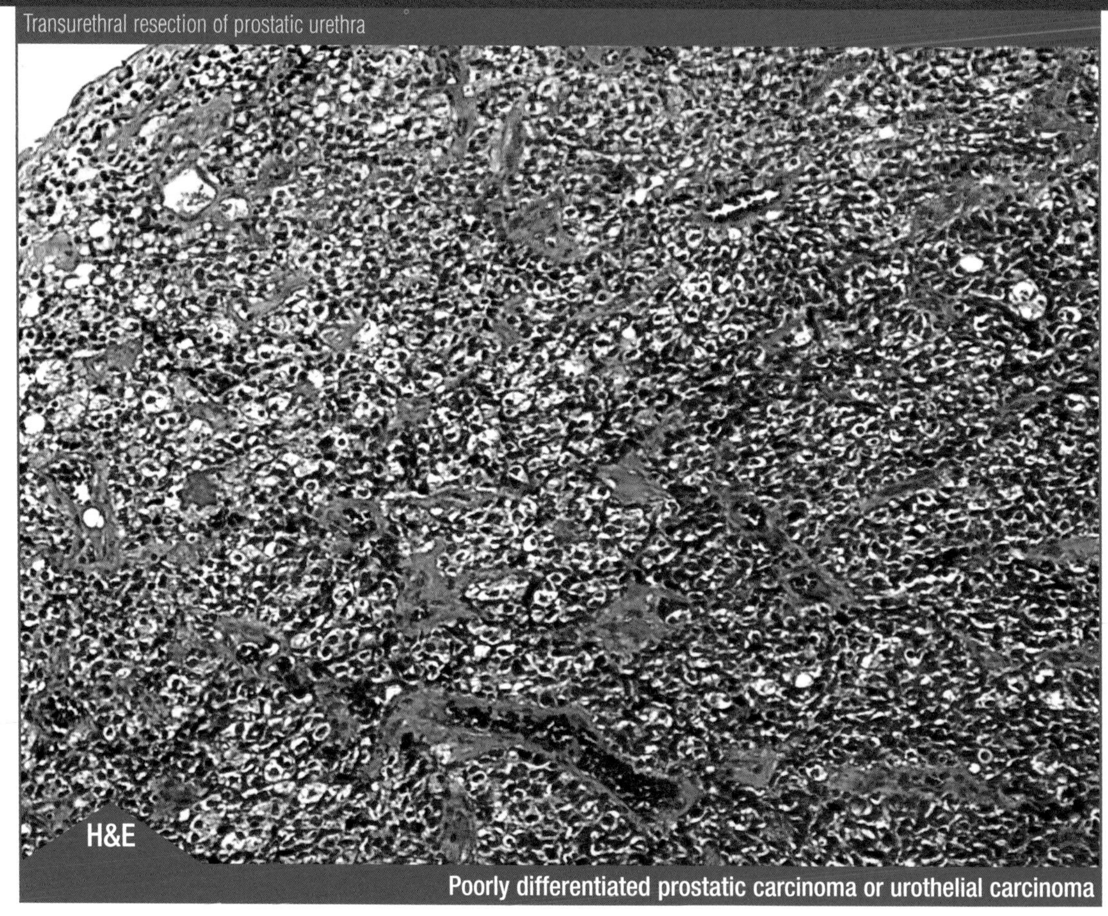

Poorly differentiated prostatic carcinoma or urothelial carcinoma

Prostatic Adenocarcinoma vs Urothelial Carcinoma		
	PSA	CEA
Prostatic Adenocarcinoma	+	–
Urothelial Carcinoma	–	+

Helpful Hints

Urothelial carcinomas may show glandular differentiation and come into the differential diagnosis of prostatic carcinomas. On the other hand, poorly differentiated prostatic carcinomas may show solid areas resembling transitional cell carcinomas. Almost all prostatic carcinomas are positive for **prostatic specific antigen** (**PSA**), regardless of their degree of differentiation. Those exceptional prostatic tumors that do not stain for prostatic specific antigen are usually positive for **prostatic acid phosphatase**. The ductal adenocarcinomas of prostate (*the so-called endometrioid type*) always react positively for prostatic specific antigen.

Urothelial carcinomas may focally express **carcinoembryonic antigen** (**CEA**); prostatic carcinomas do not. No other purported urothelial markers are useful in practice.

Nadji 1981.

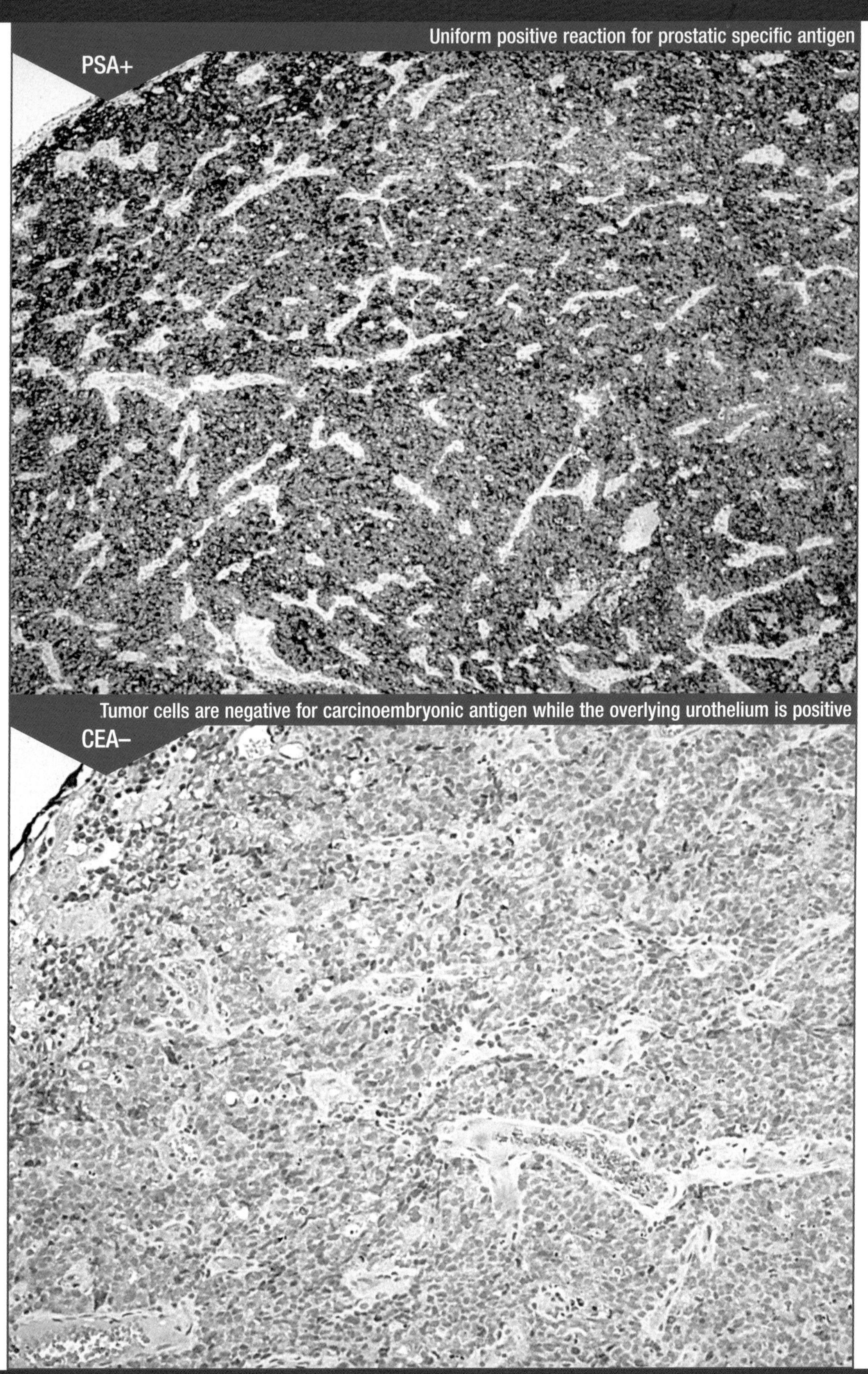

Diagnosis: Poorly Differentiated Prostatic Carcinoma

Transurethral resection of prostate

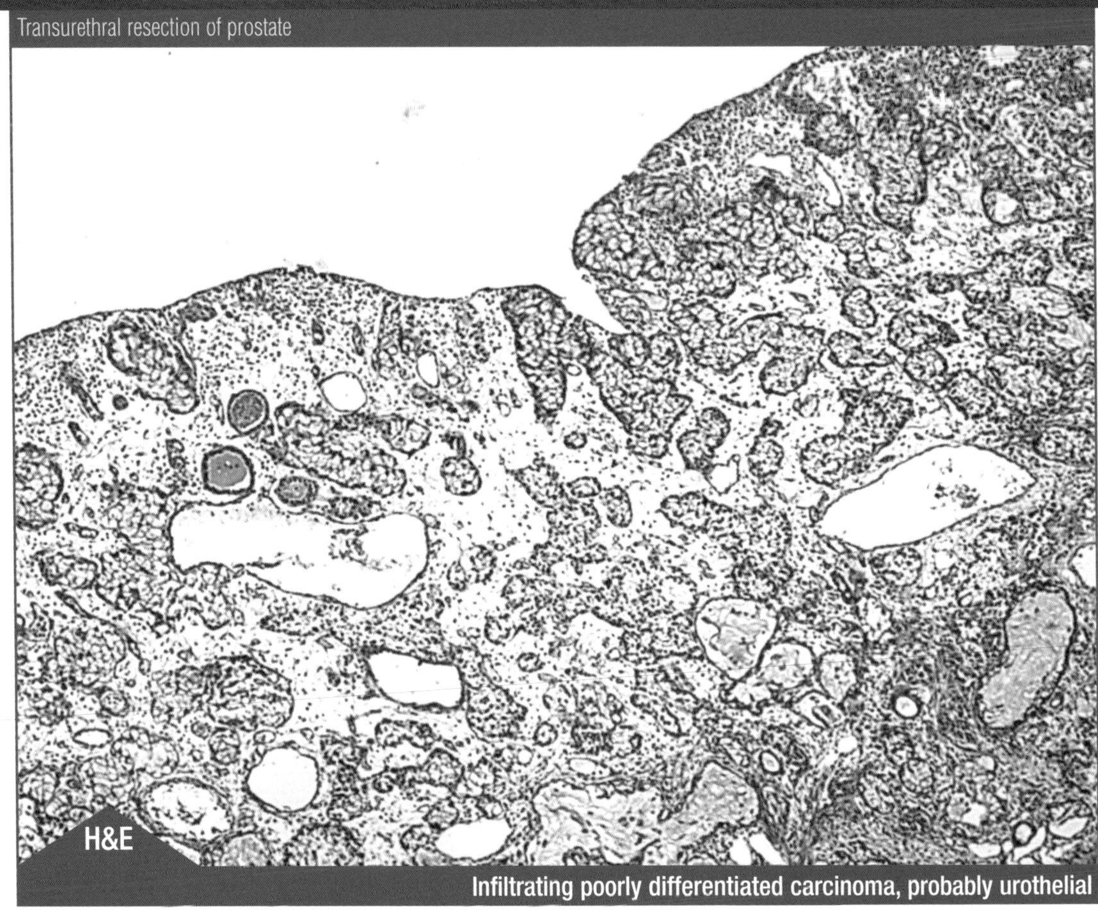

Infiltrating poorly differentiated carcinoma, probably urothelial

Prostatic Adenocarcinoma vs Urothelial Carcinoma		
	PSA	CEA
Prostatic Adenocarcinoma	+	–
Urothelial Carcinoma	–	+

Helpful Hints

Urothelial carcinomas may show glandular differentiation and come into the differential diagnosis of prostatic carcinomas. On the other hand, poorly differentiated prostatic carcinomas may show solid areas resembling transitional cell carcinomas. Almost all prostatic carcinomas are positive for **prostatic specific antigen** (**PSA**), regardless of their degree of differentiation. Those exceptional prostatic tumors that do not stain for prostatic specific antigen are usually positive for **prostatic acid phosphatase**. The ductal adenocarcinomas of prostate (*the so-called endometrioid type*) always react positively for prostatic specific antigen.

Urothelial carcinomas may focally express **carcinoembryonic antigen** (**CEA**); prostatic carcinomas do not. No other purported urothelial markers are useful in practice.

Nadji 1981.

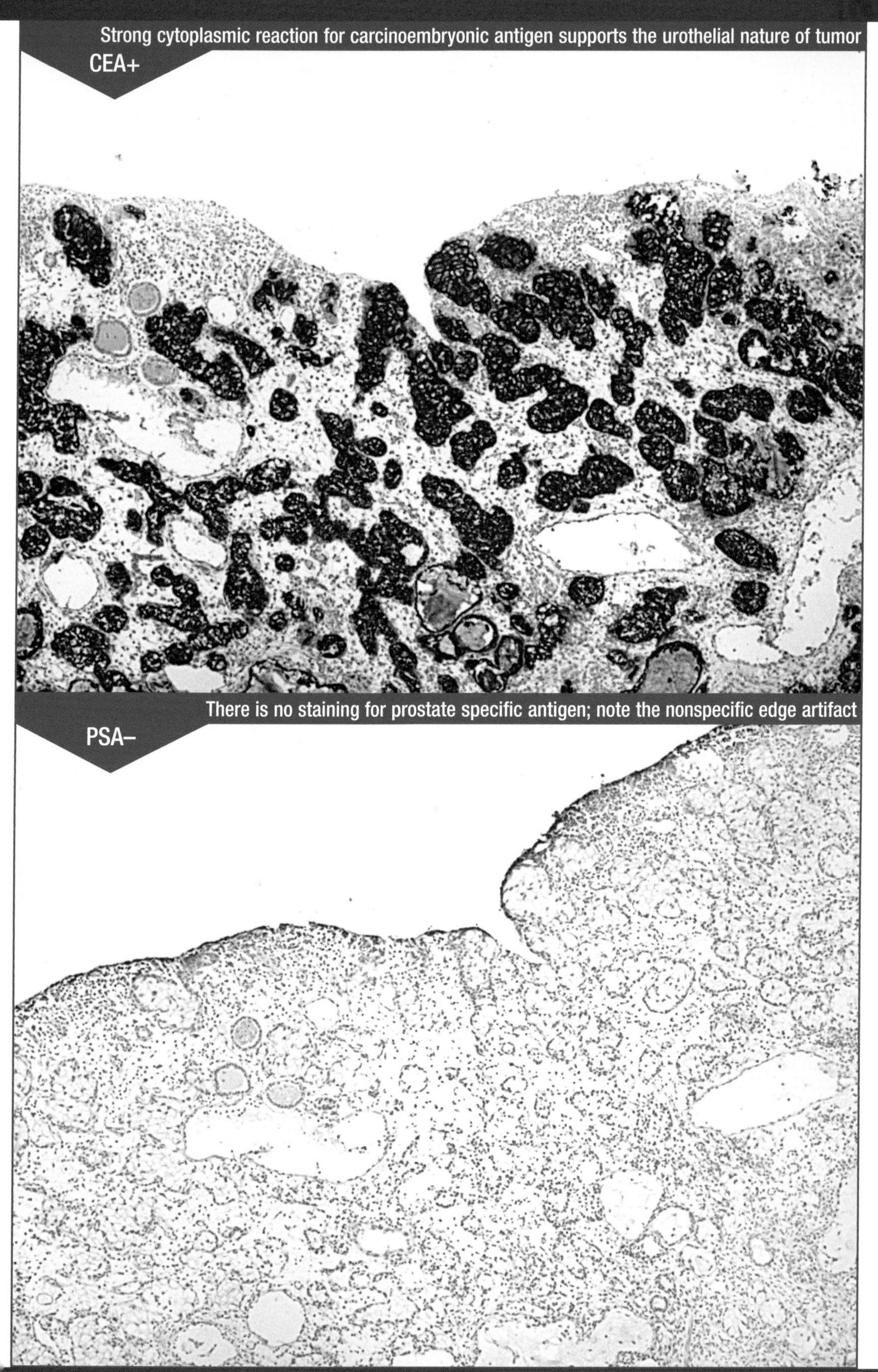

Diagnosis: Urothelial Carcinoma

Needle biopsy of prostate gland

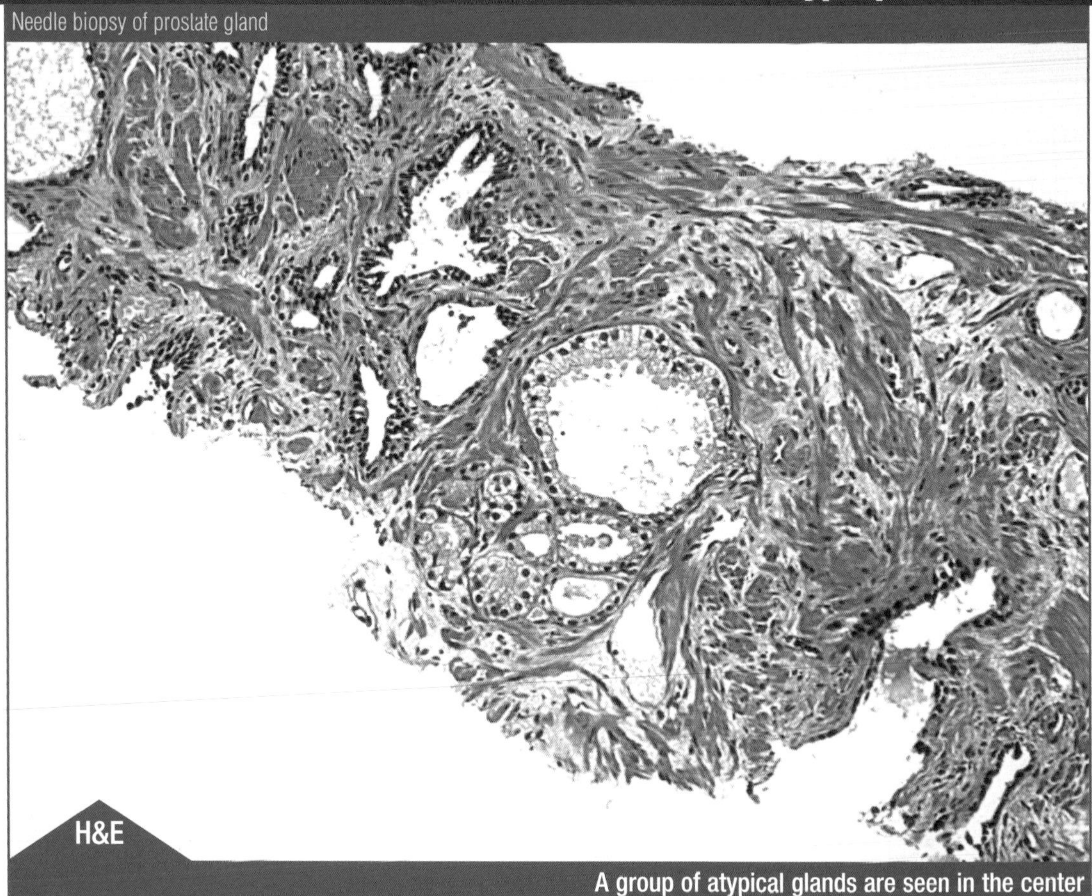

A group of atypical glands are seen in the center

Prostatic Adenocarcinoma vs Glandular Hyperplasia			
	HMWK	p63	AMACR
Prostatic Adenocarcinoma	–	–	+
Glandular Hyperplasia	+	+	–

Helpful Hints

Both **high molecular weight cytokeratin** (**HMWK**) and **p63** are markers of basal cells in prostatic glands. Their immunohistochemical localization at the base of atypical glands signals their benign nature. **P504S** (**AMACR**) stains most prostatic adenocarcinomas. It should be noted that P504S is not specific for prostatic tumors as other types of cancers may express this antigen.

Shah 2002, Magi-Galluzzi 2003.

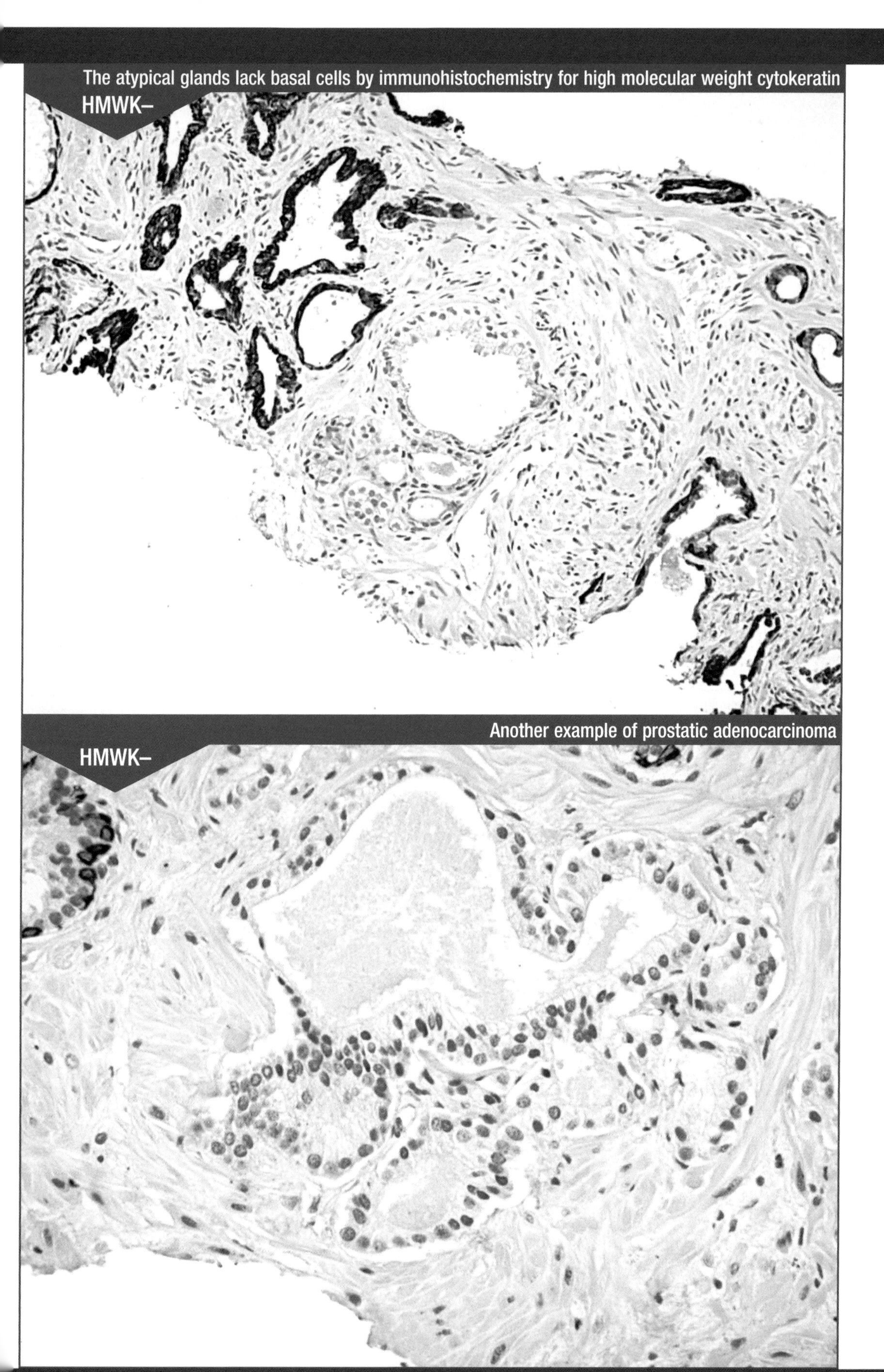

Diagnosis: Prostatic Adenocarcinoma

Needle biopsy of prostate

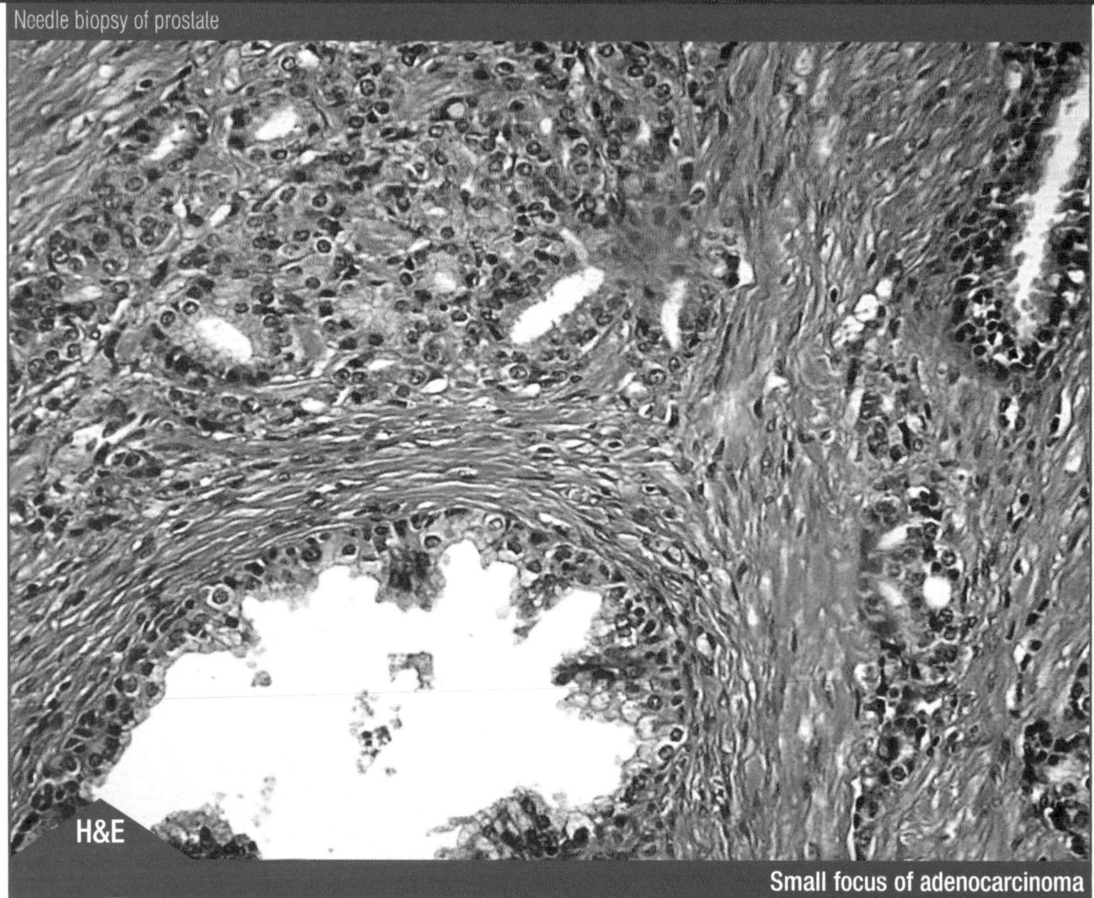

Small focus of adenocarcinoma

Prostatic Adenocarcinoma vs Glandular Hyperplasia			
	HMWK	p63	AMACR
Prostatic Adenocarcinoma	–	–	+
Glandular Hyperplasia	+	+	–

Helpful Hints

Both **high molecular weight cytokeratin** (**HMWK**) and **p63** are markers of basal cells in prostatic glands. Their immunohistochemical localization at the base of atypical glands signals their benign nature. **P504S** (**AMACR**) stains most prostatic adenocarcinomas but the benign glands either do not stain or show a different pattern of positivity (*see image*). It should be noted that P504S is not specific for prostatic tumors as other types of cancers may express this antigen.

Shah 2002, Magi-Galluzzi 2003.

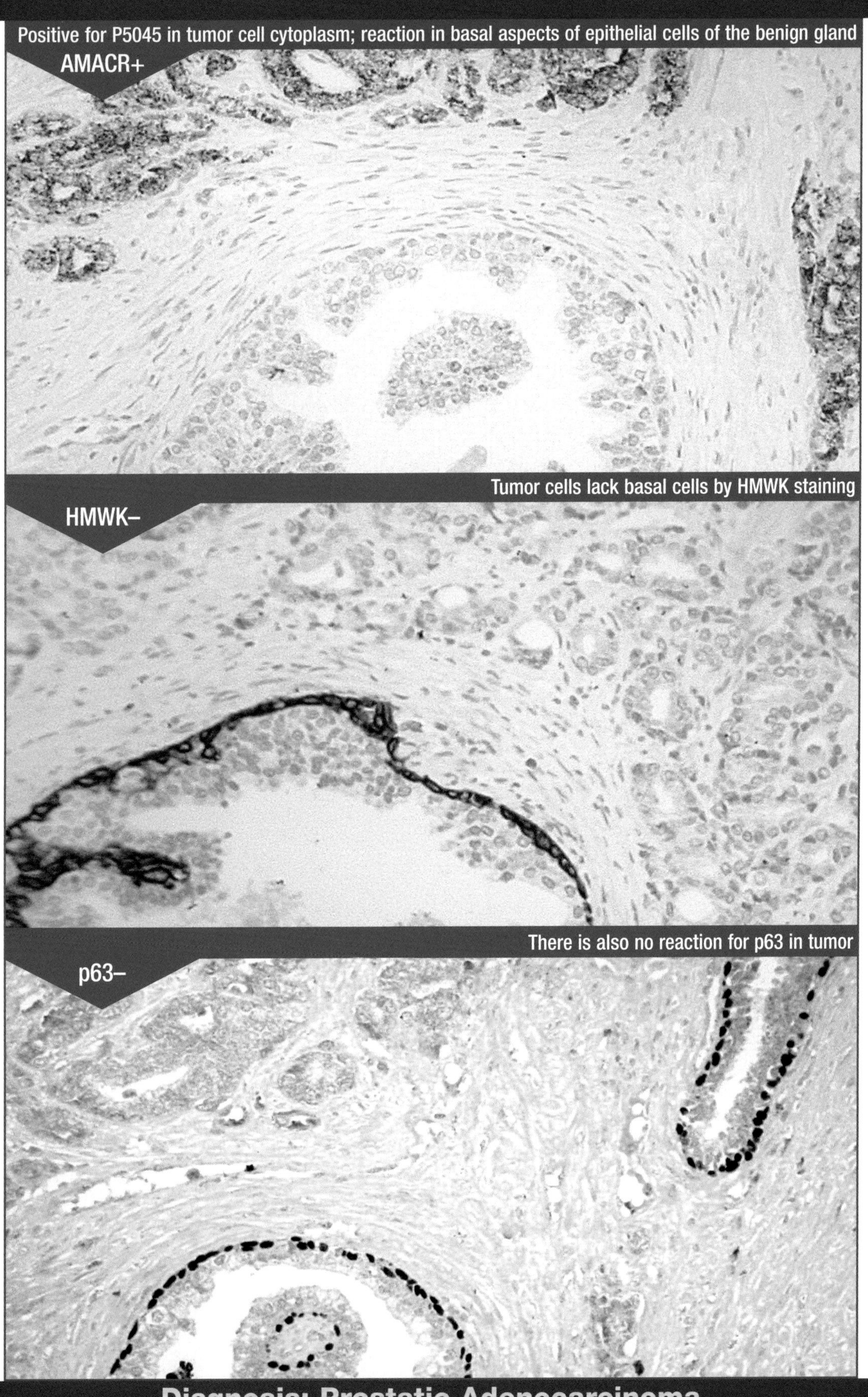

Diagnosis: Prostatic Adenocarcinoma

Rectal biopsy

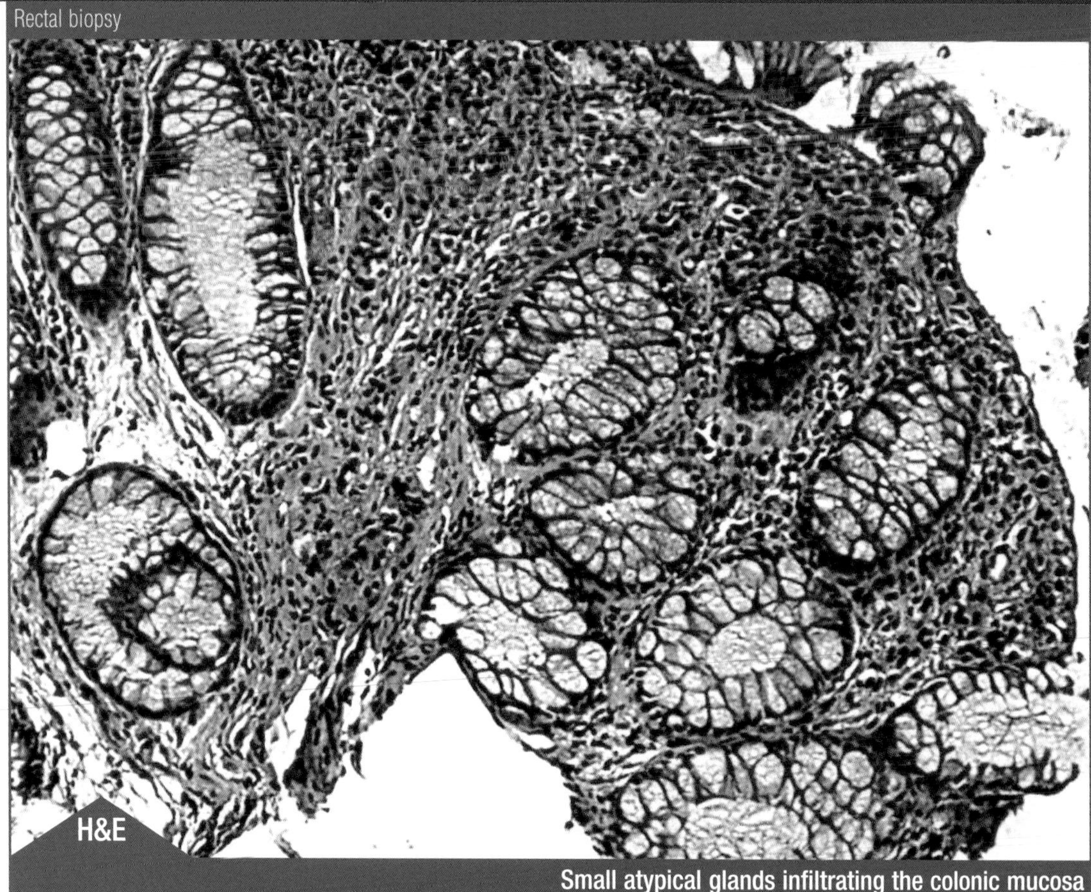

Small atypical glands infiltrating the colonic mucosa

Prostatic Adenocarcinoma vs Adenocarcinoma of Colon		
	PSA	CK20
Prostatic Adenocarcinoma	+	–
Adenocarcinoma of Colon	–	+

Helpful Hints

Extension of prostatic adenocarcinoma to colon is not uncommon and may create a diagnostic problem particularly in small mucosal biopsies. Similarly, some colorectal adenocarcinomas may extend to prostate and mimic a primary prostatic tumor. A combination of prostatic specific antigen and cytokeratin 20 will help to correctly classify these tumors in most cases.

Mai 2002.

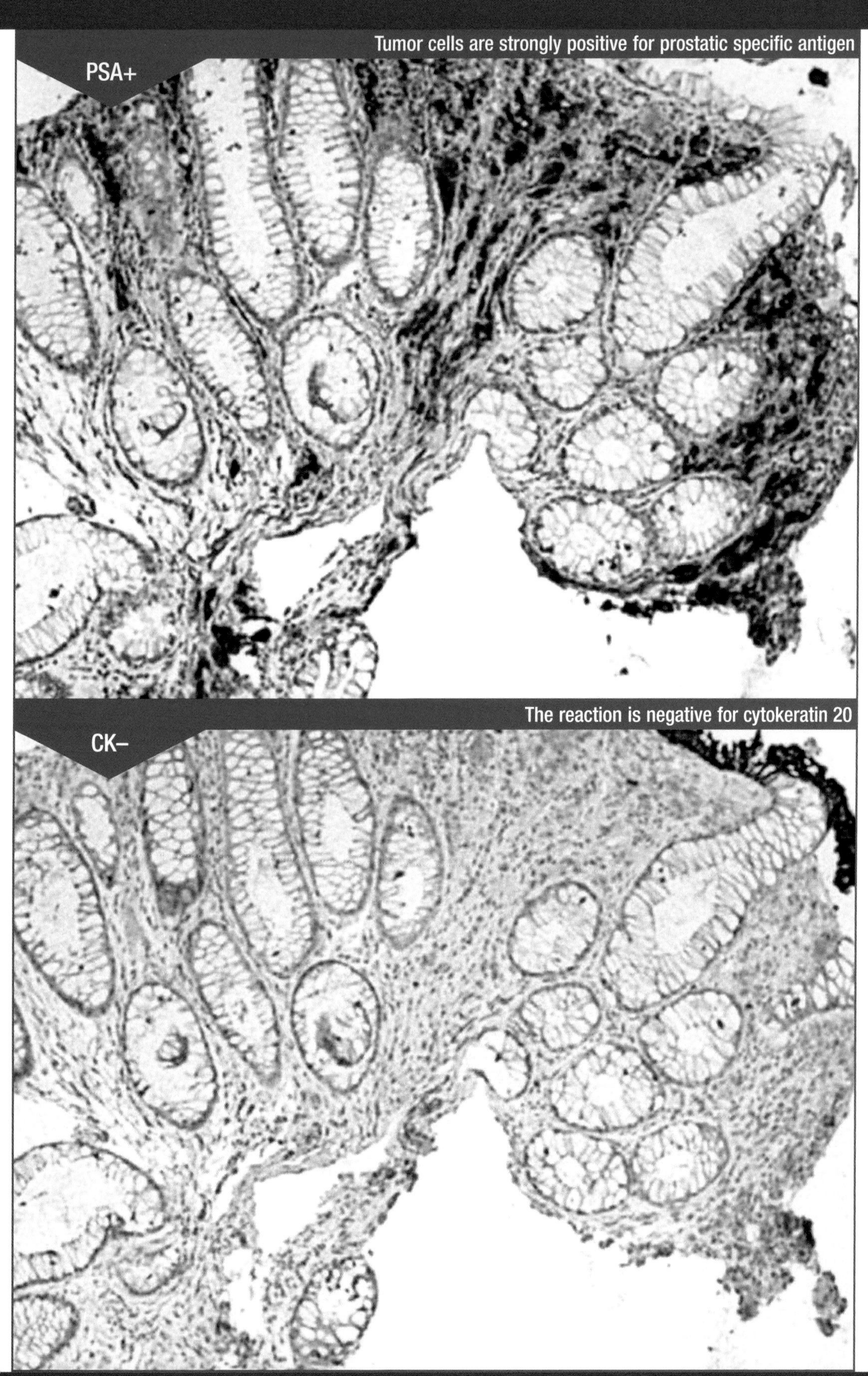

Diagnosis: Prostatic Carcinoma

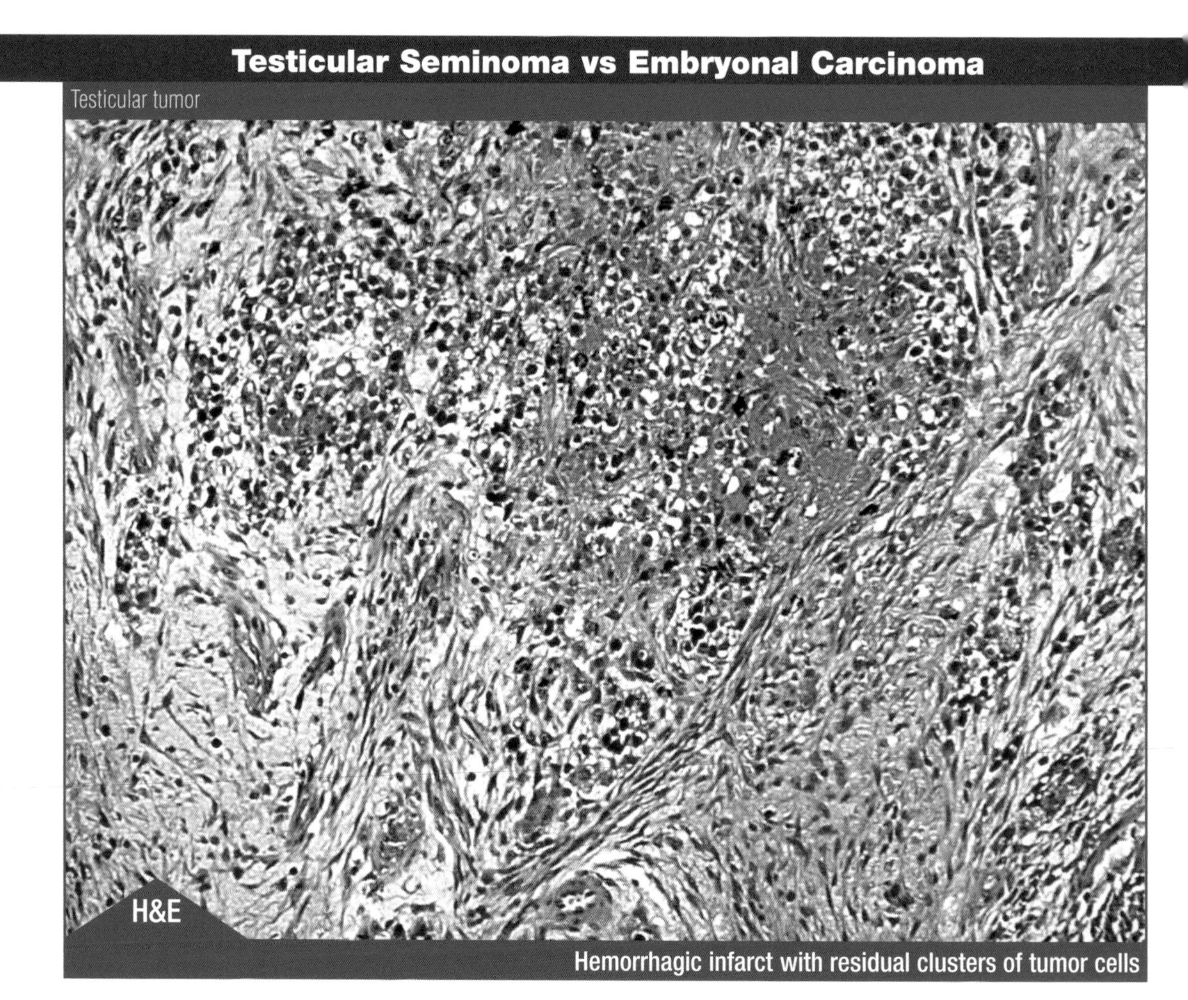

Hemorrhagic infarct with residual clusters of tumor cells

Testicular Seminoma vs Embryonal Carcinoma			
	Cytokeratin (CK)	PLAP	CD30
Testicular Seminoma	–	+	–
Embryonal Carcinoma	+	S	+

Helpful Hints

Most germ cell tumors can be identified by routine stains. Occasionally the differential diagnosis between a seminoma and embryonal carcinoma may be difficult, particularly if the sample is small or necrotic. Seminomas are usually negative for **cytokeratin** whereas embryonal carcinomas are always positive. Similarly, **CD30** is usually expressed by embryonal carcinomas but not by seminomas. **PLAP** is an excellent marker for seminomas and intratubular germ cell tumors, but it is also expressed by embryonal carcinomas. The yolk sac and trophoblastic elements of embryonal carcinomas react positively for **alpha fetoprotein** and **beta HCG**.

Pallesen 1988, Niehans 1988.

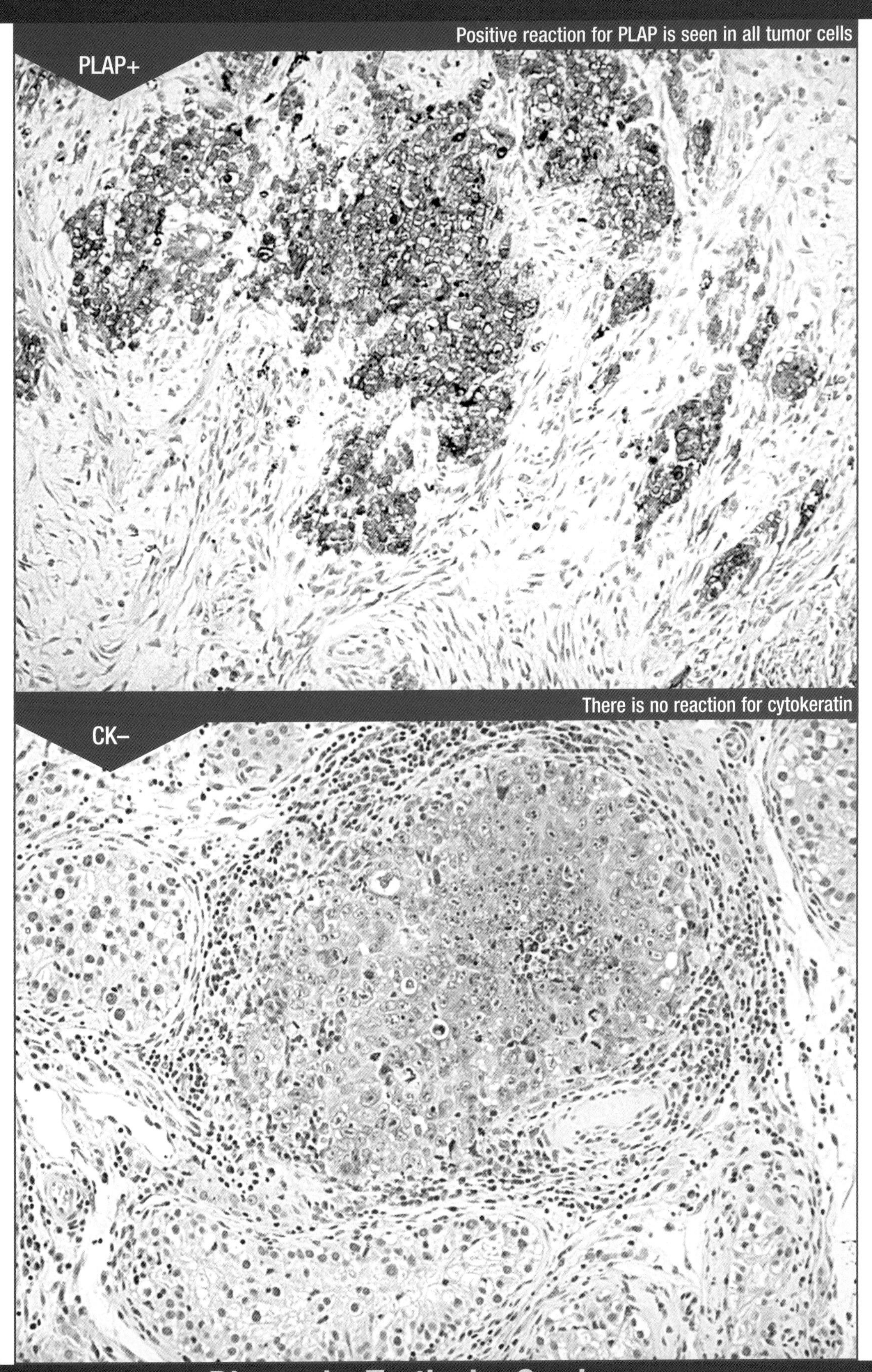

Diagnosis: Testicular Seminoma

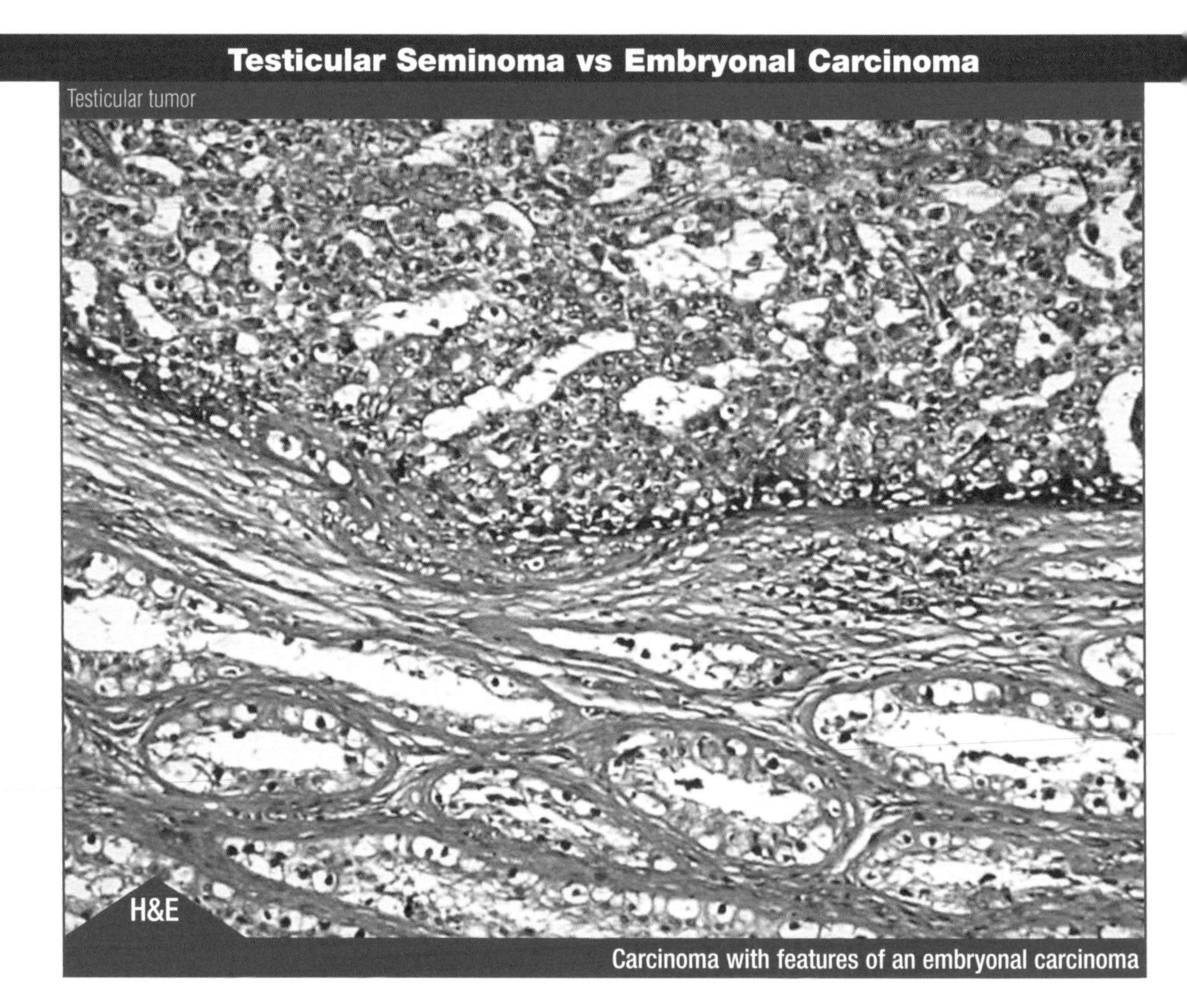

Carcinoma with features of an embryonal carcinoma

Testicular Seminoma vs Embryonal Carcinoma			
	Cytokeratin (CK)	PLAP	CD30
Testicular Seminoma	–	+	–
Embryonal Carcinoma	+	S	+

Helpful Hints

Most germ cell tumors can be identified by routine stains. Occasionally the differential diagnosis between a seminoma and embryonal carcinoma may be difficult, particularly if the sample is small or necrotic. Seminomas are usually negative for **cytokeratin** whereas embryonal carcinomas are always positive. Similarly, **CD30** is usually expressed by embryonal carcinomas but not by seminomas. **PLAP** is an excellent marker for seminomas and intratubular germ cell tumors, but it is also expressed by embryonal carcinomas. The yolk sac and trophoblastic elements of embryonal carcinomas react positively for **alpha fetoprotein** and **beta HCG**.

Pallesen 1988, Niehans 1988.

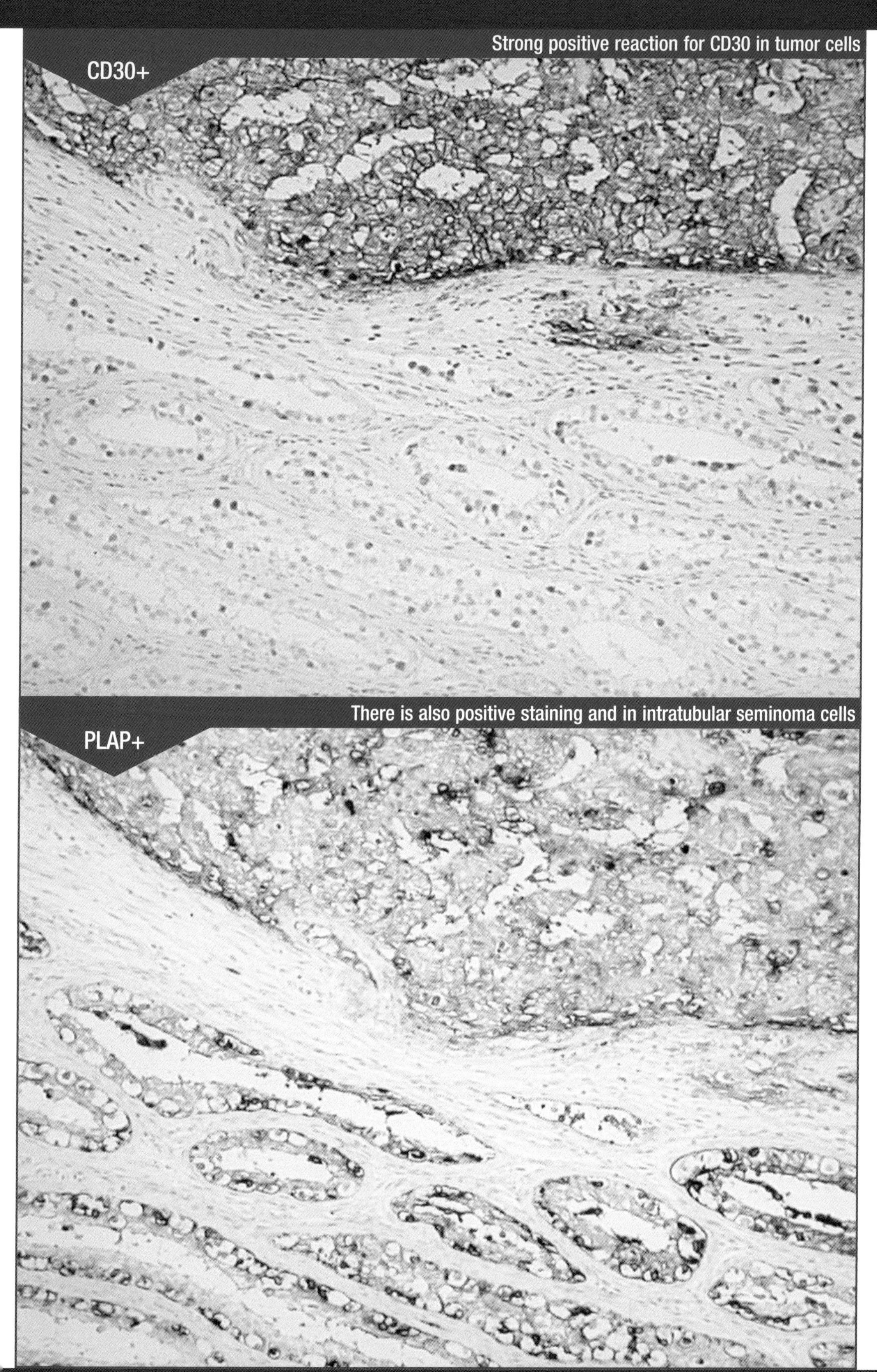
Strong positive reaction for CD30 in tumor cells
CD30+
There is also positive staining and in intratubular seminoma cells
PLAP+
Diagnosis: Embryonal Carcinoma + Intratubular Seminoma

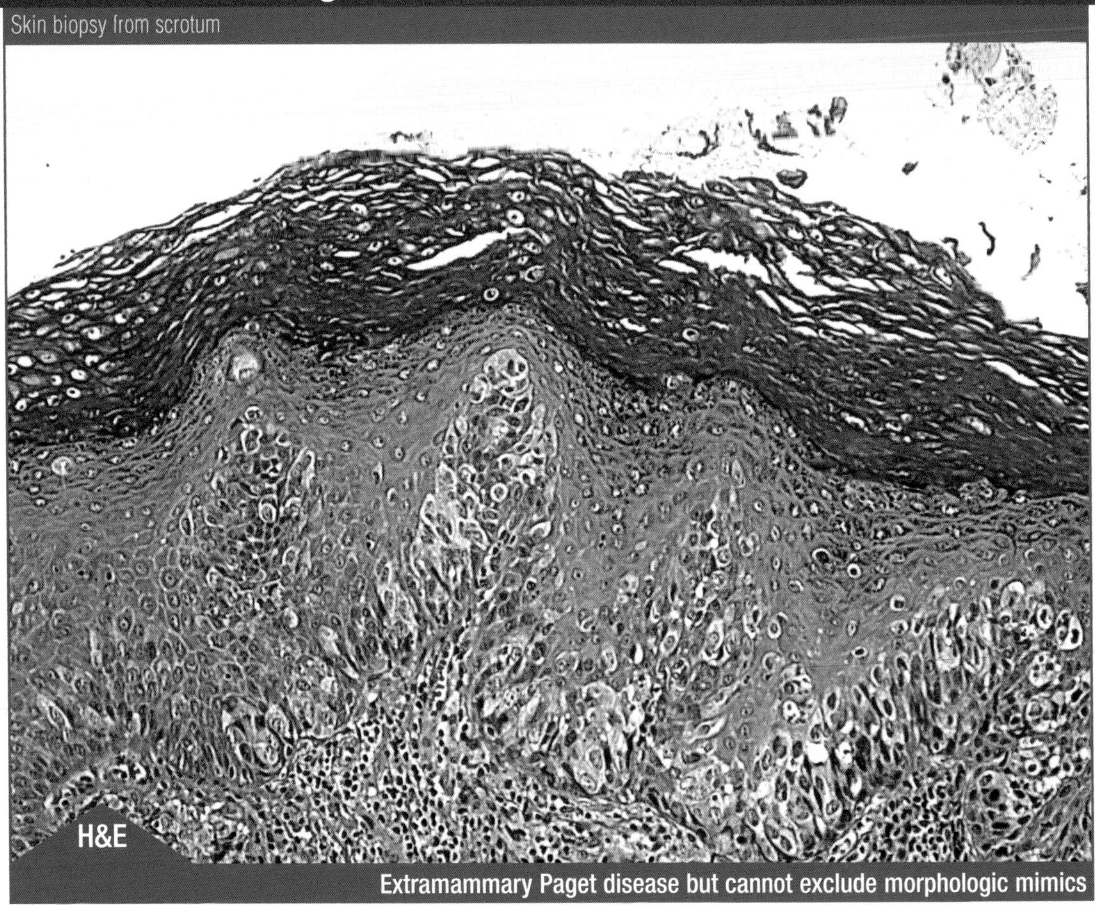

Extramammary Paget disease but cannot exclude morphologic mimics

Paget Disease vs Bowen Disease	CK7	EMA
Paget Disease	+	+
Bowen Disease	–	–

Helpful Hints

Low molecular cytokeratins in general and **cytokeratin 7** (**CK7**) in particular, are excellent markers for decoration of malignant cells in mammary and extramammary Paget disease. They are expressed by Paget cells while normal epidermis and in situ squamous cell carcinoma remain negative. **Epithelial Membrane Antigen** (**EMA**) is also useful in differentiating Paget cells from the abnormal squamous cells of in situ squamous cell carcinoma (Bowen disease).

Both markers could also be used to identify early dermal invasion in Paget disease.

Goldblum 1997a.

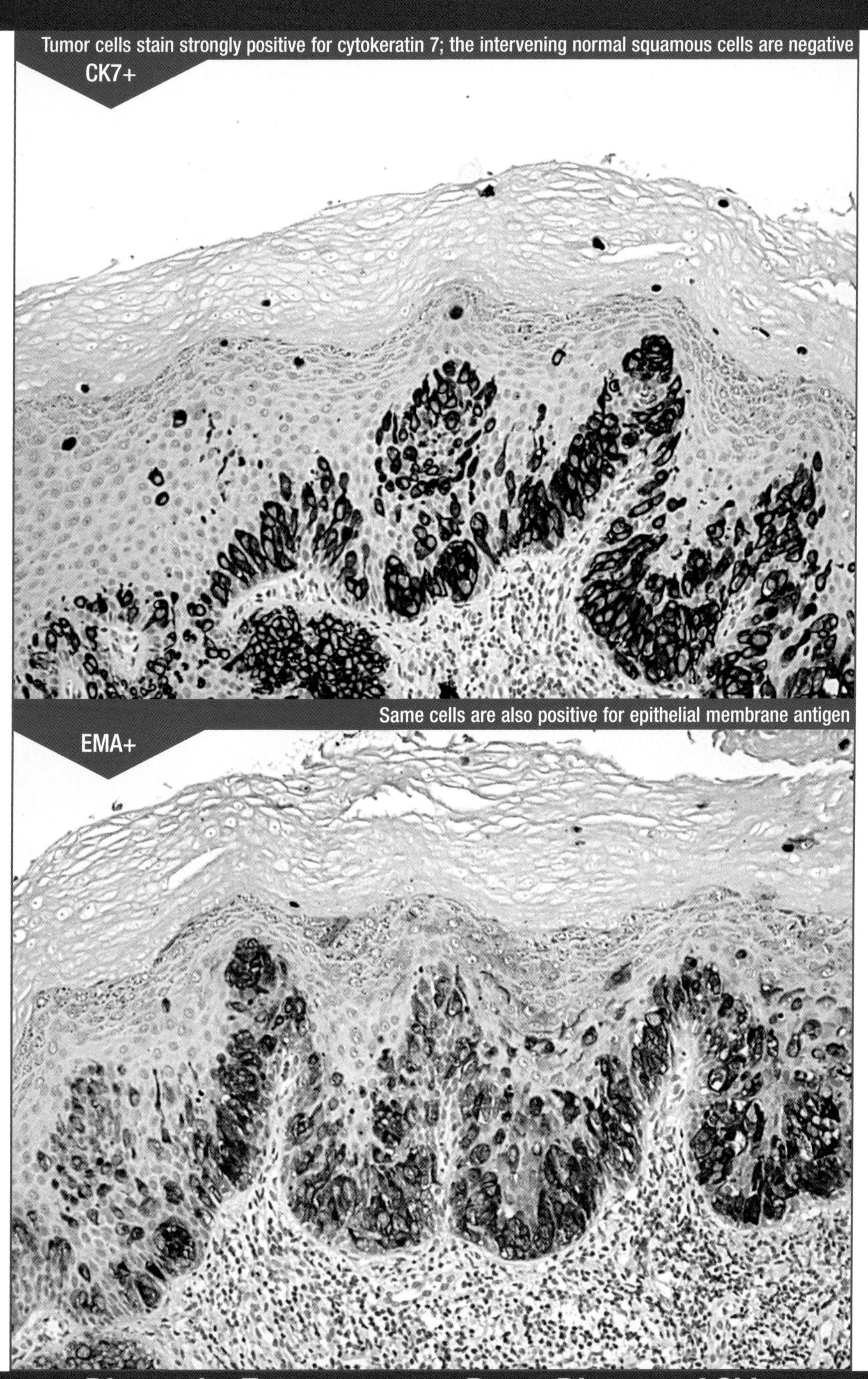

Diagnosis: Extramammary Paget Disease of Skin

Paget Disease vs In Situ Melanoma

Skin biopsy from inguinal area of an elderly female

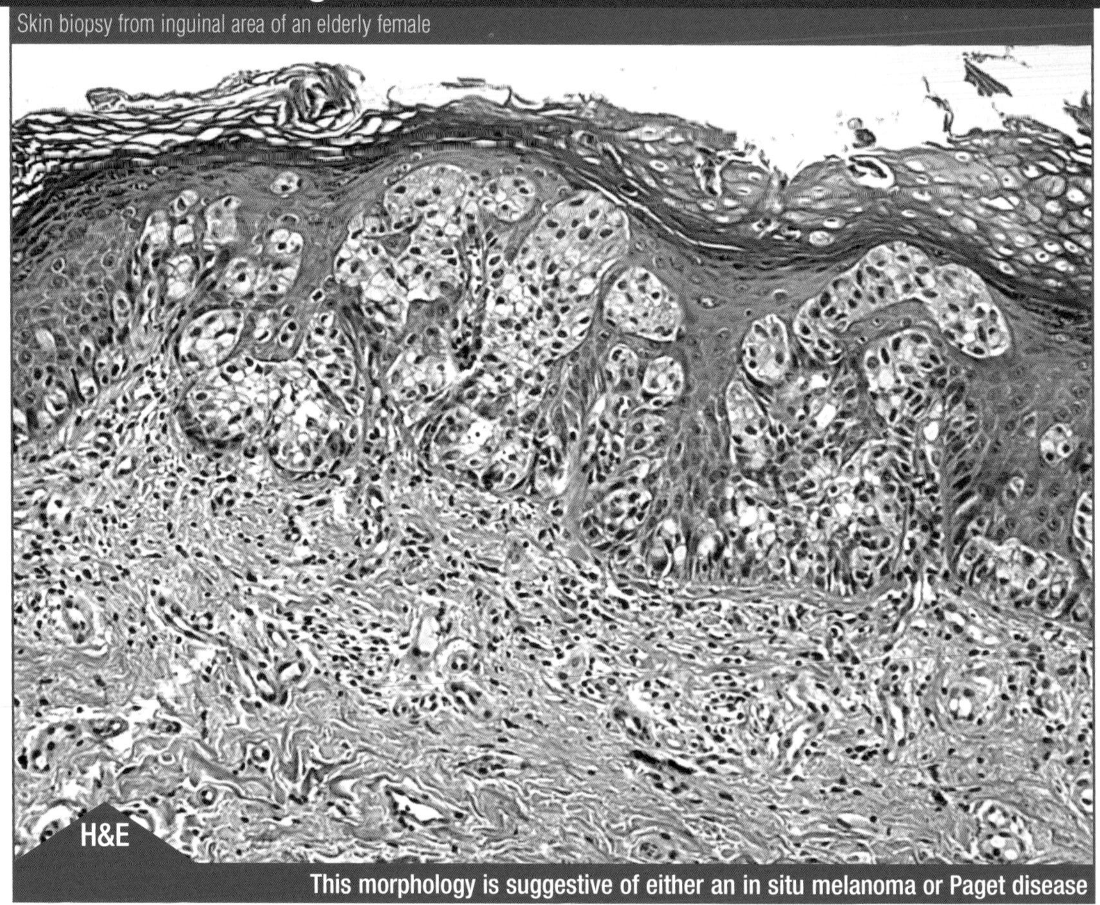

This morphology is suggestive of either an in situ melanoma or Paget disease

Paget Disease vs In Situ Melanoma			
	CK7	S100	EMA
Paget Disease	+	−	+
In Situ Melanoma	−	+	−

Helpful Hints

In situ malignant melanoma and Paget disease of skin may present similar morphologies. Melanoma cells are usually positive for **S100 protein** while **cytokeratin 7** (**CK7**) and **epithelial membrane antigen** (**EMA**) identify Paget cells.

If one uses a cytokeratin cocktail, melanoma cells may appear as empty spaces among positive epidermal cells.

Battles 1997.

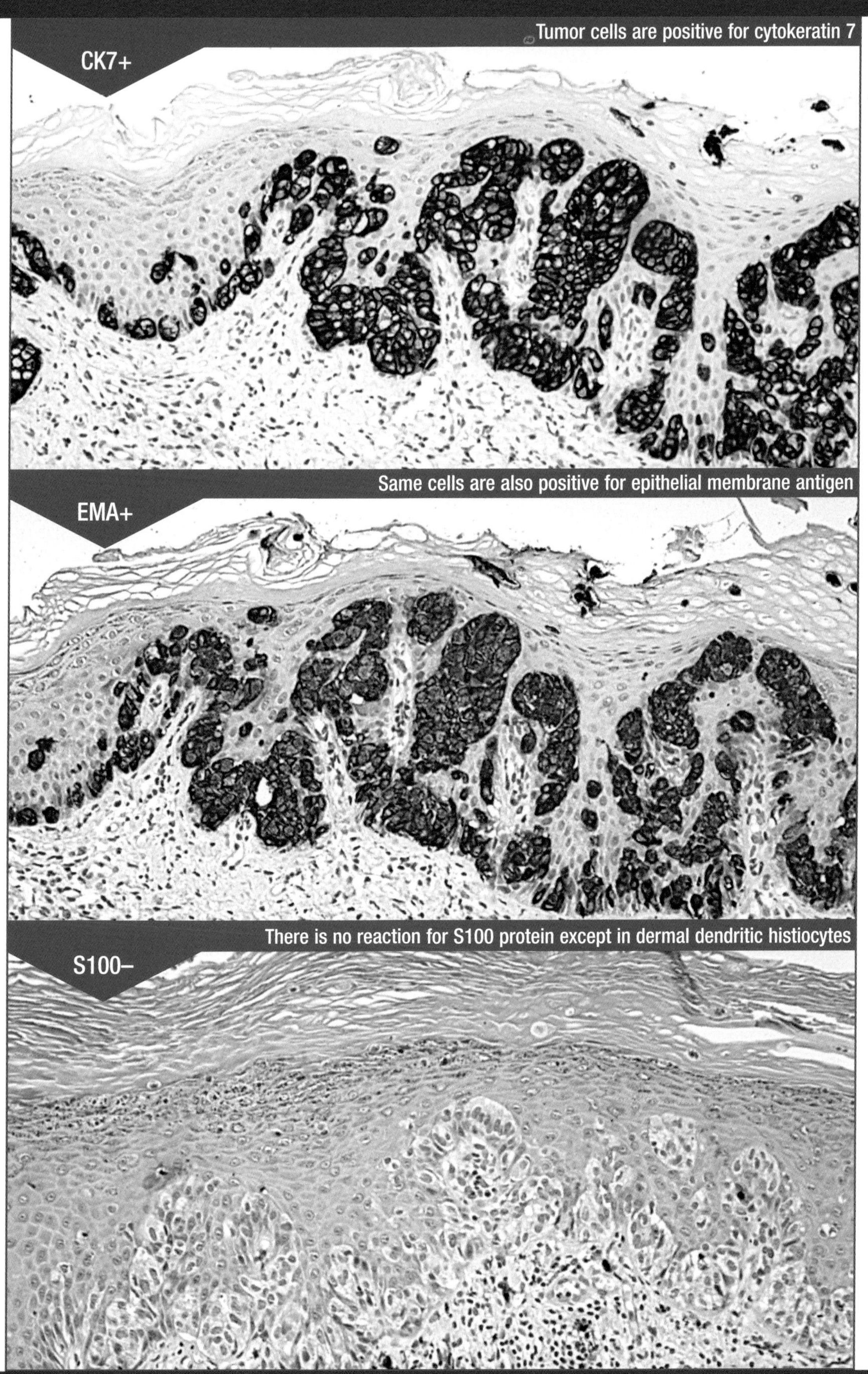

Diagnosis: Extramammary Paget Disease of Skin

Skin biopsy from dorsum of the hand

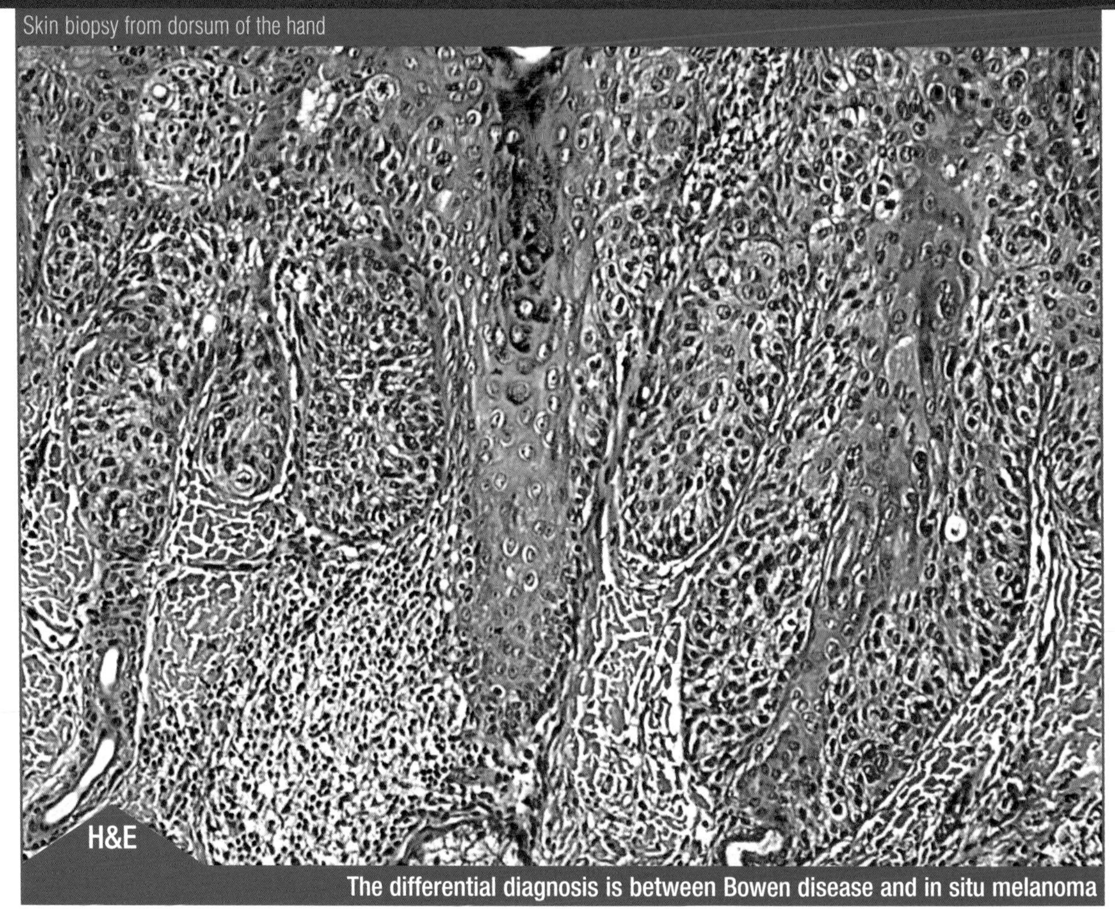

The differential diagnosis is between Bowen disease and in situ melanoma

Bowen Disease vs In Situ Melanoma		
	Cytokeratin (CK)	S100 Protein
Bowen Disease	+	–
In Situ Melanoma	–	+

Helpful Hints

The abnormal cells in Bowen disease uniformly react positively for **cytokeratin** throughout the epidermis. This is in contrast to melanoma cells that produce empty negative images.

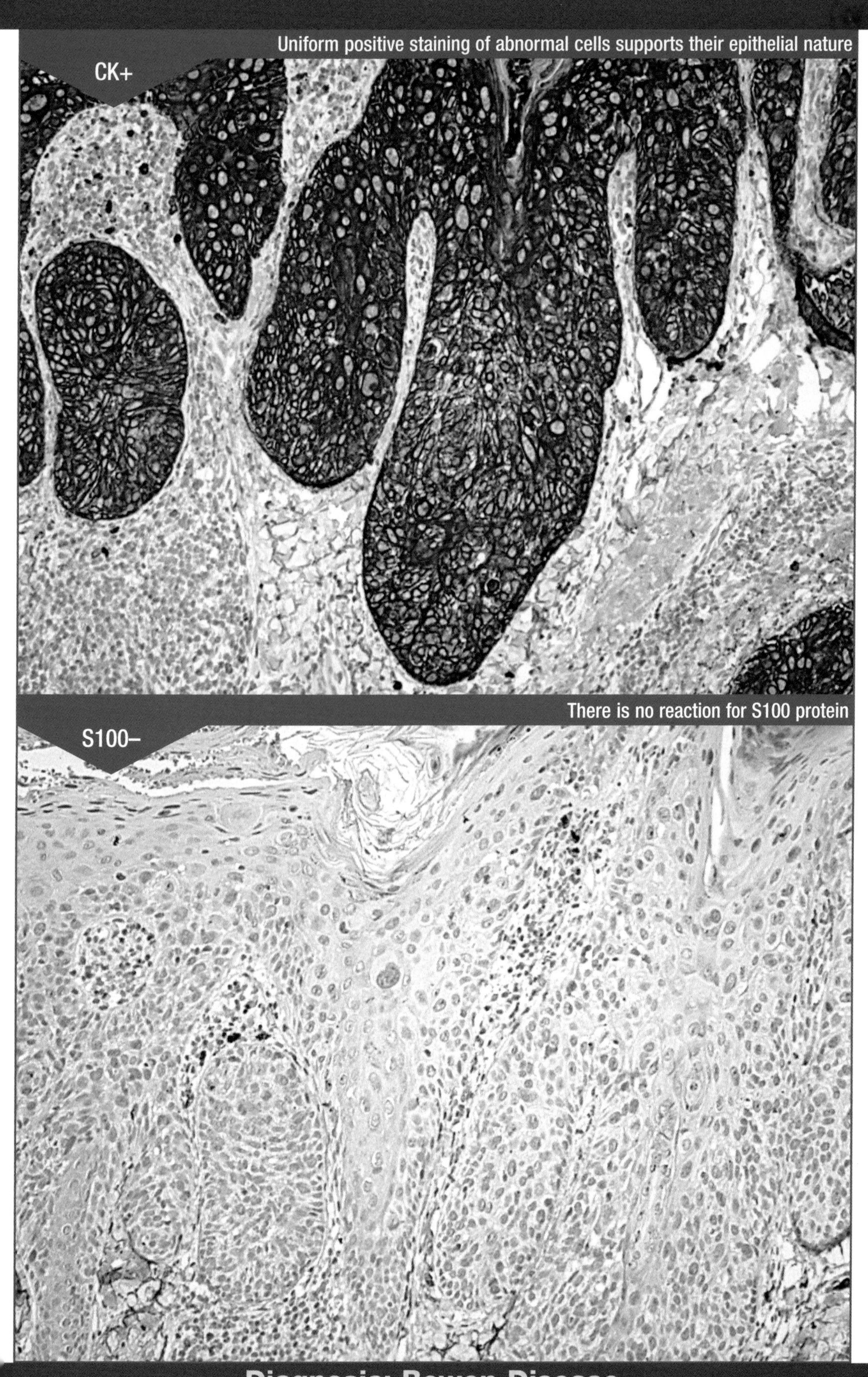

Diagnosis: Bowen Disease

Skin biopsy of scalp

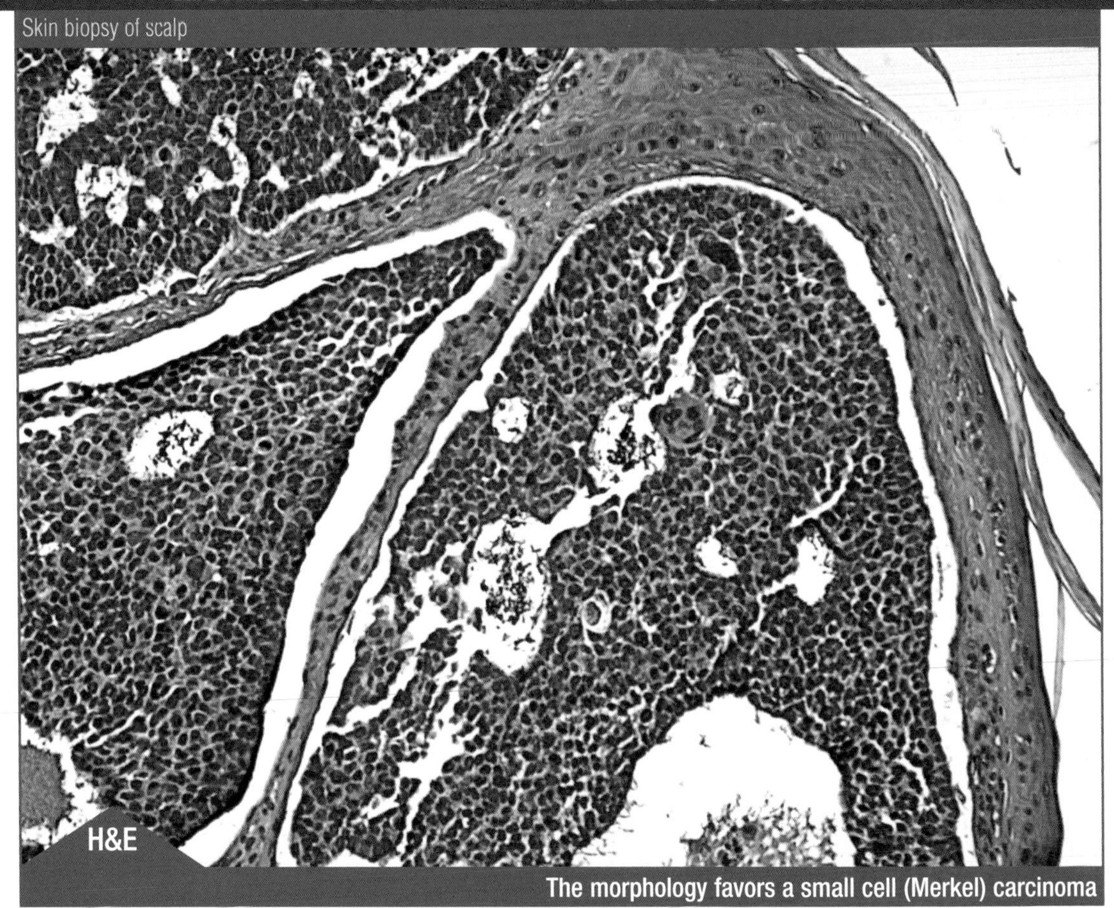

The morphology favors a small cell (Merkel) carcinoma

Merkel Cell Carcinoma vs Basal Cell Carcinoma			
	CK20	Chromogranin (Chrg)	P63
Merkel Cell Carcinoma	+	S	–
Basal Cell Carcinoma	–	–	+

Helpful Hints

While most Merkel cell carcinomas can be diagnosed with routine stain, occasionally their differential diagnosis from basal cell carcinomas may create a problem. All Merkel cell carcinomas express **cytokeratin 20** in a characteristic perinuclear or punctate pattern. Basal cell carcinomas are negative for this marker. **Chromogranin**, when positive (about 50% of cases), further supports the diagnosis of a Merkel cell carcinoma.

On the other hand, all basal cell carcinomas are positive for **p63** while Merkel cell cancers are usually negative.

Scott 1999, Reis-Filho 2002.

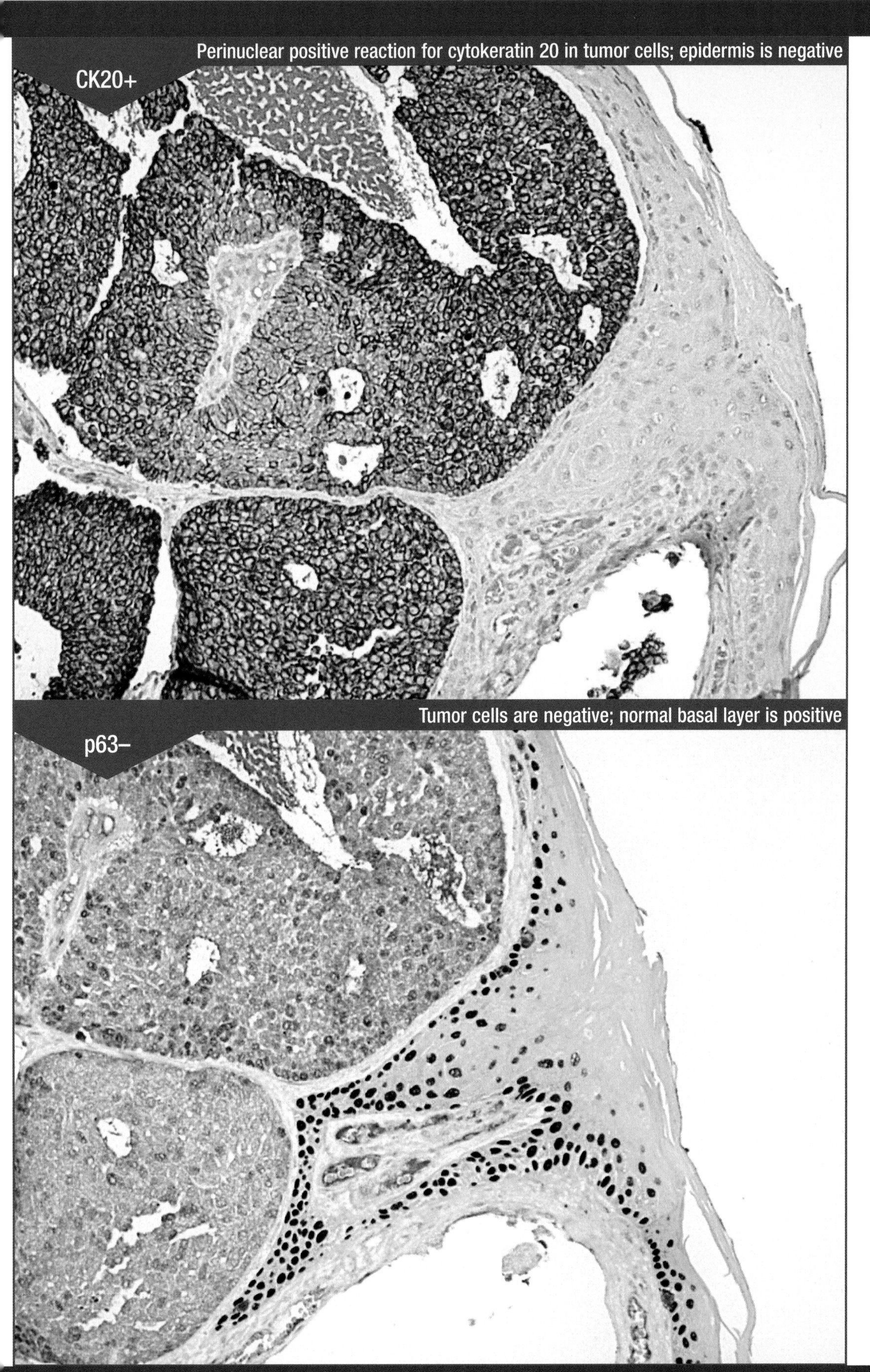

Diagnosis: Merkel Cell Carcinoma

Merkel Cell Carcinoma vs Small Cell Lung Carcinoma

Skin biopsy from shoulder; no history of lung cancer

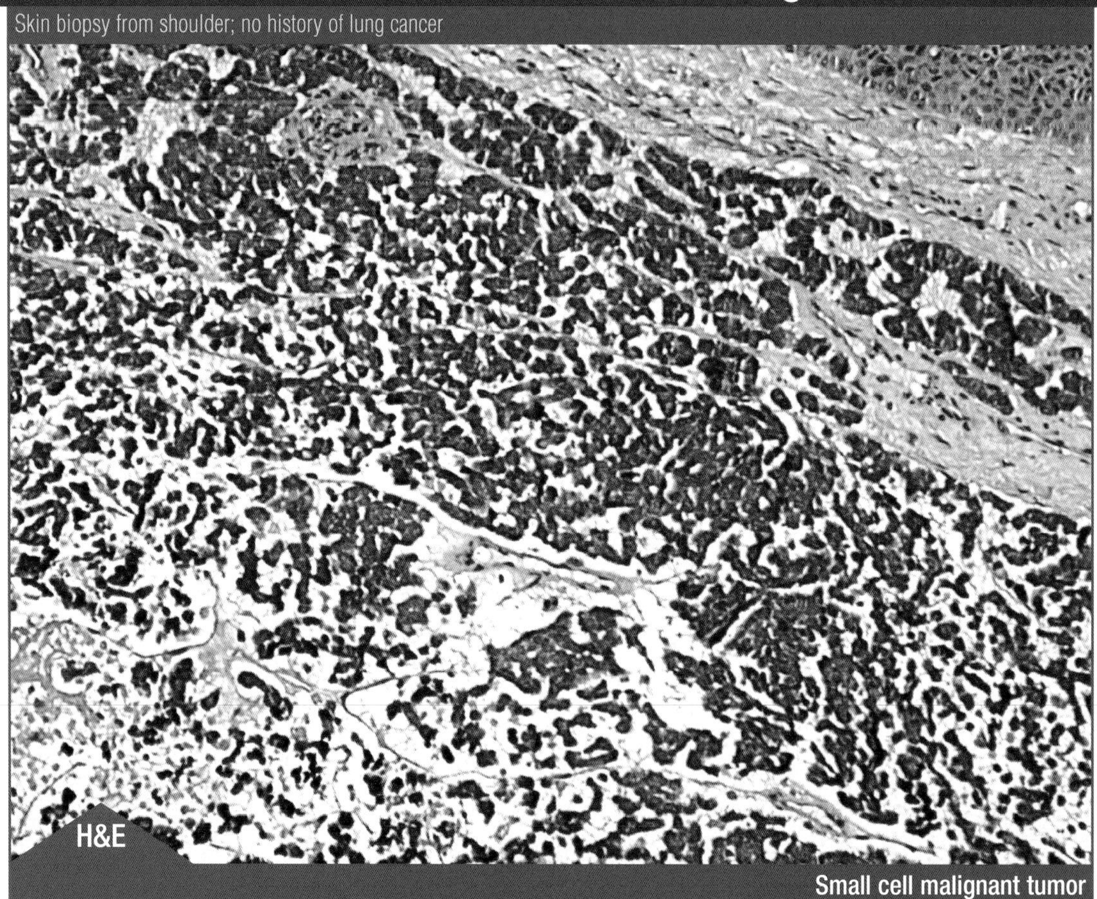

Small cell malignant tumor

Merkel Cell Carcinoma vs Small Cell Lung Carcinoma		
	CK20	TTF-1
Merkel Cell Carcinoma	+	–
Small Cell Lung Carcinoma	–	+

Helpful Hints

The majority of small cell carcinomas of the lung are positive for **TTF-1** while Merkel cell carcinomas are negative. Conversely, while Merkel cell carcinomas are always diffusely positive for **cytokeratin 20**, small cell carcinomas of the lung are usually negative.

Hanly 2000.

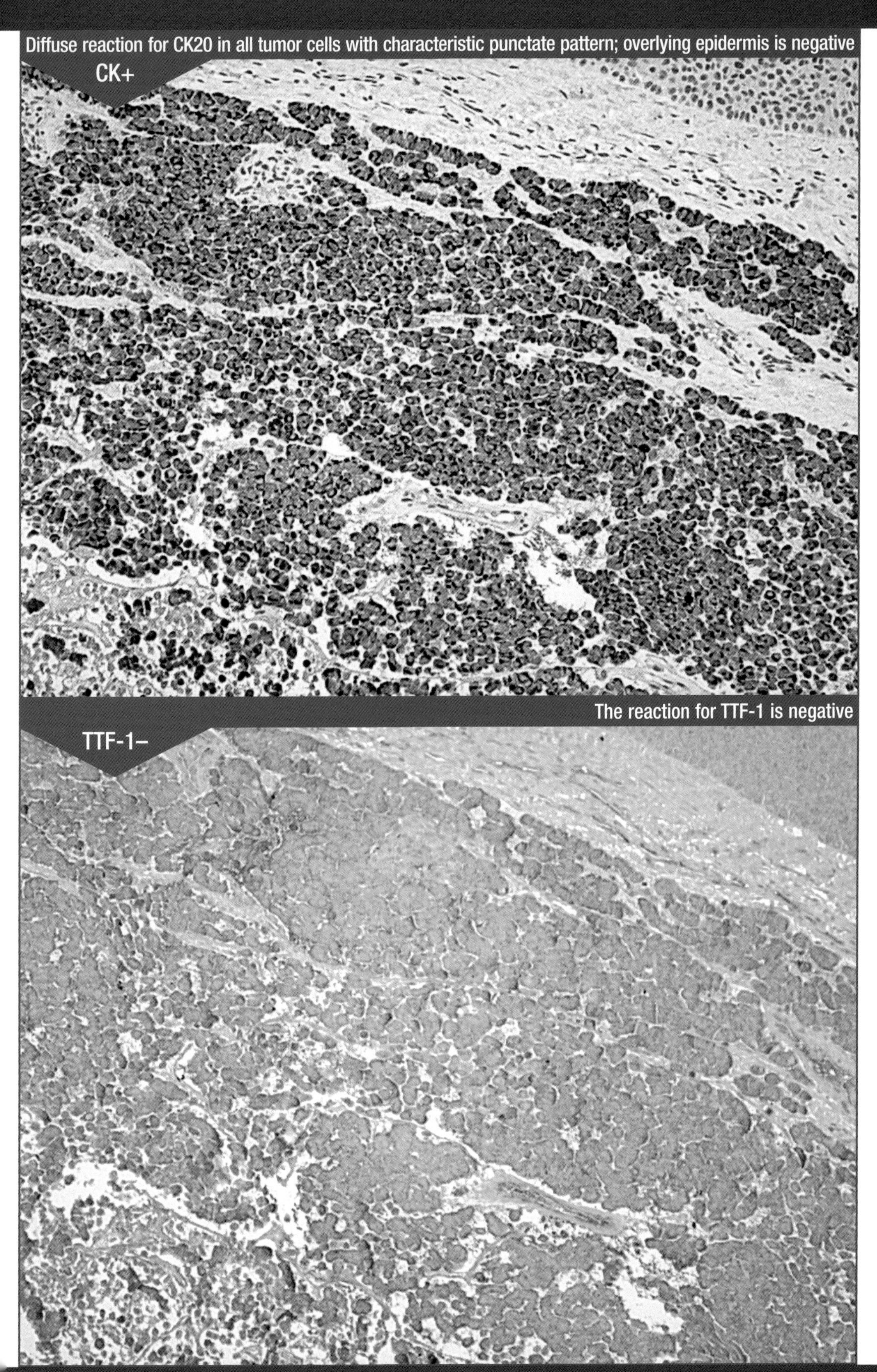
Diffuse reaction for CK20 in all tumor cells with characteristic punctate pattern; overlying epidermis is negative
CK+
The reaction for TTF-1 is negative
TTF-1–
Diagnosis: Merkel Cell Carcinoma

Merkel Cell Carcinoma vs Small Cell Lung Carcinoma

Cell block from fine needle aspiration of an axillary mass in a patient with history of skin cancer

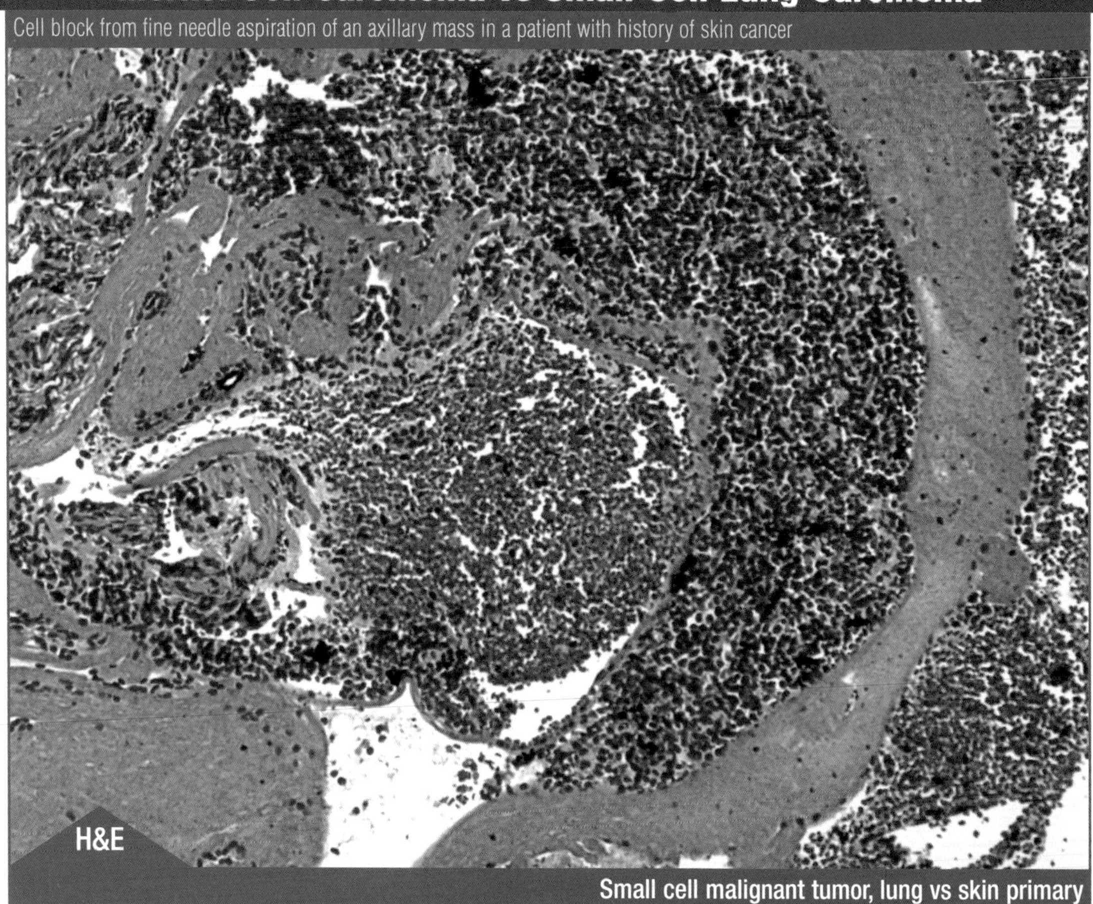

Small cell malignant tumor, lung vs skin primary

Merkel Cell Carcinoma vs Small Cell Lung Carcinoma		
	CK20	TTF-1
Merkel Cell Carcinoma	+	–
Small Cell Lung Carcinoma	–	+

Helpful Hints

The majority of small cell carcinomas of the lung are positive for **TTF-1** while Merkel cell carcinomas are negative. Conversely, while Merkel cell carcinomas are always diffusely positive for **cytokeratin 20**, small cell carcinomas of the lung are usually negative.

Hanly 2000.

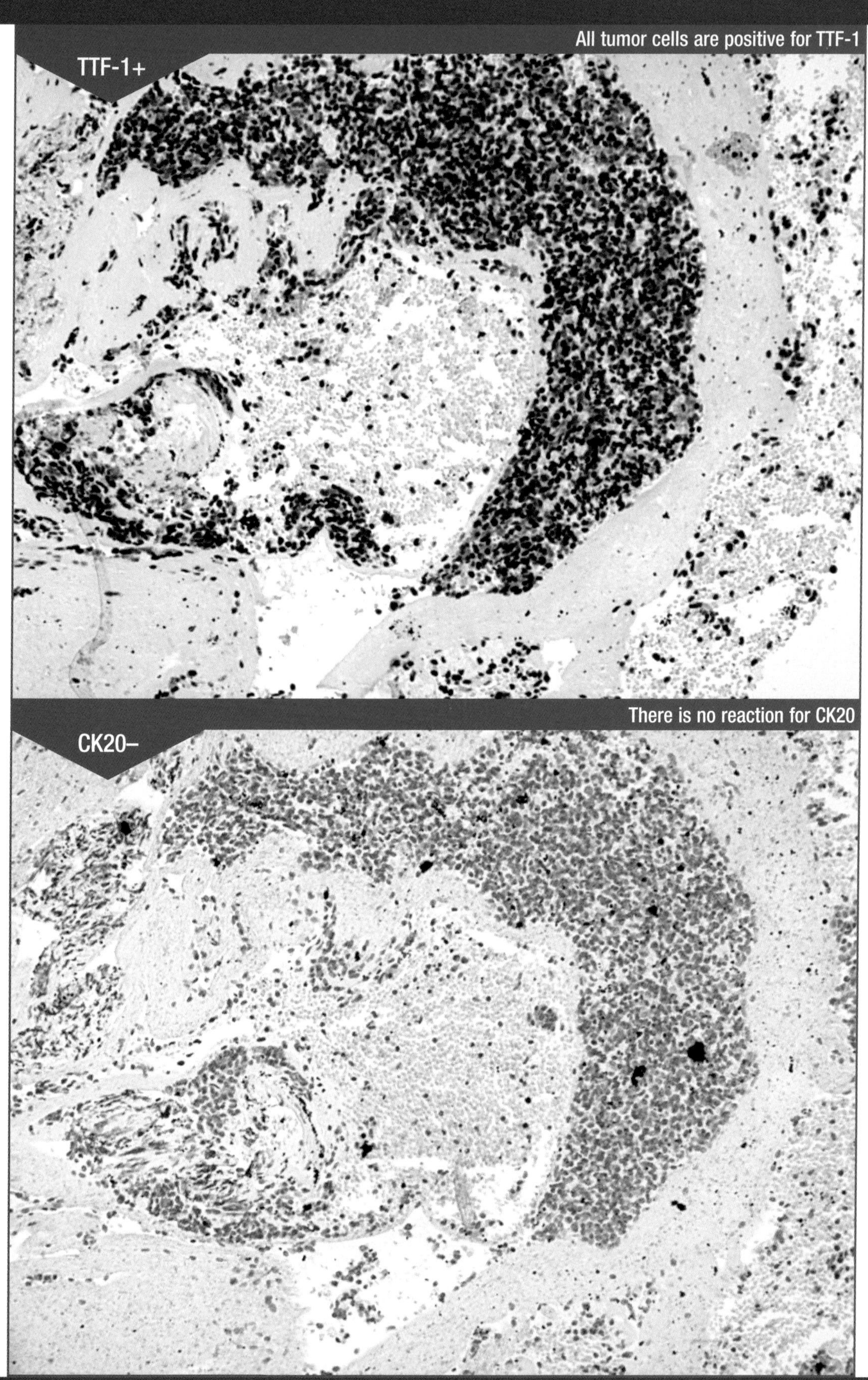

Diagnosis: Metastatic Small Cell Carcinoma of Lung

Excision of lesion in the eyelid

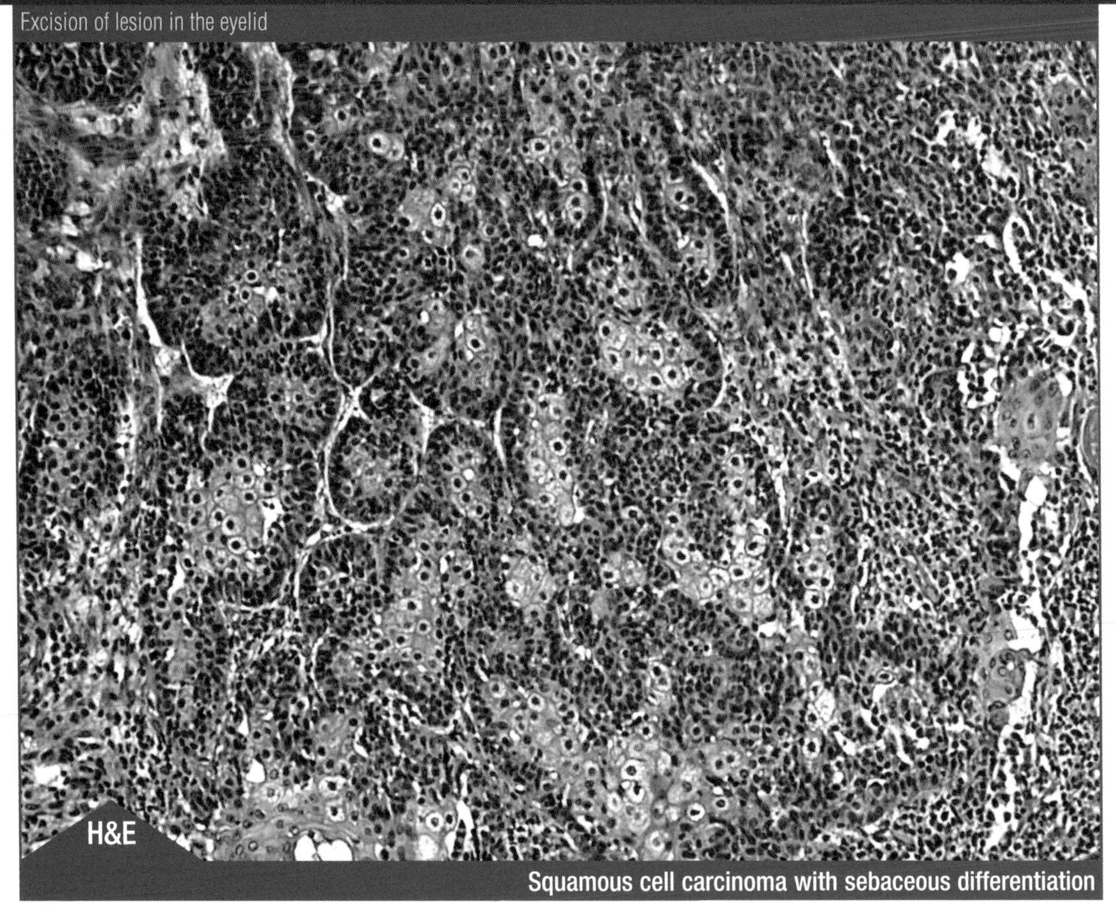

Squamous cell carcinoma with sebaceous differentiation

Sebaceous Carcinoma vs Squamous Cell Carcinoma	
	T-F Antigen
Sebaceous Carcinoma	+
Squamous Carcinoma	–

Helpful Hints

Squamous cell carcinoma with clear cells may mimic sebaceous carcinoma. The latter of course, has a more aggressive behavior, particularly when occurring in the conjunctiva.

Thomsen-Friedenreich (T-F) Antigen is expressed by normal sebaceous glands and sebaceous carcinomas, but not by squamous cell carcinoma. T-F staining in sebaceous carcinomas is usually focal and limited to the center of tumor islands where there is more sebaceous (*clear cell*) differentiation. T-F antigen is not specific for sebaceous carcinoma and may be expressed by a number of unrelated tumors.

Hassanein 2001.

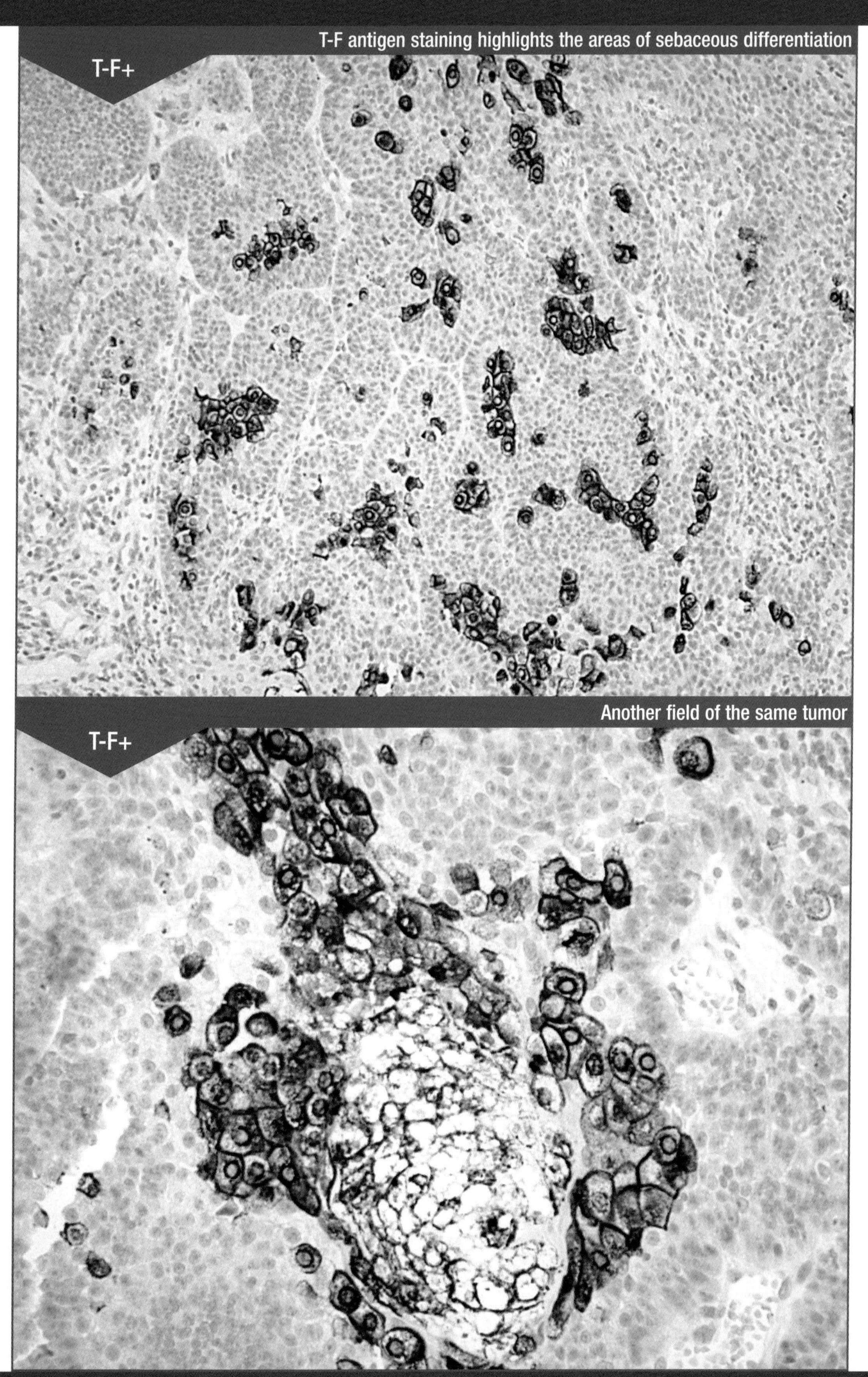
T-F antigen staining highlights the areas of sebaceous differentiation
T-F+
Another field of the same tumor
T-F+
Diagnosis: Sebaceous Carcinoma

Excision of skin lesion in the upper chest

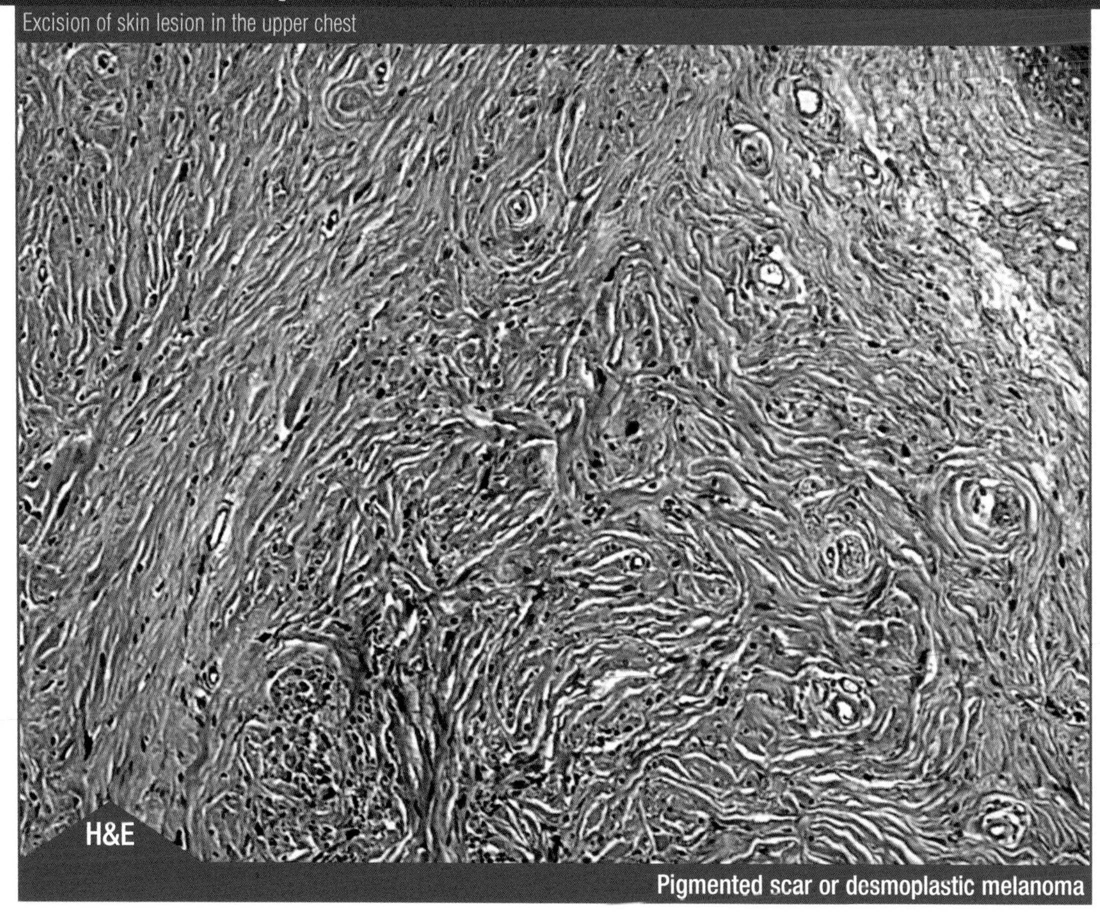

Pigmented scar or desmoplastic melanoma

Desmoplastic Melanoma vs Dermal Fibrous Scar	
	S100 Protein
Desmoplastic Melanoma	+
Dermal Fibrous Scar	–

Helpful Hints

Unlike spindle cell melanomas which morphologically resemble other malignant spindle cell neoplasms, desmoplastic melanomas present with a bland morphology that at times is indistinguishable from dermal scars. This may become more problematic when the lesion is in the area of previous punch or shave biopsy. Positivity for **S100 protein**, which at times may only be nuclear, separates desmoplastic melanomas from scars.

Other melanocytic markers such as **HMB-45**, **Melan-A**, etc, are of no value in the diagnosis of desmoplastic melanomas.

Busam 2005..

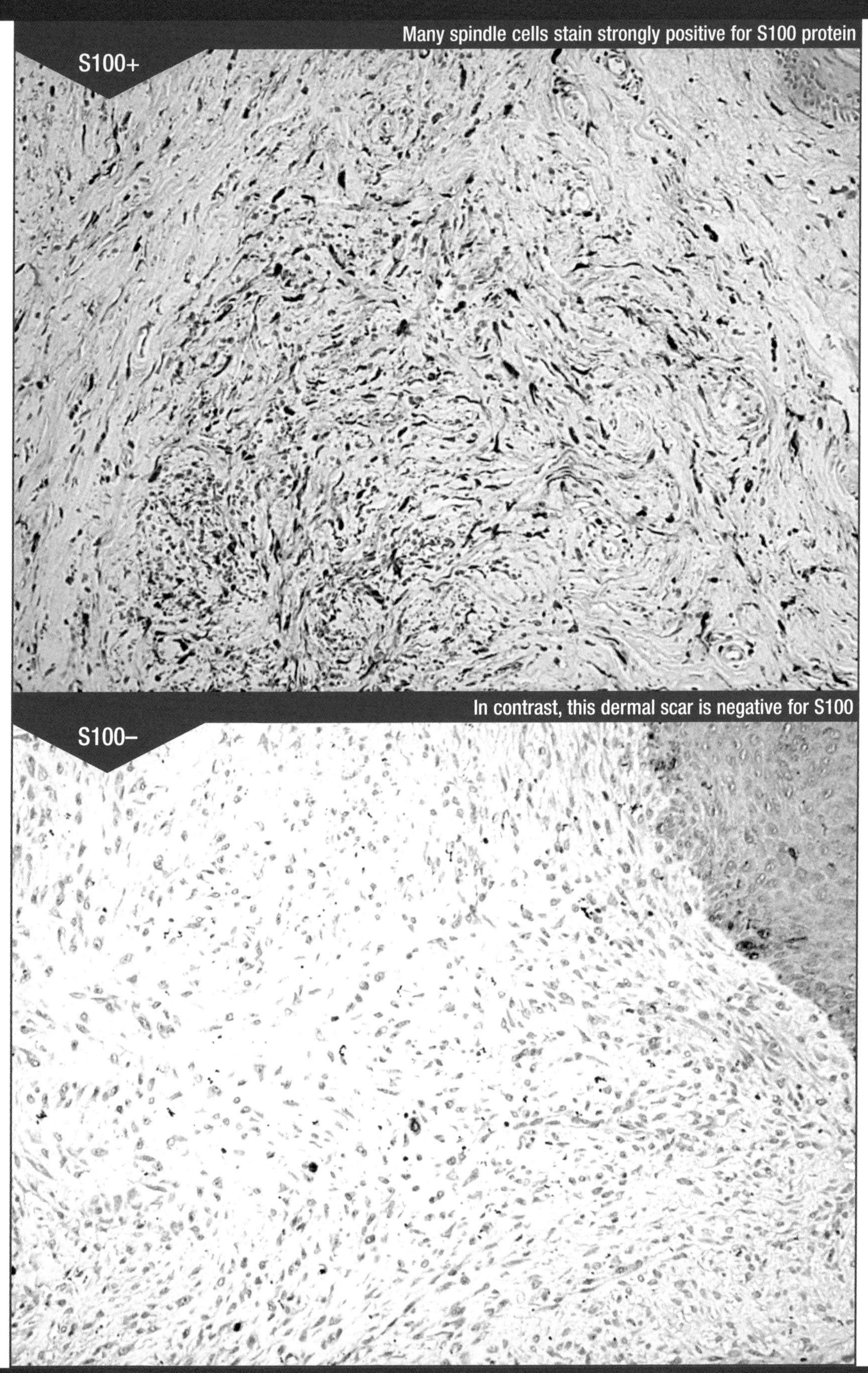

Diagnosis: Desmoplastic Malignant Melanoma

Skin nodule

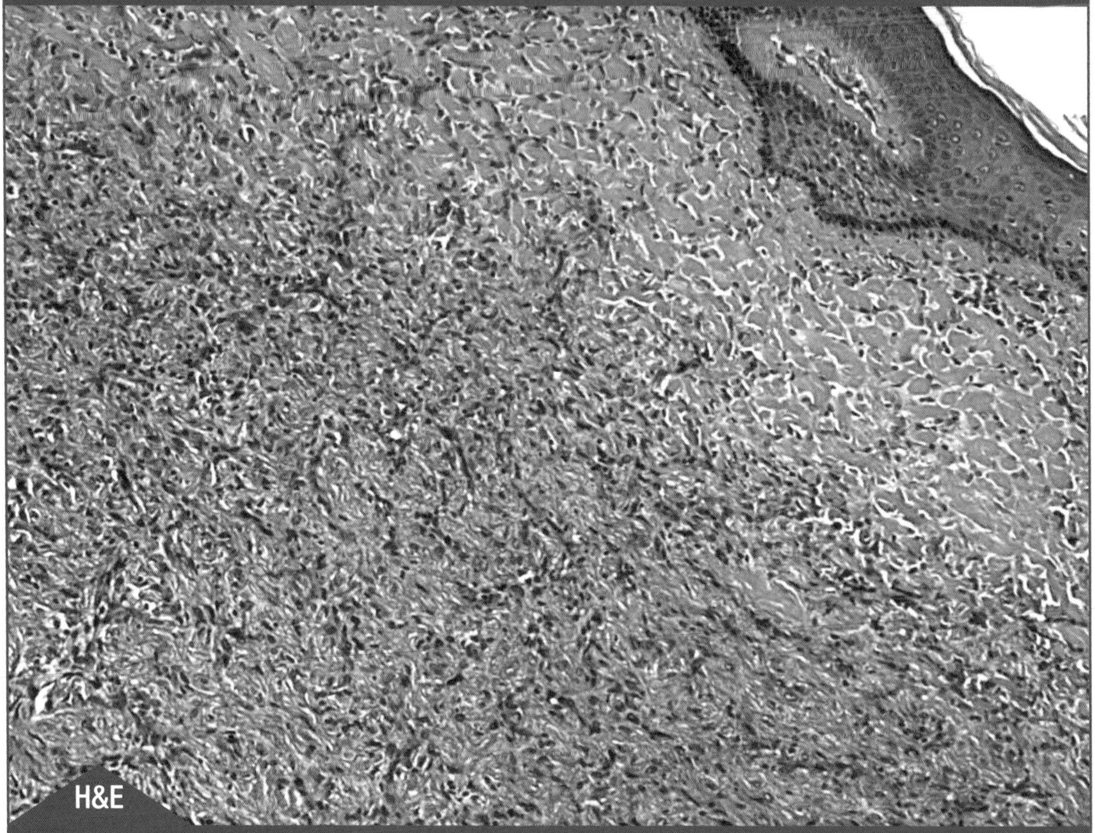

H&E

The morphology is fairly typical of a dermatofibroma

Dermatofibroma vs Dermatofibrosarcoma		
	Factor XIIIa	CD34
Dermatofibroma	+	–
Dermatofibrosarcoma	–	+

Helpful Hints

This differential diagnosis is not uncommon, particularly when the biopsy is small and does not include deep dermis. The staining for the above two markers usually resolves the problem. One should note, however, that both **Factor XIIIa** and **CD34** may react with fibroblasts at the periphery of these lesions. Interpretation therefore, should be based on the staining reaction in the center of tumor.

It has been shown that the proliferative activity of dermatofibrosarcoma protuberans is much greater than that of dermatofibroma. To that end, one could use a high **Ki-67** proliferative index to favor dermatofibrosarcoma protuberans.

Hsi 1996, Goldblum 1997b.

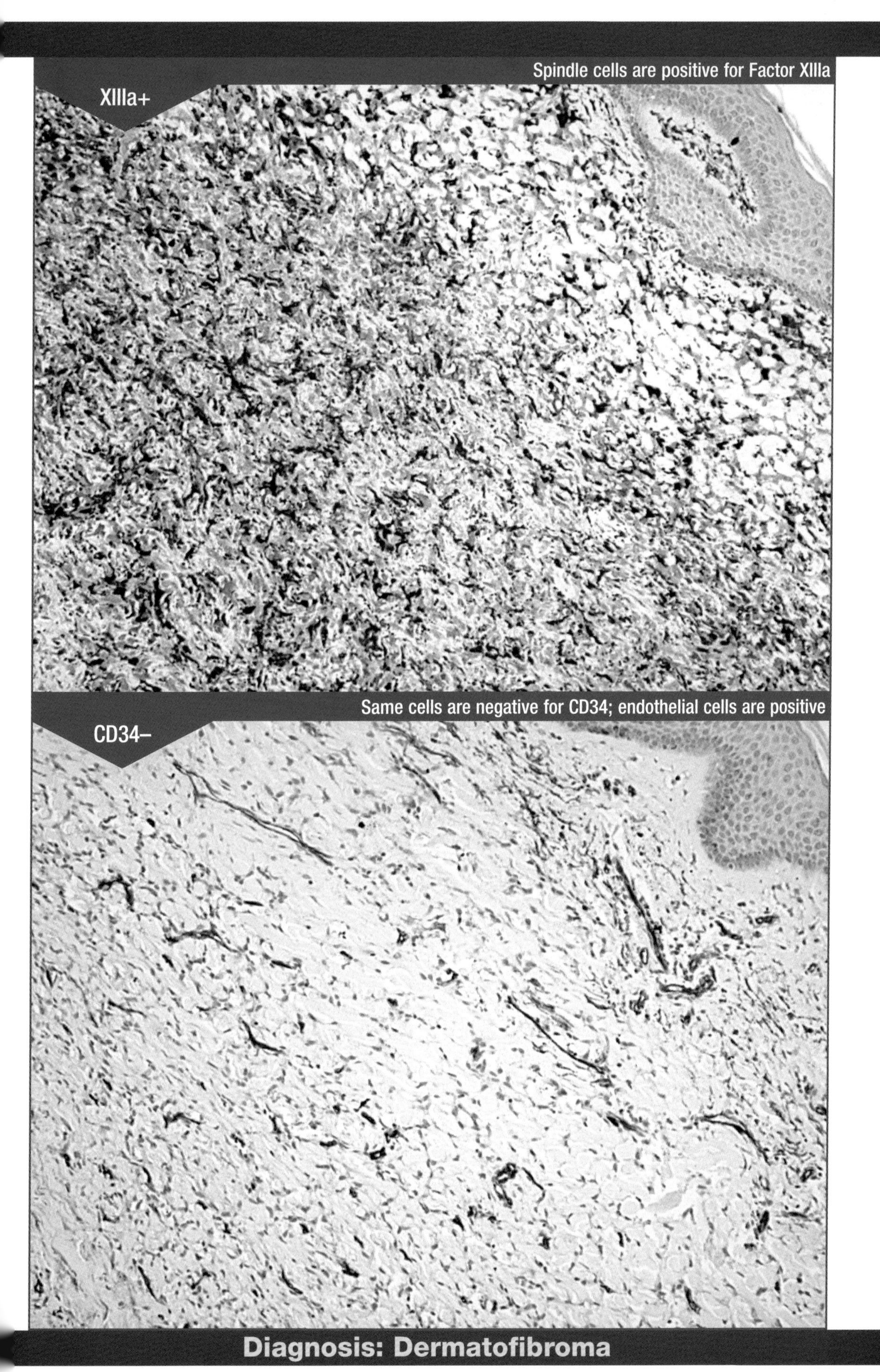
Spindle cells are positive for Factor XIIIa
XIIIa+
Same cells are negative for CD34; endothelial cells are positive
CD34–
Diagnosis: Dermatofibroma

Excision of a nodule in the thigh

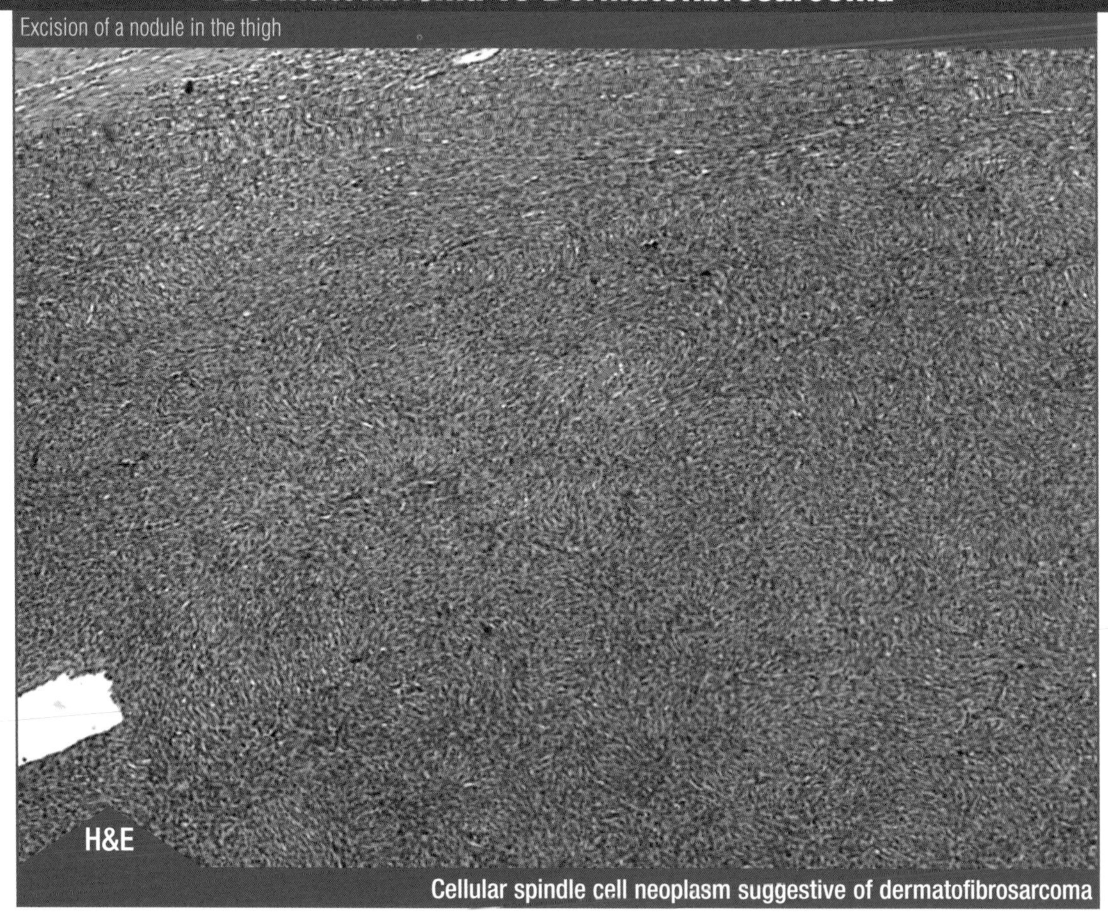

Cellular spindle cell neoplasm suggestive of dermatofibrosarcoma

Dermatofibroma vs Dermatofibrosarcoma		
	Factor XIIIa	CD34
Dermatofibroma	+	–
Dermatofibrosarcoma	–	+

Helpful Hints

This differential diagnosis is not uncommon, particularly when the biopsy is small and does not include deep dermis. The staining for the above two markers usually resolves the problem. One should note, however, that both **Factor XIIIa** and **CD34** may react with fibroblasts at the periphery of these lesions. Interpretation therefore, should be based on the staining reaction in the center of tumor.

It has been shown that the proliferative activity of dermatofibrosarcoma protuberans is much greater than that of dermatofibroma. To that end, one could use a high **Ki-67** proliferative index to favor dermatofibrosarcoma protuberans.

Hsi 1996, Goldblum 1997b.

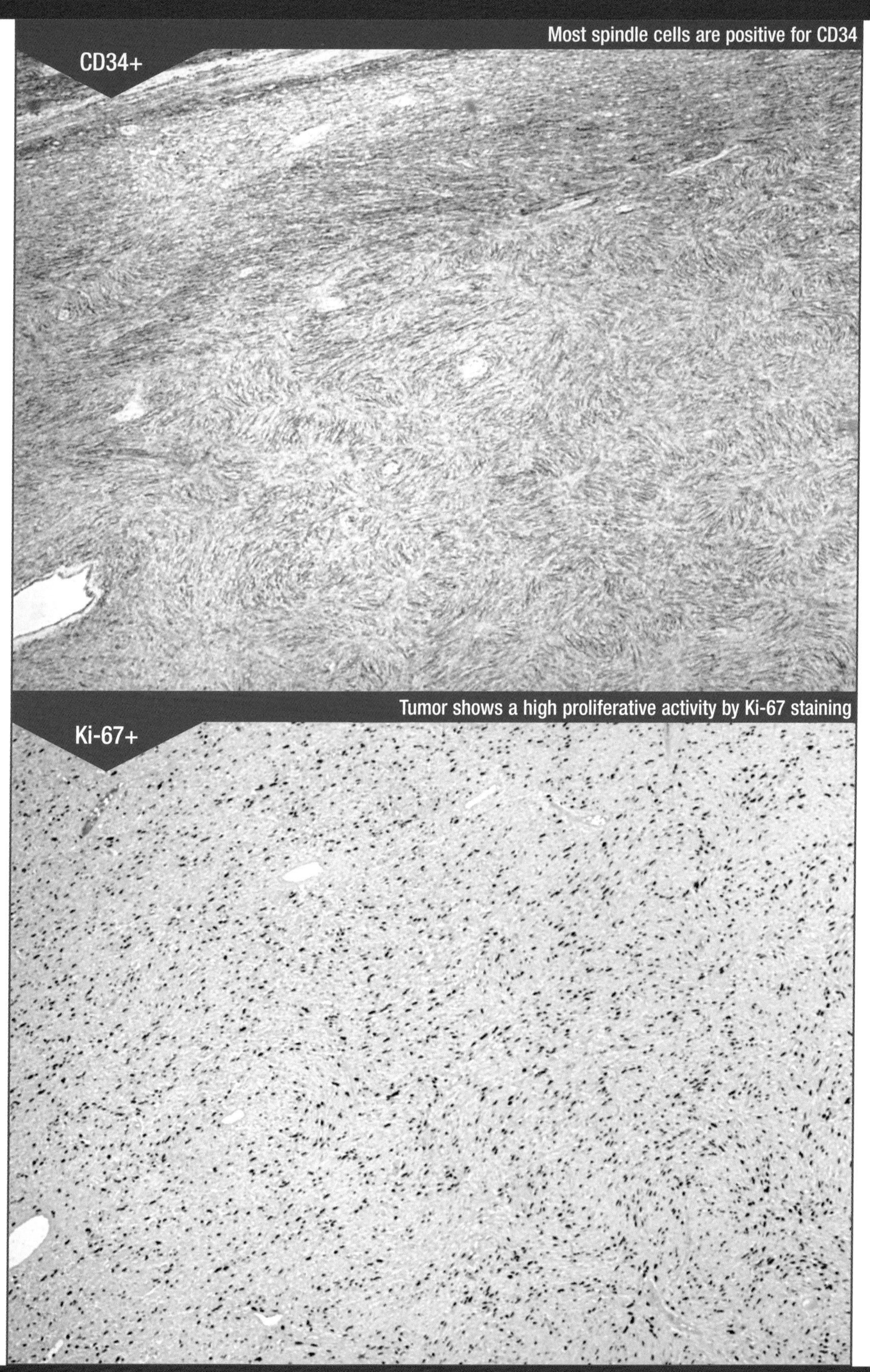
Most spindle cells are positive for CD34
CD34+
Tumor shows a high proliferative activity by Ki-67 staining
Ki-67+
Diagnosis: Dermatofibrosarcoma Protuberans

Excision of skin nodule in the parotid area

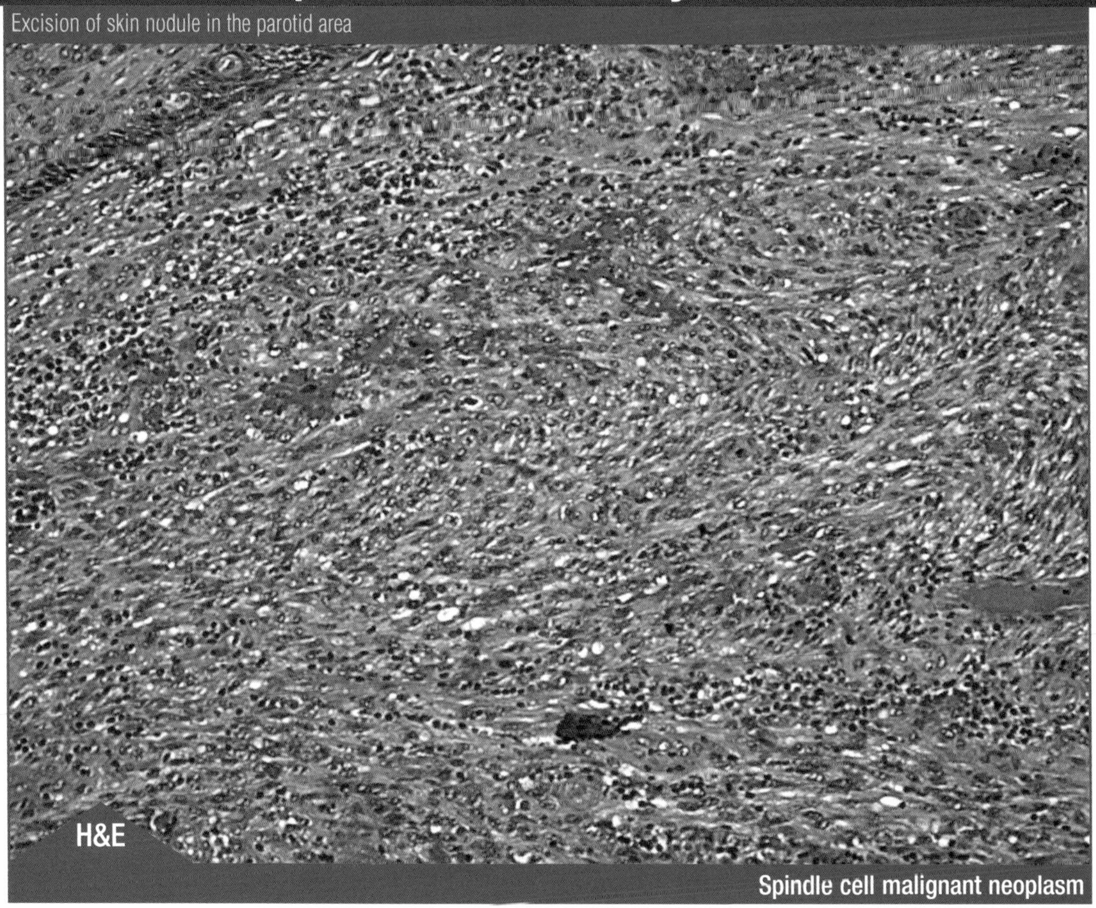

Spindle cell malignant neoplasm

Kaposi Sarcoma vs Leiomyosarcoma	CD31	vWF	H-Caldesmon (HCD)
Kaposi Sarcoma	+	+	−
Leiomyosarcoma	−	−	+

Helpful Hints

Both **CD31** and **Factor VIII-related antigen** (**vWF**) stain Kaposi sarcomas. With Factor VIII-related antigen the reaction is stronger in cells immediately adjacent to the blood channels while the intervening spindle cells may exhibit only a focal punctate staining. Most Kaposi sarcomas also stain positively for D2-40.

Most smooth muscle tumors express **H-Caldesmon** (**HCD**) but only 50% of extrauterine smooth muscle neoplasms are positive for desmin. Muscle specific actin and smooth muscle actin are not helpful because they may be present in a number of non-muscle neoplasms including Kaposi sarcoma.

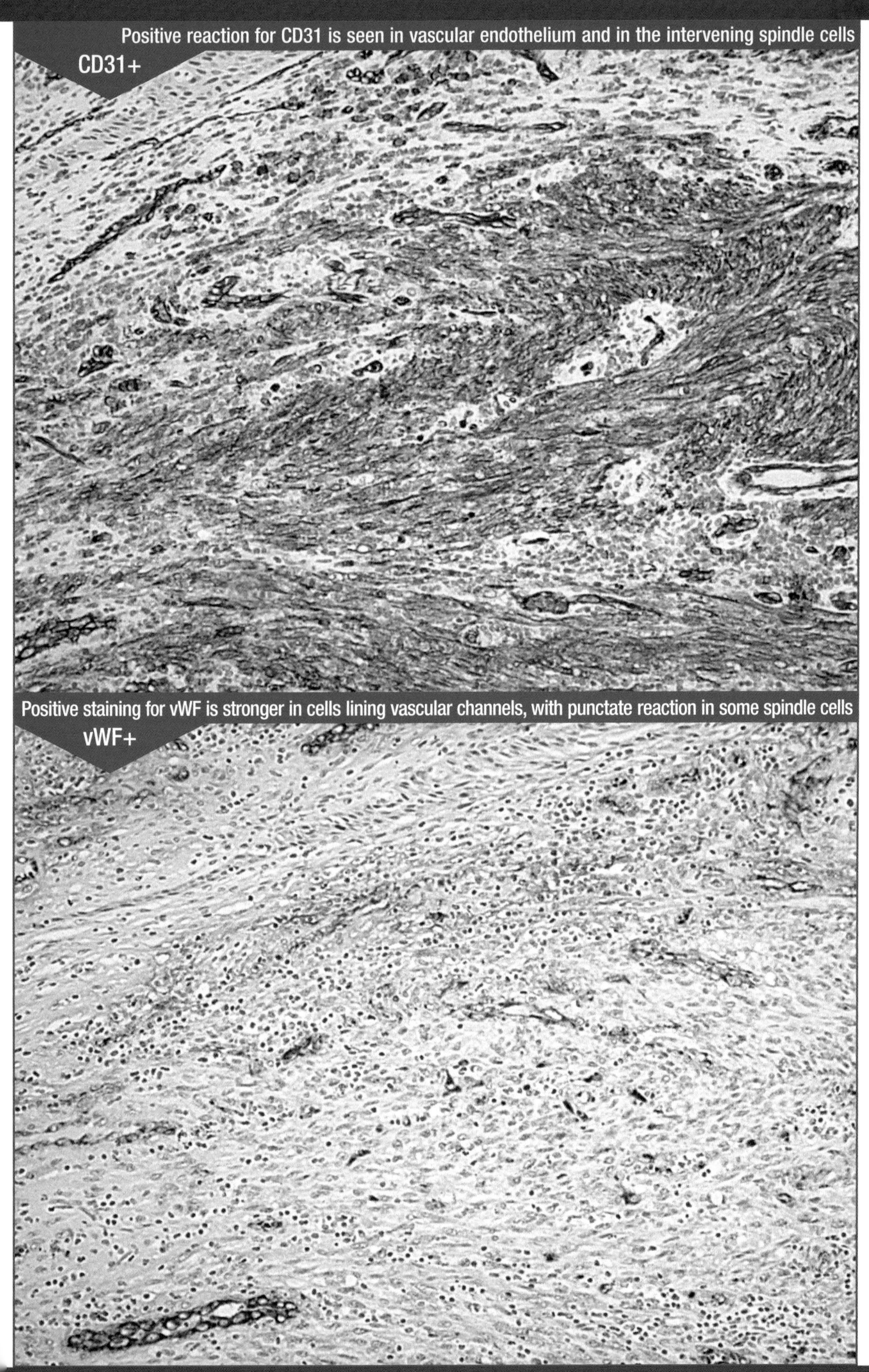
Positive reaction for CD31 is seen in vascular endothelium and in the intervening spindle cells
CD31+
Positive staining for vWF is stronger in cells lining vascular channels, with punctate reaction in some spindle cells
vWF+
Diagnosis: Kaposi Sarcoma

Excision of skin nodule in the popliteal area of an elderly female

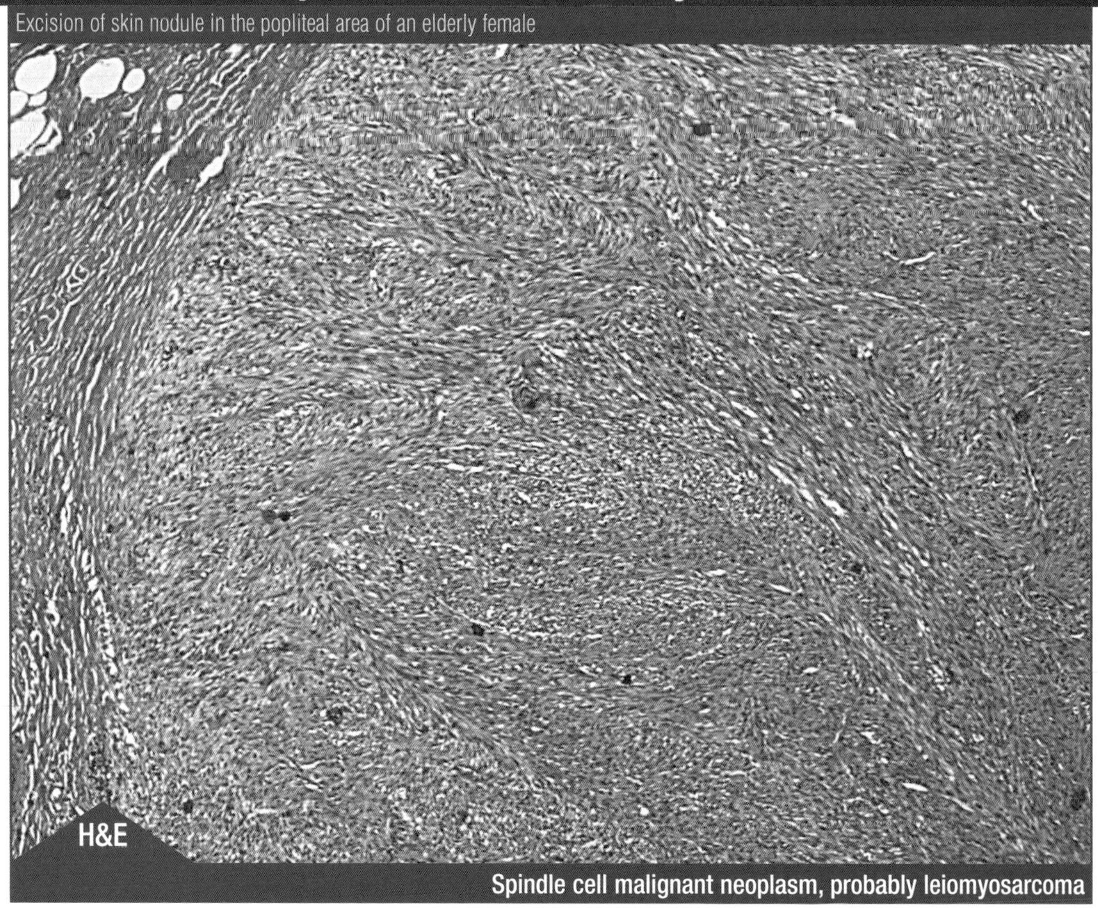

Spindle cell malignant neoplasm, probably leiomyosarcoma

Kaposi Sarcoma vs Leiomyosarcoma	CD31	vWF	H-Caldesmon (HCD)
Kaposi Sarcoma	+	+	–
Leiomyosarcoma	–	–	+

Helpful Hints

Both **CD31** and **Factor VIII-related antigen** (**vWF**) stain Kaposi sarcomas. With Factor VIII-related antigen the reaction is stronger in cells immediately adjacent to the blood channels while the intervening spindle cells may exhibit only a focal punctate staining. Most Kaposi sarcomas also stain positively for D2-40.

Most smooth muscle tumors express **H-Caldesmon** (**HCD**) but only 50% of extrauterine smooth muscle neoplasms are positive for desmin. Muscle specific actin and smooth muscle actin are not helpful because they may be present in a number of non-muscle neoplasms including Kaposi sarcoma.

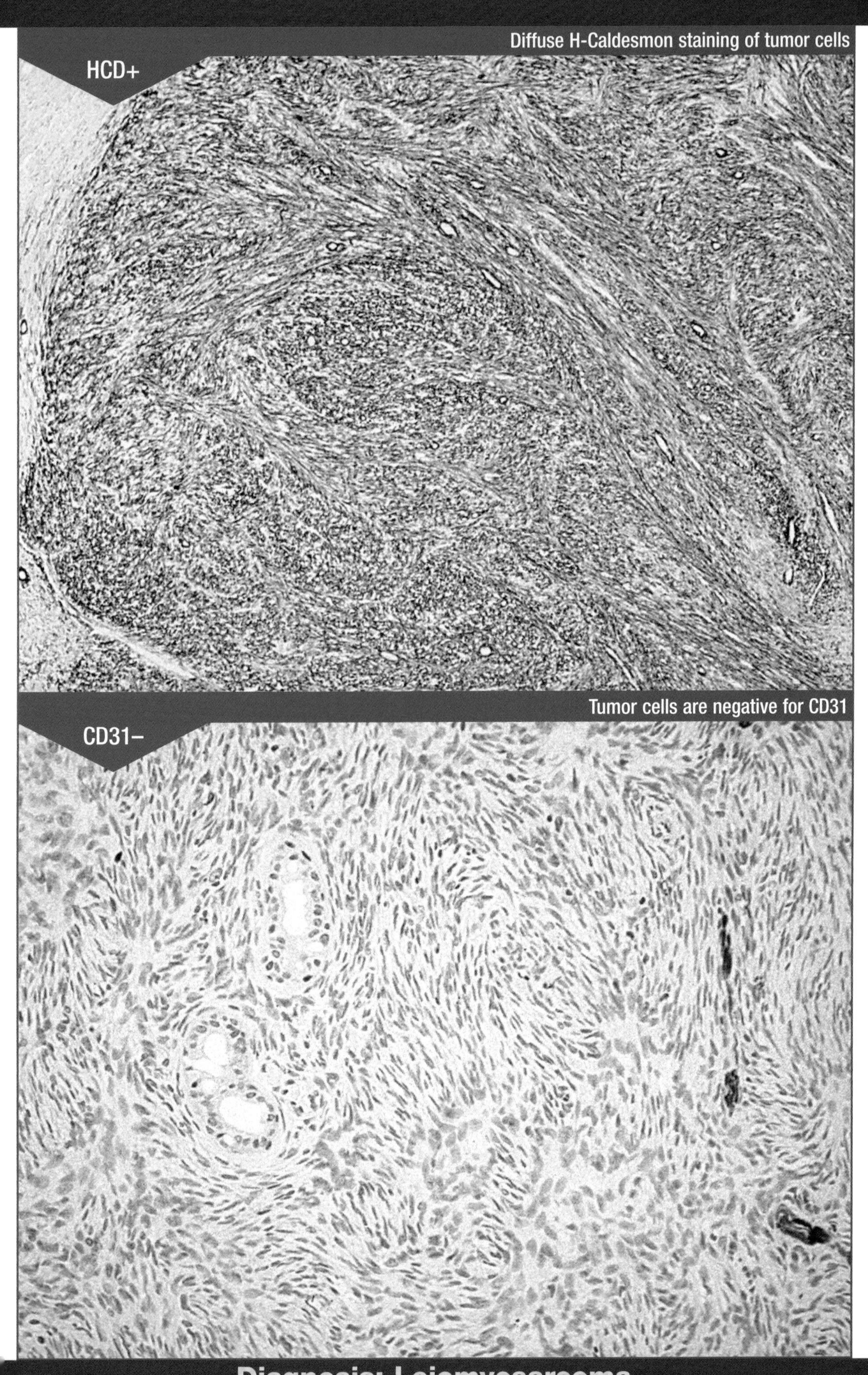

Diagnosis: Leiomyosarcoma

Excision of a nodule in the earlobe

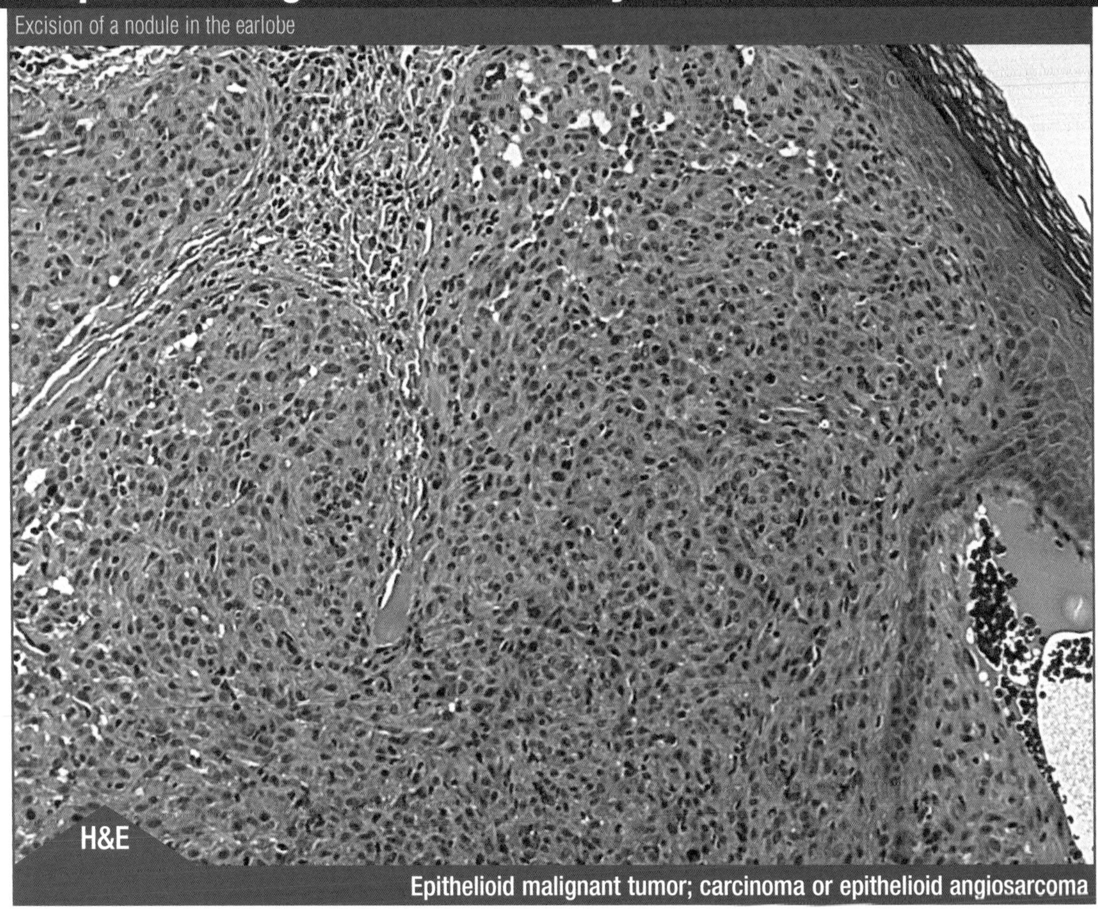

Epithelioid malignant tumor; carcinoma or epithelioid angiosarcoma

Epithelioid Angiosarcoma vs Poorly Differentiated Carcinoma		
	CD31	Cytokeratin (CK)
Epithelioid Angiosarcoma	+	S
Poorly Differentiated Carcinoma	–	+

Helpful Hints

Angiosarcomas could morphologically mimic squamous cell carcinoma of the skin, particularly the acantholytic variant. **CD31** is the marker of choice since it is positive in angiosarcoma but not in squamous cell carcinoma. **Cytokeratin** positivity, on the other hand, may be seen in epithelioid endothelial neoplasms

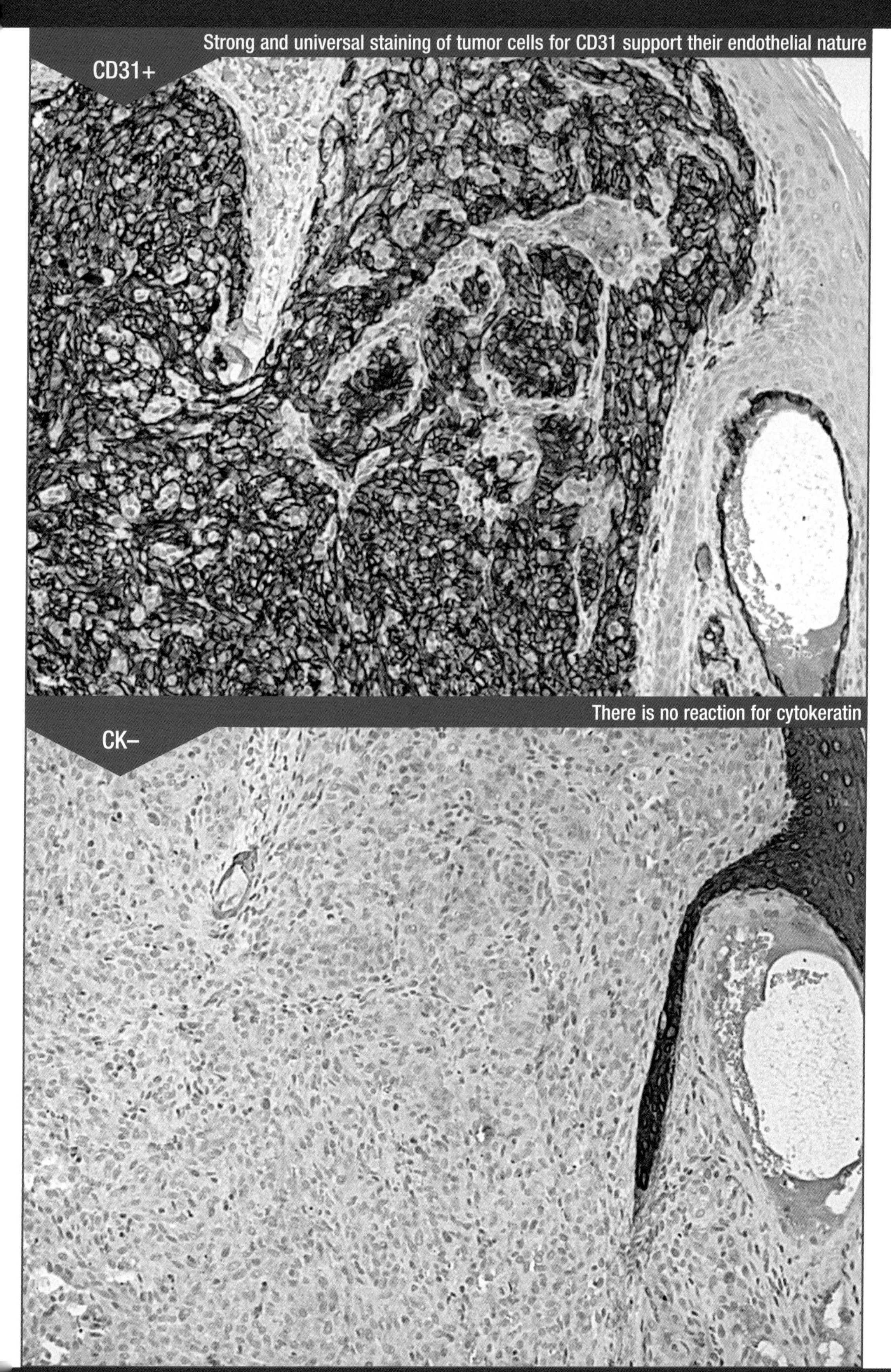

Diagnosis: Angiosarcoma

Biopsy of a vulvar lesion

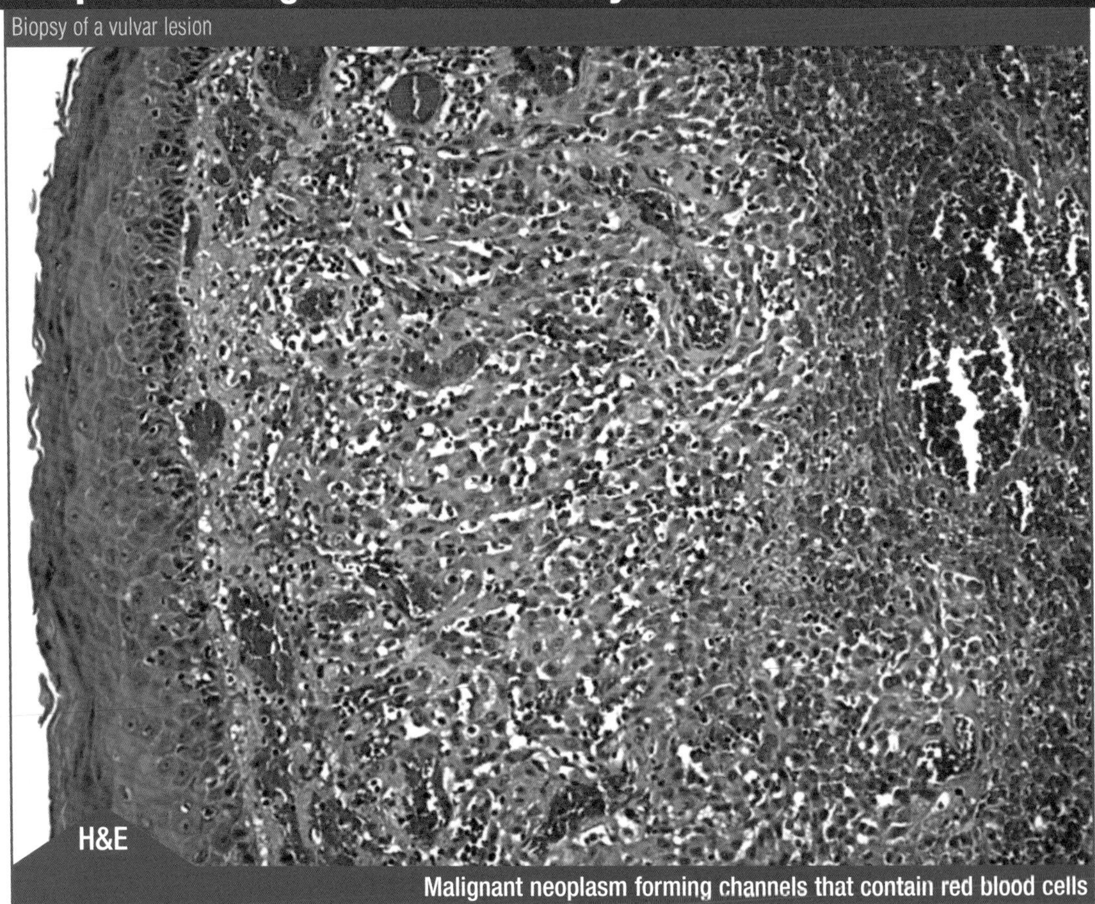

Malignant neoplasm forming channels that contain red blood cells

Epithelioid Angiosarcoma vs Poorly Differentiated Carcinoma		
	CD31	Cytokeratin (CK)
Epithelioid Angiosarcoma	+	S
Poorly Differentiated Carcinoma	–	+

Helpful Hints

Angiosarcomas could morphologically mimic squamous cell carcinoma of the skin, particularly the acantholytic variant. **CD31** is the marker of choice since it is positive in angiosarcoma but not in squamous cell carcinoma. **Cytokeratin** positivity, on the other hand, may be seen in epithelioid endothelial neoplasms

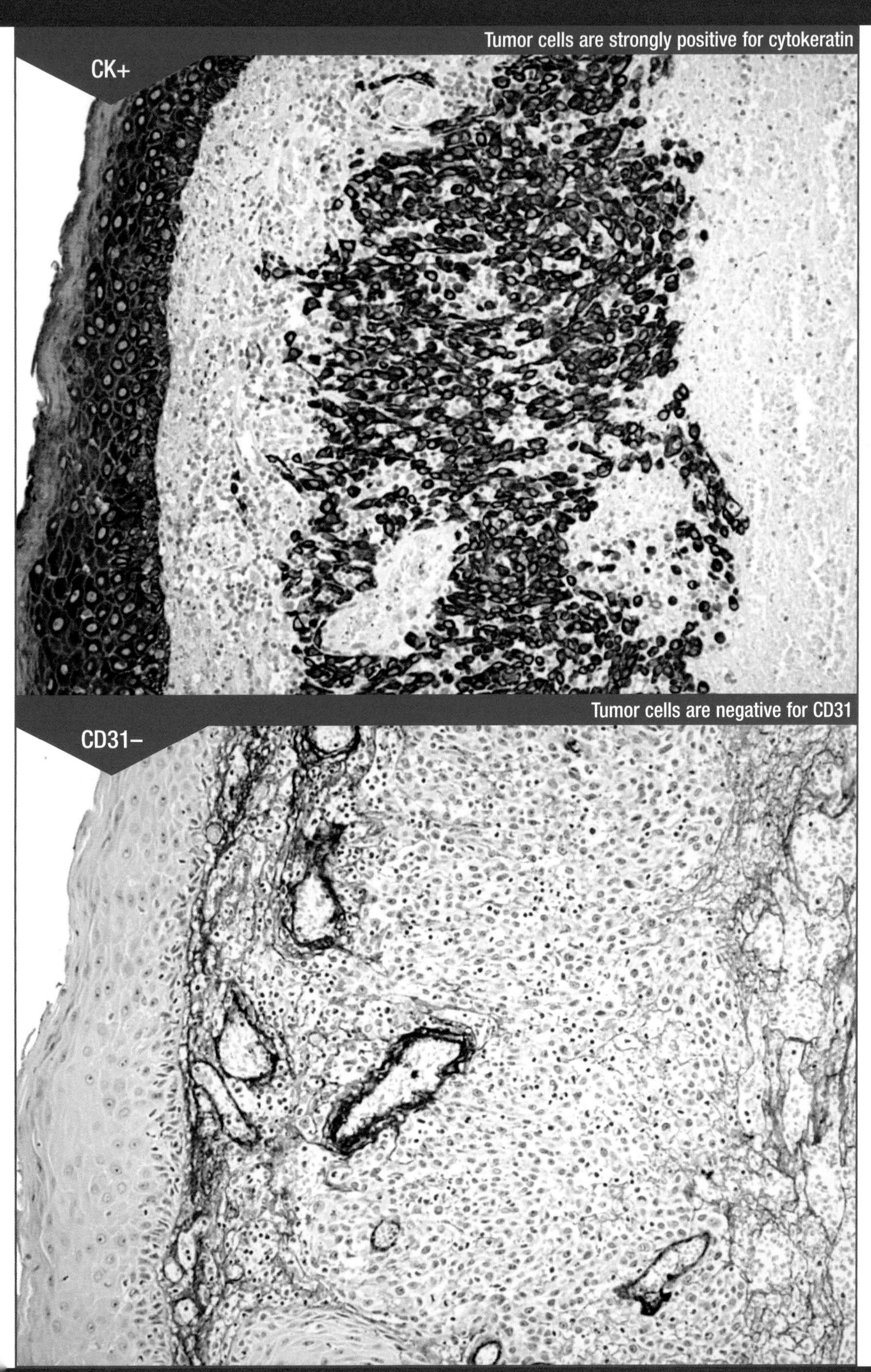

Diagnosis: Squamous Cell Carcinoma, Acantholytic Type

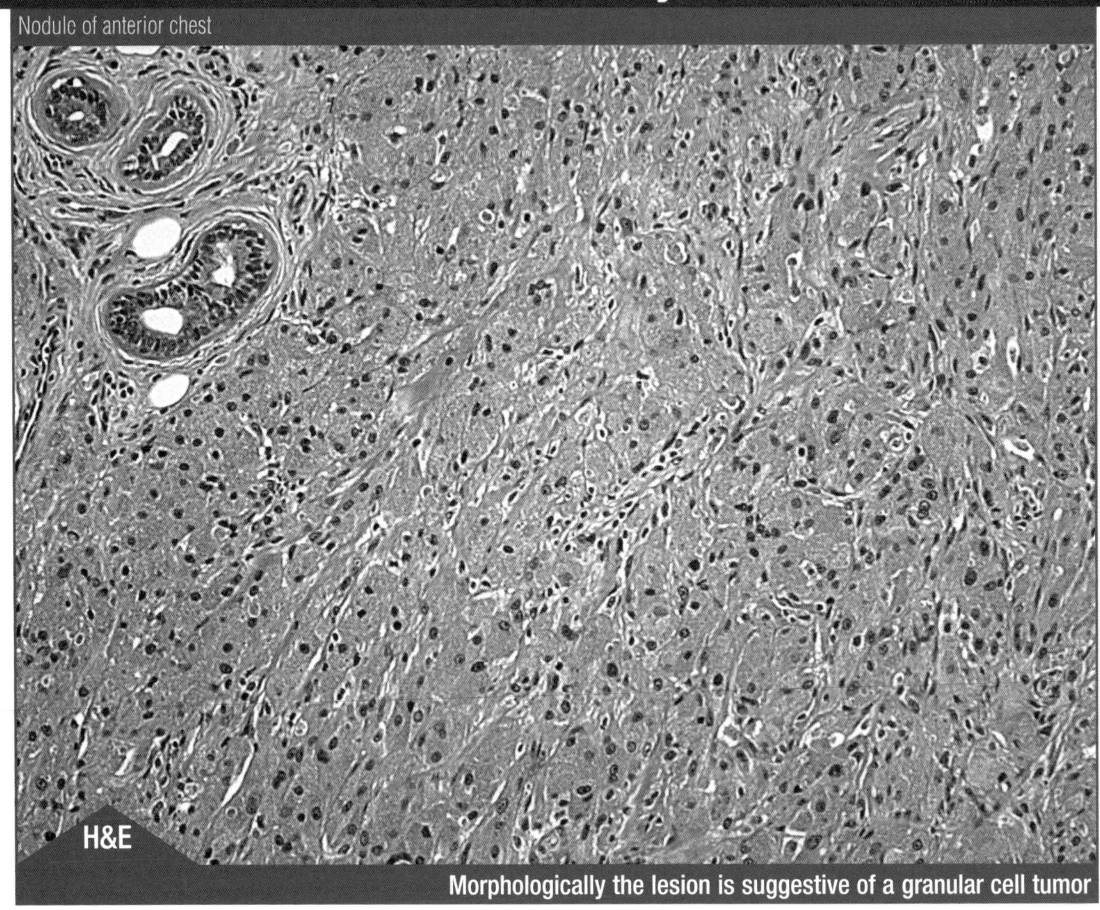

Morphologically the lesion is suggestive of a granular cell tumor

Granular Cell Tumor vs Histiocytic Skin Reaction		
	S100 Protein	CD68
Granular Cell Tumor	+	S
Histiocytic Skin Reaction	–	+

Helpful Hints

S100 protein is expressed by all granular cell tumors. One should however, observe nuclear staining for this antigen as evidence of a true positive reaction. Histiocytic skin reactions of skin may sometimes mimic granular cell tumors. These lesions are always positive for **CD68**. Granular cell tumors may also express CD68 and therefore, positivity for S100 protein is more informative.

Ordonez 1999.

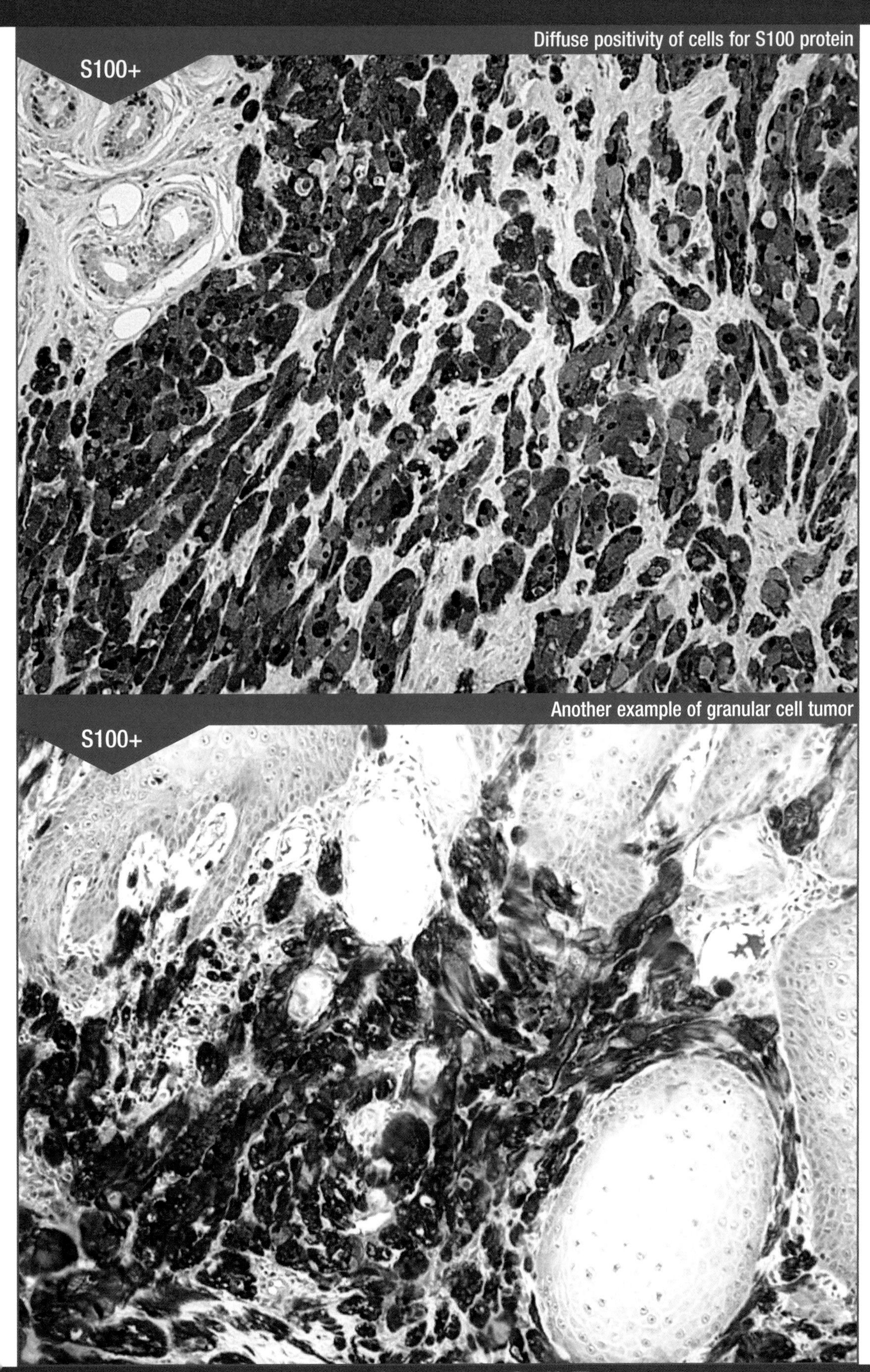

Diagnosis: Granular Cell Tumor

Skin nodule in the face

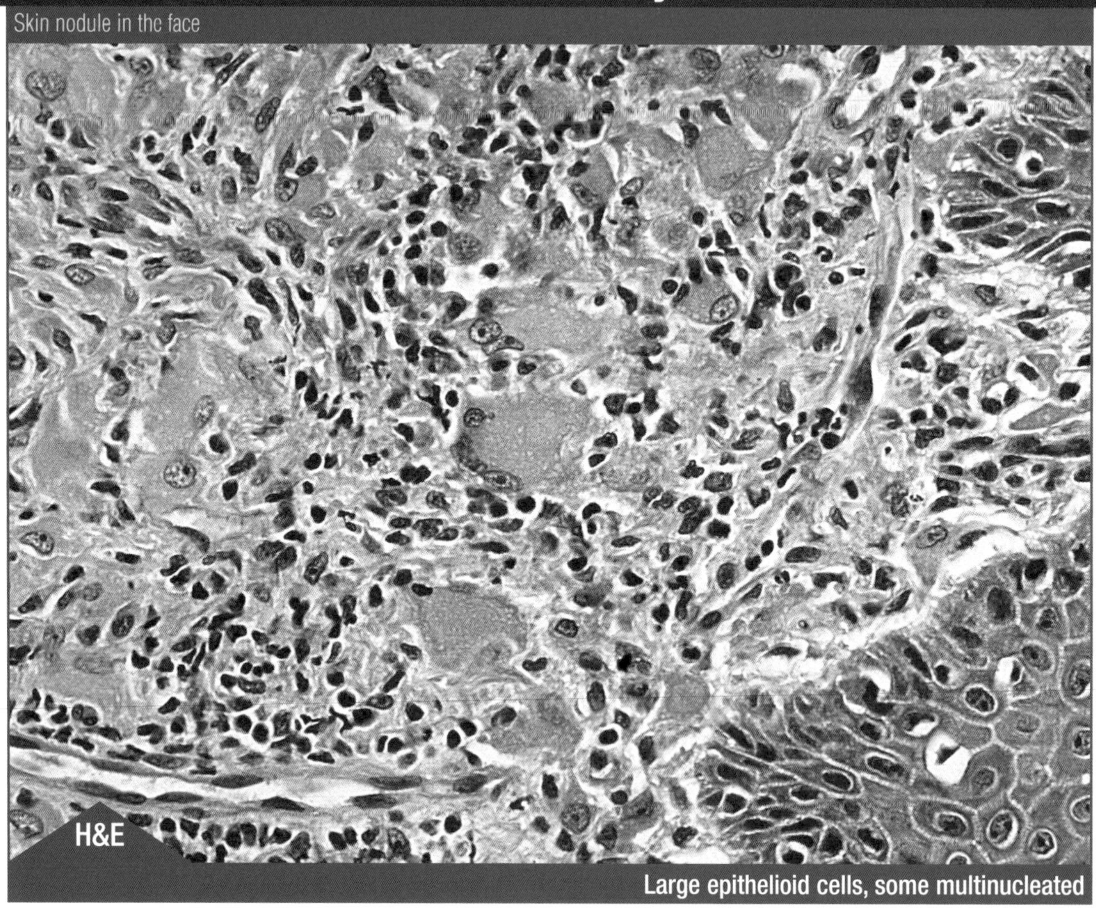

Large epithelioid cells, some multinucleated

Granular Cell Tumor vs Histiocytic Skin Reaction		
	S100 Protein	CD68
Granular Cell Tumor	+	S
Histiocytic Skin Reaction	–	+

Helpful Hints

S100 protein is expressed by all granular cell tumors. One should however, observe nuclear staining for this antigen as evidence of a true positive reaction. Histiocytic skin reactions of skin may sometimes mimic granular cell tumors. These lesions are always positive for **CD68**. Granular cell tumors may also express CD68 and therefore, positivity for S100 protein is more informative.

Ordonez 1999.

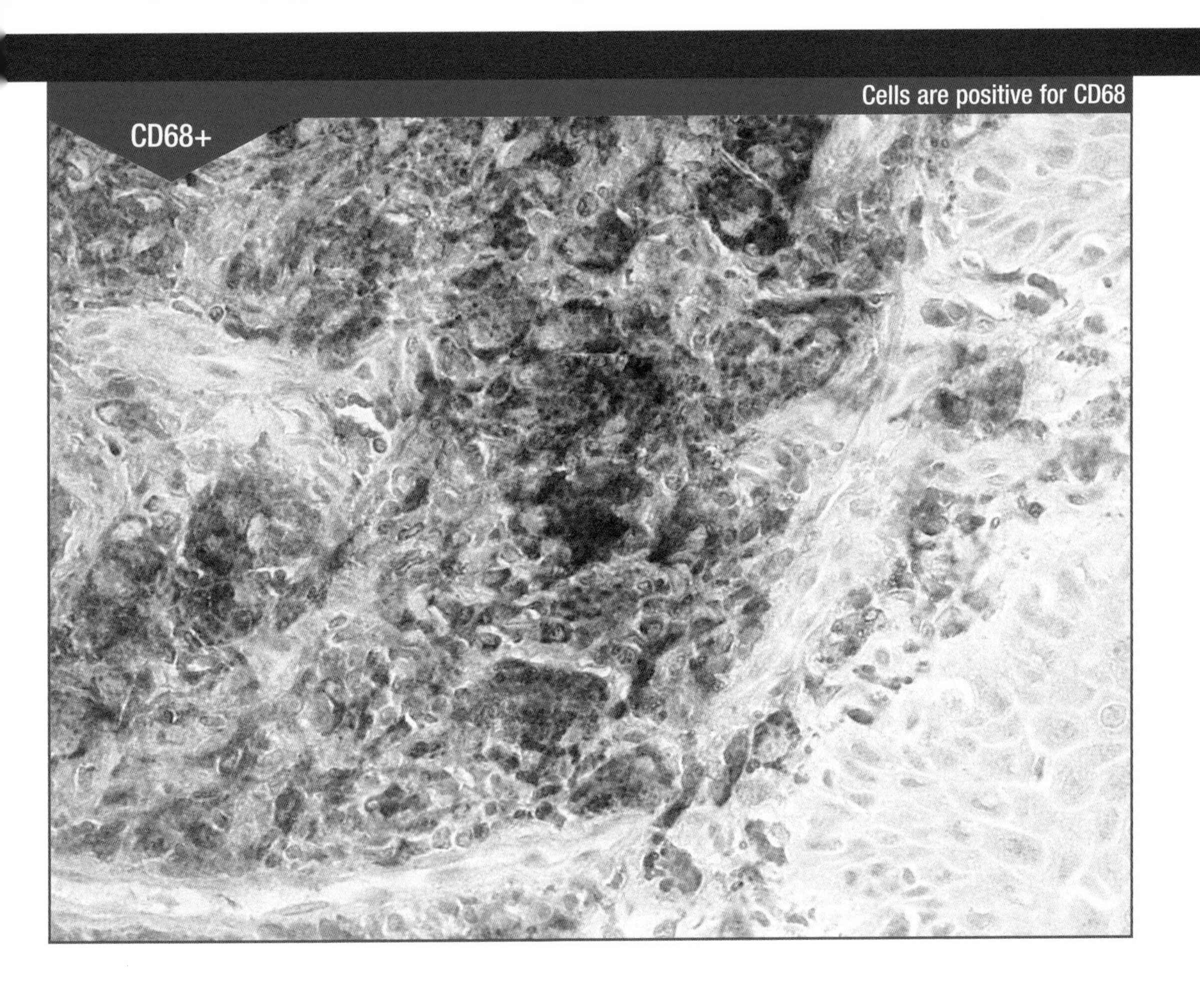

agnosis: Histiocytic Skin Reaction to a Foreign Body *(by History)*

Skin biopsy from a finger

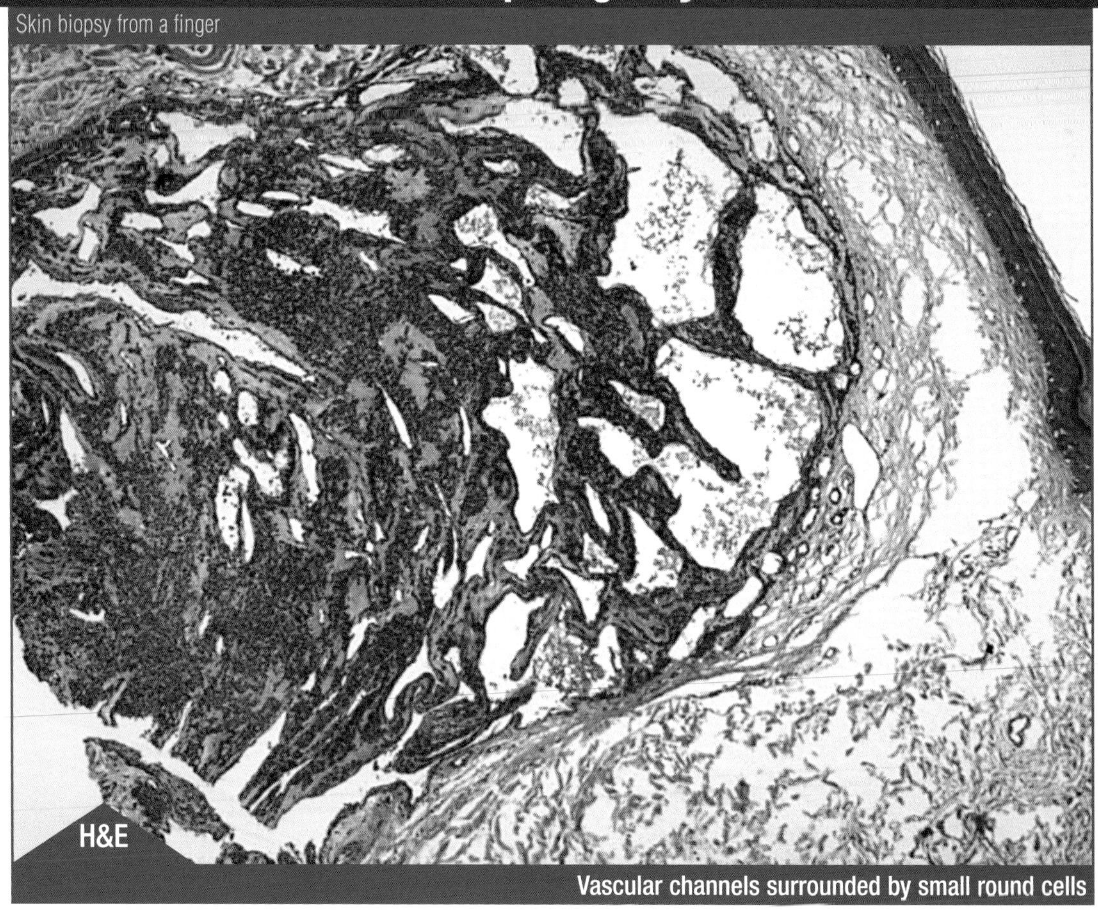

Vascular channels surrounded by small round cells

Glomus Tumor vs Morphologically Similar Lesions		
	MSA	H-Caldesmon (HCD)
Glomus Tumor	+	+
Morphologically Similar Lesions	–	-

Helpful Hints

The diagnosis of a glomus tumor, particularly when it only contains few typical perivascular glomus cells, may be difficult. Both **H-Caldesmon** and **Muscle Specific Actin** (**MSA**) stain glomus cells. **Desmin**, on the other hand, is not always expressed by these cells and is less helpful.

Liapi-Avgeri 1994.

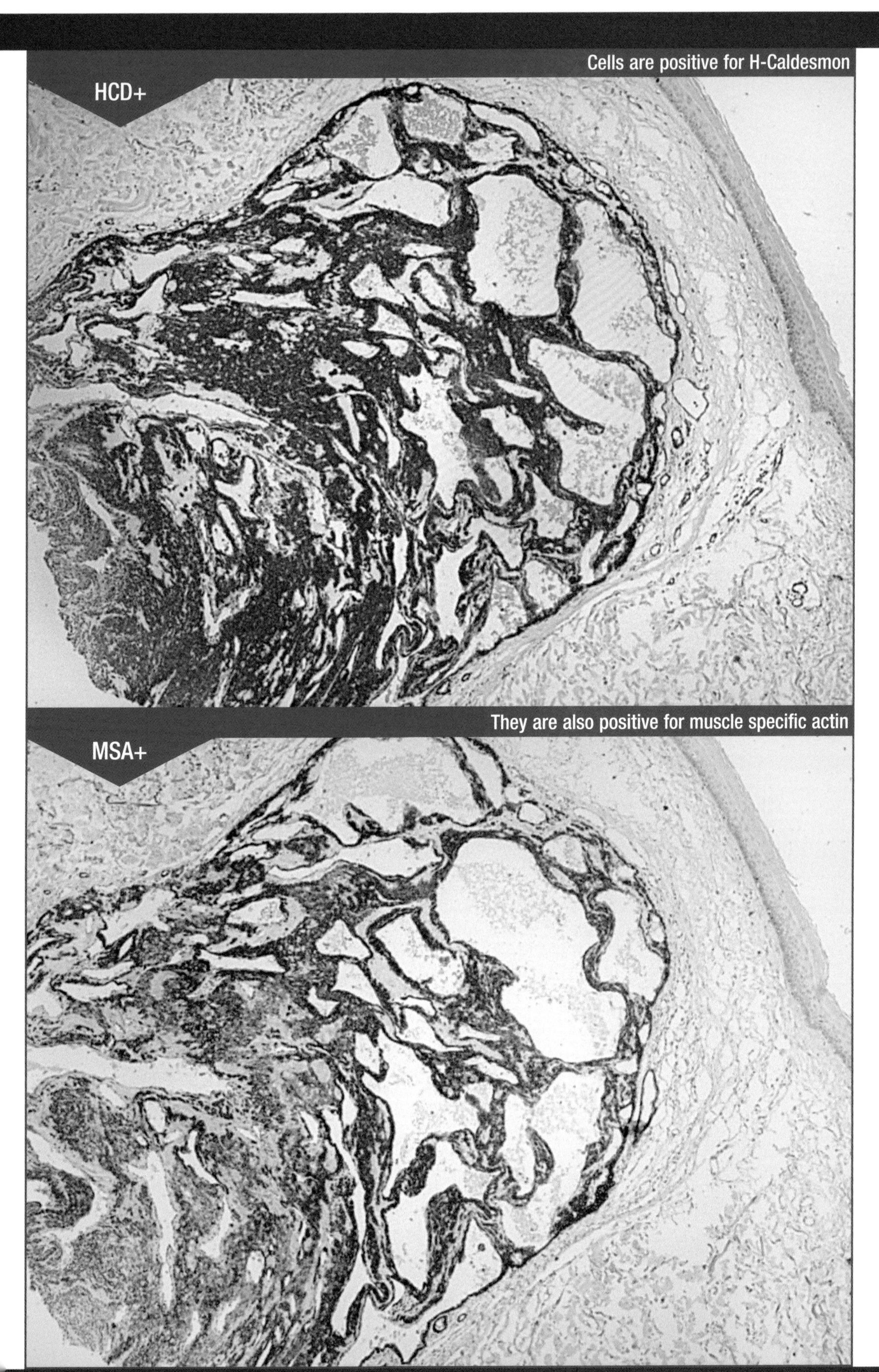

Diagnosis: Glomus Tumor (Glomangioma)

Skin biopsy from the chest wall

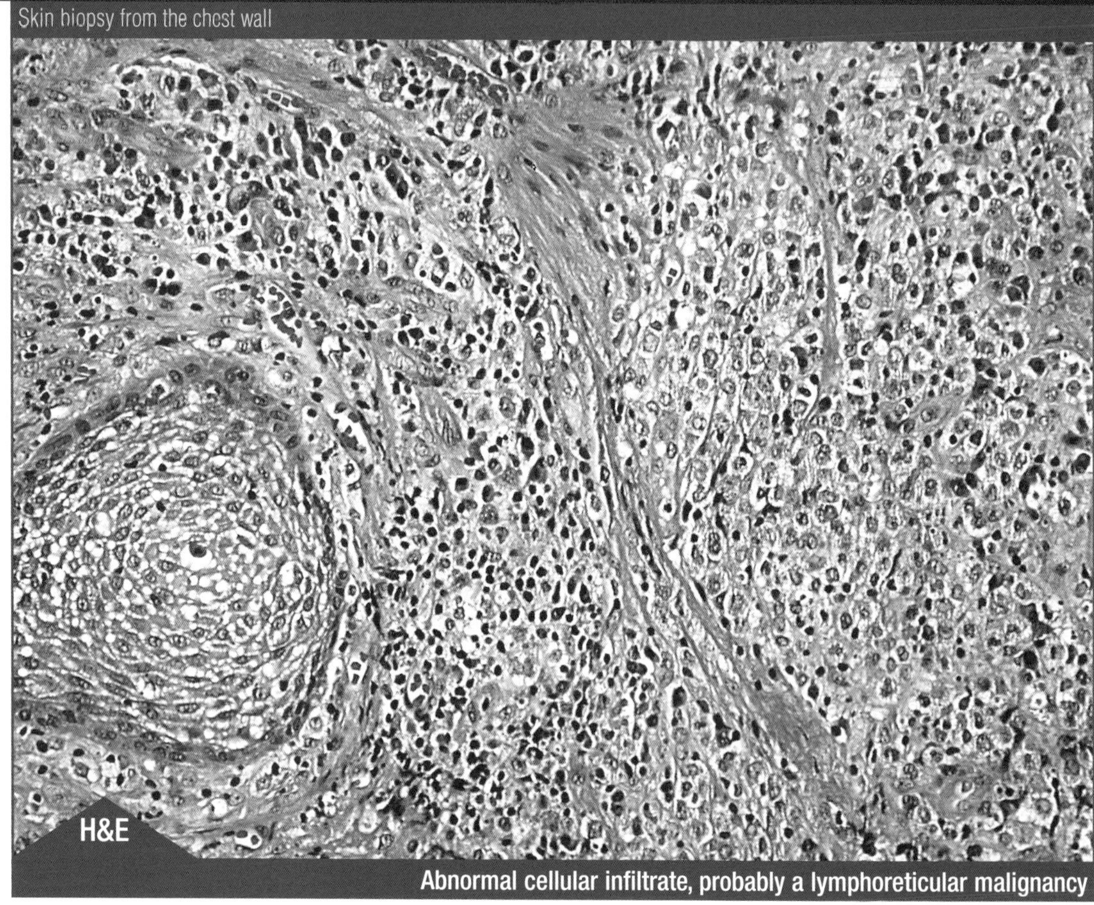

Abnormal cellular infiltrate, probably a lymphoreticular malignancy

Myeloid Leukemic Infiltrate vs Malignant Lymphoma		
	Myeloperoxidase (MPO)	CD3/CD20/CD30
Leukemic Infiltrate	+	–
Malignant Lymphoma	–	+

Helpful Hints

Subclassification of lymphoreticular malignancies of skin is usually limited to identification of cutaneous B and T cell lymphomas. Myelomonocytic leukemic infiltrates of skin are relatively rare and are usually positive for **Myeloperoxidase** (**MPO**). The number of myeloperoxidase positive cells however, may vary from case to case. Muramidase could also be used instead of, or in conjunction with myeloperoxidase.

Cutaneous T cell lymphomas of skin are positive for **CD3** and in certain subtypes for **CD30**; B cell lymphomas express **CD20**.

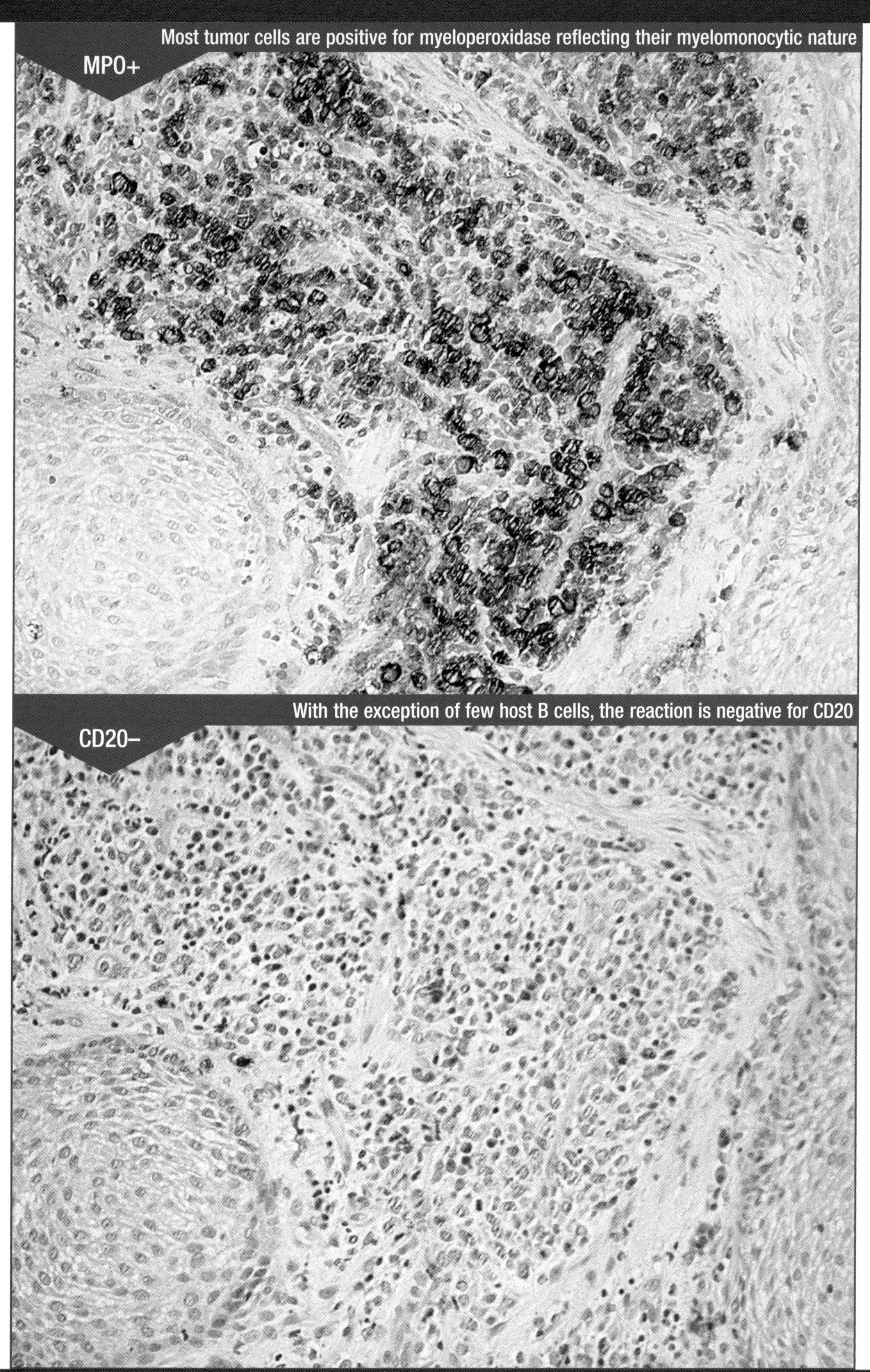

Diagnosis: Myeloid Leukemic Infiltrate of Skin

Multiple skin nodules

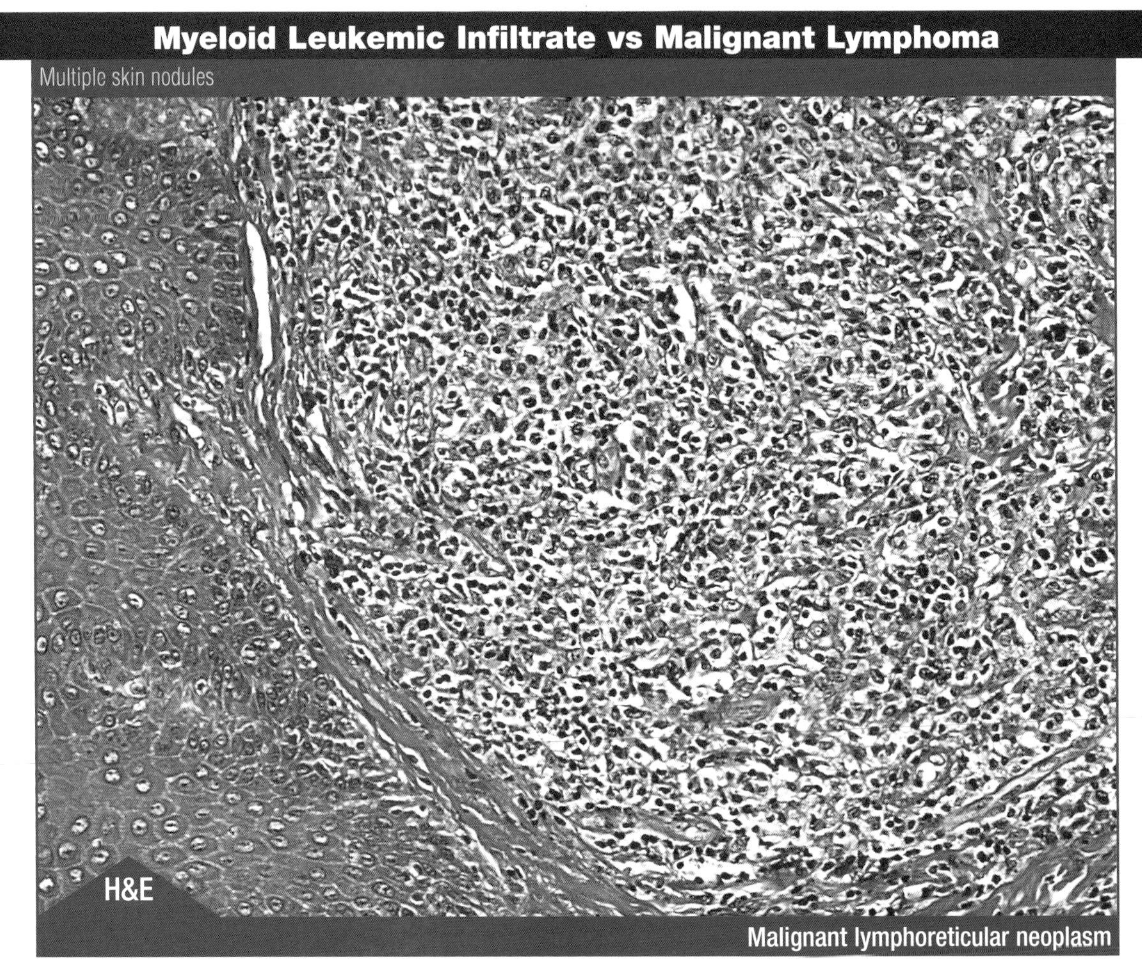

Malignant lymphoreticular neoplasm

Myeloid Leukemic Infiltrate vs Malignant Lymphoma		
	Myeloperoxidase (MPO)	CD3/CD20/CD30
Leukemic Infiltrate	+	–
Malignant Lymphoma	–	+

Helpful Hints

Subclassification of lymphoreticular malignancies of skin is usually limited to identification of cutaneous B and T cell lymphomas. Myelomonocytic leukemic infiltrates of skin are relatively rare and are usually positive for **Myeloperoxidase** (**MPO**). The number of myeloperoxidase positive cells however, may vary from case to case. Muramidase could also be used instead of, or in conjunction with myeloperoxidase.

Cutaneous T cell lymphomas of skin are positive for **CD3** and in certain subtypes for **CD30**; B cell lymphomas express **CD20**.

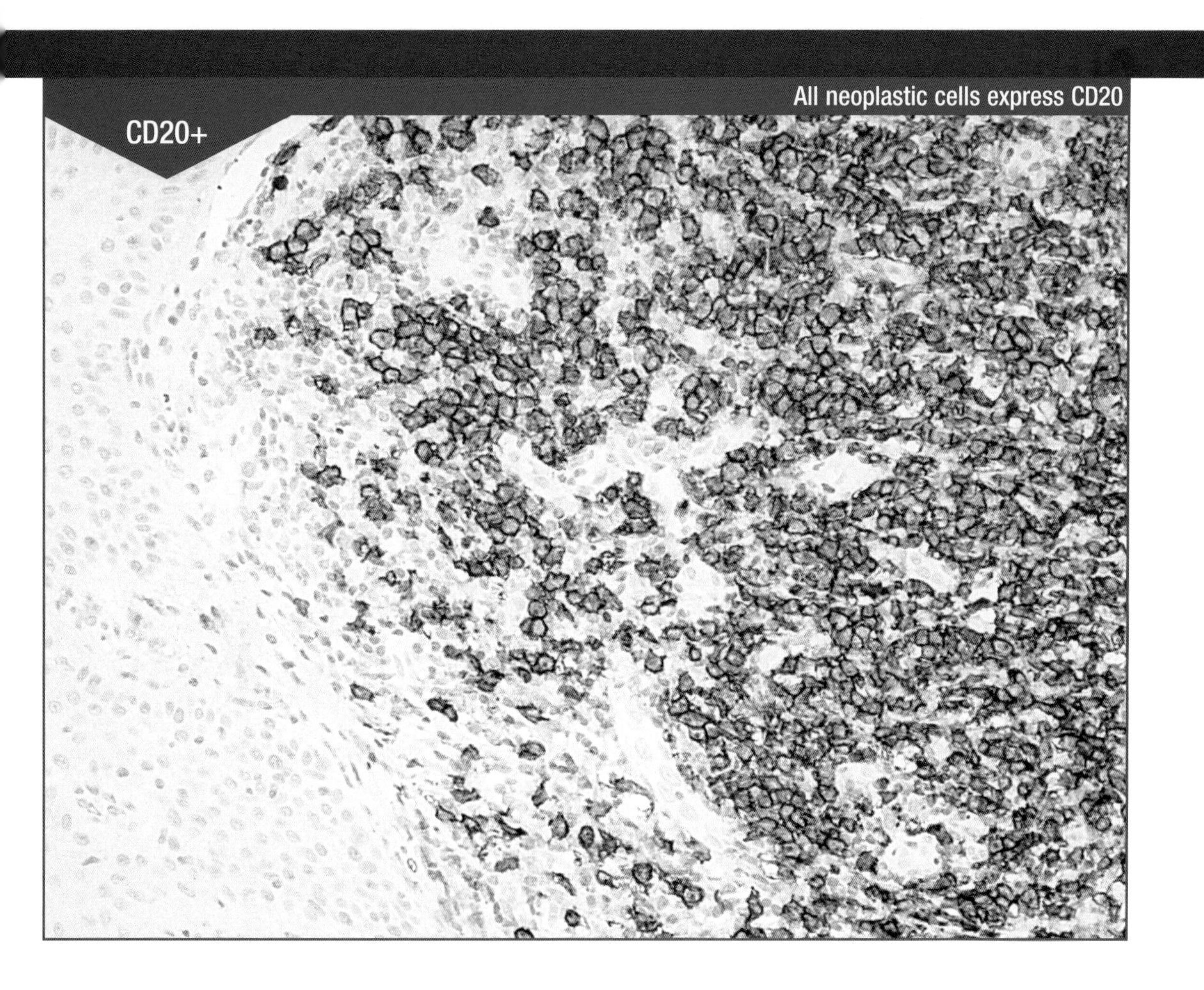

Diagnosis: Malignant Large B Cell Lymphoma

Skin biopsy of a patient clinically suspected to have mast cell disease

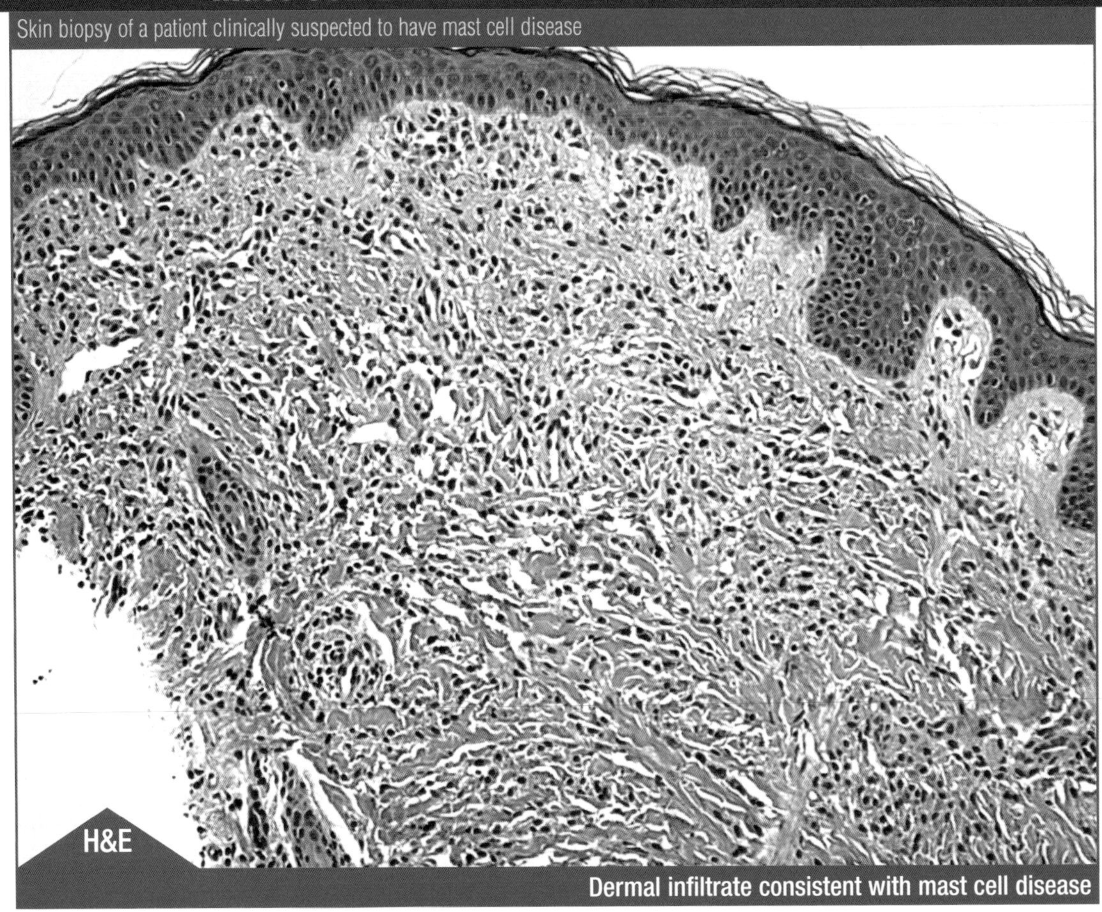

Dermal infiltrate consistent with mast cell disease

Mast Cell Disease vs Other Cell Infiltrates		
	Tryptase	CD117 (KIT)
Mast Cell Disease	+	+
Other Cell Infiltrates	–	–

Helpful Hints

Normal and neoplastic mast cells express **Mast Cell Tryptase** whereas other lymphoreticular cell infiltrates are negative. **CD117** (**KIT**) is also expressed by normal and neoplastic mast cells and may help in confirming the diagnosis of mast cell disease.

Walls 1990.

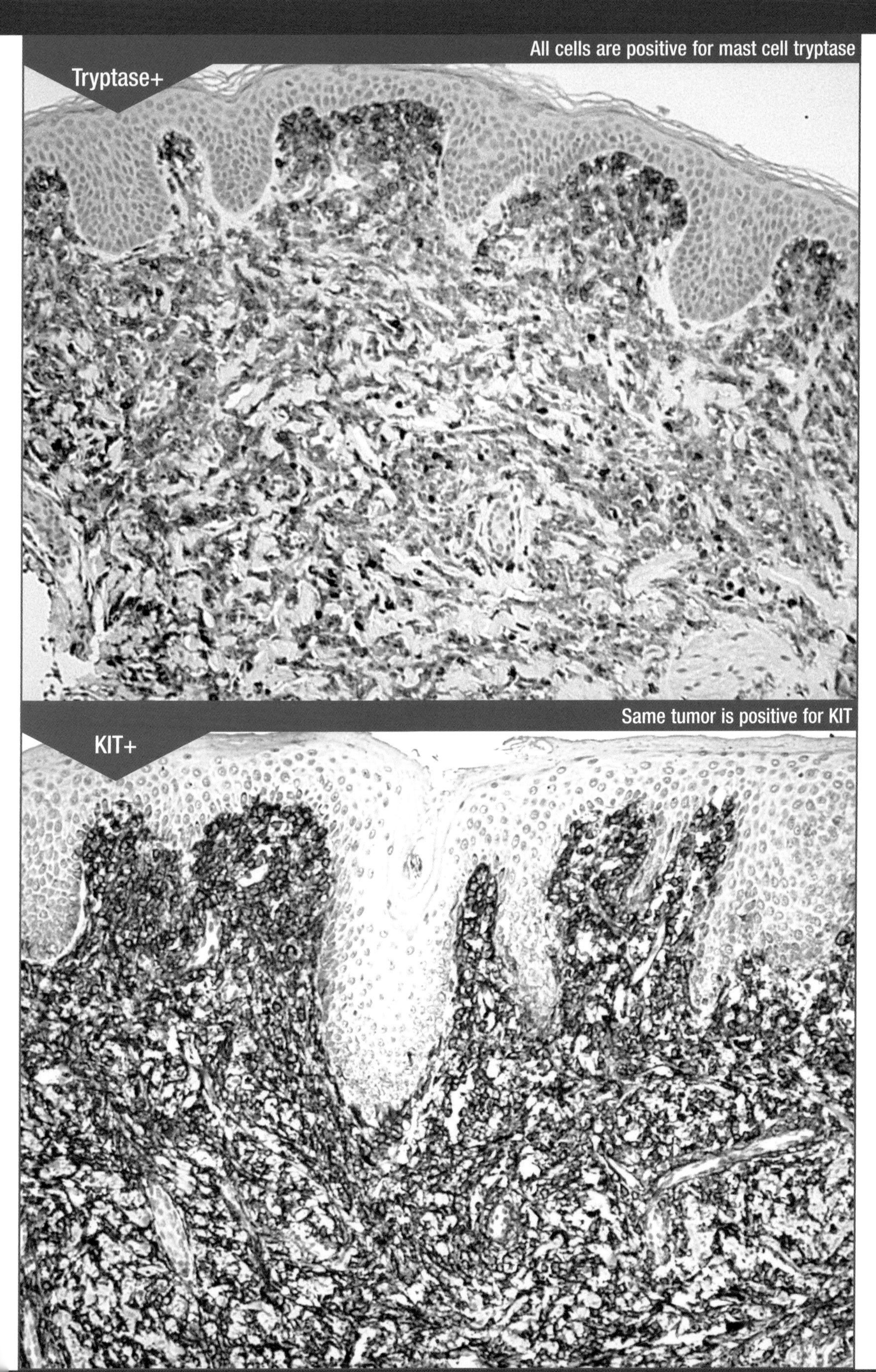

Diagnosis: Mast Cell Disease

Skin biopsy of the inguinal area

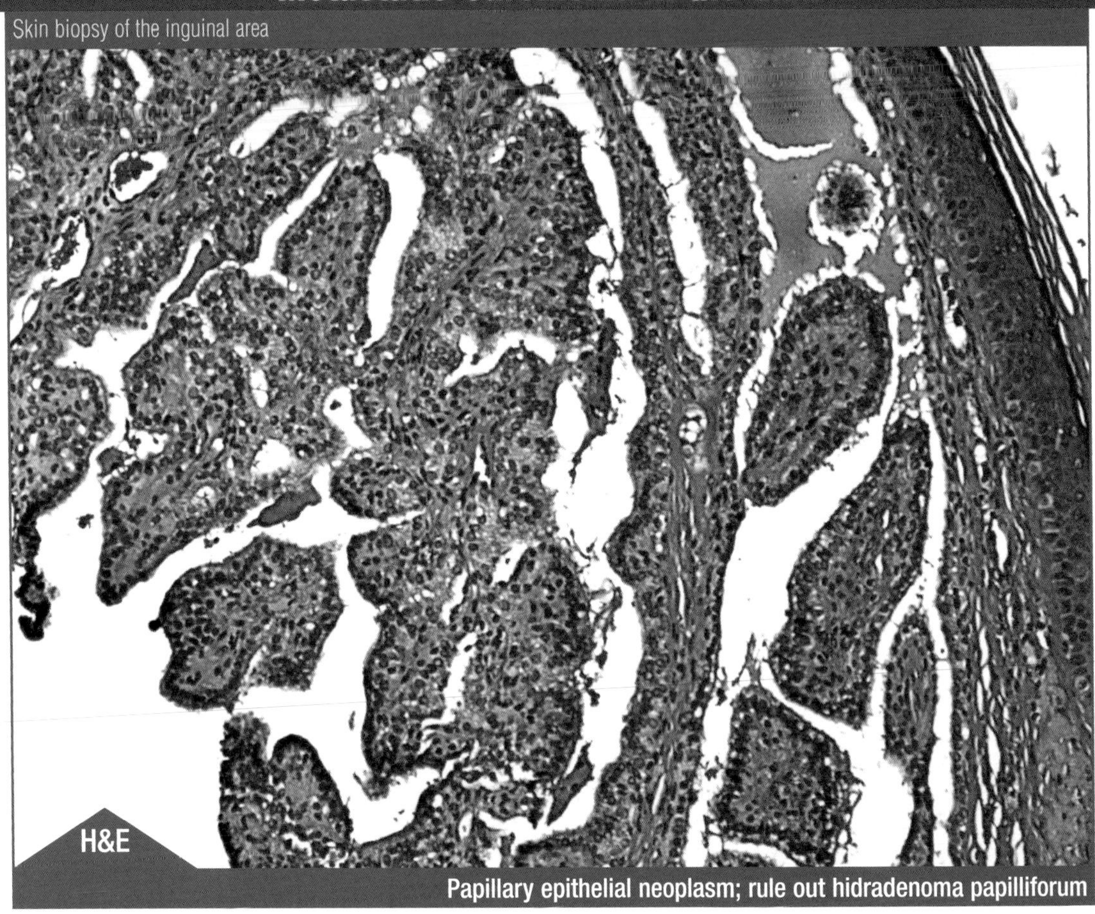

Papillary epithelial neoplasm; rule out hidradenoma papilliforum

Helpful Hints

Depending on the clinical history, histomorphology and availability of specific markers, the site of origin of a number of metastatic tumors in the skin can be determined by using one or more antibodies. Here are some examples.

1.	Metastatic adenocarcinoma of lung	TTF-1
2.	Metastatic carcinoma of breast	Estrogen Receptor
3.	Metastatic renal cell carcinoma	Renal Cell Antigen
4.	Metastatic thyroid carcinoma	Thyroglobulin, TTF-1
5.	Metastatic colonic adenocarcinoma	Cytokeratin 20

(Some skin appendage tumors also have been reported to be positive for estrogen receptor.)

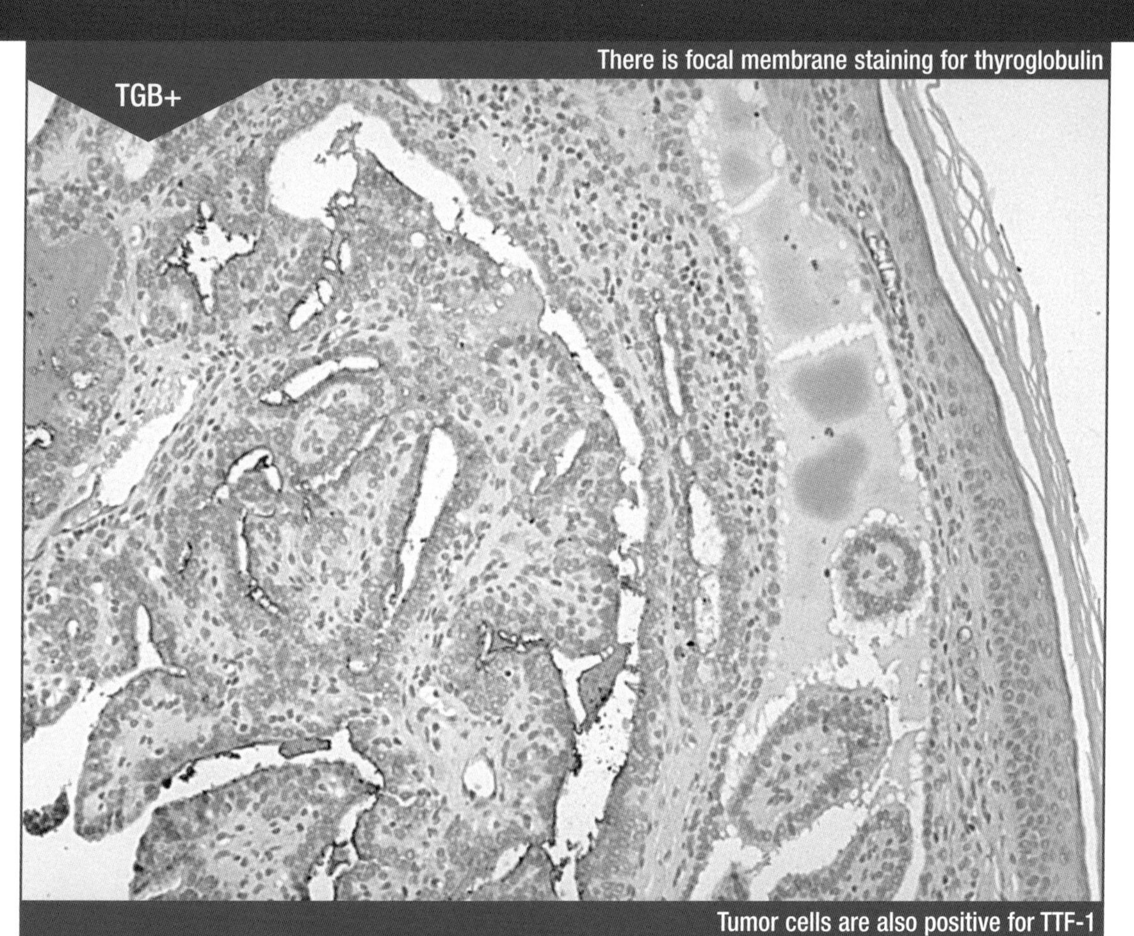

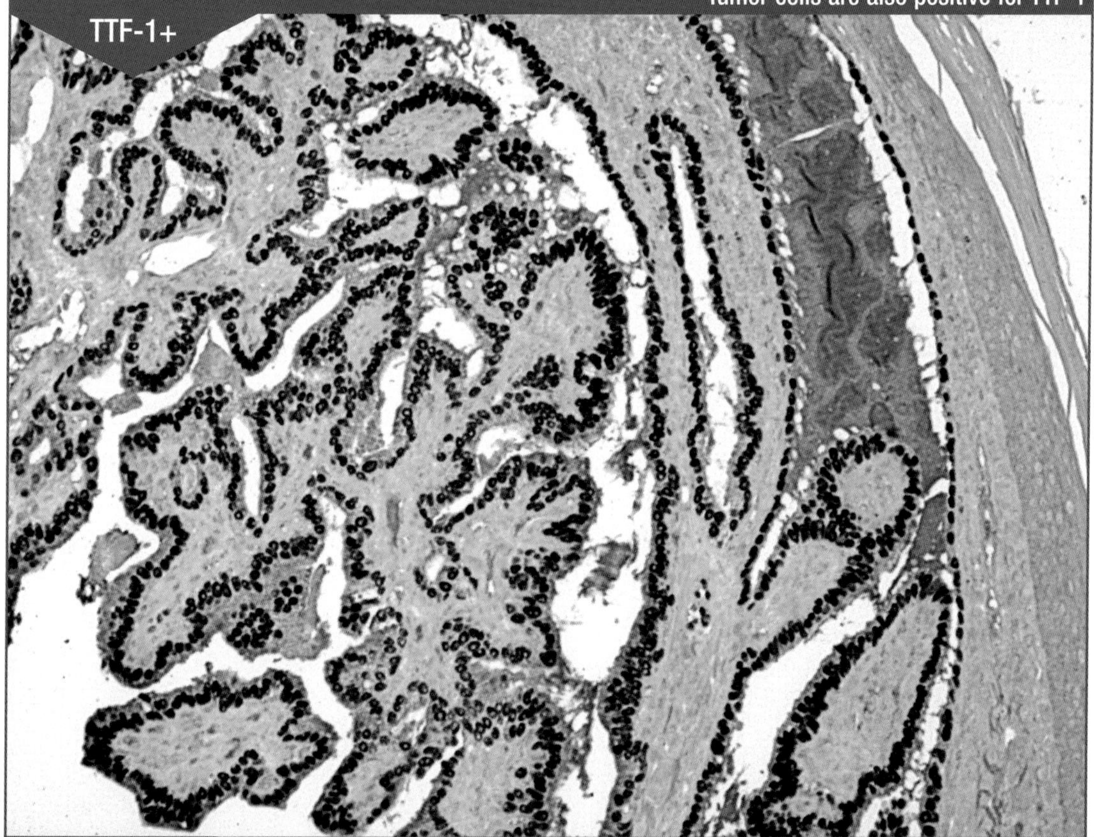

Diagnosis: Metastatic Papillary Thyroid Carcinoma

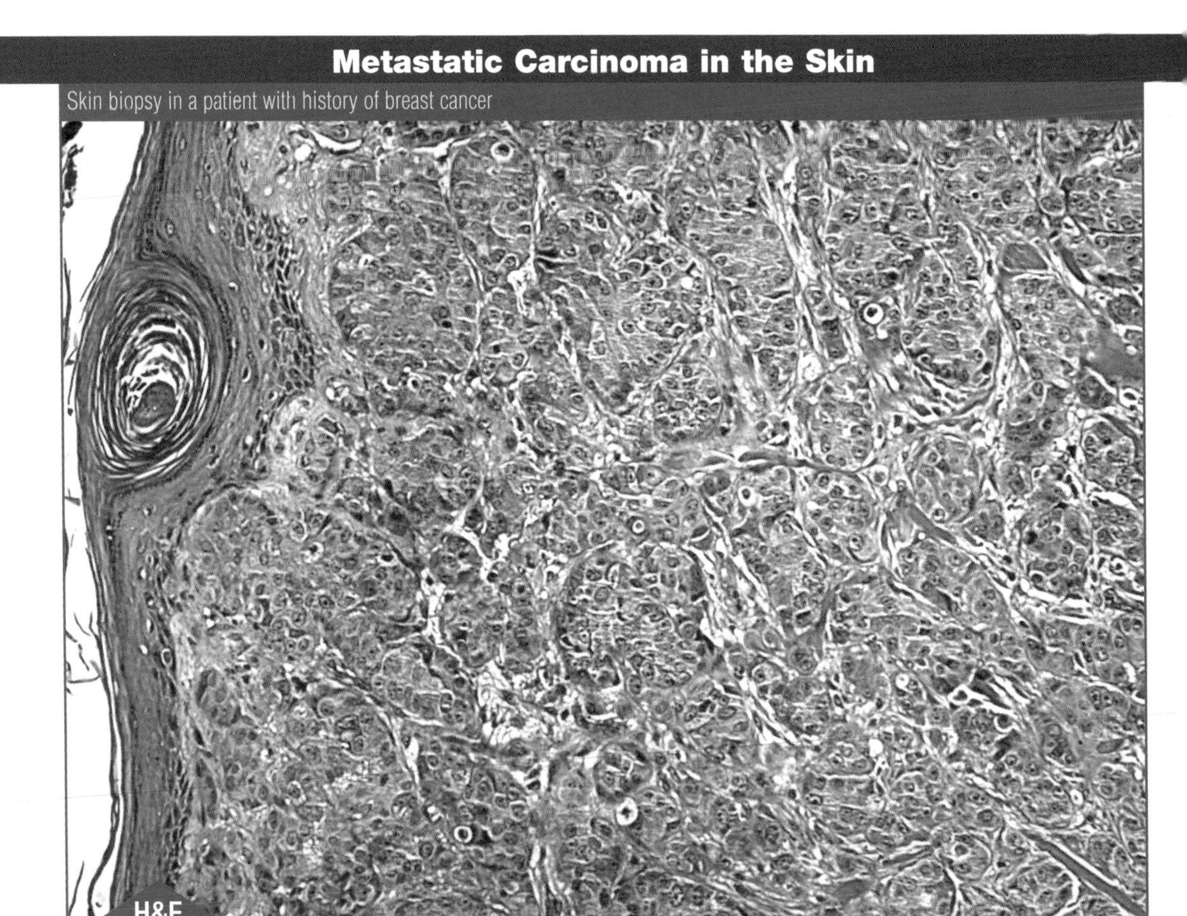

Helpful Hints

Depending on the clinical history, histomorphology and availability of specific markers, the site of origin of a number of metastatic tumors in the skin can be determined by using one or more antibodies. Here are some examples.

1.	Metastatic adenocarcinoma of lung	TTF-1
2.	Metastatic carcinoma of breast	Estrogen Receptor
3.	Metastatic renal cell carcinoma	Renal Cell Antigen
4.	Metastatic thyroid carcinoma	Thyroglobulin, TTF-1
5.	Metastatic colonic adenocarcinoma	Cytokeratin 20

(Some skin appendage tumors also have been reported to be positive for estrogen receptor.)

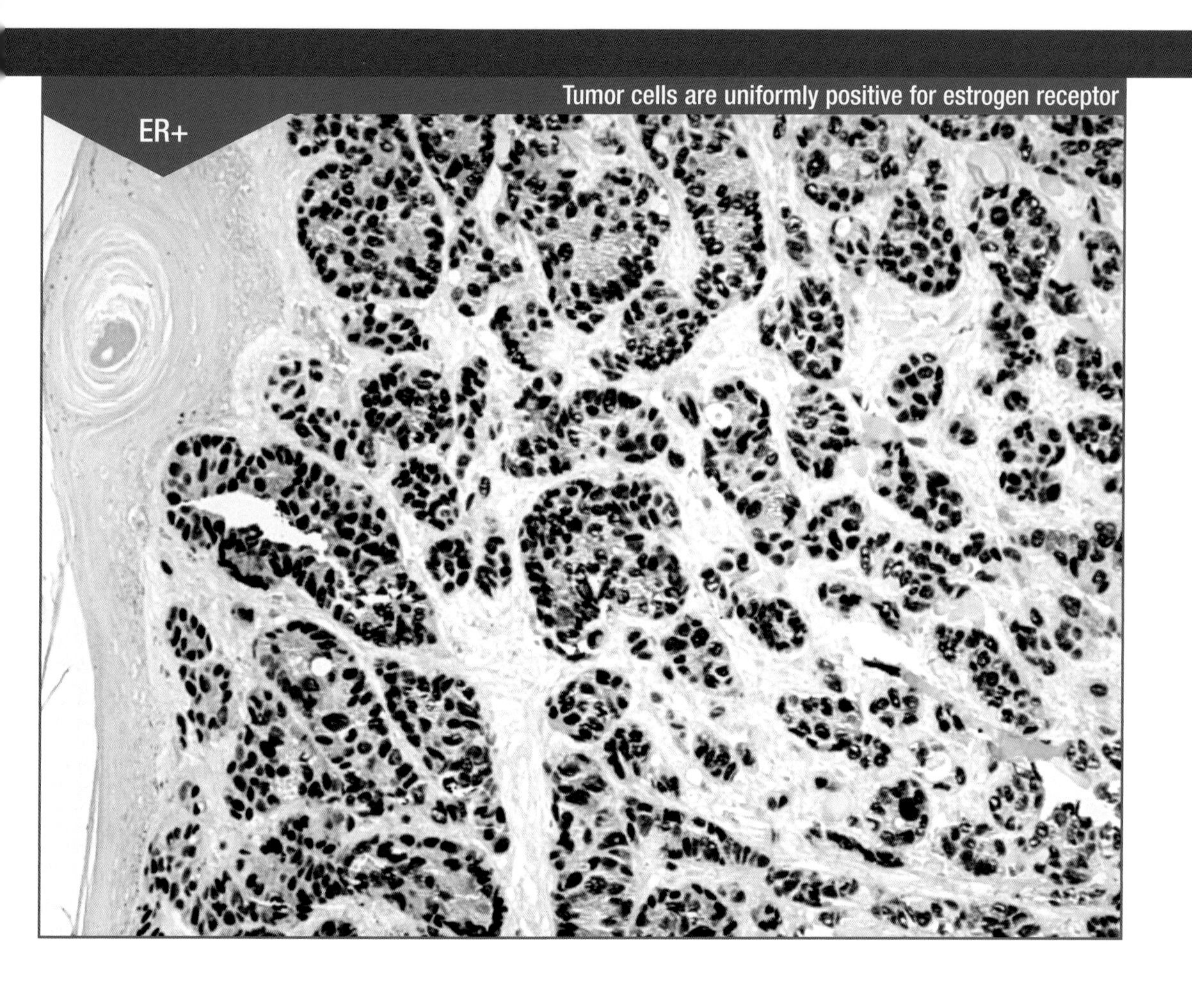

Diagnosis: Metastatic Breast Carcinoma

Metastatic Carcinoma in the Skin

Skin biopsy from the shoulder area in a patient without prior history of cancer

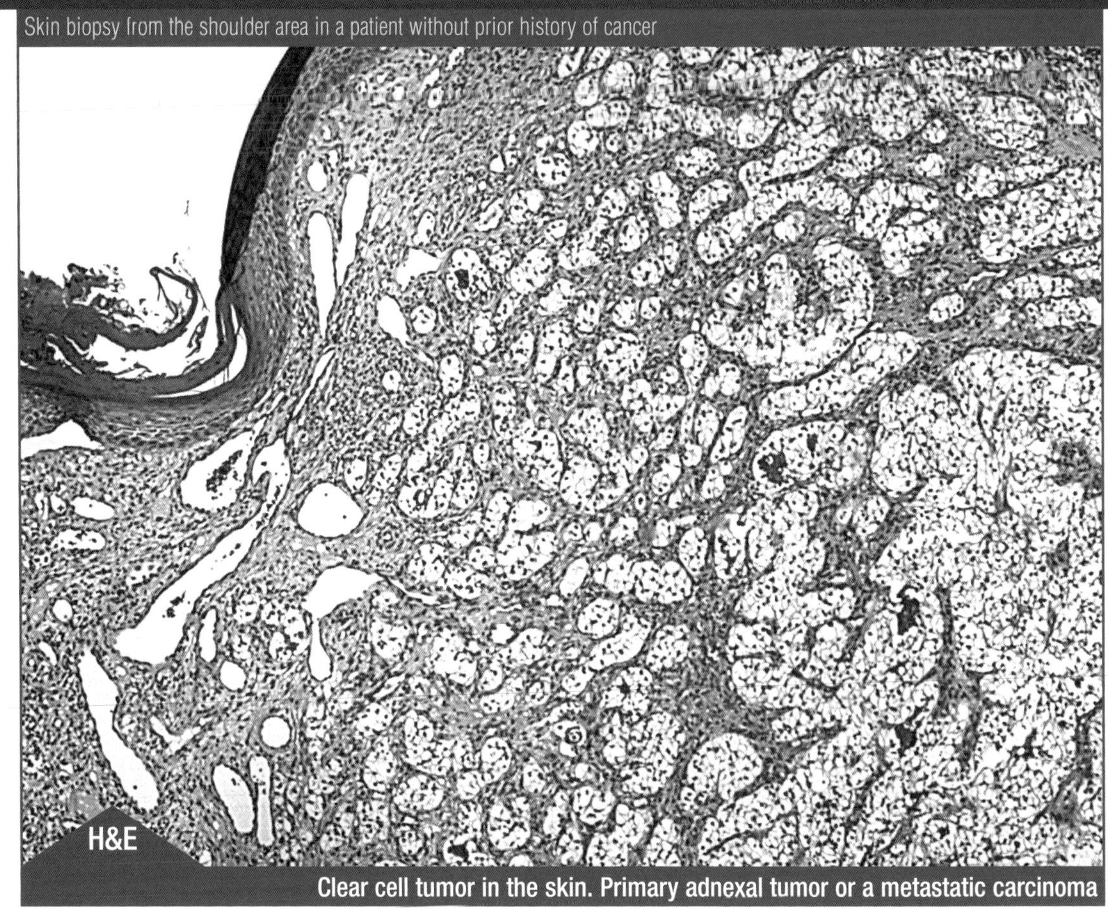

Clear cell tumor in the skin. Primary adnexal tumor or a metastatic carcinoma

Helpful Hints

Depending on the clinical history, histomorphology and availability of specific markers, the site of origin of a number of metastatic tumors in the skin can be determined by using one or more antibodies. Here are some examples.

1.	Metastatic adenocarcinoma of lung	TTF-1
2.	Metastatic carcinoma of breast	Estrogen Receptor
3.	Metastatic renal cell carcinoma	Renal Cell Antigen
4.	Metastatic thyroid carcinoma	Thyroglobulin, TTF-1
5.	Metastatic colonic adenocarcinoma	Cytokeratin 20

(Some skin appendage tumors also have been reported to be positive for estrogen receptor.)

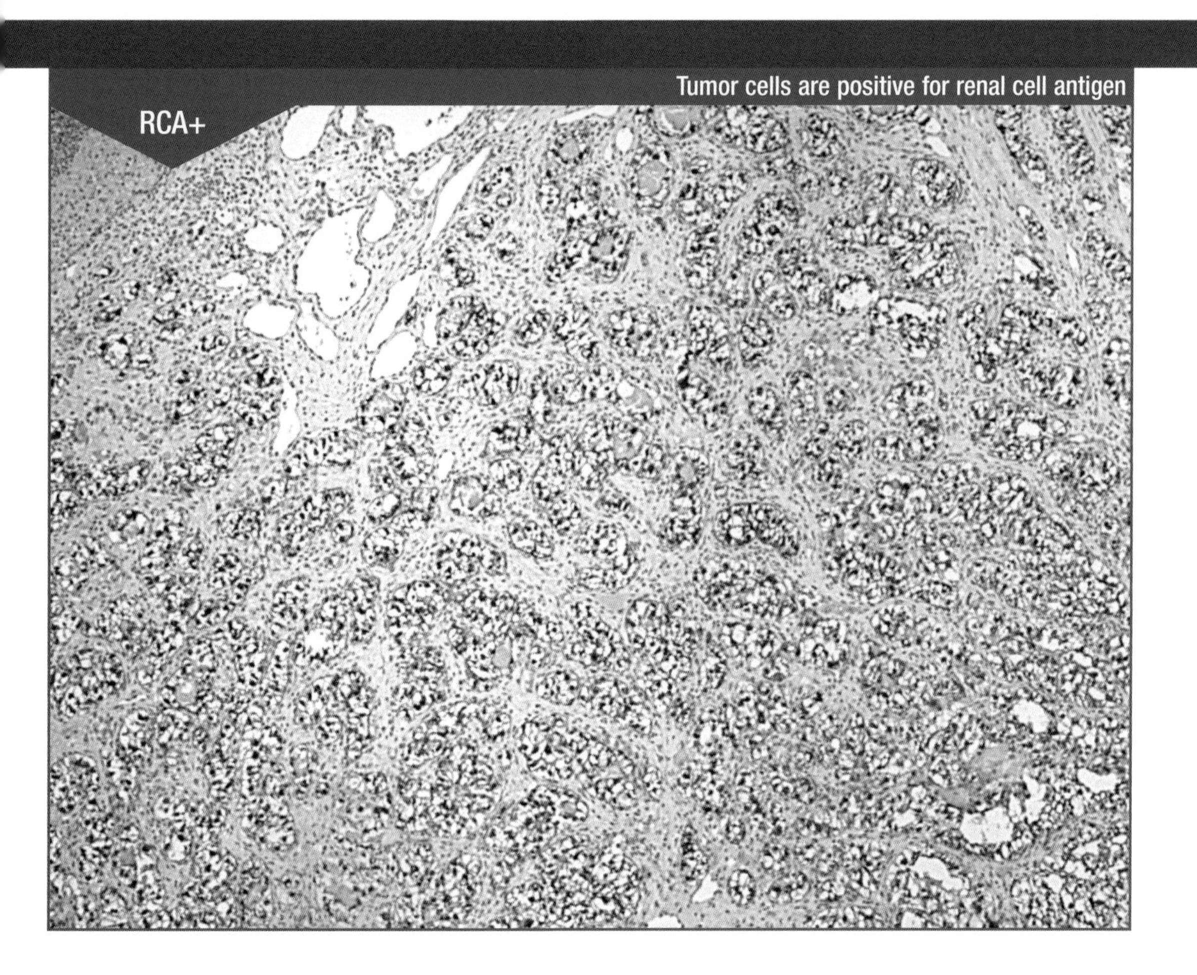

Diagnosis: Metastatic Renal Cell Carcinoma

Intracranial Tumor

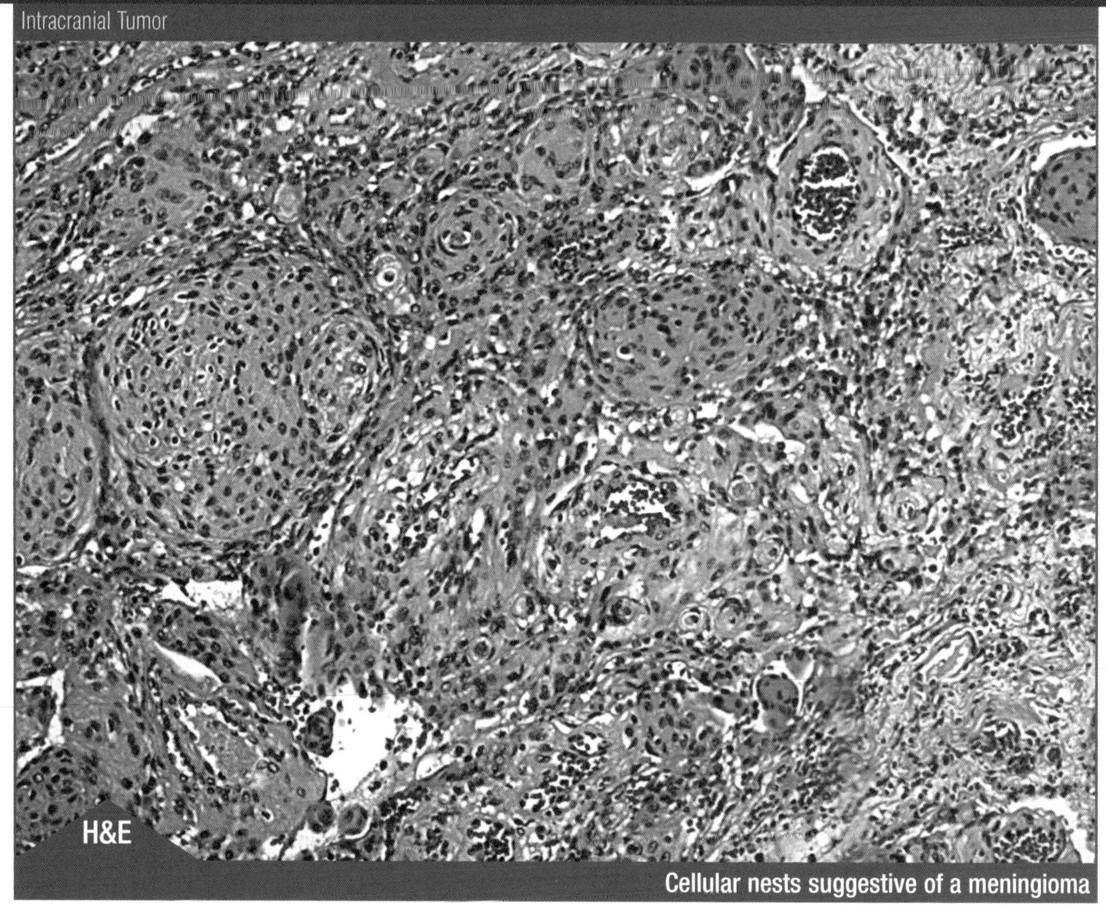

Cellular nests suggestive of a meningioma

Meningioma vs Schwannoma		
	EMA	Progesterone Receptor (PR)
Meningioma	+	+
Schwannoma	–	–

Helpful Hints

Meningiomas always express **progesterone receptor** (**PR**); the expression of **estrogen receptor** (**ER**) in these tumors is variable. The extent of progesterone receptor staining in meningiomas correlates with tumor aggressiveness; high grade tumors are only focally positive.

Epithelial Membrane Antigen (**EMA**) is commonly positive in meningiomas, but the diffuse cytoplasmic localization of this antigen is different than its usual well-defined membrane pattern seen in epithelial tumors.

Meningiomas are also positive for S100 protein, but this marker is also found in schwannomas and gliomas.

Khalid 1994.

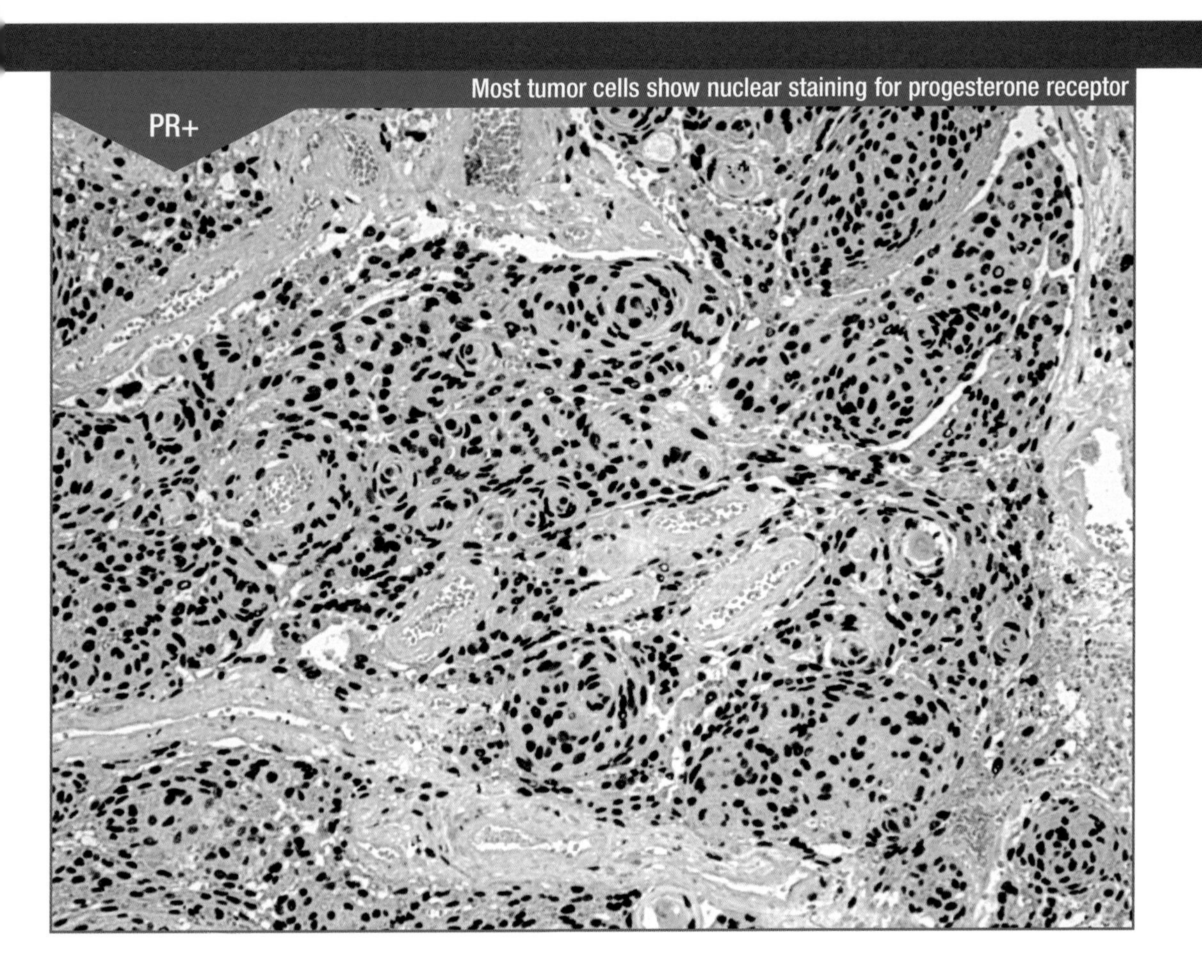

Diagnosis: Meningioma

Solitary mass in the frontal lobe

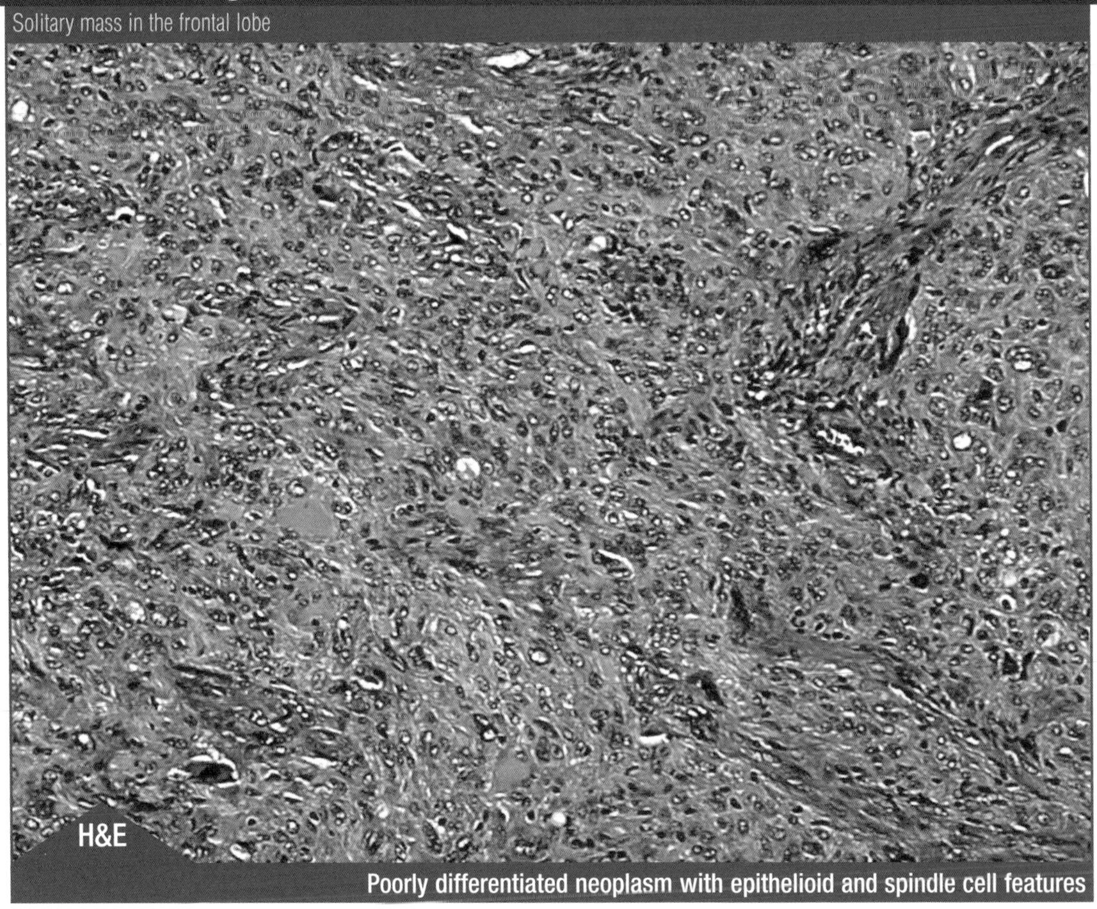

Poorly differentiated neoplasm with epithelioid and spindle cell features

High Grade Glioma vs Metastatic Carcinoma		
	GFAP	Cytokeratin (CK)
High Grade Glioma	+	–
Metastatic Carcinoma	–	+

Helpful Hints

All gliomas regardless of their degree of differentiation express **Glial Fibrillary Acidic Protein** (**GFAP**). Metastatic carcinomas, on the other hand, are positive for **cytokeratin** but negative for GFAP. All metastatic tumors to central nervous system elicit a reactive gliosis in their periphery or between tumor islands. These reactive astrocytes are GFAP-positive but the pattern of their distribution is indicative of their reactive nature.

Depending on the suspected site of origin of a metastatic carcinoma in central nervous system, one may have to add appropriate markers (ie, Estrogen Receptor for breast, TTF-1 for lung, etc.)

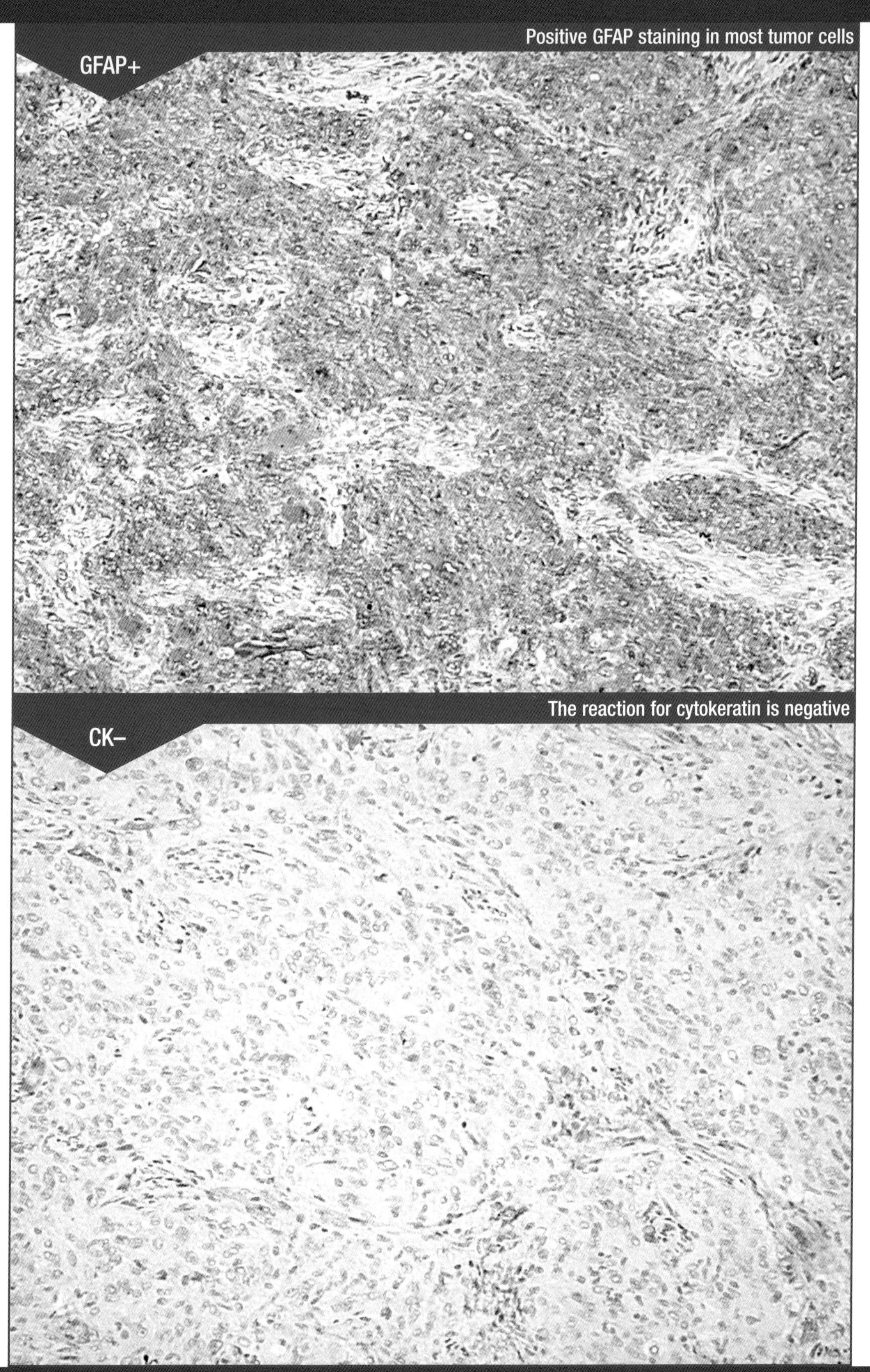

Diagnosis: High-Grade Glioma

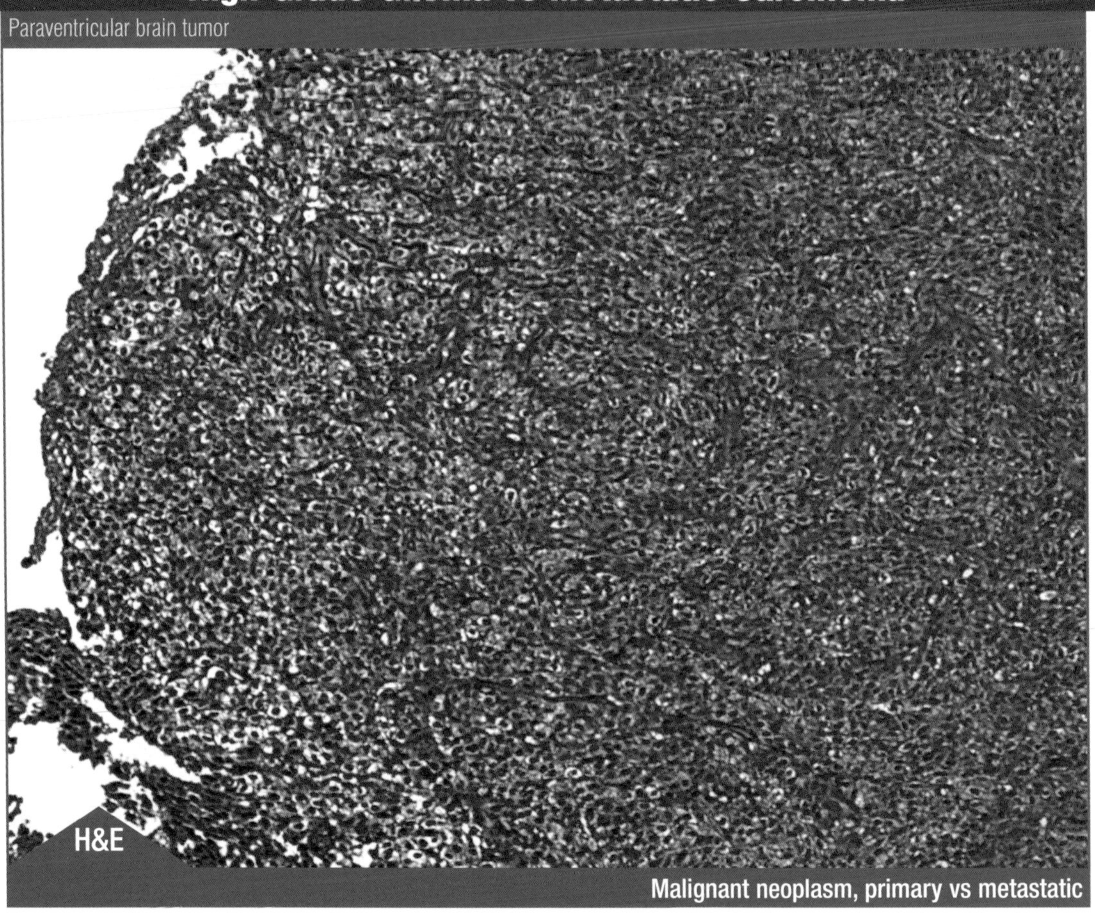

Malignant neoplasm, primary vs metastatic

High Grade Glioma vs Metastatic Carcinoma		
	GFAP	Cytokeratin (CK)
High Grade Glioma	+	–
Metastatic Carcinoma	–	+

Helpful Hints

All gliomas regardless of their degree of differentiation express **Glial Fibrillary Acidic Protein** (**GFAP**). Metastatic carcinomas, on the other hand, are positive for **cytokeratin** but negative for GFAP. All metastatic tumors to central nervous system elicit a reactive gliosis in their periphery or between tumor islands. These reactive astrocytes are GFAP-positive but the pattern of their distribution is indicative of their reactive nature.

Depending on the suspected site of origin of a metastatic carcinoma in central nervous system, one may have to add appropriate markers (ie, Estrogen Receptor for breast, TTF-1 for lung, etc.)

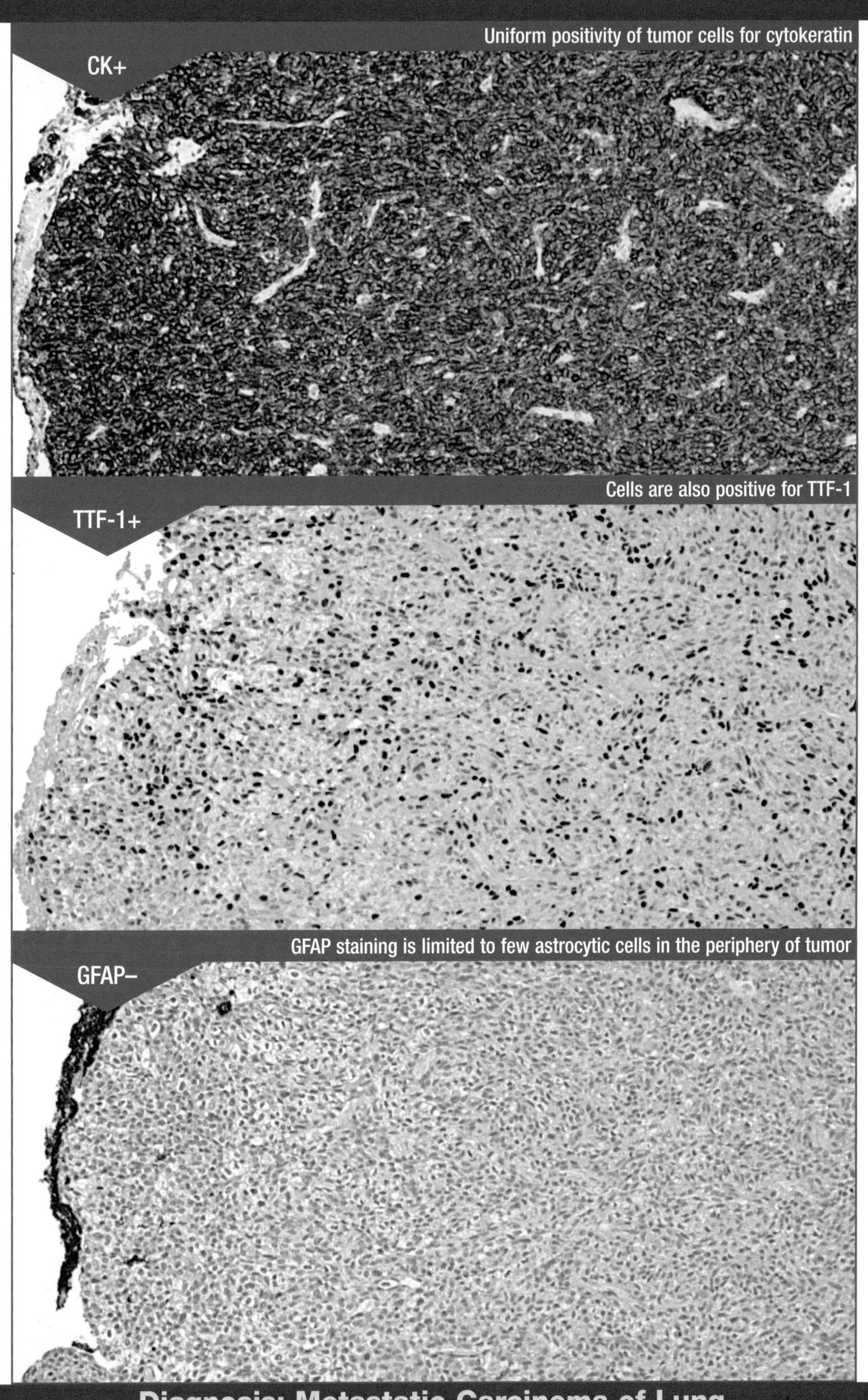

Diagnosis: Metastatic Carcinoma of Lung

High Grade Glioma vs Metastatic Melanoma

Brain tumor in a patient with history of malignant melanoma

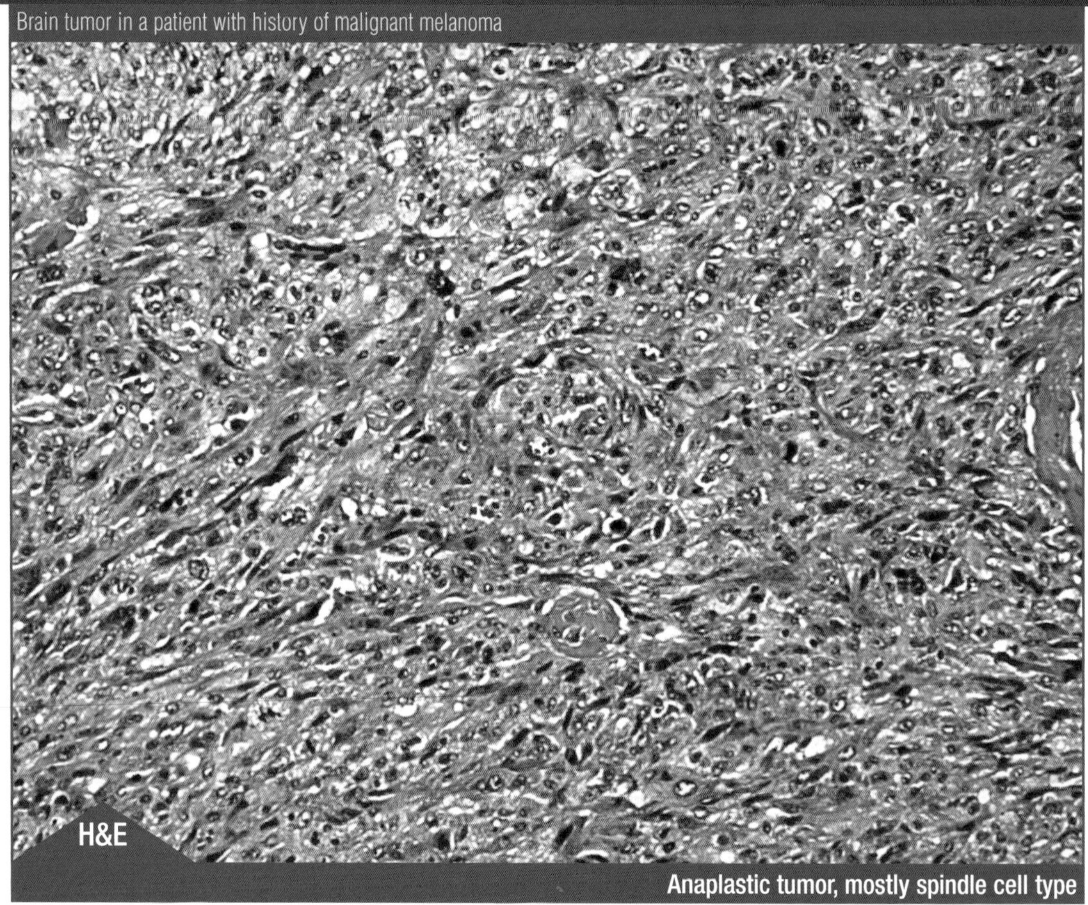

Anaplastic tumor, mostly spindle cell type

High Grade Glioma vs Metastatic Melanoma		
	GFAP	HMB-45
High Grade Glioma	+	–
Metastatic Melanoma	–	+

Helpful Hints

All gliomas regardless of their degree of differentiation express **Glial Fibrillary Acidic Protein** (**GFAP**). When metastatic melanoma is suspected in central nervous system, one should not use **S100 protein** as it is positive in gliomas as well. **HMB-45**, and if needed, **Melan-A** may help with that differential diagnosis.

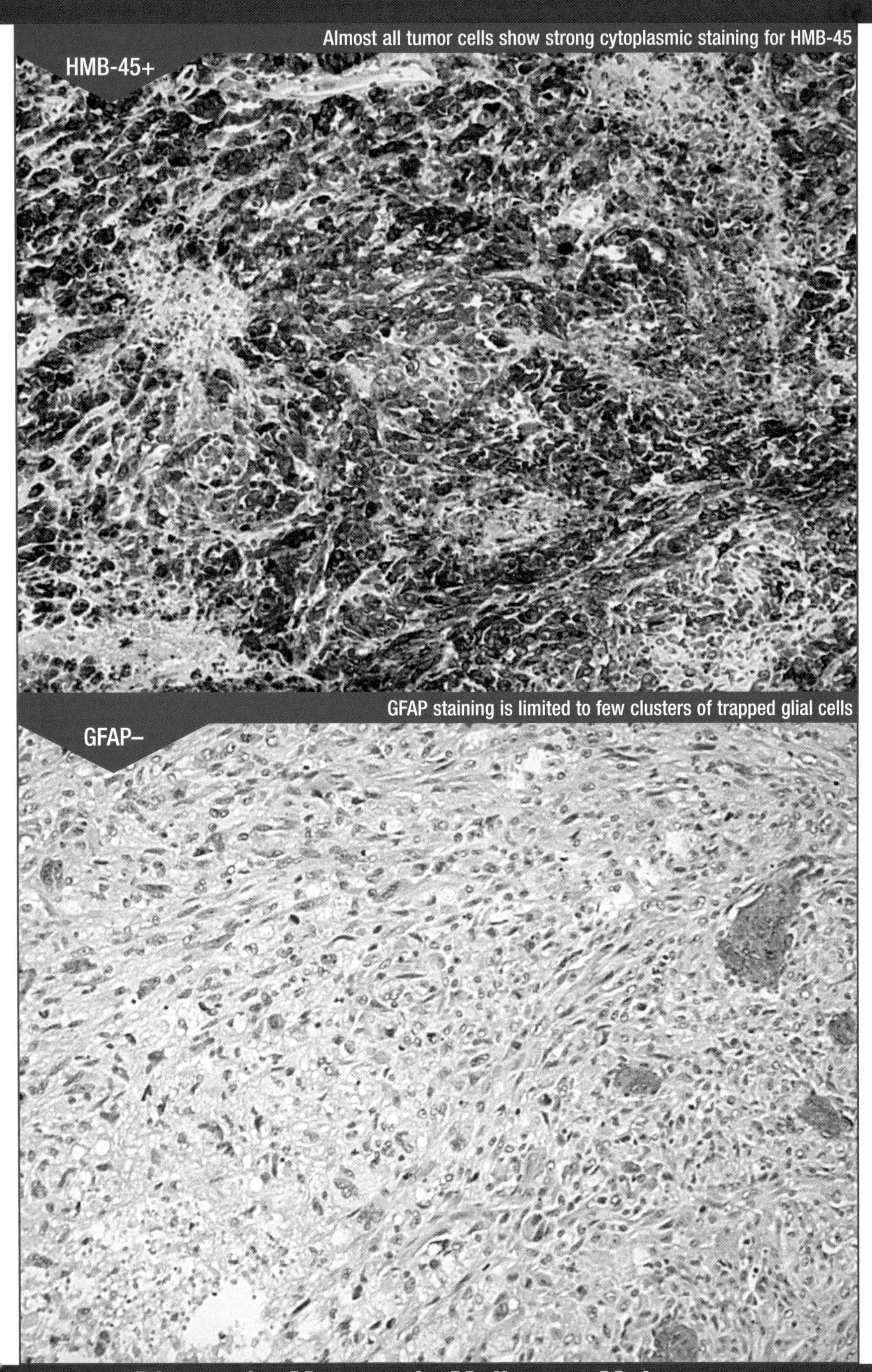

Diagnosis: Metastatic Malignant Melanoma

References

Acs G, Lawton TJ, Rebbeck TR, LiVolsi VA, Zhang PJ. Differential expression of E-cadherin in lobular and ductal neoplasms of the breast and its biologic and diagnostic implications. *Am J Clin Pathol* 115:85-98, 2001.

Albores-Saavedra J, Nadji M, Civantos F, Morales AR. Thyroglobulin in carcinoma of the thyroid: an immunohistochemical study. *Hum Pathol* 14:62-6, 1983.

Amann G, Zoubek A, Salzer-Kuntschik M, Windhager R, Kovar H. Relation of neurological marker expression and EWS gene fusion types in MIC2/CD99-positive tumors of the Ewing family. *Hum Pathol* 30:1058-64, 1999.

Battles OE, Page DL, Johnson JE. Cytokeratins, CEA, and mucin histochemistry in the diagnosis and characterization of extramammary Paget's disease. *Am J Clin Pathol* 108:6-12, 1997.

Bilal H. Handra-Luca A, Bertrand JC, Fouret PJ. P63 is expressed in basal and myoepithelial cells of human normal and tumor salivary gland tissues. *J Histochem Cytochem* 51:133-9, 2003.

Blessing K, Sanders D, Grant JJ. Comparison of immunohistochemical staining of the novel antibody Melan-A with S100 protein and HMB-45 in malignant melanoma and melanoma variants. *Histopathology* 32:139-46, 1998.

Busam KJ, Jungbluth AA. Melan-A, a new melanocytic differentiation. *Adv Anat Pathol* 6:12-8, 1999.

Busam KJ. Cutaneous desmoplastic melanoma. *Adv Anat Pathol* 12:92-102, 2005.

Chan JK, Cheuk W, Shimizu M. Anaplastic lymphoma kinase expression in inflammatory pseudotumors. *Am J Surg Pathol* 25:761-8, 2001.

Choi YL, Oh YL, Kim SH, Park CK, Ahn G. Comparative study of non-functional islet cell tumors and pancreatic solid and papillary neoplasms: biological behavior and immunohistochemistry. *Pathol Int* 52:358-66, 2002.

Civantos F, Albores-Saavedra J, Nadji M, Morales AR: Clear cell variant of thyroid carcinoma. *Am J Surg Pathol* 8:187-192, 1984.

Cochran AJ, Lu HF, Li PX, Saxton R, Wen DR. S-100 protein remains a practical marker for melanocytic and other tumours. *Melanoma Res* 3:325-30, 1993.

Comin CE, Novelli L, Boddi V, Paglierani M, Dini S. Calretinin, thrombomodulin, CEA and CD15: a useful combination of immunohistochemical markers for differentiating pleural epithelial mesothelioma from peripheral pulmonary adenocarcinoma. *Hum Pathol* 32:529-36, 2001.

Cui S, Hano H, Harada T, Takai S, Masui F, Ushigome S. Evaluation of new monoclonal anti-MyoD1 and anti-myogenin antibodies for the diagnosis of rhabdomyosarcoma. *Pathol Int* 49:62-68, 1999.

Dabbs DJ. *Diagnostic Immunohistochemistry, 2nd Ed* New York: Churchill-Livingstone, 2002.

Dan'ura T, Kawai A, Morimoto Y, Naito N, Yoshida A, Inoue H. Apoptosis and expression of its regulatory proteins in soft tissue sarcomas. *Cancer Lett* 178:167-74, 2002.

Deavers MT, Malpica A, Ordonez NG, Silva EG. Ovarian steroid cell tumors: an immunohistochemical study including a comparison of calretinin with inhibin. *Int J Gynecol Pathol* 22:162-7, 2003.

Devaney K, Wenig BM, Abbondanzo SL. Olfactory neuroblastoma and other round cell lesions of the sinonasal region. *Mod Pathol* 9:658-63, 1996

Devoe K, Weidner N. Immunohistochemistry of small round-cell tumors. *Semin Diagn Pathol* 17:216-24, 2000.

DeYoung BR, Swanson PE, Argenyi ZB, Ritter JH, Fitzgibbon JF, Stahl DJ, Hoover W, Wick MR. CD31 immunoreactivity in mesenchymal neoplasms of the skin and subcutis: report of 145 cases and review of putative immunohistologic markers of endothelial differentiation. *J Cutan Pathol* 22:215-22, 1995.

Duval JV, Savas L, Banner BF. Expression of cytokeratins 7 and 20 in carcinomas of the extrahepatic biliary tract, pancreas, and gallbladder. *Arch Pathol Lab Med* 124:1196-200, 2000.

Feinmesser M, Sulkes A, Morgenstern S, Sulkes J, Stern S, Okon E. HLA-DR and beta 2 microglobulin expression in medullary and atypical medullary carcinoma of the breast: histopathologically similar but biologically distinct entities. *J Clin Pathol* 53:286-91, 2000.

Fetsch PA, Powers CN, Zakowski MF, Abati A. Anti-alpha-inhibin: marker of choice for the consistent distinction between adrenocortical carcinoma and renal cell carcinoma in fine-needle aspiration. *Cancer* 87:168-72, 1999.

Fisher C. Synovial sarcoma. *Ann Diagn Pathol* 2:401-21, 1998.

Folpe AL, Schmidt RA, Chapman D, Gown AM. Poorly differentiated synovial sarcoma: immunohistochemical distinction from primitive neuroectodermal tumors and high-grade malignant peripheral nerve sheath tumors. *Am J Surg Pathol* 22:673-82, 1998.

Frisman, DM. ImmunoQuery Web Site. *http://www.ipox.org* [last accessed April 11, 2006].

Ghanem MA, Van der Kwast TH, Den Hollander JC, Sudaryo MK, Oomen MH, Noordzij Ma, Van den Heuvel MM, Nassef SM, Nijman RM, Van Steenbrugge GJ. Expression and prognostic value of Wilms' tumor 1 and early growth response 1 proteins in nephroblastoma. *Clin Cancer Res* 6:4265-71. 2000.

Goldblum JR. Hart WR. Vulvar Paget's disease: a clinicopathologic and immunohistochemical study of 19 cases. *Am J Surg Pathol* 21:1178-87, 1997a.

Goldblum JR, Tuthill RJ. CD34 and factor-XIIIa immunoreactivity in dermatofibrosarcoma protuberans and dermatofibroma. *Am J Dermatopathol* 19:147-53, 1997b.

Hamilton-Dutoit SJ, Lou H, Pallesen G. The expression of placental alkaline phosphatase (PLAP) and PLAP-like enzymes in normal and neoplastic human tissues. An immunohistological survey using monoclonal antibodies. *APMIS* 98:797-811, 1990.

Hanly AJ, Elgart GW, Jorda M, Smith J, Nadji M. Analysis of thyroid transcription factor-1 and cytokeratin 20 separates Merkel cell carcinoma from small cell carcinoma of lung. *J Cutan Pathol* 27:118-20, 2000.

Hassanein AM, Al-Quran SZ, Kantor GR, Pauporte M, Telang GH, Spielvogel RL. Thomsen-Friedenreich (T) antigen: a possible tool for differentiating sebaceous carcinoma from its simulators. *Appl Immunohistochem Mol Morphol* 9:250-254, 2001.

Hisaoka M, Wei-Qi S, Jian W, Morio T, Hashimoto H. Specific but variable expression of h-caldesmon in leiomyosarcomas: an immunohistochemical reassessment of a novel myogenic marker. *Appl Immunohistochem Mol Morphol* 9:302-8, 2001

Hofbauer GF, Kamarashev J, Geertsen R, Boni R, Dummer R. Tyrosinase immunoreactivity in formalin-fixed, paraffin-embedded primary and metastatic melanoma: frequency and distribution. *J Cutan Pathol* 25:204-9,1998.

Hsi ED, Nickoloff BJ. Dermatofibroma and dermatofibrosarcoma protuberans: an immunohistochemical study reveals distinctive antigenic profiles. *J Dermatol Sci* 11:1-9, 1996.

Jorda M, De MB, Nadji M. Calretinin and inhibin are useful in separating adrenocortical neoplasms from pheochromocytomas. *Appl Immunohistochem Mol Morphol* 10:67-70, 2002.

Kahn HJ, Marks A. A new monoclonal antibody, D2-40 for detection of lymphatic invasion in primary tumors. *Lab Invest* 82:1255-7, 2002.

Khalid H. Immunohistochemical study of estrogen receptor-related antigen, progesterone and estrogen receptors in human intracranial meningiomas. *Cancer* 74:679-85, 1994.

Klimstra DS, Heffess CS, Oertel JE, Rosai J. Acinar cell carcinoma of the pancreas. A clinicopathologic study of 28 cases. *Am J Surg Pathol* 16:815-37, 1992.

Koelma IA, Nap M, Rodenburg CJ, Fleuren GJ. The value of tumour marker CA 125 in surgical pathology. *Histopathology* 11:287-94, 1987.

Koshida K, Wahren B. Placental-like alkaline phosphatase in seminoma. *Urol Res* 18:87-92, 1990.

Lae ME, Roche PC, Jin L, Lloyd RV, Nascimento AG. Desmoplastic small round cell tumor: a clinicopathologic, immunohistochemical, and molecular study of 32 tumors. *Am J Surg Pathol* 26:823-35, 2002

Lau SK, Desrochers MJ, Luthringer DJ. Expression of thyroid transcription factor-1, cytokeratin 7, and cytokeratin 20 in bronchioloalveolar carcinomas: an immunohistochemical evaluation of 67 cases. *Mod Pathol* 15:538-42, 2002a.

Lau SK, Luthringer DJ, Eisen RN. Thyroid transcription factor-1: a review. *Appl Immunohistochem Mol Morphol* 10:97-102, 2002b.

Lau SK, Prakash S, Geller SA, Alsabeh R. Comparative immunohistochemical profile of hepatocellular carcinoma, cholangiocarcinoma, and metastatic adenocarcinoma. *Hum Pathol* 33:1175-81, 2002c.

Li MK, Folpe AL. CDX-2, a new marker for adenocarcinoma of gastrointestinal origin. *Adv Anat Pathol* 11:101-5, 2004.

Liapi-Avgeri G, Karabela-Bouropoulou V, Agnanti N. Glomus tumor: a histological, histochemical and immunohistochemical study of the various types. *Pathol Res Pract* 190:2-10, 1994.

Loy TS, Calaluce RD, Keeney GL. Cytokeratin immunostaining in differentiating primary ovarian carcinoma from metastatic colonic adenocarcinoma. *Mod Pathol* 9:1040-4, 1996.

Magi-Galluzzi C, Luo J, Isaacs WB, Hicks JL, de Marzo AM, Epstein JI. Alpha-methylacyl-CoA racemase: a variably sensitive immunohistochemical marker for the diagnosis of small prostate cancer foci on needle biopsy. *Am J Surg Pathol* 27:1128-33, 2003.

Mai KT, Landry DC, Collins JP. Secondary colonic adenocarcinoma of the prostate histologically mimicking prostatic ductal adenocarcinoma. *Tumori* 88:341-4, 2002.

McCluggage WG, Jenkins D. p16 immunoreactivity may assist in the distinction between endometrial and endocervical adenocarcinoma. *Int J Gynecol Pathol* 22:231-5, 2003.

McComb RD, Jones TR, Pizzo SV, Bigner DD. Specificity and sensitivity of immunohistochemical detection of factor VIII/von Willebrand factor antigen in formalin-fixed paraffin-embedded tissue. *J Histochem Cytochem* 30:371-7, 1982.

McComb RD, Jones TR, Pizzo SV, Bigner DD. Specificity and sensitivity of immunohistochemical detection of factor VIII/von Willebrand factor antigen in formalin-fixed paraffin-embedded tissue. *J Histochem Cytochem* 30:371-7, 1982.

McNutt NS. The S100 family of multipurpose calcium-binding proteins. *J Cutan Pathol* 25:521-9, 1998.

Meis-Kindblom JM, Kindblom LG. Angiosarcoma of soft tissue: a study of 80 cases. *Am J Surg Pathol* 22:683-97, 1998.

Miettinen M. Keratin immunohistochemistry: update of applications and pitfalls. *Pathol Ann* 28:113-43, 1993.

Miettinen M, Fetsch JF. Distribution of keratins in normal endothelial cells and a spectrum of vascular tumors: implications in tumor diagnosis. *Hum Pathol* 31:1062-7, 2000a.

Miettinen M, Limon J, Niezabitowski A, Losata J. Patterns of keratin polypeptides in 110 biphasic, monophasic, and poorly differentiated synovial sarcomas. *Virchows Arch* 437:275-83, 2000b.

Miettinen M, Lasota J. Gastrointestinal stromal tumors: definition, clinical, histological, immunohistochemical, and molecular genetic features and differential diagnosis. *Virchows Arch* 438:1-12, 2001.

Moldvay J, Jackel M, Bogos K, Soltesz I, Agocs L, Kovacs G, Schaff Z. The role of TTF-1 in differentiating primary and metastatic lung adenocarcinomas. *Pathol Oncol Res* 10:85-8, 2004.

Nadji M, Tabei SZ, Castro A, Chu TM, Murphy GP, Wang MC, Morales AR. Prostatic-specific antigen: an immunohistologic marker for prostatic neoplasms. *Cancer* 48:1229-32, 1981.

Nadji M, Ganjei P. Immunocytochemistry in diagnostic cytology: a 12-year perspective. *Am J Clin Pathol* 94:470-5, 1990.

Nadji M, Gomez-Fernandez C, Ganjei-Azar P, Morales AR. Immunohistochemistry of estrogen and progesterone receptors reconsidered: experience with 5,993 breast cancers. *Am J Clin Pathol* 123:21-7, 2005.

Negri G. Egarter-Vigl E. Kasal A. Romano F. Haitel A. Mian C. p16INK4a is a useful marker for the diagnosis of adenocarcinoma of the cervix uteri and its precursors: an immunohistochemical study with immunocytochemical correlations. *Am J Surg Pathol* 27:187-93, 2003.

Nicholson AG, Goldstraw P, Fisher C. Synovial sarcoma of the pleura and its differentiation from other primary pleural tumours: a clinicopathological and immunohistochemical review of three cases. *Histopathology* 3:508-13, 1998.

Niehans GA, Manivel JC, Copland GT, Scheithauer BW, Wick MR. Immunohistochemistry of germ cell and trophoblastic neoplasms. *Cancer* 62:1113-23, 1988.

Nogales FF, Isaac MA, Hardisson D, Bosincu L, Palacios J, Ordi J, Mendoza E, Manzarbeitia F, Olivera H, O'Valle F, Krasevic M, Marquez M. Adenomatoid tumors of the uterus: an analysis of 60 cases. *Int J Gynecol Pathol* 21:34-40, 2002.

O'Hara BJ, Paetau A, Miettinen M. Keratin subsets and monoclonal antibody HBME-1 in chordoma: immunohistochemical differential diagnosis between tumors simulating chordoma. *Hum Pathol* 29:119-26, 1998.

Ordonez NG, Mackay B. Granular cell tumor: a review of the pathology and histogenesis. *Ultrastruct Pathol* 23:207-22, 1999.

Pallesen G. Hamilton-Dutoit SJ. Ki-1 (CD30) antigen is regularly expressed by tumor cells of embryonal carcinoma. *Am J Pathol* 133:446-50, 1988.

Pileri SA, Grogan TM, Harris NL, Banks P, Campo E, Chan JK, Favera RD, Delsol G, De Wolf-Peeters C, Falini B, Gascoyne RD, Gaulard P, Gatter KC, Isaacson PG, Jaffe ES, Kluin P, Knowles DM, Mason DY, Mori S, Muller-Hermelink HK, Piris MA, Ralfkiaer E, Stein H, Su IJ, Warnke RA, Weiss LM. Tumours of histiocytes and accessory dendritic cells: an immunohistochemical approach to classification from the International Lymphoma Study Group based on 61 cases. *Histopathology* 41:1-29, 2002.

Poppema S, Lai R, Visser L, Yan XJ. CD45 (leukocyte common antigen) expression in T and B lymphocyte subsets. *Leuk Lymphoma* 20:217-22, 1996.

Reis-Filho JS, Torio B, Albergaria A, Schmitt FC. p63 expression in normal skin and usual cutaneous carcinomas. *J Cutan Pathol* 29:517-23, 2002.

Reis-Filho JS, Milanezi F, Paredes J, Silva P, Pereira EM, Maeda SA, de Carvalho LV, Schmitt FC. Novel and classic myoepithelial/stem cell markers in metaplastic carcinomas of the breast. *Appl Immunohistochem Mol Morphol* 11:1-8, 2003.

Riley JK, Sliwkowski MX. CD20: a gene in search of a function. *Sem Oncol* 27:17-24, 2000.

Ring NP, Addis BJ. Thymoma: an integrated clinicopathological and immunohistochemical study. *J Pathol* 149:327-37, 1986.

Romaguera R, Rodriguez M, Bruce J, Zuluaga T, Viciana A, Penalver M, Nadji M. Molar gestations and hydropic abortions differentiated by p57 immunostaining. *Fetal Pediatr Pathol* 23:181-190, 2005.

Sawady J, Mendelsohn G, Sirota RL, Taxy JB. The intrathyroidal hyperfunctioning parathyroid gland. *Mod Pathol* 2:652-7, 1989.

Sawh RN, Malpica A, Deavers MT, Liu J, Silva EG. Benign cystic mesothelioma of the peritoneum: a clinicopathologic study of 17 cases and immunohistochemical analysis of estrogen and progesterone receptor status. *Hum Pathol* 34:369-74, 2003

Schorge JO, Lea JS, Elias KJ, Rajanbabu R, Coleman RL, Miller DS, Ashfaq R. P16 as a molecular biomarker of cervical adenocarcinoma. *Am J Obstet Gynecol* 190:668-73, 2004.

Schroder S, Padberg BC, Achilles E, Holl K, Dralle H, Kloppel G. Immunocytochemistry in adrenocortical tumours: a clinicomorphological study of 72 neoplasms. *Virchows Arch* 420:65-70, 1992.

Scott MP, Helm KF. Cytokeratin 20: a marker for diagnosing Merkel cell carcinoma. *Am J Dermatopathol* 21:16-20, 1999.

Shah RB. Zhou M. LeBlanc M. Snyder M. Rubin MA. Comparison of the basal cell-specific markers, 34betaE12 and p63, in the diagnosis of prostate cancer. *Am J Surg Pathol* 26:1161-8, 2002.

Sikri KL, Varndell IM, Hamid QA, Wilson BS, Kameya T, Ponder BA, Lloyd RV, Bloom SR, Polak JM. Medullary carcinoma of the thyroid. An immunocytochemical and histochemical study of 25 cases using eight separate markers. *Cancer* 56:2481-91, 1985.

Sim SJ. Ro JY. Ordonez NG. Park YW. Kee KH. Ayala AG. Metastatic renal cell carcinoma to the bladder: a clinicopathologic and immunohistochemical study. *Mod Pathol* 12:351-5, 1999.

Sturtz CL. Dabbs DJ. Angiomyolipomas: the nature and expression of the HMB45 antigen. *Mod Pathol* 7:842-5, 1994.

Tan D, Li Q, Deeb G, Ramnath N, Slocum HK, Brooks J, Cheney R, Wiseman S, Anderson T, Loewen G. Thyroid transcription factor-1 expression prevalence and its clinical implications in non-small cell lung cancer: a high-throughput tissue microarray and immunohistochemistry study. *Hum Pathol* 34:597-604, 2003.

Taylor CR, Cote RJ. *Immunomicroscopy–A Diagnostic Tool for the Surgical Pathologist.* Philadelphia: Saunders, 1986.

Thomas JA, Iliescu V, Crawford DH, Ellouz R, Cammoun M, de-The G. Expression of HLA-DR antigens in nasopharyngeal carcinoma: an immunohistological analysis of the tumour cells and infiltrating lymphocytes. *Int J Cancer* 33:813-9, 1984.

Thomas Jo, Nijjar J, Turley H, Micklem K, Gatter KC. NB 84: a new monoclonal antibody for the recognition of neuroblastoma in routinely processed material. *J Pathol* 163:69-75, 1991.

Tobita K, Kijima H, Chino O, Dowaki S, Kashiwagi H, Tanaka M, Ohtani Y, Inokuchi S, Makuuchi H. Pancreatic acinar cell carcinoma with endocrine differentiation: immunohistochemical and ultrastructural analyses. *Anticancer Res* 2:2131-4, 2001.

Toki T, Shimizu M, Takagi Y, Ashida T, Konishi I. CD10 is a marker for normal and neoplastic endometrial stromal cells. *Int J Gynecol Pathol* 21:41-7, 2002.

Truong LD, Rangdaeng S, Cagle P, Ro JY, Hawkins H, Font RL. The diagnostic utility of desmin: a study of 584 cases and review of the literature. *Am J Clin Pathol* 93:305-14, 1990.

van de Rijn M, Lombard CM, Rouse RV. Expression of CD34 by solitary fibrous tumors of the pleura, mediastinum, and lung. *Am J Surg Pathol* 18:814-20, 1994.

Vera-Sempere FJ, Burgos JS, Botella MS, Morera C. Immunohistochemical expression of Bcl-2 oncoprotein in EBV-associated nasopharyngeal carcinoma correlated to histological type and survival. *Histol Histopathol* 12:9-18, 1997.

Walls AF, Jones DB, Williams JH, Church MK, Holgate ST. Immunohistochemical identification of mast cells in formaldehyde-fixed tissue using monoclonal antibodies specific for tryptase. *J Pathol* 162:119-26, 1990.

Wang X, Mori I, Tang W, Nakamura M, Nakamura Y, Sato M, Sakurai T, Kakudo K. p63 expression in normal, hyperplastic and malignant breast tissues. *Breast Cancer* 9:216-9, 2002.

Wick MR. Immunohistology of neuroendocrine and neuroectodermal tumors. *Semin Diagn Pathol* 17:194-203, 2000.

Wick MR, Graeme-Cook FM. Pancreatic neuroendocrine neoplasms: a current summary of diagnostic, prognostic, and differential diagnostic information. *Am J Clin Pathol* 115:28-45, 2001.

Wieneke JA, Thompson LD, Heffess CS. Adrenal cortical neoplasms in the pediatric population: a clinicopathologic and immunophenotypic analysis of 83 patients. *Am J Surg Path* 27:867-81, 2003.

Wilander E, Lundquist M, Oberg K. Gastrointestinal carcinoid tumours. Histogenetic, histochemical, immunohistochemical, clinical and therapeutic aspects. *Prog Histochem Cytochem* 19:1-88, 1989.

Yi ER, Strong CR, Piao Z, Perucho M, Weidner N. Epithelioid gastrointestinal stromal tumor with PDGFR activating mutation and immunoreactivity. *Appl Immunohistochem Mol Morphol* 13:157-161, 2005.

Yoshida SO, Imam A. Monoclonal antibody to a proximal nephrogenic renal antigen: immunohistochemical analysis of formalin-fixed, paraffin-embedded human renal cell carcinomas. *Cancer Res* 49:1802-9, 1989.

Zhu XQ, Shi YF, Cheng XD, Zhao CL, Wu YZ. Immunohistochemical markers in differential diagnosis of endometrial stromal sarcoma and cellular leiomyoma. *Gynecol Oncol* 92:71-9, 2004.

A

B

C

E

F

G

K

L

M

R

S

T

U

V

W

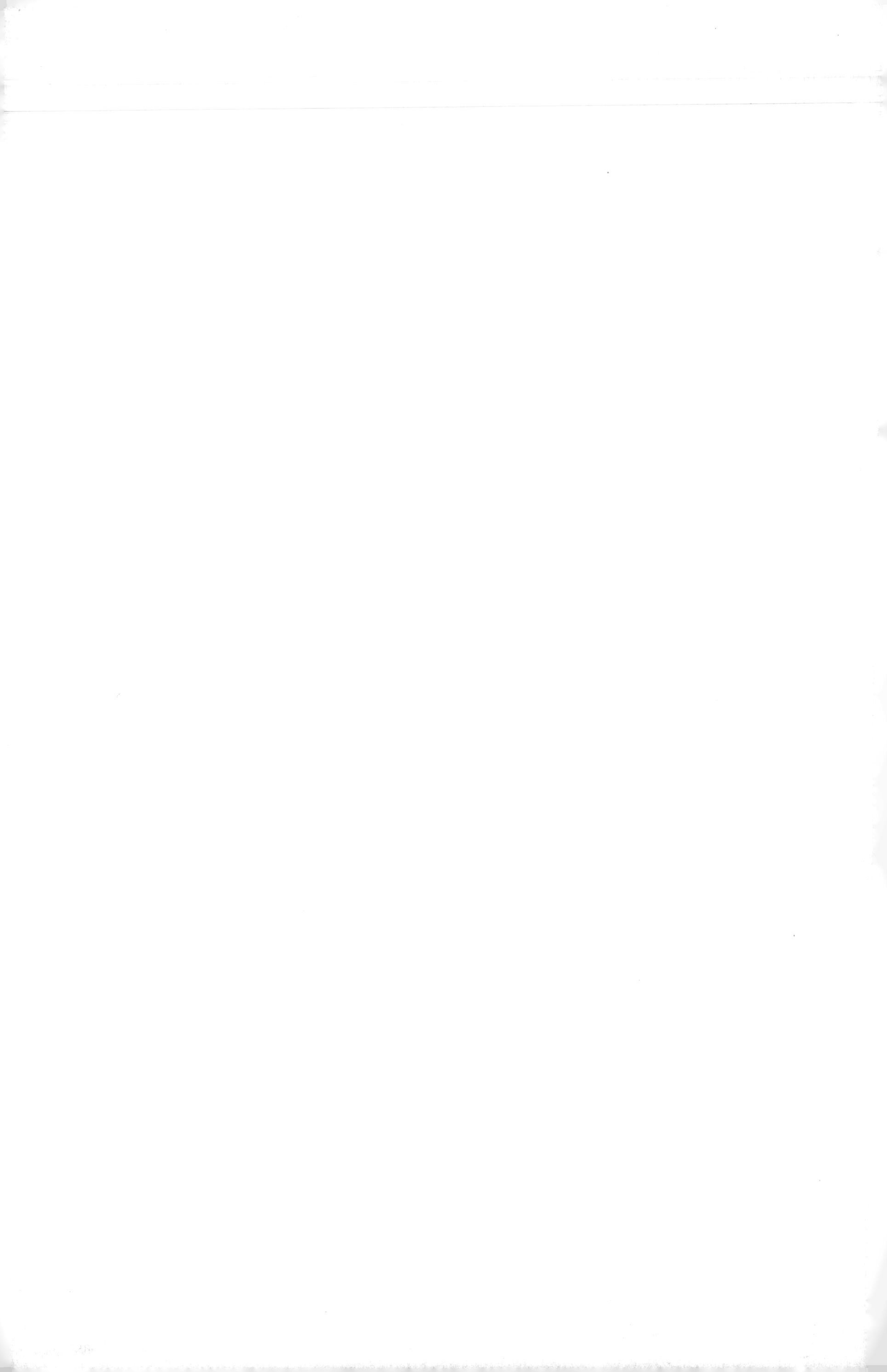